Dietitian's Handbook of Enteral and Parenteral Nutrition

Second Edition

Edited by

Annalynn Skipper, MS, RD, FADA, CNSD

Co-Director
Nutrition Consultation Service
Rush-Presbyterian-St. Luke's Medical Center
Chicago, Illinois
Assistant Professor
Department of Clinical Nutrition
Rush University
Chicago, Illinois

AN ASPEN PUBLICATION®
Aspen Publishers, Inc.
Gaithersburg, Maryland
1998

Library of Congress Cataloging-in-Publication Data

Dietitian's handbook of enteral and parenteral nutrition/edited by
Annalynn Skipper.—2nd ed.
p. cm.
Includes bibliographical references and index.
ISBN 0-8342-0920-9
1. Enteral feeding—Handbooks, manuals, etc.   2. Parenteral
feeding—Handbooks, manuals, etc.   I. Skipper, Annalynn.
RM225.D54   1998
615.8'55—dc21
97-40065
CIP

Orders: (800) 638-8437
Customer Service: (800) 234-1660

About Aspen Publishers • For more than 35 years, Aspen has been a leading professional publisher in a variety of disciplines. Aspen's vast information resources are available in both print and electronic formats. We are committed to providing the highest quality information available in the most appropriate format for our customers. Visit Aspen's Internet site for more information resources, directories, articles, and a searchable version of Aspen's full catalog, including the most recent publications: **http://www.aspenpub.com**
Aspen Publishers, Inc. • The hallmark of quality in publishing
Member of the worldwide Wolters Kluwer group.

Aspen Publishers, Inc., is not affiliated with
the American Society of Parenteral and Enteral Nutrition.

Editorial Services: Ruth Bloom
Library of Congress Catalog Card Number: 97-40065
ISBN: 0-8342-0920-9

Printed in the United States of America

1 2 3 4 5

To my mother,
Louise Skipper

Table of Contents

Contributors

Stacey J. Bell, DSc, RD
Instructor in Surgery
Harvard Medical School
Boston, Massachusetts

Peter L. Beyer, MS, RD
Associate Professor
Dietetics and Nutrition
University of Kansas Medical Center
Kansas City, Kansas

Bruce R. Bistrian, MD, PhD
Professor of Medicine
Harvard Medical School
Chief, Nutrition and Infection
    Laboratory
Department of Medicine
Beth Israel Deaconess Hospital
Boston, Massachusetts

Pamela J. Charney, MS, RD, CNSD
Clinical Nutrition Manager
University of Chicago Hospitals
Chicago, Illinois

**Paula M. Charuhas, MS, RD,
    FADA, CD, CNSD**
Research Dietitian
Department of Clinical Nutrition
Division of Clinical Research
Fred Hutchinson Cancer Research
    Center
Seattle, Washington

Sara Reek DiCecco, MS, RD
Clinical Dietitian
Department of Dietetics
Mayo Rochester Hospitals
Rochester, Minnesota

John M. Draganescu, MD
Gastroenterologist
Darby, Pennsylvania

Judith A. Fish, MMSc, RD, CNSD
Nutrition Support Clinician
Cleveland Clinic Foundation
Cleveland, Ohio

Janet A. Furman, RD, CNSD
Nutrition Support Dietitian
Nutrition Consultation Service
Rush-Presbyterian-St. Luke's Medical
    Center
Lecturer
Department of Clinical Nutrition
Rush University
Chicago, Illinois

**Michele M. Gottschlich, PhD,
    RD, CNSD**
Director, Nutrition Services
Shriners Hospitals for Children
Cincinnati Burns Institute
Cincinnati, Ohio

Leah M. Gramlich, MD, FRCP(C)
Assistant Professor of Medicine
University of Alberta
Director, Nutrition Support Service
Royal Alexander Hospital
Department of Medicine
Division of Gastroenterology
Edmonton, Alberta, Canada

**Cynthia Hamilton, MS, RD,
    CNSD**
Nutrition Support Dietitian
Cleveland Clinic Foundation
Hyperalimentation Department
Cleveland, Ohio

**Jeanette M. Hasse, PhD, RD,
    FADA, CNSD**
Transplant Nutrition Specialist
Baylor Institute of Transplantation
    Sciences
Baylor University Medical Center
Dallas, Texas

Judith C. Hestnes
Dietetics Student
Simmons College
Boston, Massachusetts

**Wanda Hain Howell, PhD, RD,
    CNSD**
Associate Professor
University of Arizona
Department of Nutritional Sciences
Tucson, Arizona

**Anne Marie B. Hunter, MS, RD,
    CNSD**
Director, Clinical Nutrition Services
St. John's Regional Medical Center
Joplin, Missouri

**Andrea M. Hutchins, MS, RD,
    CNSD**
Assistant Clinical Specialist
University of Minnesota
Department of Food Science and
    Nutrition
St. Paul, Minnesota

**Carol S. Ireton-Jones, PhD, RD,
    CNSD, FACN**
Principle
Preferred Nutrition Therapists
Carrollton, Texas

**Polly Lenssen, MS, RD, CD,
    FADA**
Assistant Director
Clinical Nutrition
Fred Huchinson Cancer Research
    Center
Seattle, Washington

Carol Liftman, MS, RD
Renal Dietitian
Franklin Dialysis Center
Pennsylvania Hospital
Philadelphia, Pennsylvania

William H. Lipshutz, MD
Head, Section of Gastroenterology
Pennsylvania Hospital
Clinical Professor of Medicine
University of Pennsylvania
Philadelphia, Pennsylvania

Laura E. Matarese, MS, RD, FADA, CNSD
Manager, Nutrition Support Dietetics
Cleveland Clinic Foundation
Hyperalimentation Department
Cleveland, Ohio

Theresa Mayes, RD
Clinical Dietitian
Shriners Hospitals for Children
Cincinnati Burns Institute
Cincinnati, Ohio

David L. Paskin, MD
Chairman
Department of Surgery
Pennsylvania Hospital
Clinical Professor of Surgery
University of Pennsylvania
Philadelphia, Pennsylvania

Natalie B. Ratz, MS, RD
Pediatric/Neonatal Nutrition
  Support Dietitian
Nutrition Consultation Service
Rush-Presbyterian-St. Luke's Medical
  Center
Chicago Illinois

Denise B. Schwartz, MS, RD, FADA, CNSD
Nutrition Support Specialist
Providence Saint Joseph Medical
  Center
Burbank, California

Eva Politzer Shronts, MMSc, RD, CNSD
Associate Director
Nutrition Support Service
Department of Surgery
Assistant Clinical Professor
College of Pharmacy
University of Minnesota
Minneapolis, Minnesota

Annalynn Skipper, MS, RD, FADA, CNSD
Co-Director
Nutrition Consultation Service
Rush-Presbyterian-St. Luke's Medical
  Center
Assistant Professor
Department of Clinical Nutrition
Rush University
Chicago, Illinois

Barbara J. Visocan Klein, MS, RD, FADA
House of Delegates/Practice
  Operations Team
The American Dietetic Association
Chicago, Illinois

Joanne E. Wade, MS
Associate Dean
Chief Operating Officer
Biological Sciences Division
University of Chicago
Chicago, Illinois

Christine Wanke, MD
Assistant Professor of Medicine
Harvard Medical School
Division of Infectious Disease
Beth Israel Deaconess Hospital
Boston, Massachusetts

Nancy H. Westbrook, RD, MMSc, LD, CNSD
Director, Professional Services
Shands HomeCare
Tampa, Florida

Marion F. Winkler, MS, RD, CNSD
Surgical Nutrition Specialist
Department of Surgery
Nutritional Support Service
Rhode Island Hospital
Clinical Teaching Associate of
  Surgery
Brown University
Providence, Rhode Island

Ka Wong, RD, CNSD
Nutrition Support Dietitian
Department of Dietetics and Food
  Service
Temple University Hospital and
  Health Sciences Center
Philadelphia, Pennsylvania

Preface

In the eight years since the first edition of *Dietitian's Handbook of Enteral and Parenteral Nutrition,* the amount of knowledge in nutrition support has expanded exponentially. A growing body of research is now available to support practice. Enteral feeding has progressed from witchcraft to science. Transitional feeding has advanced from an abstract concept to a small body of literature. Evolving knowledge of the influence of nutritional modifications on the disease process has moved enteral and parenteral feeding into the realm of nutritional pharmacology. Dietitians have proven their value as primary providers of nutrition support and have expanded their role accordingly.

The second edition of *Dietitian's Handbook of Enteral and Parenteral Nutrition* is designed to reflect these and many other changes. While providing a practical approach, this text is designed to support introductory level nutrition support for critical care nutrition courses and to serve as a practical reference.

Revisions to the first edition are based on reviews by teachers who adopted it, comments by practicing nutrition support dietitians, and my experiences using the text to teach a graduate course in critical care nutrition. All chapters have been updated; almost all have undergone substantial revision.

The chapters on nutritional assessment, macronutrient requirements, indirect calorimetry, and enteral nutrition have been completely rewritten. The chapter on home care has been revised to focus on regulatory and economic issues in addition to clinical ones.

Eight new chapters have been added, and the contributions of seventeen new authors incorporated. Consistent with the growing body of literature establishing indications for nutrition support, the chapter entitled "Nutrition Support: Indications and Efficacy" has been added. To address issues related to diabetes and glucose control, a separate chapter on pancreatic function has been included. Four new chapters entitled "Bone Marrow Transplantation," "HIV and AIDS," "Solid

Organ Transplantation," and "Burns" have been included to meet needs that did not exist when the first edition was written. The chapter entitled "Surgery and Wound Healing" recognizes that surgical patients form the basis of nutrition support practice. Finally, there is enough literature to support a brief chapter entitled "Transitional Feeding," which can be used to develop institutional protocol.

One of the most challenging editorial tasks is incorporating unique information about specific patient populations into a standardized format. Some inconsistencies are unavoidable. It is hoped that the different viewpoints offered by the experts who contributed to this text will be used to stimulate academic debate and ultimately advance practice.

Annalynn Skipper, MS, RD, FADA, CNSD
Chicago, Illinois

Acknowledgments

No task of this magnitude is completed alone. I am grateful to many for their support of my editorial and professional efforts. Mike Brown at Aspen envisioned a series of books on nutrition, and during the last ten years has made it a reality. He deserves a tremendous amount of credit for disseminating nutrition knowledge. Many others as Aspen contributed to this effort including Sandy Cannon, Mary Anne Langdon, Ruth Bloom, and Nick Radhuber. Reviewers were Jorge E. Albina, MD; Kary Caba, RD, CNSD; Janet Furman, RD, CNSD; Wissam Hasnain, RD; Kerri Hood, PharmD; Eugenia Kennedy, PharmD; Song Mi Lee; Susan Manchester, RD, LDN, CNSD; Carol O'Neil, RD; Kevin Roggins, MD; Christine Watkins, RN, MSN, CNSN; and Dana Weinstein, MNS, RD, CNSD.

Just as my colleagues at Pennsylvania Hospital supported me through the first edition of this text, my colleagues at Rush-Presbyterian-St. Luke's Medical Center have done likewise. Rebecca Dowling has provided a wonderful example and opportunities to expand my teaching and professional skills. Linda Lafferty has challenged me with new experiences and along with Maureen Murtaugh and Christy Tangney has encouraged my academic career. Carol Cotner has supported my teaching efforts. Ellis Pool, Diana Berry, and Brenda Kirkland made me laugh during rough spots. Mary Gregoire has always taken time to listen.

The staff of the Nutrition Consultation Service at Rush are some of the best nutrition support dietitians and pharmacists anywhere. Their interest in nutrition support practice, the broad scope of skills they maintain, and their inquisitive nature foster a challenging intellectual environment. During my career, I also have had the privilege of working with a number of graduate students in Clinical Nutrition, residents in surgery and medicine, and nutrition support fellows. Their intellectual curiosity and energy stimulate scientific inquiry and advancement of practice.

As in the first edition, I would also like to thank my parents, John D. and Louise Skipper, who insisted that I acquire the skills necessary for this undertaking and provided me with the background to bring it to completion. Finally, I would like to thank Joe for his unflagging encouragement.

Introduction

Over the past 30 years, the science and art of nutritional support has developed, grown, and matured. During this time, artificial nutrients in the form of intravenous hyperalimentation have been provided to patients unable or unwilling to consume them via conventional means. The development of parenteral nutrition also focused attention on the medical necessity of nutritional support and catalyzed the rapid development and widespread use of medical nutrition therapy. Appropriate use of parenteral nutrition demanded that techniques for nutritional assessment of hospitalized patients be evaluated and applied. With the commitment and creativity of hundreds of patients, physicians, nurses, dietitians, pharmacists, and others, nutritional support has evolved into a sophisticated, multidisciplinary effort.

Although malnutrition upon hospital admission remains a major problem, patients who otherwise would remain unfed and potentially malnourished may now be adequately treated. Nutritional assessment of hospitalized adult and pediatric patients continues to evolve. Nutritional assessment is no longer used solely to identify candidates for nutritional support; ever more sophisticated methods are also used to measure the response to increasingly complex nutritional therapy. Thirty years ago, existing nutritional assessment methodologies, used primarily in epidemiological surveys, were applied to hospitalized patients. These methods required critical scientific review and interpretation to ensure that their application achieved medical and scientific credibility. Many of these methods continue to be in widespread use; others have fallen from favor, and new methods have taken their place. Research into more specific, rapid, and cost-effective methodologies for nutritional assessment continues.

Safe and effective methods of administering parenteral and enteral nutrient solutions are available. Advances in biomedical technology have revolutionized and enhanced our ability to provide nutritional support to patients who otherwise would not be able to ingest adequate nutrients. The development of specially designed intravenous catheters, venous access discs, enteral feeding catheters, and parenteral and enteral pumps has resulted in the precise access to delivery systems necessary to provide optimal nutrition to critically or chronically ill patients.

Many parenteral and enteral nutrient solutions have been developed over the past three decades, ranging from those that can be used in a broad spectrum of clinical conditions to those that are disease-specific. Researchers and clinicians have teamed with industry to identify, design, evaluate, and manufacture nutrient sources that can be modulated to achieve a specific nutrient composition and profile. The result is the ability to provide nutrient solutions specially designed for individual clinical and nutritional requirements.

Early in the development of parenteral nutrition, a solution of macronutrients— primarily dextrose and protein with added known vitamins, electrolytes, and trace elements—was thought to provide total nutritional support. As the application of parenteral nutrition broadened, clinicians and researchers learned a great deal about the vitamin, trace element, and macronutrient needs of patients receiving enteral and parenteral nutrients both in the hospital and at home. Clinicians and researchers also learned that, in certain disease states, increased amounts of micronutrients (eg, biotin and manganese) were necessary to prevent further deficiencies and physiologic complications. In organ-specific diseases, the amino acid profile can now be manipulated to improve the assimilation of nutrients, thereby enhancing the body's ability to utilize them. The addition of lipids as a source of fuel and essential fatty acids further expanded the application of peripheral parenteral nutrition. Today, although researchers continue to investigate the optimal source of carbohydrate and lipid in both central and peripheral parenteral nutrition, available solutions can provide maximal nutritional support to hospitalized patients. Clinicians' ability to measure energy expenditure and substrate utilization with indirect calorimetry has further refined knowledge about nutrient requirements, resulting in the obsolescence of the term *hyperalimentation*. Research defining the advantages of enteral feeding has led to an explosion in the use of enteral feeding products.

Specialized nutritional support has fostered the multidisciplinary concept of health care. The core team of physicians, dietitians, nurses, and pharmacists has expanded to include dietetic technicians, physical therapists, and social workers. The expertise of each profession is integrated in assessing, managing, and monitoring patients so as to provide the safest, most efficient, and most cost-effective nutritional support. The multidisciplinary concept enhances the collegial relationships of these professionals, resulting in unique opportunities for improving patient care. This multidiscipinary vehicle for providing nutritional care has been so successful that regulatory agencies have mandated it.

The education and credentialing of practitioners is essential to providing the highest-quality health care. Techniques of nutritional assessment and support have become increasingly sophisticated as research and clinical experience continue to define and resolve issues related to the pathophysiology of disease and the impact of nutrition. With these advances comes the responsibility to teach the health care community not only the technical and clinical applications but the potential benefits and costs to society. A thorough understanding of the science of medical nutrition and the art of its application is required in the current cost-conscious clinical setting.

This book represents the experience of professionals who practice the fine art of nutritional support, who contribute to clinical research as a means of improving patient care, and who further the knowledge of the health care community. It presents a practical approach, supported by clinical experience and research, to the provision of nutritional support. Clearly, dietitians have made a unique contribution to the growth and development of nutritional support. This book is evidence of the expertise that clinical dietitians demonstrate in the provision of optimal nutritional support and of their commitment to educating the health care community about the field of specialized nutritional support.

Joanne E. Wade, MS
Associate Dean
Chief Operating Officer
Biological Sciences Division
University of Chicago
Chicago, Illinois

PART I

Selection of Candidates for Nutrition Support

CHAPTER 1

Nutritional Screening and Assessment

Pamela J. Charney

INTRODUCTION

Inappropriate feeding (either over- or underfeeding) can lead to multiple adverse outcomes, including hepatic and pulmonary effects, excess lipogenesis, or prolonged inadequate intake. Additionally, the benefits of aggressive nutrition support (particularly parenteral) appear to be realized most often in patients with the most severe deficits.[1] Therefore, it is imperative that nutrition support clinicians develop skills to assess nutritional status quickly and accurately in a wide variety of clinical conditions in order to optimize the provision of specialized nutrition support.

Recognizing the importance of nutrition in all phases of health care, regulatory agencies have begun requiring nutritional assessment for all at-risk patients very shortly after admission. Many facilities have developed nutritional risk screening programs in order to identify at-risk patients quickly and allow for timely, effective, comprehensive nutritional assessment for patients most likely to benefit from aggressive nutrition support.

In a landmark article, Butterworth first noted the incidence of untreated malnutrition in hospitalized patients.[2] Since then, others have reported the prevalence of malnutrition in hospitalized patients; the rate of malnutrition varies, depending on the setting and parameters used to identify it.[3–5] Weinsier et al[6] evaluated the nutritional status of 134 consecutive admissions to a medical service at admission, and then weekly starting after 2 weeks of hospitalization. Serum vitamin levels, hematological values, anthropometric measurements, and serum albumin levels were measured at admission and during the follow-up period. On admission, 48% of the patients had a score that indicated a high likelihood of malnutrition. On follow-up, patients' nutritional status worsened; this was associated with a longer hospitalization and increased mortality.[6] A follow-up study at the same hospital 12 years later reported no change in the percentage of patients admitted with a high likeli-hood of malnutrition; however, patients' nutritional status improved with hospi-talization, suggesting greater awareness of the nutritional needs of hospitalized patients and more rapid initiation of nutrition therapy.[7]

Malnourished patients may be at greater risk for complications including longer length of stay and more infections, leading to increased hospital costs. Protein deple-tion, as determined by prompt in vivo neutron activation analysis and tritiated water dilution technique, was associated with a significantly higher incidence of postopera-tive pneumonia as well as a longer length of stay in patients undergoing major gas-trointestinal surgery.[8] Other parameters associated with malnutrition—such as serum albumin (Alb) levels, weight loss, and immune dysfunction—have been linked to increased morbidity and mortality, mainly in hospitalized surgical patients.[9–12]

MALNUTRITION

The extremes of over- and undernutrition are easily recognizable. Mild to mod-erate nutritional deficits that develop over time may be well tolerated and show no overt signs until illness or stress lead to the expression of clinically evident malnu-trition. Often, changes in body composition, including loss of lean body mass and increase in body fat, occur prior to obvious weight loss. It is important for clini-cians to identify not only the presence of deficits, but also the extent of loss (par-ticularly loss of lean body mass) and the time frame over which the loss occurred in order to develop an effective plan for repletion.

Traditionally, two forms of malnutrition have been identified. These two forms, marasmus and kwashiorkor, were first described in malnourished children in un-derdeveloped countries. A third type of malnutrition has been identified in pa-tients with severe illness; this is a combination of marasmus- and kwashiorkor-type malnutrition (see Table 1–1).

Marasmic malnutrition is probably the most easily identified form of malnutri-tion. Individuals with marasmus appear cachectic and wasted due to long-term deficits of all nutrients, especially energy and protein. The normal adaptive re-sponse to uncomplicated starvation is to utilize body energy stores while preserv-ing lean body mass, leading to a wasted appearance. Metabolic rate is decreased in an attempt to conserve energy. Hormonal changes include decreased insulin levels leading to mobilization of energy stores. Skeletal muscle and fat stores provide the majority of energy during long-term starvation. Levels of serum proteins such as albumin are maintained until late in the course of starvation, making them poor markers of nutritional status in individuals with pure marasmus. Uncomplicated starvation tends to be well tolerated until more than 30% of initial body weight is lost or stress or illness occurs.

In contrast to marasmic malnutrition, kwashiorkor appears to be the result of a protein deficit out of proportion to deficits of other nutrients; this form of malnu-

Table 1–1 Metabolic Physiology

Characteristic Finding	Starvation (Marasmus)	Metabolic Response to Injury (Protein-Energy Malnutrition)
Energy needs	Decreased	Increased
Primary fuel (RQ)	Lipids (0.75)	Mixed (0.85)
Insulin	Decreased	Increased (resistance)
Ketones	Present	Absent
Counterregulatory hormones	Basal	Increased
Total-body water	Decreased	Increased
Proteolysis	Decreased	Accelerated
Glycogenolysis	Increased	Accelerated
Lipolysis	Increased	Increased
Body stores		
Skeletal muscle	Reduced	Reduced
Fat	Reduced	Reduced
Visceral protein	Preserved	Increased liver/immune
Refeeding response	Net anabolism	None (unless reversed)
Weight (lean tissue) loss	Gradual	Accelerated
Typical setting	Chronic diseases (cardiac, COPD, etc)	Hospitalized/ICU patient

RQ = respiratory quotient; COPD = chronic obstructive pulmonary disease; ICU = intensive care unit.

Source: Reprinted with permission from Zaloga, *Nutrition in Critical Care,* p. 13, © 1994, Mosby-Year Book, Inc.

---

trition has mainly been identified in malnourished children in underdeveloped countries. Williams used the term *kwashiorkor* in the mid-1930s to describe an edematous form of protein energy malnutrition seen in some countries in Africa.[13] These individuals develop edema and hypoalbuminemia. Body weight may be normal or only slightly decreased due to edema. Insulin levels are not decreased in kwashiorkor; this leads to deposition of essential amino acids in muscle, making them unavailable for hepatic protein synthesis. Hypoalbuminemia develops as the shortage of amino acids available for protein synthesis becomes severe. Additionally, fatty liver may be seen due to lack of beta-lipoprotein synthesis.[14] Pure kwashiorkor is rarely, if ever, seen in a clinical setting in developed countries.

Combination marasmus/kwashiorkor is often referred to as hypoalbuminemic malnutrition and is often seen when individuals with or without chronic malnutrition experience some form of acute stress. Classification systems for determining marasmic or kwashiorkor-like malnutrition have been developed (see Table 1–2). During

Table 1–2 Classification of Malnutrition

Type of Malnutrition	% Ideal Weight	Creatinine Height Index (%)	Skin Test (mm)
Marasmus			
Moderate	60–80	60–80	—
Severe	<60	<60	<5*

	Serum Albumin (g/dL)	Serum Transferrin mg/100 mL	Total Lymphocyte Count mm³	Skin Test (mm)
Kwashiorkor-like				
Moderate	2.1–3.0	100–150	800–1200	<5*
Severe	<2.1	<100	<800	<5*

Treatment of malnutrition requires characterization into two general categories that reflect their
  1. different consequences in terms of morbidity and mortality
  2. different treatment modalities
  3. different pathogenesis

Furthermore, these *diseases* should be coded so that they appear on hospital discharge summaries and in health planning statistics.

ICDA—International Classification
Protein malnutrition—Kwashiorkor-like   No. 267
Nutritional marasmus   No. 268
Other nutrition disorders—unspecified   No. 269.9

*On all three skin tests.

Source: Reprinted with permission from G.L. Blackburn et al., *Journal of Parenteral and Enteral Nutrition,* Vol. 1, No. 1, pp. 1–12, © 1977, A.S.P.E.N.

---

uncomplicated stress or surgery, the stress response lasts 24 to 72 hours. If complications occur and the stress response lasts more than 5 to 7 days, catabolism and protein loss may have serious consequences in the absence of appropriate nutrition support. The acute stress response is characterized by production of inflammatory mediators and counterregulatory hormones leading to inflammation, fever, increased vascular permeability, increased gluconeogenesis, and changes in hepatic protein synthesis. There is no compensatory reduction in metabolic rate, and gluconeogenesis is not halted by glucose infusion. Hepatic synthesis of the acute-phase reactants occurs at the expense of skeletal muscle, with loss of as much as 20 to 30 grams of nitrogen per day. Peripheral insulin resistance leads to hyperglycemia not responsive to exogenous insulin. These patients seem to be at greatest risk for nutrition-related complications, as compensatory mechanisms may have been exhausted by long-term inadequate nutrition. A significant increase in length of hospital stay has been noted in patients with this type of malnutrition.[15]

COMPONENTS OF NUTRITIONAL ASSESSMENT

A complete history and physical exam, as well as diet history, are vital in assessing nutritional status, because many factors may lead to altered nutrient intake and utilization (see Exhibit 1–1). While the presence of malnutrition is unmistakable in the cachectic patient, those who are initially overweight may suffer significant nutritional deficits before overt signs appear. Changes in skin—including dryness, rashes, ulceration, or cracking—may be due to nutritional deficiencies as well as other medical or environmental factors (see Table 1–3). The presence of edema should alert the clinician to potential fluid overload leading to dilution of certain serum protein levels and alterations in body weight not due to increased lean body mass. Dehydration may lead to falsely elevated serum levels of albumin and other proteins. Another important piece of information from the history and physical exam is the patient's medication history. In many cases, there exists the potential for drug-nutrient interactions and altered nutrient intake or utilization. Gastrointestinal status and function, surgical history, allergies, and chronic medical conditions as well as changes in functional status are also important and should

---

Exhibit 1–1 Components of Nutritional Screening and Assessment

History and Physical Examination
- medical history
- surgical history
- diagnosis
- medications
- current intake
- physical examination

Anthropometric Measurements
- height
- weight
- skinfold measurements
- urinary measurements of creatinine and 3-methylhistidine
- bioelectric impedance analysis

Biochemical Measurements
- albumin
- transferrin
- prealbumin
- retinol-binding protein
- insulin-like growth factor-1 (IGF-1)
- fibronectin

Functional Tests
- muscle strength
- hand grip dynamometry

Immune Function
- skin testing
- total lymphocyte count

Table 1–3 Physical Examination of Nutritional Status

System	Symptoms
General	Weight loss (% of usual and ideal body weight), triceps skinfold, midarm muscle circumference
Skin	Pallor, xerosis, follicular hyperkeratosis, pellagrous or flaky paint dermatitis, petechiae, ecchymosis, perifollicular hemorrhage
Hair	Dyspigmentation, thinning, straightening, easy pluckability
Head	Parotid enlargement, temporal wasting
Eyes	Bitot's spots, angular palpebratus, conjunctival and scleral xerosis, corneal vascularization, keratomalacia
Mouth	Angular stomatitis, cheilosis, spongy gums, poor dentition, glossitis, magenta tongue, tongue fissuring, atrophic lingual papillae
Heart	Cardiomegaly, congestive heart failure
Abdomen	Hepatomegaly, ascites
Extremities	Edema, muscle atrophy, koilonychia
Nervous system	Weakness, calf tenderness, loss of deep tendon reflexes

Source: Reprinted with permission from F. Bozzetti, *Journal of Parenteral and Enteral Nutrition,* Vol. 11, No. 5, pp. 115S–121S, © 1987, A.S.P.E.N.

be noted. Patients with recent multiple admissions to the hospital may be at increased risk for developing nutritional deficits. It is also important to note socioeconomic factors, such as access to food and social support systems. The dietitian should become skilled in interpreting all data from the history and physical exam in order to determine changes due to nutritional deficiencies.

It is important to gather data on recent and long-term nutrient intake. The current "gold standard" for determining intake is observed intake of known quantities of food. Because this is only feasible in well-controlled metabolic ward studies, a more practical method is needed for assessing intake of individual patients. Diet records involve self-recording of intake over a specified period of time, usually 3 to 8 days. Food-frequency questionnaires provide information about usual intake over a specific time period, while a 24-hour recall obtains information on recent intake. Without careful attention to methodology, accuracy may be compromised in all these methods.[16] Often, a complete 24-hour recall is combined with an abbreviated food frequency in order to obtain a more complete indication of the adequacy of intake prior to hospitalization. A "calorie count," often for 3 days, is commonly used to determine adequacy of intake during hospitalization; however, this method provides no information on intake prior to hospitalization. Additionally, calorie counts may lack accuracy, depending on methods used for collecting and interpreting intake data. The time required to collect and interpret data may lead to unnecessary delays in initiating appropriate nutrition therapy. Nutritional assessment may often be completed based on the patient's history and physical while other data are being collected and analyzed. Sound clinical judgment allows for assessment to be completed while calorie-count data are being collected and analyzed.

Anthropometric Assessment

The goal of anthropometric assessment is to determine actual or estimated body composition, specifically lean body mass and fat stores. Techniques used for anthropometric assessment range from simple, inexpensive methods such as measurement of height and weight, to more complicated, expensive direct measurements of body composition such as dual-energy X-ray absorptiometry. Methods commonly used in clinical practice have included measurement of height, weight, skinfold, urinary creatinine excretion, and bioelectric impedance analysis.

Actual measurement of height is a simple procedure that is often overlooked in clinical practice. Clinicians should measure the patient's height if at all possible in order to avoid inaccuracies introduced by use of a stated height in the assessment process. Loss of height occurs in many individuals as part of the aging process. Alternate methods to estimate height can be used for patients who are unable to stand. Knee height has been shown to correlate with stature and can be measured using a knee-height caliper. Recumbent height may also be used, although this method is less accurate.

Clinicians have known for many years that weight loss may act as an indicator of increased risk for postoperative complications.[17] Various standards for evaluating weight are available, but the most commonly used are the Metropolitan Height-Weight Tables, which present the weight ranges associated with lowest mortality.[18] Clinicians should remember that these tables were developed using healthy, young adults (age 25 to 59 years) who could afford to purchase life insurance. Asians, African Americans, and other ethnic groups were not well represented. Additionally, approximately 10% of the data for the 1983 tables were self-reported, leading to potential errors and inaccuracies.[19] For these reasons, the tables should be used with caution in evaluating nutritional status.[20]

Rather than comparing a patient's current weight to some desirable or ideal weight, it is probably more appropriate to compare current weight to the patient's usual weight. Loss of as little as 5% of usual body weight has been associated with decreased survival in patients with various types of cancer; in fact, weight loss is part of the staging process for some cancers.[10] Patients who had a self-reported weight loss of more than 10 pounds within 6 months prior to admission for elective surgical procedures had significantly increased mortality rates compared to patients who had not lost weight.[21] Unintentional weight loss may be associated with factors that may increase mortality, such as age or poorer health.[22] Researchers have noted that the significance of weight loss as a prognostic indicator increases when weight loss is combined with impairment in functional status.[23]

Many factors may influence weight measurements. In critical care settings, usual weight may not be available initially, so the first weight measurement often includes significant amounts of resuscitation fluids. Fluid shifts are fairly common in critically ill patients and can lead to significant inaccuracies in weight measurements. An additional 1 L of fluid can add approximately 1 kg to weight measurements, so the presence of ascites or significant edema should be noted. Scales that are not calibrated properly or interobserver differences in technique may also lead to inaccurate weight measurement. Gain or loss of more than 0.5 kg over 24 hours in the absence of significant fluid shifts may signify measurement error and should be rechecked. Significant weight change has been defined as loss of more than 10% of usual weight over 6 months or less (see Table 1–4).

Measurement of skinfold thicknesses has been used to estimate body fat, because much of the body's adipose tissue lies in the subcutaneous tissue. Although many anatomical sites have been used for assessment of skinfold thickness, the triceps skinfold (TSF) is probably most commonly used in clinical practice due to accessibility. Midarm muscle circumference (MAMC), calculated using the TSF and arm circumference measurements, provides an estimate of muscle protein stores. Skinfold measurements are quick, easy, and noninvasive. Careful attention must be paid to technique, as considerable intra- and interindividual variation in measurement has been reported.[24] Percentage of body fat as determined from

---

Table 1–4 Evaluation of Weight Change*

Time	Significant Weight Loss	Severe Weight Loss
1 week	1–2%	>2%
1 month	5%	>5%
3 months	7.5%	>7.5%
6 months	10%	>10%

*Values charted are for percent weight change:

$$\text{Percent weight change} = \frac{(\text{Usual weight} - \text{Actual weight})}{(\text{Usual weight})} \times 100$$

Source: Reprinted with permission from G.L. Blackburn et al., *Journal of Parenteral and Enteral Nutrition,* Vol. 1, No. 1, pp. 1–12, © 1977, A.S.P.E.N.

skinfold measurements was found to overestimate fat mass in lean individuals and underestimate it in obese subjects when compared to bioelectric impedance analysis (BIA).[25] Fluid retention in critically ill patients also makes evaluation of MAMC difficult.[26] Additionally, although several standards for evaluation of results are available, most were developed in nonhospitalized populations and may not be applicable to hospitalized patients. Poor correlation was found between two commonly used standards when tested in healthy volunteers and patients with malignant and nonmalignant gastrointestinal pathology.[27] Individual differences in fat distribution may limit accuracy of interpretation of results.[28] Skinfold measurements may be most appropriate for use in long-term population studies due to the longer time (often greater than 3 to 4 weeks) required to see clinically significant changes and the lack of precision required to monitor individual patients.[29,30]

BIA measures the electrical impedance of body tissues, which allows for estimation of total body water. Because almost all body water is contained in fat-free mass, body fat can then be estimated from impedance measurements.[31,32] BIA is most often measured by use of tetrapolar electrodes placed on the dorsal surfaces of the hand and foot.[33] Under most conditions, BIA provides reasonable estimates of body fat and fat-free mass. However, measurements may be compromised in situations where there are alterations in body water distribution, including critical illness.

Urinary Measurements

Urinary measurement of creatinine and 3-methylhistidine (3-MeHis) excretion has been used as a mechanism for estimating body protein status. Creatinine is the metabolic product of creatine metabolism in the muscle and is excreted unchanged in the urine. It has been estimated that 1 g of urinary creatinine represents approximately 18 kg of fat-free muscle; thus, measurement of 24-hour urine excretion of creatinine should reflect muscle mass.[34] The creatinine-height index (CHI) has been used to express creatinine excretion as a percentage of that expected for individuals matched for height and sex.[35] These data were obtained from healthy, young adults. As there is an age-related decrease in creatinine excretion, the tables have been modified to account for age.[36] Difficulties in the use of CHI in nutritional assessment include the need for an accurate 24-hour urine collection and the time required to complete the assay.

Another measure of body protein status is urinary 3-MeHis excretion. Like creatinine, 3-MeHis is a byproduct of muscle metabolism that is excreted entirely in the urine. Thus, 3-MeHis provides a measure of protein breakdown.[37] Urinary excretion of 3-MeHis was found to correlate with response to parenteral nutrition in a group of malnourished patients.[38] As with creatinine, 3-MeHis is not commonly used in nutritional assessment due to the need for a complete 24-hour urine collection and the expense of completing the test.

Biochemical Assessment of Nutritional Status

Meaurement of serum albumin is inexpensive and easily done, leading to its widespread use in nutritional screening and assessment. In addition to its role as a marker of nutritional status, albumin functions in maintaining oncotic pressure and as a carrier protein for many substances, including hormones, fatty acids, amino acids, metals, and drugs. Several studies have shown that decreased albumin levels act as a marker for increased length of stay as well as increased risk for complications and death.[39,40] In a small group of critically ill, intensive care unit patients, albumin levels less than 2.5 g/dL predicted survival.[41] In a cohort study, Alb level was an independent risk factor for mortality in elderly individuals.[42]

Serum levels of albumin must be interpreted with caution in acute care settings. Normal or nearly normal levels are maintained in patients with marasmic-type malnutrition due to previously described compensatory mechanisms. For this reason, it is not uncommon for wasted individuals to be incorrectly described as having "adequate visceral protein stores" when a more appropriate description would be "compensated chronic malnutrition." Due to a large body pool (5 g/kg) and a long half-life of approximately 20 days, albumin levels do not reflect acute changes in nutritional status. For these reasons, albumin alone should not be used as a nutritional assessment parameter.

Albumin levels often decrease rapidly following surgery or trauma. Causes of postoperative hypoalbuminemia include increased levels of the counterregulatory stress hormones and an inflammatory response. In human volunteers, simulation of the endocrine response to surgery by infusion of the counterregulatory hormones epinephrine, glucagon, and hydrocortisone did not lead to hypoalbuminemia; this finding led investigators to conclude that postoperative hypoalbuminemia was most likely caused by vascular redistribution mediated by cytokines.[43] Infusion of interleukin-1β led to decreased albumin synthesis in an animal study potentially indicating cytokine regulation of postoperative hypoalbuminemia.[44] In these situations, hypoalbuminemia may reflect disease severity rather than nutritional status. Additionally, albumin levels alone cannot be used as an index of adequacy of feeding, because changes occur very slowly during the recovery period.

Due to a shorter half-life and smaller body pool, transferrin levels are frequently used in assessing nutritional status in acute care settings. Transferrin is a 77,000 molecular weight protein with a half-life of 8 to 10 days. Because transferrin is an iron-transport protein, its levels are affected by iron status. Transferrin levels increase in the face of iron deficiency, transfusion, or massive blood loss. Levels are also affected by the presence of infection. As direct measurement of transferrin may not be readily available in the clinical setting, equations have been developed for estimating transferrin from total iron-binding capacity (TIBC).[45]

$$\text{Serum transferrin} = (\text{TIBC} \times 0.76) + 18$$

Transferrin levels calculated from TIBC were found to predict nutritional status best in populations; they lacked sensitivity and specificity to determine nutritional status in individual patients.[46] Serum transferrin measurements predicted spontaneous fistula closure in a retrospective study.[47] If transferrin levels are to be used for nutritional assessment, it would be prudent to use actual levels rather than those calculated from TIBC; if calculated levels are used, equations used should be established for the lab performing the tests.

Prealbumin (TBPA) (or transthyretin) is synthesized in the liver; it functions in transport of thyroxine and binds to retinol-binding protein in order to prevent its renal loss. Due to a short half-life and small body pool, TBPA levels have been reported to be a sensitive indicator of response to refeeding. Additionally, hepatic TBPA synthesis appears to be extremely sensitive to changes in energy and protein intake.[48] Studies in malnourished children found that TBPA levels responded to refeeding before changes were seen in serum Alb levels.[49] Energy restriction led to a decrease in TBPA levels in a group of obese women; levels were restored within 72 hours of increasing the energy content of the diet.[50] Currently, because of its rapid response to refeeding, TBPA level is used mainly as a marker of response to nutrition therapy.[51,52]

Other, less commonly used biochemical markers of nutritional status include retinol-binding protein (RBP), fibronectin, and insulin-like growth factor-1 (IGF-1). RBP has a half-life of approximately 10 to 12 hours and may therefore reflect more acute changes in protein metabolism. RBP functions in vitamin A transport, leading to decreased levels with vitamin A deficiency. While RBP has been shown to reflect protein repletion in a group of premature infants,[53] it is not commonly used as a nutritional assessment parameter.

Fibronectin is a glycoprotein that exists in both soluble and insoluble forms. The soluble form assists in immune function by attaching to foreign particles and making them more easily recognizable by phagocytes, while the insoluble form has structural functions. Levels have been shown to decrease after 7 days of starvation and return to normal levels after 5 days of refeeding in obese subjects.[54] Researchers reported that 2 to 3 weeks of total parenteral nutrition (TPN) led to a statistically significant increase in fibronectin levels in malnourished patients with gastrointestinal disorders and in patients with anorexia nervosa. However, the authors of this study noted that interpretation of these results in individual patients may be complicated because only a few patients had fibronectin levels that were lower than normal limits when TPN was started.[55] Authors of another study reported that individual fibronectin levels did not predict survival in septic intensive care unit patients.[56] Others have found that fibronectin levels were able to predict outcome in malnourished patients receiving parenteral nutrition.[57]

IGF-1 is a growth factor with anabolic actions found in the serum. Levels of IGF-1 have been found to correlate with nitrogen balance and response to feeding but not with outcome in malnourished or critically ill patients.[58,59] IGF-1 levels were found to significantly correlate with nitrogen balance after 7 days of enteral nutrition support in a group of critically ill trauma patients.[60] The use of IGF-1 in nutritional assessment has not been evaluated.

Markers of anemia such as serum hemoglobin and hematocrit have been used in evaluation of nutritional status. The nutritional anemias are those caused by iron deficiency as well as folate and vitamin B_{12} deficiency. Although repletion of the iron, folate, or vitamin B_{12} treats the anemia, the cause of the condition is most often not related to nutritional status; rather, it is caused by blood loss, disease, or malabsorption. The use of hemoglobin or hematocrit alone is not sufficient to determine nutritional status.

Immune Function

Researchers and clinicians have known for many years that malnutrition leads to alterations in immune function. Deficits in cell-mediated immunity, bactericidal function, complement, and secretory IgA function have been described.[61] The interactions between nutritional status and immune function are complex and may involve deficiencies in energy and protein intake as well as vitamin, mineral, and trace element status.[62] It is hoped that treatment of malnutrition will lead to improvement in immune function. Indicators of immune function that are clinically applicable include delayed cutaneous hypersensitivity and total lymphocyte (TLC) count.

Testing for delayed cutaneous hypersensitivity (DCH) has been used as a measure of cellular immunity. Common recall antigens are injected intradermally, and response is typically measured at 24, 48, or 72 hours. A positive response is often interpreted as greater than 5 mm induration at one of the measurement points. Researchers found that reduced immune response as measured by DCH testing predicted sepsis-related mortality in patients undergoing elective gastrointestinal surgery.[63] Others have found that in patients with malignant diseases of the gastrointestinal tract, clinical judgment alone was more effective than DCH in predicting postoperative septic complications.[64] Problems with the use of DCH include low specificity of response and inability to identify other than obvious malnutrition.[65,66] In addition, many nonnutritional factors may influence DCH testing (see Exhibit 1–2). As with other objective measurements of nutritional status, the time required for results (up to 72 hours) may limit the usefulness of DCH testing in clinical practice.

TLC has been used as an indirect measure of immune status as well as nutritional status. Levels of TLC less than $1500/mm^3$ have been used as markers of compromised immune function. The prognostic significance of TLC can be increased when it is used in conjunction with another parameter, such as albumin. By itself, TLC lacks the sensitivity and specificity needed to determine nutritional status, because levels are affected by many nonnutritional factors.

Monocyte function, as measured by major histocompatability complex class II responses, has been studied in malnourished surgical patients. Malnourished sur-

Exhibit 1–2 Nonnutritional Influences on Skin Test Response

Technical
- antigen source and batch
- preparation and storage
- method of administration
- site of test
- booster effect
- criteria of positivity
- reader variability

Patient Factors
- age
- race
- geographic location
- prior exposure to antigen
- circadian rhythm
- psychologic state

Diseases—Benign
- infections
  — viral
  — bacterial
  — fungal
- metabolic
  — uremia
  — liver diseases
- inflammatory
  — Crohn's disease
  — ulcerative colitis
  — sarcoid

- immune alterations
  — congenital
    1. DiGeorge's syndrome
    2. thymic aplasia
  — acquired
    1. systemic lupus erythematosus (SLE)
    2. rheumatoid arthritis
- trauma, burns, hemorrhage

Diseases—Malignant
- most solid tumors, especially advancing stages
- lymphomas
- leukemias
- prior malignancy, especially squamous cancer, lymphoma

Iatrogenic
- drugs
  — immunosuppressants
  — most antineoplastics
  — antiinflammatory
  — anticoagulants
  — H₂ blockers (cimetidine)
  — aspirin
- X-ray therapy
- general anesthesia
- surgery

Source: Reprinted with permission of P. Twomey et al., *Journal of Parenteral and Enteral Nutrition,* Vol. 6, No. 1, pp. 50–58, A.S.P.E.N.

gical patients were found to have a decreased response to interferon gamma when compared to well-nourished, disease-matched control patients. Response was improved after 5 days of TPN.[67] Other measures of immune function (such as response to concanavalin A or phytohemagglutinin or levels of various immunoglobulins) have been used for research purposes, but are not commonly used in clinical practice.

Functional Assessment of Nutritional Status

Ideally, tests of nutritional status assess the impact of nutritional deficits on functional status. Measures of muscle strength, such as hand-grip dynamometry, test functional status. Animal studies have found decreases in muscle function, including loss of force and increased fatigability, after both acute and chronic starvation.[68] Similar findings in humans who were fed a 400-kcal diet were reported to be a result of cellular alterations including changes in muscle enzyme content, amino acid levels, and cellular ultrastructure.[69] Hand-grip strength proved to be a better predictor of postoperative complications than skinfold measurements, Alb levels, and weight loss in patients undergoing abdominal surgery.[70] Hand-grip strength was found to be a sensitive predictor of postoperative complications and increased length of hospitalization in a group of patients having elective surgery.[71] Researchers found that forearm muscle dynamometry is a better predictor of complications and mortality in patients with gastrointestinal cancer than is the Prognostic Nutritional Index (PNI).[72] Techniques for measurement of muscle strength are simple to perform and relatively inexpensive, results are readily available, and functional status seems to reflect nutritional status; therefore, some assessment of functional status should be included in nutritional assessment.

INDEXES USED IN NUTRITIONAL ASSESSMENT

Because no single parameter is universally accepted in assessment of nutritional status, attempts have been made to develop indexes to improve the sensitivity and specificity of individual parameters. Among the first of these was the PNI, which was developed to identify patients at risk of postoperative, nutrition-related complications. The PNI was developed based on data collected in 161 patients prior to elective surgical procedures. A linear predictive model was determined as follows:

$$PNI (\%) = 158 - 16.6 \text{ (Alb g/dL)} - 0.78 \text{ (TSF mm)} - 0.20 \text{ (transferrin}$$
$$\text{mg/100 mL)} - 5.8 \text{ (delayed hypersensitivity)}$$

It was found that the incidence of complications and death increased with increases in the PNI.[73] The model was validated in 100 patients undergoing elective gastrointestinal surgery.[74] The PNI was further tested in a group of patients undergoing surgery for head and neck cancer and was found to predict patients who were at risk for increased morbidity and mortality.[75] While the PNI appears to show promise in determining patients at high risk for nutrition-related complications from surgery, it is not commonly used in clinical practice, mainly due to the need for laboratory tests that may not be readily available (transferrin) and the need to wait at least 24 hours for skin test results.

The Instant Nutritional Assessment (INA) was developed as a simple method to assess nutritional status quickly; it uses only albumin and TLC. Researchers who conducted a retrospective analysis of 500 admissions reported a statistically significant increase in complications and deaths if albumin or both albumin and TLC were abnormal.[76] Further testing of the INA in intensive care unit patients showed that patients with abnormalities in both albumin and TLC had significantly higher morbidity and mortality than did patients with normal levels.[77] Others have confirmed these results.[78] Because alterations in both albumin and TLC may be due to many factors other than nutritional status, it may be best to use the INA as a screening tool to identify those patients who may require more in-depth nutritional assessment.

Subjective global assessment (SGA) uses components of the history and physical exam as well as the diet history to determine nutritional status. Baker et al were first to demonstrate that subjective assessment of nutritional status correlated with more objective parameters in predicting infection, antibiotic use, and length of stay.[79] Components of the SGA include weight changes, changes in nutrient intake, gastrointestinal function and functional status, as well as an assessment of the metabolic demands of the primary illness (see Exhibit 1–3). Patients are classified as well nourished, moderately malnourished, or severely malnourished based on the examiner's subjective rating. The technique for SGA is easily taught to clinicians and is simple and inexpensive to perform.[75] Adequate training is important to ensure interobserver reproducibility. Detsky et al have suggested combining albumin levels with SGA to better predict postoperative complications.[80]

Other indexes include the Prognostic Inflammatory and Nutritional Index (PINI), which includes markers of the inflammatory response as well as nutritional status. Nutritional markers used include Alb and TBPA; the inflammatory markers were C-reactive protein (CRP) and alpha$_1$-acid glycoprotein (AGP).

$$\text{PINI} = \frac{\text{AGP (mg/dL)} \times \text{CRP (mg/L)}}{\text{Alb (g/L)} \times \text{TBPA (mg/L)}}$$

Higher PINI values are associated with greater risk, as levels of AGP and CRP are increased during stress or infection and Alb and TBPA are low.[81] Researchers found that although PINI decreased during enteral feeding in a group of trauma patients, the index did not predict survival.[82] The use of the PINI may be somewhat limited by the availability of lab values in a timely fashion for rapid assessment of nutritional status.

RECOMMENDATIONS FOR NUTRITIONAL RISK SCREENING

Patients admitted to the hospital today are more acutely ill than in the past. Therefore, timely nutritional risk screening is needed in order to identify patients who require more comprehensive nutritional assessment. Nutritional risk screening should be simple, quick, and inexpensive to perform and should maintain an acceptable degree of accuracy in identifying at-risk patients. Ideally, nutritional risk screening should be completed at admission in order to ensure availability of needed data and to minimize redundancy in information gathering and documen-

Exhibit 1–3 Features of Subjective Global Assessment (SGA)

*(Select appropriate category with a checkmark, or
enter numerical value where indicated by #.)*

History

1. Weight change

   Overall loss in past 6 months: amount = # _____ kg; % loss = # _____.

   Change in past 2 weeks: _____ increase

   _____ no change

   _____ decrease

2. Dietary intake change (relative to normal)

   _____ No change

   _____ Change _____ duration = # _____ weeks.

   _____ type: _____ suboptimal solid diet _____ full liquid diet

   _____ hypocaloric liquids _____ starvation

3. Gastrointestinal symptoms (that persisted for > 2 weeks)

   _____ none _____ nausea _____ vomiting _____ diarrhea _____ anorexia

4. Functional capacity

   _____ No dysfunction (eg, full capacity)

   _____ Dysfunction _____ duration = # _____ weeks

   _____ type: _____ working suboptimally

   _____ ambulatory

   _____ bedridden

5. Disease and its relation to nutritional requirements

   Primary diagnosis (specify) _____

   Metabolic demand (stress): _____ no stress _____ low stress

   _____ moderate stress _____ high stress

Physical

(For each trait specify: 0 = normal, 1+ = mild, 2+ = moderate, 3+ = severe):

   # _____ loss of subcutaneous fat (triceps, chest)

   # _____ muscle wasting (quadriceps, deltoids)

   # _____ ankle edema

   # _____ sacral edema

   # _____ ascites

SGA Rating

(Select one):

   _____ A = Well nourished

   _____ B = Moderately (or suspected of being) malnourished

   _____ C = Severely malnourished

Source: Reprinted with permission from A.S. Detsky et al., *Journal of Parenteral and Enteral Nutrition,* Vol. 11, pp. 8–13, © 1987, A.S.P.E.N.

tation. Information gathered as part of the admission process often includes height, weight, and diagnosis. These data, combined with quick questions concerning unintentional weight loss and changes in functional status could serve as an initial screen (see Exhibit 1–4). Patients who are determined to be at-risk can be referred to the dietitian for more comprehensive nutritional assessment. In this

Exhibit 1–4 Examples of Nutritional Risk Screening Form

Example 1: Clinical Nutrition—Screening and Needs Assessment

Patient has been screened. Appears to be at risk for malnutrition.

Diet Rx: _____

Ht.: _____ Wt.: _____ IBW: _____ %IBW: _____ UBW: _____

Significant unintentional weight loss: _____ over _____ weeks/months

Patient reports appetite as: Poor _____ Fair _____ Good _____

Nutrition counseling: Requested _____ Declined _____

Nourishments ordered: _____

_____ Refer patient to the dietitian for a complete nutritional assessment.

_____

_____

_____

Example 2: Clinical Nutrition—Screening and Needs Assessment

The patient has been screened. Appears to be at low risk for malnutrition.

INSTRUCTION: Requested _____ Declined _____ Snacks ordered _____

ASSESSMENT:

_____ Will monitor the patient's intake on daily meal rounds.

_____ Further nutrition intervention is available upon request.

_____ The patient has been referred to the dietitian for nutrition counseling.

_____

_____

_____

Signature: _____ Food and Nutrition Coordinator

Courtesy of Rush-Presbyterian-St. Luke's Medical Center, Chicago, Illinois.

way, nutritional screening is completed at admission, and nutrition therapy can be initiated within 24 to 48 hours of admission.

RECOMMENDATIONS FOR NUTRITIONAL ASSESSMENT

The goals of nutritional assessment are to determine the presence and duration of nutritional deficits, to estimate current body composition, to determine the effect of metabolic stress on nutritional status, and to provide baseline information for determining the effectiveness of therapy. It has been shown that clinical judgment compares favorably with objective measures in assessment of nutritional status.[83] Biochemical and anthropometric measures of nutritional status have been found to be unreliable without clinical assessment.[84] Due to the need for rapid, accurate assessment of patients' nutritional status, nutritional assessment should provide information on a timely basis. Clinicians no longer have the luxury of waiting for the results of objective tests and need to rely on sound clinical judgment. Protocols developed for nutritional assessment should include information concerning weight status and unintentional weight loss prior to admission, some measure of functional status, nutrient intake and problems interfering with normal intake, physical assessment for signs and symptoms of nutrient deficiencies, and evaluation of current and chronic illnesses and their impact on nutritional status. Although somewhat lacking in sensitivity and specificity, Alb levels may be available for assessment of severity of illness and long-term adequacy of intake. Albumin levels may also function as a predictor of survival in some situations. Albumin levels should always be evaluated critically, however. Other biochemical markers, such as transferrin or TBPA, may not improve the accuracy of the nutritional assessment but may provide baseline information needed to monitor effectiveness of nutrition therapy.

REFERENCES

1. The Veterans Affairs Total Parenteral Nutrition Study Group. Perioperative total parenteral nutrition in surgical patients. *N Engl J Med.* 1991;325:525–532.
2. Butterworth C. The skeleton in the hospital closet. *Nutr Today.* 1974;9:4–8.
3. Pettigrew RA, Hill GL. Indicators of surgical risk and clinical judgement. *Br J Surg.* 1986;73:47–51.
4. Klidjian AM, Archer TJ, Foster KJ, Karran SJ. Detection of dangerous malnutrition. *J Parenter Enter Nutr.* 1982;6:119–121.
5. Bistrian BR, Blackburn GL, Hallowell E, Heddle R. Prevalence of malnutrition in general surgical patients. *JAMA.* 1974;230:858–860.
6. Weinsier RL, Hunker EM, Krumdieck CL, Butterworth CE. Hospital malnutrition: a prospective evaluation of general medical patients during the course of hospitalization. *Am J Clin Nutr.* 1979;32:418–426.

7. Coats KG, Morgan SL, Bartolucci AA, Weinsier RL. Hospital-associated malnutrition: a reevaluation 12 years later. *J Am Diet Assoc.* 1993;93:27–33.

8. Windsor JA, Hill GL. Risk factors for postoperative pneumonia: the importance of protein depletion. *Ann Surg.* 1988;208:209–214.

9. Reinhardt GF, Myscofski JW, Wilkens DB, Dobrin PB, et al. Incidence and mortality of hypoalbuminemic patients in hospitalized veterans. *J Parenter Enter Nutr.* 1980;4:357–359.

10. DeWys WD, Begg C, Lavin PT, Band PR, et al. Prognostic effect of weight loss prior to chemotherapy in cancer patients. *Am J Med.* 1980;69:491–497.

11. Christou NV, Meakins JL, MacLean LD. The predictive role of delayed hypersensitivity in preoperative patients. *Surg Gynecol Obstet.* 1981;152:297–301.

12. Dempsey DT, Mullen JT, Buzby GP. The link between nutritional status and clinical outcome: can nutritional intervention modify it? *Am J Clin Nutr.* 1988;47:352–356.

13. Williams CD. A nutritional disease of childhood associated with a maize diet. *Arch Dis Child.* 1933;8:423–433.

14. Coward WA, Lunn PG. The biochemistry and physiology of kwashiorkor and marasmus. *Br Med Bull.* 1981;37:19–24.

15. McClave S, Mitoraj T, Thielmeier K, Greenburg R. Differentiating subtypes of protein calorie malnutrition: incidence and clinical significance in a university hospital setting. *J Parenter Enter Nutr.* 1992;16:337–342.

16. Karkeck J. Improving the use of dietary survey methodology. *J Am Diet Assoc.* 1987;87:869–871.

17. Studley HO. Percentage of weight loss. A basic indicator of surgical risk in patients with chronic peptic ulcer. *JAMA.* 1936;106:458–460.

18. *1983 Metropolitan Height and Weight Tables. Statistical Bulletin.* Metropolitan Life Insurance Company; 1983.

19. Pirie P, Jacobs D, Jeffery R, Hannan P. Distortion in self-reported height and weight data. *J Am Diet Assoc.* 1981;78:601–606.

20. Robinett-Weiss N, Hixson ML, Keir B, Sieberg J. The Metropolitan height-weight tables: perspectives for use. *J Am Diet Assoc.* 1984;84:1480–1481.

21. Seltzer MH, Slocum BA, Cataldi-Betcher EL, Fileti C, et al. Instant nutritional assessment: absolute weight loss and surgical mortality. *J Parenter Enter Nutr.* 1982;6:218–221.

22. Meltzer A, Everhart JE. Unintentional weight loss in the United States. *Am J Epidemiol.* 1995;142:1039–1046.

23. Windsor JA, Hill GL. Weight loss with physiologic impairment: a basic indicator of surgical risk. *Ann Surg.* 1988;207:290–296.

24. Heymsfield S, McManus C, Seitz S, Nixon D, et al. Anthropometric assessment of adult protein-energy malnutrition. In: Wright R, Heymsfield S, eds. *Nutritional Assessment of the Adult Hospitalized Patient.* Boston: Blackwell Scientific Publications; 1984:27–82.

25. Vansant G, Van Gaal L, Deleeuw I. Assessment of body composition by skinfold anthropometry and bioelectric impedance technique: a comparative study. *J Parenter Enter Nutr.* 1994;18:427–429.

26. Green CJ, Campbell IT, McClelland P, Hutton JL, et al. Energy and nitrogen balance and changes in midupper-arm circumference with multiple organ failure. *J Nutr.* 1995;11:739–746.

27. Thuluvath PJ, Triger DR. How valid are our reference standards of nutrition? *J Nutr.* 1995;11:731–733.

28. Gray GE, Gray LK. Anthropometric measurements and their interpretation: principles, practices, and problems. *J Am Diet Assoc.* 1980;77:534–538.

29. Jensen MD. Research techniques for body composition assessment. *J Am Diet Assoc.* 1992; 92:454–460.

30. Collins JP, McCarthy ID, Hill GL. Assessment of protein nutrition in surgical patients: the value of anthropometrics. *Am J Clin Nutr.* 1979;32:1527–1530.

31. *Bioelectrical Impedance Analysis in Body Composition Measurement.* Technology assessment conference statement. Bethesda, MD: National Institutes of Health; 1994.

32. Lukaski HC. Methods for the assessment of human body composition: traditional and new. *Am J Clin Nutr.* 1987;46:537–556.

33. Heitmann BL. Impedance: a valid method in assessment of body composition? *Eur J Clin Nutr.* 1994;48:228–240.

34. Heymsfield SB, Arteaga C, McManus C, Smith J, et al. Measurement of muscle mass in humans: validity of the 24-hour urinary creatinine method. *Am J Clin Nutr.* 1983;37:478–494.

35. Bistrian BR, Blackburn GL, Sherman M, Scrimshaw NS. Therapeutic index of nutritional depletion in hospitalized patients. *Surg Gynecol Obstet.* 1975;141:512–516.

36. Walser M. Creatinine excretion as a measure of protein nutrition in adults of varying age. *J Parenter Enter Nutr.* 1987;11:73S–78S.

37. Ballard FJ, Tomas FM. 3-methylhistidine as a measure of skeletal muscle protein breakdown in human subjects: the case for its continued use. *Clin Sci.* 1983;65:209–215.

38. Kim CW, Okada A, Itakura T, Takagi Y, et al. Urinary excretion of 3-methylhistidine as an index of protein nutrition in total parenteral nutrition. *J Parenter Enter Nutr.* 1988;12:198–204.

39. Herrmann F, Safran C, Levkoff S, Minaker K. Serum albumin on admission as a predictor of death, length of stay, and readmission. *Arch Intern Med.* 1992;152:125–130.

40. Rudman D, Feller AG, Nagraj HS, Jackson DL, et al. Relation of serum albumin concentration to death rate in nursing home men. *J Parenter Enter Nutr.* 1987;11:360–363.

41. Apelgren KN, Rombeau JL, Twomey PL, Miller RA. Comparison of nutritional indices and outcome in critically ill patients. *Crit Care Med.* 1982;10:305–307.

42. Corti MC, Guralnik JM, Salive ME, Sorkin JD. Serum albumin level and physical disability as predictors of mortality in older persons. *JAMA.* 1994;272:1036–1042.

43. Smeets HJ, Kievit J, Harinck HIJ, Frölich M, et al. Differential effects of counterregulatory stress hormones on serum albumin concentrations and protein catabolism in healthy volunteers. *J Nutr.* 1995;11:423–427.

44. Ballmer PE, McNurlan MA, Grant I, Garlick PJ. Down-regulation of albumin synthesis in the rat by human recombinant interleukin-1β or turpentine and the response to nutrients. *J Parenter Enter Nutr.* 1995;19:266–271.

45. Stromberg BV, Davis RJ, Danziger LH. Relationship of serum transferrin to total iron binding capacity of nutritional assessment. *J Parenter Enter Nutr.* 1982;6:392–394.

46. Roza AM, Tuitt D, Shizgal HM. Transferrin—a poor measure of nutritional status. *J Parenter Enter Nutr.* 1984;8:523–528.

47. Kuvshinoff BW, Brodish RJ, McFadden DW, Fischer JE. Serum transferrin as a prognostic indicator of spontaneous closure and mortality in gastrointestinal cutaneous fistulas. *Ann Surg.* 1993;217:615–623.

48. Ingenbleek Y, Young V. Transthyretin (prealbumin) in health and disease: nutritional implications. *Ann Rev Nutr.* 1994;14:495–533.

49. Smith FR, Suskind R, Thanangkul O, Leitzmann C, et al. Plasma vitamin A, retinol-binding protein and prealbumin concentrations in protein-calorie malnutrition, III: response to varying dietary treatments. *Am J Clin Nutr.* 1975;28:732–738.

50. Shetty PS, Jung RT, Watrasiewicz KE, James WPT. Rapid-turnover transport proteins: an index of subclinical protein-energy malnutrition. *Lancet.* 1979;10:230–232.

51. Tuten MB, Wogt S, Dasse F. Utilization of prealbumin as a nutritional parameter. *J Parenter Enter Nutr.* 1985;9:709–711.

52. Winkler MF, Gerrior SA, Pomp A, Albina JE. Use of retinol-binding protein and prealbumin as indicators of the response to nutrition therapy. *J Am Diet Assoc.* 1989;89:684–687.

53. Helms RA, Dickerson RN, Ebbert ML, Christensen ML, et al. Retinol-binding protein and prealbumin: useful measures of protein repletion in critically ill, malnourished infants. *J Pediatr Gastroenterol Nutr.* 1986;5:586–592.

54. Scott RL, Sohmer PR, MacDonald MG. The effect of starvation and repletion on plasma fibronectin in man. *JAMA.* 1982;248:2025–2027.

55. Sandstedt S, Cederblad G, Larsson J, Schlidt B, et al. Influence of total parenteral nutrition on plasma fibronectin in malnourished subjects with or without inflammatory response. *J Parenter Enter Nutr.* 1984;8:493–496.

56. Rubli E, Bussard S, Frei E, Lundsgaard-Hansen P, et al. Plasma fibronectin and associated variables in surgical intensive care patients. *Ann Surg.* 1983;197:310–317.

57. McKone TK, Davis AT, Dean RE. Fibronectin: a new nutritional parameter. *Am Surg.* 1985;51:336–339.

58. Hawker FH, Stewart PM, Baxter RC, Borkman M, et al. Relationship of somatomedin-C/insulin-like growth factor I levels to conventional nutritional indices in critically ill patients. *Crit Care Med.* 1987;15:732–736.

59. Clemmons DR, Underwood LE, Dickerson RN, Brown RO, et al. Use of plasma somatomedin-C/insulin-like growth factor measurements to monitor the response to nutritional repletion in malnourished patients. *Am J Clin Nutr.* 1985;41:191–198.

60. Mattox TW, Brown RO, Boucher BA, Buonpane EA, et al. Use of fibronectin and somatomedin-C as markers of enteral nutrition support in traumatized patients using a modified amino acid formula. *J Parenter Enter Nutr.* 1988;12:592–596.

61. Chandra RK. Nutrition, immunity, and infection: present knowledge, and future directions. *Lancet.* 1(8326 Pt. 1):688–691, March 26, 1983.

62. Chandra R, Kumari S. Effects of nutrition on the immune system. *J Nutr.* 1994;10:207–210.

63. Christou NV, Rodriguez JT, Chartrand L, Giannas B, et al. Estimating mortality risk in preoperative patients using immunologic, nutritional, and acute-phase response variables. *Ann Surg.* 1989;210:69–77.

64. Ottow RT, Bruining HA, Jeekel JI. Clinical judgment versus delayed hypersensitivity skin testing for the prediction of postoperative sepsis and mortality. *Surg Gynecol Obstet.* 1984;159:475–477.

65. Twomey P, Ziegler D, Rombeau J. Utility of skin testing in nutritional assessment: a critical review. *J Parenter Enter Nutr.* 1982;6:50–58.

66. Griffith CDM, Ross AHM. Delayed hypersensitivity skin testing in elective colorectal surgery and relationship to postoperative sepsis. *J Parenter Enter Nutr.* 1984;8:279–280.

67. Welsh F, Farmery S, Ramsden C, Guillou P, et al. Reversible impairment in monocyte major histocompatibility complex class II expression in malnourished surgical patients. *J Parenter Enter Nutr.* 1996;16:344–348.

68. Russell DM, Atwood HL, Whittaker JS, Itakura T, et al. The effect of fasting and hypocaloric diets on the functional and metabolic characteristics of rat gastrocnemius muscle. *Clin Sci.* 1984;67:185–194.

69. Russell DM, Walker PM, Leiter LA, Sima AF, et al. Metabolic and structural changes in skeletal muscle during hypocaloric dieting. *Am J Clin Nutr.* 1984;39:503–513.

70. Klidjian AM, Poster KJ, Kammerling RM. Relation of anthropometric and dynamometric variables to serious postoperative complications. *Br Med J.* 1980;281:899–901.

71. Hunt DR, Rowlands BJ, Johnston D. Hand grip strength: a simple prognostic indicator in surgical patients. *J Parenter Enter Nutr.* 1985;9:701–704.

72. Kalfarentzos F, Spiliotis J, Velimezis G, Dougenis D, et al. Comparison of forearm muscle dynamometry with nutritional prognostic index as a preoperative indicator in cancer patients. *J Parenter Enter Nutr.* 1989;13:34–36.

73. Mullen J, Buzby G, Waldman T, Gertner M, et al. Prediction of operative morbidity and mortality by preoperative nutritional assessment. *Surg Forum.* 1979;30:80–82.

74. Buzby GP, Mullen JL, Matthews DC, Hobbs CL, et al. Prognostic nutritional index in gastrointestinal surgery. *Am J Surg.* 1980;139:160–167.

75. Hooley R, Levine H, Flores TC, Wheeler T, et al. Predicting postoperative head and neck complications using nutritional assessment. *Arch Otolaryngol.* 1983;109:83–85.

76. Seltzer MH, Bastidas JA, Cooper DM, Engler P, et al. Instant nutritional assessment. *J Parenter Enter Nutr.* 1979;3:157–159.

77. Seltzer MH, Fletcher HS, Slocum BA, Engler PE. Instant nutritional assessment in the intensive care unit. *J Parenter Enter Nutr.* 1981;5:70–72.

78. Winters JO, Leider ZL. The value of instant nutritional assessment in predicting postoperative complications and death in gastrointestinal surgical patients. *Am J Surg.* 1983;49:533–535.

79. Baker JP, Detsky AS, Wesson DS, Wolman SL, et al. Nutritional assessment: a comparison of clinical judgment and objective measurements. *N Engl J Med.* 1982;306:969–972.

80. Detsky AS, Baker JP, O'Rourke K, Johnston N, et al. Predicting nutrition associated complications for patients undergoing gastrointestinal surgery. *J Parenter Enter Nutr.* 1987;11:440–446.

81. Ingenbleek Y, Carpentier YA. A prognostic inflammatory and nutritional index scoring critically ill patients. *Int J Vitam Nutr Res.* 1985;55:91–101.

82. Vehe KL, Brown RO, Kuhl DA, Boucher BA, et al. The prognostic inflammatory and nutritional index in traumatized patients receiving enteral nutrition support. *J Am Coll Nutr.* 1991;10:355–363.

83. Lupo L, Pannarale O, Altomare D, Memeo V, et al. Reliability of clinical judgement in evaluation of the nutritional status of surgical patients. *Br J Surg.* 1993;80:1553–1556.

84. Neithercut WD, Smith ADS, McAllister J, La Ferla G. Nutritional survey of patients in a general surgical ward: is there an effective predictor of malnutrition? *J Clin Pathol.* 1987;40:803–807.

CHAPTER 2

Nutrition Support: Indications and Efficacy

Laura E. Matarese and Cynthia Hamilton

INTRODUCTION

Recent technological advances in health care have provided clinicians with an unprecedented ability to improve and maintain nutritional integrity, regardless of the severity of the illness. Patients, who just 30 years ago would have died of malnutrition and its consequences, are routinely nourished today by enteral and parenteral therapies that have become relatively commonplace. However, these therapies are not totally innocuous and carry potential risks and complications. Questions arise not only about safety, but also about efficacy and cost. Many issues must be addressed such as reimbursement, allocation of limited resources, and access. In the absence of scientific evidence, there is the potential for misuse of these therapies. Generally as a new therapy becomes available, too many inappropriate patients receive it; then no one receives it; eventually, the appropriate patients receive it. The careful evaluation of these therapies is therefore essential if they are to be used safely and appropriately.

Our knowledge base has grown to the point that, in most cases, we know what to give, how much to give, and in what form. But the operational questions still prevail: when to give it and to whom. The risk-benefit ratio needs to be evaluated; that is, the relative benefit derived from this therapy needs to be evaluated in terms of the necessary expenditures of personnel, time, and money as well as the potential complications associated with providing the therapy. It is important to define those instances where nutrition support is essential for optimal patient care and those instances in which nutrition support may be withheld without detriment to patients. In many instances, the answer may not be clear-cut.

The potential economic impact of enteral and parenteral therapies, particularly parenteral nutrition, is very apparent; the benefits are not. The costs include not only solutions, bags, tubing, and infusion pumps, but also personnel time, laboratory tests, and radiology fees. These costs may be in addition to the cost of the hospital room. Although the number and frequency of complications associated with nutrition support are low, they do occur and must be considered in the calculation of total costs.

How does one quantify the benefits of nutrition support? Does the provision of nutrition support have to result in improved outcome—such as decreased morbidity and mortality, reduced complication rates, or decreased length of hospital stay? Or is it enough to demonstrate an improvement in nutritional markers? Should one consider subjective criteria such as feelings of well-being and improved quality of life? And, what are the alternatives? Should one compare nutrition support to starvation or semistarvation with intravenous fluids and electrolytes? Certainly, there is no clinical state that benefits from malnutrition. But the question remains, does nutrition make any difference at all? Does nutrition support alter the course of an illness in some quantifiable way? Or does nutrition support merely correct malnutrition? Is nutrition support worth the time, money, and potential risks? This chapter outlines the data for the indications and efficacy of nutrition support.

MALNUTRITION

Dr. Charles Butterworth's landmark article, "The Skeleton in the Hospital Closet" published in 1974, was the first to call attention to the extent and impact of hospital-related malnutrition.[1] His observations included significant delays in initiation of feeding, sometimes up to several weeks; absence of nutritional assessment; failure to consult the dietitian; failure to record patient weights throughout hospitalization; vitamin deficiencies and decreased wound healing; failure to prescribe vitamin and mineral supplementation; and failure to use appropriate modalities of nutrition support such as enteral and parenteral nutrition. It appeared that malnutrition was a common finding in hospitalized patients, that it contributed to increased mortality and morbidity and that it was primarily iatrogenic in nature. The impact of this article was profound, and it stimulated subsequent research concerning the incidence and implications of malnutrition in hospitalized patients.

Using well-defined indexes of malnutrition (weight/height [wt/ht], triceps skinfold [TSF], arm muscle circumference [AMC], serum albumin, and hematocrit [hct]), Bistrian et al[2,3] found a 50% incidence of malnutrition in surgical patients and 44% incidence among medical patients. Medical patients tended to experience more caloric deficits (wt/ht, TSF) than surgical patients; surgical patients had worse protein status (AMC, serum albumin) than medical patients. Mullen et al[4] in 1979 also studied the frequency of malnutrition in surgical patients but went a step further to determine if nutritional and immunologic factors were predictive of postoperative morbidity and mortality. These authors found that 35% of patients had three or more abnormal nutritional and immunologic measurements. Serum albumin, transferrin, and delayed hypersensitivity reactions had significant predictive value of postoperative morbidity and mortality.

Further studies evaluating nutritional status over the course of hospitalization and the impact on hospital length of stay (LOS) were conducted. Weinsier et al developed the likelihood of malnutrition (LOM) score, a nutritional assessment score combining weighted subjective and objective parameters.[5] Parameters included TSF, wt/ht, AMC, serum folate, serum vitamin C, albumin, total lymphocyte count, and hct. These authors reported that, of medical patients in 1976, 48% were found at admission to have a high LOM.[5] Patients with a high LOM score had a significantly longer hospital stay and increased mortality rate. Additionally, nutritional status worsened with prolonged hospital stay (greater than 2 weeks) in 69% of patients. Albumin and hct were closely associated with prolonged hospital stay, and TSF and wt/ht were closely associated with increased mortality. A reevaluation 12 years later (1988) with the same testing methods, diagnoses, and patient demographics indicated that the initial LOM score was still high at 38% of patients.[6] The LOS was the same for patients who stayed 2 weeks or more, but a smaller percentage of patients stayed 2 weeks or longer compared to the 1976 study. In addition, LOM scores showed improvement after a 2-week follow-up period (46% of patients in 1988 versus 62% in the earlier study). This evidence indicated a decreased likelihood of patients' developing malnutrition during hospitalization.

Once malnutrition became a recognized problem in hospitalized patients through documentation of incidence and its impact on mortality, morbidity, and LOS, a number of methods were developed to help identify nutritional risk and predict outcomes.

Subjective global assessment uses history and physical examination to assess nutritional status. It can be used in a variety of clinical situations to predict patients who are at high risk of developing complications such as poor wound healing.[7] However, in a study that compared subjective global assessment to objective measurements, Baker and colleagues found that malnutrition was missed in 19% of the patients who were assessed using subjective global assessment.[7]

The Prognostic Nutritional Index is a validated measure of nutritional status and gives a quantitative estimate of patients at operative risk and in need of preoperative nutrition support. It is based on serum albumin, TSF, serum transferrin, and delayed hypersensitivity skin tests.[8]

The Nutrition Risk Index was developed by the Veterans Affairs Total Parenteral Nutrition Cooperative Study Group to identify patients at nutritional risk using serum albumin, current weight, and usual weight. The formula is a sensitive and positive predictor for identifying patients at risk for complications who required laparotomy or noncardiac thoracotomy.[9]

The Prognostic Inflammatory and Nutritional Index (PINI) is a method of categorizing critically ill patients using acute-phase reactant proteins and visceral proteins. The formula categorizes patients by risk of complications or death. PINI decreases during enteral nutrition support in critically ill trauma patients.[10]

Today, clinicians who deal with malnutrition no longer simply identify and categorize malnourished patients; they focus on improving outcomes and reducing health care costs. Appropriate nutrition intervention for diagnoses that are likely to respond to treatment is indicated. Specialized nutrition modalities and their impact on outcome should be determined through nutrition intervention trials.

NUTRITION SUPPORT—ADJUNCTIVE VERSUS PRIMARY THERAPY

Nutrition support may be indicated as primary therapy whereby it alters the morbidity and mortality of a disease, or it may be considered adjunctive therapy. Adjunctive or supportive nutrition therapy is given to avoid malnutrition and the consequences of malnutrition. However, in many disease states, nutrition support has not been shown to alter the course of the disease. Only a few well-controlled studies have been done to demonstrate efficacy of nutrition support. Below is a discussion of various disease states in which nutrition support is frequently used. The discussion indicates whether nutrition support is considered adjunctive or primary therapy.

Gastrointestinal Fistulas

A fistula or connection between the intestines and the skin or other area of the body may occur postoperatively, in patients with Crohn's disease, or in patients with abdominal malignancies. Nutrition support is frequently used for patients with this condition until the fistula spontaneously closes or surgical intervention is indicated. There are no prospective, randomized trials involving the use of nutrition support in patients with fistulas. The reports have been retrospective. The reported benefits of total parenteral nutrition (TPN) include decreased intestinal secretions, decreased fistula drainage, and spontaneous closure. A review of 404 patients with gastrointestinal (GI) fistulas noted an increase in the spontaneous closure rate from 10% in patients without TPN to 31% in patients who received TPN.[11]

Short Bowel Syndrome

The most obvious effect of TPN as a therapeutic modality has been with patients with short bowel syndrome. For these patients, TPN is considered lifesaving and primary therapy. Patients with this condition can develop malnutrition due to large amounts of diarrhea, fluid and electrolyte disturbances, and malabsorption. Patients with 2 feet or less of small bowel beyond the duodenum cannot digest and absorb nutrients by oral intake. Some patients with longer amounts of remaining small bowel may eventually be able to adapt to partial or full intake, but this could take months to years.[12]

Pancreatitis

The role of nutrition support in patients with pancreatitis is supportive. Parenteral or enteral nutrition has not been shown to improve disease activity. Acute, mild, and moderate pancreatitis is usually of short duration and generally does not warrant nutrition support. Sax et al[13] conducted a prospective, randomized, controlled trial involving 54 patients with acute pancreatitis receiving conventional therapy or conventional therapy and TPN within 24 hours; these researchers reported no differences with respect to time of initiation of liquids. Patients who received TPN had higher catheter infection rates and longer hospital stays than those who did not receive TPN. The early initiation of TPN did not result in improved outcome in this group.[13]

Kirby and Craig[14] reviewed evidence of efficacy with all types of nutrition support in pancreatitis. Noted were various complications for which TPN was used including pancreatic ascites, fistulas, pseudocysts, and necrotizing pancreatitis. These complications may lead to malnutrition due to the catabolic effects of the disease as well as a prolonged course of NPO. Kirby and Craig reported that patients in this group showed improved nutritional status when nutrition support was provided.

Acquired Immune Deficiency Syndrome

Weight loss is well documented in patients with acquired immune deficiency syndrome (AIDS). The magnitude of lean body mass depletion is significant. Kotler and colleagues reported that patients with AIDS had 54% of normal body cell mass and 66% of ideal body weight at the time of death.[15] Patients with AIDS tend to suffer from malabsorption, anorexia, decreased intake, severe diarrhea, and infections. The use of enteral feedings with percutaneous endoscopic gastrostomy (predicted calorie needs plus 500 kcals/day) resulted in increased weight, body cell mass, body fat, and serum albumin in this group of patients.[16] Patients receiving TPN also demonstrated increased weight, body fat, and body cell mass if no evidence of systemic infection was present. However, patients with systemic infections showed a net loss of body cell mass when fed with parenteral nutrition.[17] Although enteral and parenteral nutrition are effective in replenishing lean tissues in the absence of active infections, there are no studies showing decreased morbidity and mortality. For patients with AIDS, all aspects of nutrition support—

including potential benefits, potential risks, and costs—should be reviewed with the patient or family before initiating therapy.

Cancer

Malnutrition in cancer may occur secondary to the course of the disease or to treatment side effects. Improved nutritional indexes and improvement in overall performance in patients with GI obstruction or treatment toxicity have been observed with the use of enteral or parenteral nutrition.[18] However, patients with cancer cachexia have not shown the same improvements.[19] Additionally, in a prospective randomized trial of TPN after major pancreatic resection for malignancy, Brennan et al[20] found no benefit in the use of adjuvant parenteral nutrition. Patients who received TPN had significantly more infections (particularly abdominal abscess formation) compared to patients who did not receive TPN.

Koretz[21] reviewed 15 prospective, randomized clinical trials with TPN in nonoperative cancer patients. Results were varied, with no clear evidence that improvement in nutritional status was related to improved morbidity and mortality. Some studies showed an increase in the incidence of sepsis and complication rates.[21] Klein and colleagues[22] evaluated 28 prospective controlled trials and reported results similar to Koretz.[21] In a position paper based on a meta-analysis of patients who received TPN and chemotherapy, the American College of Physicians reported that parenteral nutrition had no significant effects on survival or remission; the authors also observed an increase in the infection rate. The overall conclusion was that TPN may be harmful.[23]

Perioperative Total Parenteral Nutrition

Preoperative malnutrition is associated with a higher rate of postoperative complications and mortality. However, studies have not shown perioperative nutrition support to reduce complications to the same level as that found in well-nourished patients undergoing the same procedures.[24]

Postoperative surgical complications (prolonged ileus, abdominal abscess, anastomotic leak, wound dehiscence) may be indications for early postoperative feedings, especially if a prolonged period of inadequate intake (greater than 5 days) is anticipated. Frequently, the clinician must use appropriate judgment regarding when to start nutrition support for operative patients to prevent malnutrition.

Critical Care, Burns, and Trauma

The metabolic response to severe injury includes the release of various mediators of metabolism such as glucagon, catecholamines, and glucocorticosteroids as well as the production of cytokines including tumor necrosis factor, interleukin-1, and interleukin-6. This leads to hypermetabolism, hypercatabolism, and protein-calorie malnutrition. The efficacy of nutrition support in this group of patients has been difficult to prove due to the heterogeneity of the group, as well as other factors that influence outcomes.

Initial studies used parenteral nutrition formulas enriched with branched-chain amino acids (BCAA) compared with standard amino acid formulas. Improved nitrogen balance was observed, but no effect on outcome was evident.[25]

The use of supplemental enteral nutrition formulas (enriched with glutamine, arginine, omega-3 fatty acids) in a limited number of randomized clinical trials has shown immunoregulatory effects, decreased length of stay, and decreased infectious complications in GI malignancies and burn patients.[26,27] Bone marrow transplant patients have also shown a decrease in the incidence of infections and a decrease in LOS when given TPN with supplemental glutamine.[28] Additional prospective, randomized studies using these specialized formulas are indicated.

The route of nutrition support in critically ill patients appears to be an important factor in outcome. One study comparing TPN with enteral nutrition demonstrated decreased incidence of infection with enteral nutrition.[29] A lower incidence of septic mor was seen in patients fed enterally versus parenterally after blunt and penetrating trauma.[30] The preservation of GI barriers and host defenses may be the responsible factor.[30] During prolonged critical illness, immediate nutrition support is indicated as supportive therapy.

Inflammatory Bowel Disease

Inflammatory bowel disease includes Crohn's disease and idiopathic ulcerative colitis. These diseases involve the large intestines (as with ulcerative colitis) or both the small and large intestines (as with Crohn's disease). Both of these conditions are associated with malnutrition due to malabsorption. A number of clinical trials have been conducted with these disease states using TPN and enteral formulas. Some studies have shown remission rates between 60% and 80% with TPN or elemental enteral diets in Crohn's disease.[31] However, in a meta-analysis of enteral nutrition as primary treatment in active Crohn's disease versus corticosteroids, Griffiths and colleagues found that enteral nutrition was inferior to corticosteroids.[32] In addition, these authors reported no difference in the efficacy of elemental versus nonelemental formulas.[32]

Nutrition support for patients with ulcerative colitis helps prevent nutritional deficiencies but does not seem to influence disease activity. McIntyre et al[33] studied patients with severe, acute colitis receiving intravenous steroids and either bowel rest with TPN or oral diet. No differences in operative or mortality rates were observed. Nutrition support in inflammatory bowel disease is considered adjunctive due to the lack of clinical trials showing long-term remission of disease activity.

Liver Failure

Patients with chronic liver disease are malnourished due to decreased intake, increased requirements, and malabsorption. With the progression of liver disease, nutrient metabolism becomes increasingly abnormal. The effect on amino acid metabolism may lead to hepatic encephalopathy. Enteral and parenteral products that contain decreased aromatic amino acids and enriched BCAA were designed to correct the abnormal plasma pattern of these patients. Studies using these products have not shown consistent results. In 70 patients with acute hepatic encephalopathy, no significant differences were seen between patients who received TPN with standard amino acids and patients who received TPN enriched with BCAA.[34] However, Cerra et al reported improved mortality for patients using the BCAA-enriched product compared with patients given only intravenous glucose and conventional therapy.[35]

Patients with acute alcoholic liver disease treated with supplemental intravenous amino acids or tube feeding showed improved nutritional parameters, lower mortality, and faster improvements in encephalopathy.[36,37] The goal of nutrition support in this group is to prevent or correct malnutrition, and it is supportive in nature.

Acute Renal Failure

Acute renal failure is characterized by hypercatabolism and hypermetabolism. This condition may occur after major surgery or trauma and is associated with increased mortality. Early studies using small quantities of essential amino acids with dextrose reported improved survival when compared with dextrose alone,[38] but subsequent trials have not shown any difference in rate of recovery when a balanced mixture of amino acids is used compared with the essential amino acid mixture.[39] Nutrition support should be provided to patients who remain catabolic for an extended period of time if adequate intake is not possible.

Respiratory Failure

The provision of nutrition support to patients with acute and chronic respiratory failure has been shown to improve respiratory muscle strength and endurance.[40] However, administration of excess calories has been shown to be detrimental in this group of patients and leads to excess carbon dioxide production and increased ventilatory demand, particularly with high dextrose concentrations. A reduction of the carbohydrate calories may minimize carbon dioxide production.[41] Patients with respiratory failure who are unable to consume nutrients by mouth for an extended period of time require nutrition support.

Pregnancy

There is a direct association between maternal nutrition during pregnancy and fetal outcome. Inadequate nutrition may lead to low-birth-weight infants or risk of neonatal death.[42] Nutritional deficits may occur in pregnant women with hyperemesis gravidarum or those with other illnesses affecting nutrient intake (eg, inflammatory bowel disease, cancer, pancreatitis). Both enteral and parenteral feeding have been used successfully during pregnancy to promote adequate maternal weight gain and appropriate fetal growth.[43,44]

Neurologic Impairment

Various neurologic disorders can affect the hypothalamus, pituitary, brain stem, and autonomic nervous system. These disorders can influence appetite, digestion, hormonal milieu, and basal energy expenditure. Nutritional disorders include cachexia, reduced energy expenditure (as with quadriplegia), and hypermetabolism in head injury. Other disorders affect fluid and electrolyte balance. Nutrition support in these disorders may be necessary as short-term or long-term therapy in order to prevent malnutrition. The GI tract is the preferred method of support, with TPN indicated when the GI tract is not functional.[45,46]

Eating Disorders

The most common eating disorders—anorexia nervosa and bulimia—are associated with marasmic malnutrition. These disorders are psychologically mediated and require individual, group, and family counseling. Most of these patients have functioning GI tracts and can be supported with enteral nutrition, although occasionally TPN is necessary. There are no studies comparing nutrition support with other treatment therapies. Nutrition support should be initiated for severely malnourished patients who are unable to sustain adequate intake.[47]

Pediatrics, Infants, and Neonates

Adequate nutrition for children is essential for growth, maturation, and development of organs. Malnutrition in infants and children has potential long-term consequences that may be irreversible. Because children do not have the reserves that adults have, the need for nutrition support may be immediate. In particular, low-birth-weight infants, with very little caloric reserves, are frequently provided TPN within 48 hours after birth. TPN results in a faster weight gain and return to birth weight than intravenous glucose or enteral feeding.[48,49] The use of enteral or parenteral feeding may be considered in this group, depending on the disease state and accessibility of the GI tract.

Geriatrics

With advancing age, the risk of developing serious nutritional deficiencies increases. This is due to age-related reductions in total food intake, socioeconomic status, difficulty with activities of daily living, and the presence of debilitating disease. With decreased intake, there is a reduced reserve capacity, which makes the elderly prone to severe nutritional deficiencies. The goal of nutrition support in the elderly is frequently to improve functional independence and strength.

Studies of undernourished patients in a geriatric rehabilitation unit found highly significant correlations between nutritional assessment parameters and the risk of developing complications, infections, and mortality. The best predictor of mortality was percentage of usual body weight and weight lost in the previous year of hospital admission. Complications were associated with functional status at admission, serum albumin, and the amount of weight lost in the previous year.[50,51] These data provide evidence of the importance of identification of nutritional status of the elderly and help identify candidates for aggressive nutrition support.

STANDARDS AND GUIDELINES

Practice guidelines, protocols, critical pathways, algorithms, criteria, and standards are tools that guide and evaluate clinical decision making. They are generally used to control variations in practice, to promote efficient use of health care resources, and to address potential cases of inappropriate care.[52] *Guidelines* are used by many people for a wide variety of reasons. Clinicians use them to assist in clinical decision making and improve outcomes. Guidelines work well for the "standard" patient but may not be useful for patients who are not "typical" or "standard." Institutions apply guidelines to reduce the variability in the use of resources while maintaining quality and ensuring good clinical outcomes. Individual patients may use them to become better informed when making health care decisions. Special interest groups and professional societies often develop guidelines in order to improve and standardize care.

Many of these terms have been used interchangeably in the literature. Although they have a similar purpose, the exact meaning of each term is different. This terminology has been standardized for use in quality assurance and quality improvement programs.[53] *Standards of practice* are statements of the practitioner's responsibility for providing quality of nutrition care. These standards of practice are designed to be used by the individual practitioner to guide and evaluate personal performance. *Practice guidelines* are systematically developed statements or specifications designed to help practitioners or to help patients/clients choose appropriate health care in "typical" clinical circumstances. These are based on the best available research and professional judgment. They should be thoroughly researched, validated, and field-tested. They should be comprehensive, specific, and manageable. Other terms that have been used interchangeably with practice guidelines include clinical standard, practice parameter, protocol, algorithm, and preferred practice pattern. There has been a tremendous growth of guideline development in the past few years with many professional organizations, federal agencies, insurers, managed care programs, and hospitals participating. The prevailing reason remains quality patient care for the best cost.

Continuous quality improvement (CQI) refers to an approach to quality management that builds on traditional quality assurance methods by emphasizing the organization and systems (rather than individuals), the need for objective data with which to analyze and improve processes, and the ideal that systems and performance can always improve even when high standards have been met. There is a strong emphasis on customer satisfaction. Other terms that have been used interchangeably with CQI include quality improvement, continuous improvement, and total quality management. This approach is never static, and the goal is to continually strive for the best.

Quality assurance refers to the certification of continuous, optimal, effective, and efficient health and nutrition care. The goal is to improve client or patient-related outcomes. It involves assessment of the quality of care and evaluation of the results. If suboptimal care is identified or desirable outcomes are not achieved, a change in practice should occur. This terminology is being phased out and replaced with quality assessment and improvement.

Quality assessment refers to the measurement of the technical and interpersonal aspects of health care and services and the outcomes of the care and service. Quality assessment provides information that may be used in CQI activities.

Criteria or *criteria sets* are predetermined elements of health care services used for quality assessment or professionally developed statements that describe desirable health care processes or outcome. *Structure* relates to institutional and provider characteristics such as budget, organizational mission, policies, staffing qualifications, specialty certification, the facility, and equipment. *Process* refers to the sequence of activities, procedures, or functions used by practitioners and managers in the delivery of health care. *Outcomes* are observable end results or changes in client, patient, or customer health and nutritional status.

An *indicator* is a measurement tool used to monitor and evaluate the quality of important governance, management, and support functions and important aspects of patient care. Indicators serve as screens or flags that direct attention to specific performance issues within a health care organization, which should then become the subject of more intensive review. Indicators focus on key functions; treatment processes; and other high-volume, high-frequency, high-risk, and problematic aspects of care or service. Indicators are not intended to be direct measures of quality; instead, they describe events, complications, or outcomes.

Guidelines are created by a variety of methods (see Exhibit 2–1). Many are based on the opinions of "experts" by informal consensus. Guidelines are sometimes developed by formal consensus, which generally involves an exhaustive and critical review of the scientific literature. This may or may not involve assessing the quality of the evidence used. In some instances, an attempt is made to include an evaluation of the strength of the supporting material, thus enabling evidence-based guideline development.

American Gastroenterological Association Guidelines

The American Gastroenterological Association published two sets of guidelines, one on parenteral nutrition in 1989[54] and one on enteral nutrition in 1995[55]

Exhibit 2–1 Guideline Development

1. Identify specific clinical area.
2. Conduct comprehensive literature review.
3. Review the benefits and risks of each intervention.
4. Review significant patient outcomes.
5. Determine the most important clinical criteria.
6. Develop the guidelines.
7. Have experts review guidelines.
8. Revise guidelines.
9. Test and validate guidelines.
10. Implement guidelines.
11. Conduct periodic review and revision of guidelines.

(see Table 2–1). The prevailing theme throughout the parenteral guidelines is that the decision to institute TPN should be made on the basis of (1) the degree of malnutrition, (2) the anticipated length of disability, and (3) the state of metabolic stress. Enteral nutrition should be used whenever possible.

The guidelines for the use of enteral nutrition[55] presented recommendations for providing safe and effective enteral nutrition to adult patients. The guidelines addressed general indications for enteral nutrition, methods of enteral feeding administration, complications of tube feeding, specialized enteral formulations, and the role of nutrition support teams in providing enteral nutrition.

Georgetown Guidelines

In 1990, the Program on Technology and Health Care of the Georgetown University School of Medicine convened an invited forum to assess the appropriate uses of safety, effectiveness, and cost of TPN as well as ethical and legal issues.[56] Enteral nutrition was not addressed except as an alternative to TPN. The group established guidelines for specific disease states after conducting a review of the scientific literature and reaching a consensus (see Table 2–1).

American Society for Parenteral and Enteral Nutrition Guidelines

These guidelines were prepared by a committee of members of the American Society for Parenteral and Enteral Nutrition[57] and approved by the society's board of directors (see Table 2–1). They encompass both enteral and parenteral nutrition. The authors of this document attempted to code the strength of the evidence in the literature that was used to support each practice guideline.

Evaluating Guidelines

Clinicians should exercise caution when comparing guidelines from different groups, because these guidelines were prepared at different times with differences in the availability of data. But in each case, the prevailing theme is to use enteral nutrition whenever possible and to use TPN only in cases of malnutrition and anticipation of prolonged NPO status.

Table 2–1 Guidelines for Parenteral and Enteral Nutrition

Disease	American Gastroenterological Association	Georgetown	American Society for Parenteral and Enteral Nutrition
Short bowel syndrome	TPN as sole nutrition support or until enteral nutrition is tolerated	Not addressed	Home TPN may be needed for patients with <60 cm small bowel or only the duodenum
Inflammatory bowel disease (IBD)	TPN indicated with severe IBD to reverse malnutrition and its complications	Defined formula diets preferable to TPN in Crohn's disease. Reserve TPN for enteral failure or acute flare-ups. TPN useful as adjunctive therapy in chronic ulcerative colitis	Enteral nutrition preferable whenever possible. TPN may be of benefit in acute ulcerative colitis in preparation for surgery or with failure of enteral nutrition
Chronic intestinal disorders (eg, scleroderma, Whipple's disease, radiation enteritis, pseudo-obstruction)	Use of TPN debatable; defined formula diets should be tried first	Not addressed	Patients with active pseudo-obstruction benefit from TPN
GI fistulas	May aid in fistula closure along with antibiotics/medications to decrease fistula output	Not addressed	Not addressed

Postoperative complications	No data to support a decrease in postoperative complications with TPN	Routine use of TPN not justified; reserve for correction of malnutrition	TPN may be indicated for malnourished patients; TPN may be indicated for mildly malnourished patients expected to be NPO for more than 1 week
Preoperative support	No data to demonstrate any advantage of preoperative TPN	Routine use of TPN not justified; reserve for correction of malnutrition	TPN should be used for malnourished patients requiring major operations for 7–10 days; not indicated for mild malnutrition
Pancreatitis	Data conflicting; routine use of TPN not recommended	Patients with severe necrotizing pancreatitis may benefit from TPN; reserve for patients requiring bowel rest	Enteral nutrition should be used whenever possible; TPN should be used for enteral failures; lipid emulsions can be used for patients with triglycerides <400 mg/dL
Burns/trauma	TPN recommended for prolonged ileus or abdominal injuries	Not addressed	Not addressed
Cancer	TPN or enteral nutrition recommended to make patient a better candidate for treatment	TPN appropriate for severely malnourished patients or those in whom enteral nutrition cannot be used within 10–14 days TPN not indicated in terminal disease	Enteral and parenteral nutrition may benefit severely malnourished patients who are receiving oncologic therapy; TPN is unlikely to benefit patients with advanced cancer unresponsive to chemotherapy or radiation therapy

continues

Table 2–1 continued

Disease	American Gastroenterological Association	Georgetown	American Society for Parenteral and Enteral Nutrition
Neurologic and pulmonary disease	Use enteral route whenever possible Use TPN only if enteral nutrition is contraindicated	Not addressed	Use enteral route whenever possible; adjust total calories to prevent overfeeding in pulmonary disease
Neonates and infants	TPN warranted to prevent malnutrition, especially for low-birth-weight infants whose GI tract is not fully developed	TPN indicated to maintain growth and development in the absence of or with insufficient enteral nutrition	Specialized nutrition support indicated to sustain normal growth and development and promote catch-up growth
Acute renal failure	Not addressed	TPN may be useful	Provide balanced mixture of essential and nonessential amino acids; use of only essential amino acids generally not recommended
Hepatic dysfunction	Not addressed	TPN indicated in nutritionally compromised patients who are unable to tolerate enteral nutrition; for those who cannot tolerate 60–80 g amino acids due to grade-3 and grade-4 hepatic encephalopathy, a BCAA-enriched TPN solution is recommended	Most patients without hepatic encephalopathy (HE) can tolerate standard amino acids; in the presence of HE, a specialized liver enteral or parenteral solution may be used to meet protein requirements

Critical care	Not addressed	TPN may be of benefit in patients who were previously well nourished but cannot be enterally fed within 5 to 7 days or in malnourished patients in whom TPN would be of benefit prior to the hypermetabolic phase	Enteral feedings should be used whenever possible; TPN should be used in enteral failures
AIDS	Not addressed	Routine use of TPN is discouraged; enteral nutrition should be used whenever possible	Diet with supplements should be used whenever possible; then enteral tube feedings and lastly TPN
Home TPN (HPN)	Not addressed	HPN may improve the quality of life for patients and/or decrease costs compared with hospitalization	Not addressed
Pregnancy	Not addressed	Not addressed	Enteral tube feeding or TPN may be used to prevent nutritional deficits and promote weight gain
Geriatrics	Not addressed	Not addressed	Enteral and/or parenteral nutrition should be provided according to the same guidelines used for younger adults with similar diagnoses
Eating disorders (anorexia nervosa)	Not addressed	Not addressed	Provide nutrition support in severe malnutrition with poor oral intake; TPN should be used for enteral nutrition failure

NUTRITION SUPPORT EFFICACY

Veterans Affairs Cooperative Study

The Veterans Affairs cooperative study was a multiinstitutional, prospective clinical trial, designed to test the hypothesis that perioperative TPN decreases the incidence of serious complications after major abdominal or thoracic surgery in malnourished patients.[9] The sample included 395 malnourished patients who required laparotomy or noncardiac thoracotomy. The patients were stratified according to nutritional status based on objective measurements. The degree of malnutrition ranged from borderline to severe. Patients were randomly assigned to receive either TPN for 7 to 15 days before surgery and 3 days afterwards (TPN group) or no perioperative TPN (control group). The patients were monitored for 90 days after surgery. The effect of TPN on the operative outcome depended on each patient's baseline nutritional status. Overall rates of complications and mortality were similar in the treatment and control groups. However, more complications related to infection occurred in the TPN group. Patients with mild malnutrition did not benefit from TPN, and the complications related to infection increased in well-nourished and mildly malnourished groups. This was not due to catheter-related sepsis or bacteremia, but to an increased frequency of postoperative infections such as pneumonia and wound infections. Severely malnourished patients had fewer noninfectious complications with TPN than did the control group, without an increase in infectious complications. This study demonstrates the lack of benefit of TPN in borderline malnourished patients, provides strong evidence against TPN efficacy in mildly or moderately malnourished patients, and suggests but does not confirm efficacy in severely malnourished patients. The authors concluded that the use of preoperative TPN should be limited to patients who are severely malnourished unless there are other specific indications.

Meta-Analysis

Detsky and colleagues conducted a meta-analysis of 18 controlled trials of perioperative parenteral nutrition to evaluate the usefulness of perioperative parenteral nutrition.[58] The pooled results of 11 trials suggested that TPN reduces the risk for complications from major surgery and fatalities. However, the authors noted that many of these pooled studies had flaws in the design as well as iatrogenic complications. These authors concluded that, based on the evidence available up to 1986, the routine use of perioperative TPN in unselected patients having major surgery was not justified. However, selected groups of high-risk patients may benefit from this intervention.

CONCLUSIONS

Although nutrition support remains a powerful tool in the medical armamentarium, it has not been proven to be unequivocally beneficial. Unfortunately, many of the studies to date have had flaws in experimental design, have lacked controls, have consisted of small sample sizes, and have had inappropriate patient selection or inadequate treatment regimens. Nutrition support can maintain body weight, primarily as fat and water in acute illness; improve visceral protein markers; improve the response to delayed hypersensitivity skin tests; and improve nitrogen balance. Some studies have shown improved outcome. Unstressed or even mildly stressed patients who will be eating relatively soon probably do not benefit from nutrition support, especially parenteral nutrition. However, an expanding body of literature demonstrates the safety and efficacy of early enteral nutrition.

Is nutrition support indicated for every hospitalized patient? The answer is no. There is a lack of data supporting the use of nutrition support for all hospitalized patients and a small body of literature suggesting that it may be harmful. The challenge is to determine which patients will derive the most benefit. Can clinicians determine with 100% accuracy which patients will benefit from nutrition support? The answer to this question is also no. But clinicians can determine and adhere to practice guidelines that direct and guide the type of nutrition provided, the amount, the way nutrition support is administered, and to whom.

REFERENCES

1. Butterworth CE Jr. The skeleton in the hospital closet. *Nutr Today.* 1974;9:4–8.
2. Bistrian BR, Blackburn GL, Hallowell E, Heddle R. Protein status of general surgical patients. *JAMA.* 1974;230:858–860.
3. Bistrian BR, Blackburn GL, Vitale J, Cochran D, et al. Prevalence of malnutrition in general surgical patients. *JAMA.* 1976;235:1567–1570.
4. Mullen JL, Gertner MH, Buzby GP, Goodhart GL, et al. Implications of malnutrition in the surgical patient. *Arch Surg.* 1979;114:121–125.
5. Weinsier RL, Hunker EM, Krumdieck CL, Butterworth CE. A prospective evaluation of general medical patients during the course of hospitalization. *Am J Clin Nutr.* 1979;32:418–426.
6. Coats KG, Morgan SL, Bartolucci AA, Weinsier RL. Hospital-associated malnutrition: a reevaluation 12 years later. *J Am Diet Assoc.* 1993;93:27–33.
7. Baker JP, Detsky AS, Wesson DE, Wolman SL, et al. Nutritional assessment: a comparison of clinical judgment and objective measurements. *N Engl J Med.* 1982;306:969–972.
8. Buzby GP, Mullen JL, Matthews DC, Hobbs CL, et al. Prognostic nutritional index in gastrointestinal surgery. *Am J Surg.* 1980;139:160–167.

9. The Veterans Affairs Total Parenteral Nutrition Cooperative Study Group. Perioperative total parenteral nutrition in surgical patients. *N Engl J Med.* 1991;325:525–532.

10. Ingenbleek Y, Carpentier Y. A prognostic inflammatory and nutritional index scoring critically ill patients. *Int J Vitam Nutr Res.* 1985;55:91–101.

11. Socters PB, Ebeid AM, Fischer JE. Review of 404 patients with gastrointestinal fistulas: impact of parenteral nutrition. *Ann Surg.* 1979;190:189–202.

12. Scheflan M, Gall SJ, Perrotto J, Fischer JE. Intestinal adaptation after intensive resection of small intestine and prolonged administration of parenteral nutrition. *Surg Gynecol Obstet.* 1976; 143:757–762.

13. Sax HC, Warner BW, Talamini MA, Hamilton FN, et al. Early total parenteral nutrition in acute pancreatitis: lack of beneficial effects. *Am J Surg.* 1987;153:117–124.

14. Kirby DF, Craig RM. The value of intensive nutritional support in pancreatitis. *J Parenter Enter Nutr.* 1985;9:353–357.

15. Kotler D, Tierney A, Wang J, Pierson RN. Magnitude of body-cell mass depletion and timing of death from wasting in AIDS. *Am J Clin Nutr.* 1989;50:444–447.

16. Kotler D, Tierney A, Ferraro R, Cuff P, et al. Effect of enteral alimentation and repletion of body cell mass in malnourished patients with acquired immunodeficiency syndrome. *Am J Clin Nutr.* 1991;53:149–154.

17. Kotler DP, Tierney AR, Culpepper-Morgan JA, Wang J, et al. Effect of home total parenteral nutrition on body composition in patients with acquired immunodeficiency syndrome. *J Parenter Enter Nutr.* 1990;14:454–458.

18. Burt ME, Gorschboth CM, Brennan MF. A controlled, prospective, randomized trial evaluating the metabolic effects of enteral and parenteral nutrition in the cancer patient. *Cancer.* 1982;49:1092–1105.

19. Brennan MF. Uncomplicated starvation versus cancer cachexia. *Cancer Res.* 1977;37:2359–2364.

20. Brennan MF, Pisters PWT, Posner M, Quesada O, et al. A prospective randomized trial of total parenteral nutrition after major pancreatic resection for malignancy. *Ann Surg.* 1994;220:436–444.

21. Koretz RL. Parenteral nutrition: is it oncologically logical? *J Clin Oncol.* 1984;2:534–538.

22. Klein S, Simes J, Blackburn G. TPN and cancer clinical trials. *Cancer.* 1986;58:1378–1386.

23. American College of Physicians. Position paper: parenteral nutrition in patients receiving cancer chemotherapy: a meta-analysis. *Ann Intern Med.* 1989;110:734–736.

24. Mullen JL, Buzby GP, Waldman MT, Gertner MH, et al. Prediction of operative morbidity and mortality by preoperative nutritional assessment. *Surg Forum.* 1979;30:80–82.

25. Cerra FB, Blackburn G, Hirsch J, Mullen K, et al. The effect of stress level, amino acid formula, and nitrogen dose on nitrogen retention in traumatic septic stress. *Ann Surg.* 1987;205:282–287.

26. Daly JM, Lieberman M, Goldfine J, Shou J, et al. Enteral nutrition with supplemental arginine, RNA, and omega-3 fatty acids in patients after operation: immunologic, metabolic, and clinical outcome. *Surgery.* 1992;112:56–67.

27. Gottschlich MM, Jenkins M, Warden GD, Baumer T, et al. Differential effects of three enteral dietary regimens on selected outcome variables in burn patients. *J Parenter Enter Nutr.* 1990;14:225–236.

28. Ziegler TR, Young LS, BenFell K, Scheltinga M, et al. Clinical and metabolic efficacy of glutamine-supplemented parenteral nutrition after bone marrow transplantation. *Ann Intern Med.* 1992;116:821–828.

29. Moore FA, Moore EE, Jones TN, McCroskey BL, et al. TEN vs. TPN following major abdominal trauma: reduced septic morbidity. *J Trauma.* 1989;29:916–923.

30. Kudsk KA, Croce MA, Fabian TC, Minard G, et al. Enteral versus parenteral feeding: effects on septic morbidity after blunt and penetrating abdominal trauma. *Ann Surg.* 1992;215:503–511.

31. Greenberg GR, Fleming CR, Jeejeebhoy KN, Rosenberg IH, et al. Controlled trial of bowel rest and nutritional support in the management of Crohn's disease. *Gut.* 1988;29:1309–1315.

32. Griffiths AM, Ohlsson A, Sheraman PM, Sutherland LR. Meta-analyis of enteral nutrition as a primary treatment of active Crohn's disease. *Gastroenterology.* 1995;108:1056–1067.

33. McIntyre PB, Powell-Tuck J, Wood SR, Lennard-Jones JE, et al. Controlled trial of bowel rest in the treatment of severe acute colitis. *Gut.* 1986;27:481–485.

34. Michel H, Bories P, Aubin JP, Pomier-Layrargues G, et al. Treatment of acute hepatic encephalopathy in cirrhotics with a branched-chain amino acids enriched versus a conventional amino acids mixture: a controlled study of 70 patients. *Liver.* 1985;5:282–289.

35. Cerra FB, Cheung NK, Fischer JE, Kaplowitz N, et al. Disease-specific amino acid infusion (F080) in hepatic encephalopathy: a prospective, randomized, double-blind controlled trial. *J Parenter Enter Nutr.* 1985;9:288–295.

36. Nasrallah SM, Galambos JT. Amino acid therapy for alcoholic hepatitis. *Lancet.* 1980;2:1276–1277.

37. Kearns PJ, Young H, Garcia G, Blaschke T, et al. Accelerated improvement of alcoholic liver disease with enteral nutrition. *Gastroenterology.* 1992;102:200–205.

38. Abel RM, Beck CH, Abbott WM, Ryan JA, et al. Improved survival from acute renal failure after treatment with intravenous essential L-amino acids and glucose. *N Engl J Med.* 1973;288:695–699.

39. Mirtallo J, Schneider P, Mavko K, Ruberg RL, et al. A comparison of essential and general amino acid infusions in the nutritional support of patients with compromised renal function. *J Parenter Enter Nutr.* 1982;6:109–113.

40. Arora NS, Rochester DF. Effect of body weight and muscularity on human diaphragm muscle mass, thickness, and area. *J Appl Physiol.* 1982;52:64–70.

41. Askanazi J, Rosenbaum SH, Hyman AZ, Silverberg PA, et al. Respiratory changes induced by the large glucose loads of total parenteral nutrition. *JAMA.* 1980;243:1444–1447.

42. Institute of Medicine. *Nutrition During Pregnancy.* Washington, DC: National Academy Press; 1990.

43. Barclay BA. Experience with enteral nutrition in the treatment of hyperemesis gravidarum. *Nutr Clin Pract.* 1990;5:153–155.

44. Levine MG, Esser D. Total parenteral nutrition for the treatment of severe hyperemesis gravidarum: maternal nutritional effects and fetal outcome. *Obstet Gynecol.* 1988;72:102–107.

45. Hadley MN, Graham TW, Harrington T. Nutritional support and neurotrauma: a critical review of early nutrition in forty-five acute head injury patients. *Neurosurg.* 1986;19:367–373.

46. Graham TW, Zadrozny DB, Harrington T. The benefits of early jejunal hyperalimentation in the head-injured patient. *Neurosurg.* 1991;25:729–735.

47. Kamal N, Chami T, Anderson A, Rosell FA, et al. Delayed gastrointestinal transit times in anorexia nervosa and bulimia nervosa. *Gastroenterology.* 1991;101:1320–1324.

48. Driscoll JM, Heird WC, Schullinger JN, Gongaware RD, et al. Total intravenous alimentation in low-birth weight infants: a preliminary report. *J Pediatr.* 1972;81:145–153.

49. Anderson TL, Muttart CR, Bieber MA, Nicholson JF, et al. A controlled trial of glucose versus glucose and amino acids in premature infants. *J Pediatr.* 1979;94:947–951.

50. Sullivan DH, Walls RC, Lipschitz DA. Protein-energy undernutrition and the risk of mortality within 1 year of hospital discharge in a select population of geriatric rehabilitation patients. *Am J Clin Nutr.* 1991;53:599–605.

51. Sullivan DH, Patch GA, Walls RC, Lipschitz DA. Impact of nutrition status on morbidity and mortality in a select population of geriatric rehabilitation patients. *Am J Clin Nutr.* 1990;50:749–758.

52. Woolf SH. Practice guidelines: a new reality in medicine: part I. *Arch Intern Med.* 1990; 150:1811–1818.

53. COP Quality Assurance Committee, The American Dietetic Association. Learning the language of quality care. *J Am Diet Assoc.* 1993;93:531–532.

54. Sitzmann JV, Pitt HA. Statement on Guidelines for Total Parenteral Nutrition. *Dig Dis Sci.* 1989;34:489–496.

55. Kirby DF, Delegge MH, Fleming CR. American Gastroenterology Association Medical Position Statement: guidelines for the use of enteral nutrition. *Gastroenterology.* 1995;108:1280–1301.

56. *Evaluating Total Parenteral Nutrition: Final Report and Core Statement of the Technology Assessment and Practice Guidelines Forum.* Washington, DC: Georgetown University School of Medicine, Program on Technology and Health Care, Department of Community and Family Medicine; November 1990.

57. Guidelines for the use of parenteral and enteral nutrition in adult and pediatric patients. *J Parenter Enter Nutr.* 1993;17:1SA–52SA.

58. Detsky AS, Baker JP, O'Rourke K, Vivek G. Perioperative parenteral nutrition: a meta-analysis. *Ann Intern Med.* 1987;107:195–203.

CHAPTER 3

Ethical Issues in Nutrition Support

Anne Marie B. Hunter

INTRODUCTION

Twentieth-century advances in the science of medicine have irrevocably altered the art, the questions, the choices, and the decisions regarding the dilemma of what constitutes acceptable human life. If the medical miracles of today had been witnessed in the past, they could only have been explained as divine or providential intervention. In the past, the art of medicine was in diagnosing the patient's illness and in providing comfort and occasionally a cure.[1]

The capabilities to resuscitate a stopped heart, to provide mechanical breathing indefinitely with a respirator, to cleanse toxic waste from the body by dialysis, and to supply food with a constant-drip formula are some of the most dramatic advances in medicine. Of these medical wonders, questions about the continued use or cessation of the delivery of feeding can be the most sensitive.

Traditionally, food and water have been considered basic needs and comfort measures in the care of persons and are symbolically based in cultural, religious, and moral traditions in our society.[2] However, the delivery of nutrition and hydration via artificial enteral and parenteral solutions and devices has opened a Pandora's box in terms of fundamental rights and needs, as well as appropriate medical treatment.

Aggressive nutrition support therapy was created with the best of intentions. It was designed to provide an alternative route and method of feeding for individuals who were unable to consume required nutrients by mouth. The technology of nutrition support afforded maintenance of adequate nutritional status and prevention or reversal of protein-calorie malnutrition. It was intended to alleviate life-threatening conditions that precluded normal digestive functioning and to allow a return to health and improvement in the quality of life as we know and experience it.

In the shadows of our enthusiastic embrace of technologic developments in medicine is the potential for misuse or abuse of these medical miracles, including nutrition support. Decisions about instituting or withdrawing feeding via enteral tubes or parenteral lines when the patient is neither terminally ill nor brain dead— such as when the patient is in irreversible coma, in a persistent vegetative state, or has cognitive impairment—are highly controversial and heatedly debated.

Many argue that nutrition and hydration are basic to human care and should always be provided and continued to preserve and protect life. Such persons do not regard nutrition support as medical treatment but rather as a means of feeding and hydrating. They believe that withholding nutrition support and hydration would lead to death by starvation and dehydration and that such death would be equivalent to euthanasia or suicide. These persons also fear that refusal to provide nutrition support will compromise the integrity of health care professionals and could set precedents for casual disregard of the viability of patients with varying forms and degrees of mental or physiologic dysfunction.

Others make a distinction between food that can be swallowed and digested via normal physiologic processes and food and fluids that are provided artificially in formulas delivered through enteral tubes and intravenous lines. These individuals view nutrition support as an extraordinary technologic means of nutrient delivery.[3] They consider it a medical treatment requiring the knowledge and art of the physician, sophisticated admixtures and equipment, and continuous monitoring of the formulations and methodology by health care professionals with expertise in the treatment. Such persons believe that, as with other medical treatments, the obligation to initiate nutrition support should be based on current medical practice, and that the obligation to continue should be based on the ability to achieve the desired result. Because they view nutrition support as a medical treatment, these individuals believe that the benefits should outweigh the actual or potential burdens that may ensue. They believe that the patient or guardian has the right to refuse initiation or continuation of artificial nutrition and hydration. These persons perceive nutrition support as "too much" care when the patient's ability to return to an acceptable level of cognitive-affective functioning is permanently impaired. This method of treatment is seen as having fulfilled its purpose; it is no longer lifesaving but rather organ-sustaining, and unnaturally postpones death. Proponents of this position argue that destiny should not be mandated by technology simply because it is available.

The dilemma concerning the practice of nutrition support illustrates the difficulty that exists in deciding whether to continue care. The issues are ethically based, morally complex, and legally perverse. The problem lies in conflicting value claims regarding care, obligation, and acceptable human life. The questions and the choices to be argued are profound and require humility, wisdom, and the feel of truth to guide the decision-making process.

This chapter considers fundamental ethical principles, reviews legal precedents, and discusses guidelines that may be useful in arriving at decisions about the appropriate use of nutrition support.

VALUES, MORALS, AND ETHICS

Human life is a gift—a gift with an inherent purpose based in values, morals, and ethics. The terms values, morals, and ethics are often used interchangeably. However, when applied in the philosophical sense, distinct differences exist in meaning and application. *Values* look descriptively at human behavior; are not necessarily right or wrong, good or bad; and measure the worth or merit that an individual places on something regardless of standards, principles, or norms.[4,5] *Morals* reflect human behavior and belief about right and wrong, good and evil, in light of a religious tradition or social consensus.[5,6] *Ethics* is a systematic discussion of morals. It is the disciplined study of the nature and justification of moral principles, decisions, and problems.[4] Ethics addresses oughtness—that is, how certain things ought or ought not to be done because they affect people.[5,7] *Applied ethics* uses normative ethical principles, arrives at an intellectual judgment about the appropriateness of an act, and takes a moral position for specific problems.[5]

Ethical Reasoning

Beauchamp and Walters[7] described a hierarchy of ethical reasoning where specific moral assertions are justified by appeal to the more general premise. This methodology uses judgments that represent particular, individual decisions justified by rules, which can be justified by principles, which are justified by ethical theories. Figure 3–1 illustrates the ascending order of justification.

Ethical principles relevant to moral issues in health care include (1) the principle of autonomy, (2) the principle of nonmaleficence, (3) the principle of beneficence, (4) the principle of veracity, (5) the principle of confidentiality, and (6) the principle of justice.[4,7,8]

The principle of autonomy is the principle of respect for persons, seeing human beings as possessing an "incalculable worth or moral dignity not possessed by other things or creatures." It acknowledges personal liberty of action with (1) the freedom to decide, (2) the freedom to act, and (3) mutual respect for the autonomy of others.[8] According to Beauchamp and Walters, to be autonomous, the person must be both "free of external control" and "in control of his or her own affairs."[7]

The principle of nonmaleficence is reflected in the Hippocratic oath; the physician is admonished not to inflict evil or harm and to prevent evil or harm when possible.[7] This principle is frequently brought to issue in decisions concerning initiation or discontinuation of nutrition support.

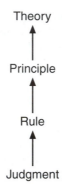

Figure 3–1 Ethical Principles.

The principle of beneficence addresses the virtue of doing and promoting good.[7] In health care, professionals are obligated to do more than refrain from inflicting harm; there is the bounden duty to do good.

The principle of veracity demands telling the truth, and the principle of confidentiality obliges respect of privacy.[7]

The principle of justice requires that like cases should be treated alike and that equals should be treated equally. The principle does not show us how to discern quality, but "merely asserts that whatever respects are under consideration, 'if' persons are equal in those respects, they should be treated alike."[7]

Ethical Conflicts and Dilemmas

Hiller[4] stated that for an *ethical conflict* to exist, (1) a real choice must exist between two possible courses of action, and (2) each possible action or its consequences must hold a significantly different value. An *ethical dilemma* occurs when the performance of an act, based on ethical principles, can be viewed as morally right by some and as morally wrong by others; where evidence on both sides is morally inconclusive, there is reason from a moral perspective why the act ought and ought not to be performed.[7]

Ethical conflicts generally fall into one of four categories: (1) good versus evil, (2) better versus worse, (3) good versus good, and (4) allocation conflicts. Good-versus-evil conflicts are the least difficult to resolve, since the outcomes are relatively obvious. Better-versus-worse situations are not as clear, because the best of possible choices may seem neither better nor worse. Good-versus-good dilemmas occur when there is good evidential reason for mutually exclusive options. Withholding or withdrawing nutrition support is an example of this type of conflict. Allocation conflicts involve the apportionment of scarce resources—saying no to some in order to say yes to others.

Decision-Making Models for Resolving Ethical Conflicts

Ethics is not an exact science. According to Maguire: "Sometimes it can only lighten the darkness slightly, but not dispel it, leaving us with an only partially guided leap in the dark."[9] In situations involving ethical conflict, determining the appropriate choice is a difficult task. Nevertheless, the resolution of ethical dilemmas can be facilitated via a systematic process of ethical analysis. Decision-making models generally approach conflict resolution either qualitatively or quantitatively, and no single method of analysis is recognized preferentially over another. The decision-making models designed by Harron, Burnside, and Beauchamp,[10] Drane,[11] and Francoeur[8] are discussed below. Harron, Burnside, and Beauchamp used a qualitative approach to ethical inquiry, as did Drane. Francoeur, however, used quantitative analysis for ethical conflict resolution.

Harron, Burnside, and Beauchamp designed a six-step process for decision making.[10] An outline of this process is shown in Exhibit 3–1.

Drane's model (Exhibit 3–2), which consists of four phases, is a qualitative approach specifically designed for making health care decisions.[11]

The Francoeur model (Exhibit 3–3) uses a mathematical decision matrix; although the approach is quantitative, the elements examined remain qualitative in nature.[8]

Judeo-Christian Influence on Ethical Issues

American society is deeply rooted in Judeo-Christian tradition, which has a marked impact on an individual's perception of the value of human life. Because this perspective is so pervasive in our culture, it must be considered when discussing issues related to medical life support.

Since the 16th century, the Roman Catholic Church has extensively studied what one is obliged to do to preserve human life.[12] The following discussion focuses on this position, since it is accepted by the majority of Christian groups.

Theology addresses those ardent, fundamental questions pertaining to human life: What is life? Who is the author of life? What is the value of life? Theology answers these questions in the context of the Divine Order of things and God's plan of salvation. Christian belief presupposes that God is the author of life, and that God alone has dominion over life. Each person is responsible for interpreting God's will and the mission of one's own life.

Richard McCormick,[13] a noted Catholic moral theologian, stated that in the Judeo-Christian perspective, "the meaning, substance and consummation of life is

Exhibit 3–1 Harron, Burnside, and Beauchamp's Six-Step Decision-Making Model

1. **Identify the problem.**
   - Base the process on perception, identification, and confirmation.
   - A real choice must exist between possible courses of action.
   - Each outcome must have a significantly different value.
2. **Analyze alternatives.**
   - Generally there are only two options: to do or not to do.
3. **Weigh competing options.**
   - Consider the consequences of each possible action and assess the most likely results.
4. **Justify by principle.**
   - Apply ethical principles to substantiate the moral reason for an act as compared with the application of ethical principles of an alternative act and the consequences.
   - Prioritize ethical principles in competition.
5. **Make a choice.**
   - Select an alternative based on a justifiable argument.
6. **Reassess the choice.**
   - Analyze retrospectively to review justification for the choice, unresolved questions, and comparison with similar cases and conclusions.

Source: Reprinted with permission from F. Harron, J. Burnside, T. Beauchamp. *Health and Human Values: A Guide to Making Your Own Decisions,* © 1983, Yale University Press.

found in terms of love of God and neighbor, human relationships and the qualities of justice, respect, concern, compassion and support."[13] McCormick went on to explain the value of human life as

> a value to be preserved precisely as a condition for other values, and therefore insofar as these other values remain attainable. Since these other values cluster around and are rooted in human relationships, it seems to follow that life is a value to be preserved only insofar as it contains some potentiality for human relationships. When in human judgment this potentiality is totally absent or would be, because of the condition of the individual, totally subordinated to the mere effort for survival, that life can be said to have achieved its potential.[13]

The Catholic moral position is firmly seated in the relative value of human life. Human life is not an absolute good, and the duty to preserve it is a limited one.[13] Pius XII stated that "life, health, all temporal activities are subordinated to spiritual ends."[14]

Exhibit 3–2 Drane's Four-Phase Health Care Decision-Making Model

1. **Phase 1: Expository, Descriptive Phase**
   - concrete elements of the case
     — *medical facts:* diagnosis, prognosis, medical alternatives, consequences of treatment or nontreatment
     — *human facts:* demographics, religion, mental status, credibility of all persons involved in the case
2. **Phase 2: Rational, Analytical Phase**
   - critical reflection of situation
     — medical ethics categories: definitions of death, informed consent, right to treatment, suicide, euthanasia
     — conceptual distinctions: act and omission, prolonging death and prolonging life
     — principles and moral guidelines: autonomy, beneficence, justice, fidelity, truth
     — legal decisions and professional codes
3. **Phase 3: Volitional, Decisional Phase**
   - ordering goods and values: prioritizing interests, preferences, goods
   - ordering the principles: weighing consequences of one principle over another
   - decision making: considering effect on all concerned
4. **Phase 4: Public, Reflective Phase**
   - making assumptions explicit: recognizing underlying beliefs and admitting influences on the decision
   - correlating reasons and feelings: correlating initial feelings about supporting one decision over another
   - organizing reasons for public communication: explaining professional choices based on publicly accepted standards of behavior

Source: Reprinted with permission from J.F. Drane. A methodology for making ethical healthcare decisions, *Health Prog,* Vol. 67, pp. 36–64.

The Catholic Church has consistently differentiated between ordinary and extraordinary means for sustaining human life as those measures proportionate to one's condition or state in life.[12] Pius XII affirmed this principle when he described the obligation of using only those means that, according to the circumstances of persons, places, time, and culture, will provide substantial benefit and that do not cause any grave burden for oneself or another.[14] The benefit derived must be proportionate to the burden imposed.

In *The Vatican's Declaration on Euthanasia,* human life is described as the fundamental basis of all goods and the necessary source and condition of "every human activity and of all society."[15] The declaration supports the principle of benefit versus burden regarding continuation of medical treatment. The withdrawal of

Exhibit 3–3 Francoeur's Six-Step Decision-Making Model

---

1. **Identify alternatives.**
   - *All possible* alternatives are considered as the effectiveness of the analysis and as a function of the number of alternatives.
2. **Determine evaluation criteria.**
   - Ethical principles have the greatest weight.
   - Economic, political, legal, and philosophical principles have lower weight.
3. **Derive value statements from criteria.**
   - Value statements are developed and assigned to criteria identified as relevant in step 2.
4. **Rank order and calculate weighting factors for value statements.**
   - Value statements are rank ordered and prioritized in order of importance.
   - Rank ordering ranges from highest priority (10) to lowest priority (1).
   - Weighting factor is calculated for each statement by:
     — sum of numbers in ordering column
     — division of order for each value statement by total number of statements
5. **Rate the alternatives.**
   - Decision matrix is constructed consisting of all possible alternatives.
   - Value statements' rank ordering and weighting factor results are listed.
   - Numerical rating factors are determined for each alternative on a scale of 10 (high) to 1 (low).
6. **Complete matrix and make a decision.**
   - Calculate a product of the rating and weighting factors.
   - All products for an alternative are added for a total sum.
   - Sum columns are reviewed for all alternatives.
   - Sum of highest ranking is most ethical conclusion.

Source: Reprinted with permission from J.F. Drane. A methodology for making ethical healthcare decisions, *Health Prog,* Vol. 67, pp. 36–64.

---

medical treatment is not viewed as euthanasia, nor is it equivalent to suicide: "On the contrary, it should be considered as an acceptance of the human condition, or a wish to avoid the application of a medical procedure disproportionate to the results that can be expected, or a desire not to impose excessive expenses on the family or community."[15] McCormick substantiated this position when he said that it is "neither inhuman nor un-Christian to say that there comes a point where an individual's condition itself represents the negation of any truly human—ie, relational—potential. When the point is reached, is not the best treatment no treatment?"[13]

It would seem then that the mere maintenance of physiologic organ function is inconsistent with the Judeo-Christian meaning of life. O'Rourke stated that "The primary role of physiological function is to support cognitive-affective function"[16] and that the ethical obligation to prolong life ceases when that life can no longer "achieve, recover, or initially develop cognitive-affective function and strive for the purpose of life."[16] The ethical obligation in those instances then becomes one of providing comfort care.

In regard to artificial nutrition and hydration, the Catholic tradition is consistent with its position on the obligation of preserving human life. Bayer concluded: "The artificial provision of food and fluid does not bind us with the same force as does the ingestion process conatural to our body."[14] Kelly carried this further when he declared: "No one is obliged to use any means—natural or artificial—if it does not offer a reasonable hope of success in overcoming that person's condition."[11] In the case of coma, once the patient is diagnosed as terminally ill, "the use of artificial means to prolong life not only need not but should not be used."[11]

Paris and McCormick, in their discussion on the Catholic tradition on the use of nutrition and hydration, stated that "bedrock teaching of theology on the meaning of life and death should guide our judgments" in this issue.[12] In those instances where nutrition and hydration are withdrawn, the purpose should be not to hasten death by starvation and dehydration, but to "spare the patient the prolongation of life when the patient can derive no benefit from such prolongation."[12]

O'Rourke stated that "withholding artificial hydration and nutrition from a patient in irreversible coma does not induce a new fatal pathology; rather it allows an already existing fatal pathology to take its natural course."[16]

Paris[17] affirmed that the application of the basic ethical principles of autonomy, beneficence, nonmaleficence, and justice must be considered in the decision-making process for issues of initiating and/or withdrawing artificial sustenance. Using these pertinent ethical principles, Nelson[18] identified three situations where the provision of artificial nutrition and hydration might be forgone ethically: (1) when the procedure is so unlikely to provide the patient with nutrients and fluids that it is futile; (2) when the patient will experience no benefit from the procedure even though it would provide sufficient nutrients and fluids to sustain biologic life; and (3) when the burdens of the procedure to the patient outweigh the benefits.

LEGAL CONSIDERATIONS IN NUTRITION SUPPORT

Historically, the termination of life support from a legal perspective has been contingent upon the determination and documentation of brain death. *Brain death* is defined as the nonfunction of the entire brain and the dependence of life systems (ie, cardiovascular and respiratory systems) on ventilators and other artificial means of support. With or without these artificial support systems, the brain-dead patient's own physiologic organ systems eventually will die.[19]

Within the past decade, the courts have been petitioned regarding the legal propriety of terminating nutrition support as a life-sustaining medical treatment in three scenarios: (1) a surrogate refusing continuation of a feeding procedure for a patient in a persistent vegetative state; (2) a surrogate refusing a feeding procedure for someone with severely diminished mental capacity; and (3) a mentally competent patient refusing nutrition and hydration as a medical treatment.[18]

The controversy exists over the patient's or surrogate's interest in determining medical procedures and in avoiding "burdensome, intrusive and ineffective treatment"[20] weighed against the state's interest in (1) preserving life and preventing suicide, (2) protecting innocent third parties, and (3) maintaining the ethical integrity of the medical profession.[1,21,22]

The state's interest in preserving life must be balanced against the individual's rights to privacy and to self-determination.[1,22] The right to privacy allows individuals to make decisions regarding "intimate details of their behavior."[1] These decisions, however, depending upon the circumstances, may be restricted by the state's interests. The right to self-determination permits every adult human being of sound mind to decide what is personally appropriate to do with his or her own body.[1]

Informed consent and substituted judgment are also considered the state's interest for decisions in matters concerned with termination of nutrition support. Informed consent mandates that any patient who is capable of making a decision has the right to be presented with the diagnosis, prognosis, alternative treatments, and risks and benefits of nonintervention. The patient has the right to decide on medical treatment, uncoerced by others or by inappropriate pressure. If the patient decides to consent or to refuse care, the decision is "legally appropriate, legally binding and morally uncontrovertible even if the result is death." Furthermore, refusal of treatment that will sustain life is not suicide if the patient's death results from an underlying disease process that is not of the patient's own doing.[23]

The substituted-judgment standard has been used in cases where the patient no longer has the capacity to make decisions regarding medical care. Substituted judgment asks the question, What would the patient want if he or she could tell us? Substituted judgment considers benefit versus burden. According to Dubler, "As the possible benefit of the treatment decreases, and the possible burden and intrusiveness of care increases, the patient's right to refuse rises and the state's interest in preserving life decreases."[1]

At this writing, the number of legal cases being argued for termination of nutrition support continues to rise. The following review is limited to the most noted cases reflecting the scenarios described earlier.

In 1986 the Massachusetts Supreme Judicial Court ruled that gastrostomy tube feeding could be discontinued on Paul Brophy, who had sustained a ruptured cerebral aneurysm that had rendered him unconscious and in a persistent vegetative state. The court authorized the patient's wife to order removal of the feeding tube. The decision was based on the following factors:

- the patient's previously expressed choice during cognitive life not to have his life maintained by artificial means, but to be allowed to die
- the patient's right to privacy and right to self-determination and individual autonomy
- the patient's right to refuse medical treatment
- the determination that maintenance of Brophy's life by artificial means would be not only intrusive but extraordinary
- the determination that discontinuing the feeding would not be equivalent to suicide, since Brophy was no longer able to swallow because of brain damage, and therefore brain damage would be the cause of death
- the charge to Mrs. Brophy of the responsibility for finding professionals willing to discontinue treatment and not ordered of those who would feel ethically and professionally compromised.[3,21,24]

Claire Conroy was an 84-year-old woman with severe organic brain syndrome, "conscious but demented," in a semifetal position with various physical ailments. In 1983, her legal guardian, a nephew, petitioned the New Jersey court to allow the removal of a nasogastric feeding tube. The patient died with the tube in place prior to a decision on appeal to the New Jersey Supreme Court. In 1985, the New Jersey Supreme Court rendered the opinion that any life-sustaining treatment, including nutrition support, could be withheld or withdrawn. The opinion was based on the following analysis:

- the existence of evidence that indicated what the patient would have chosen if she were competent, and the surrogate decision maker's choosing the treatment outcome most consistent with that evidence
- the determination that the burdens of the patient's continued life with the treatment would outweigh the benefits of that life for her
- the determination that the net burdens of continued life "clearly and markedly" would exceed whatever benefits might be obtained[18–20,22]

The Second District Court of Appeals of California ruled in 1986 that High Desert Hospital must honor Elizabeth Castner Bouvia's request not to be tube-fed. Elizabeth Bouvia, a 29-year-old woman with cerebral palsy, was neither terminally ill nor mentally incompetent. The court's ruling was based on the right of competent adults to refuse medical treatment, as well as the rights to privacy and self-determination. The court also held that caretakers were not subject to criminal liability "when honoring a competent, informed patient's refusal of medical service."[18,25]

The state of Missouri heard its first case in 1988. In this case, the Circuit Court of Jasper County authorized the removal of a gastrostomy feeding tube from Nancy Cruzan, age 31, who had been in a persistent vegetative state since January 1983 following an automobile accident. However, the order was reversed by the

Missouri State Supreme Court. The Cruzan family filed an appeal to the U.S. Supreme Court, which ruled that the feeding tube could be removed. This was done, and the patient died 12 days later.

The *Cruzan* decision had several important implications: (1) it established the right to refuse life-sustaining treatment including tube feeding; (2) it supports the concept that nutrition support is indistinguishable from other medical treatments; (3) for patients who are not competent to make decisions, and who have not left a written directive of their preferences, states may require "clear and convincing" evidence of the patient's wishes.[26]

Living Wills and Durable Powers of Attorney

In 1985, the American Bar Association approved the Uniform Rights of the Terminally Ill Act, drafted by the National Conference of Commissioners on Uniform State Laws. The act states "that an individual of sound mind and nineteen or more years of age may execute at any time a declaration governing the withholding or withdrawal of life sustaining treatment . . . that only prolongs the process of dying and is not necessary for comfort or to alleviate pain." However, the act prohibits excluding nutrition and hydration for a patient's comfort care.[27]

The "living will" enacted by many states is based on the above act. These documents, if drafted when an individual is mentally competent, are legally binding, but they generally are unclear regarding the exclusion or provision of nutrition and hydration. In fact, 15 states explicitly do not consider nutrition and hydration as extraordinary treatment; therefore, withholding or withdrawing nutrition support in those states would not be authorized, even with the existence of a living will.[23]

Durable powers of attorney have significantly more leverage than the living will. The power of attorney allows competent adults to designate an agent or agents to act in their behalf when and if their decisional capacity is irredeemable. Therefore, if a person specified that nutrition and hydration be withheld or withdrawn under certain conditions and circumstances via a power of attorney, that request would be considered legally binding, even in states that specify exclusion of nourishment. According to Mishkin, "The reason is, that an agent has the same legal powers, under a power of attorney, that the person delegating the power of attorney would have."[23] Therefore, an agent may refuse treatment on behalf of the patient based on prior knowledge of the patient's wishes.

Guidelines for Decisions To Withdraw or Withhold Nutrition Support

Hospital ethics committees can help clarify the confusion in decisions about nutrition support by being proactive rather than reactive. Supportive care guidelines and specific policies pertaining to feeding should be developed that reflect the institution's mission and philosophy.[28] These guidelines and policies should be presented to the patient, if competent, or to the guardian, if the patient is incompetent, prior to the initiation of nutrition support, and should be reviewed when "there is no reasonable hope that the patient will recover."[29]

Policies should be structured to assist patients or guardians in the decision-making process about their treatment and should address at least the following issues:

- patient autonomy
- burden/benefit
- competence/incompetence
- supportive care plans
  1. care and treatment provided to an individual "to preserve comfort, hygiene, and dignity, but not prolong life"[30]
  2. factors considered in the plans
     — do-not-resuscitate guidelines
     — fluids, intravenous therapies
     — nutrition (total parenteral nutrition, gastric feeding)
     — symptom management
     — invasive diagnostic and therapeutic procedures[29]

According to Dubler,[1] the following set of guidelines may aid in the decision-making process: (1) to ensure that health care facilities of excellence are available where decisions can be made adequately; (2) to require that the decision to refuse care be a real refusal based on the patient's wishes and not a denial of care; (3) to be aware of those instances when the patient's condition is medically futile (ie, that death will occur soon, regardless of intervention); (4) to know there is no possible benefit because there can be no improvement (ie, irreversible coma or persistent vegetative state); and (5) to recognize when there is a disproportionate burden to the patient.

Carson observed: "Feeding is an act that requires a willingness to give and a willingness to receive. When there is no willingness to receive on the part of the patient, and the giving will not make any difference in or will reduce the patient's well being, it makes sense for caregivers to find other ways to express their concern and to give care."[31]

IMPLICATIONS FOR DIETITIANS

The registered dietitian, as a member of the dietetics profession, is guided in practice and conduct by The American Dietetic Association's Code of Ethics for the Profession of Dietetics.[32] This document serves as the foundation for decisions on all levels of practice.

Guidelines for the use of enteral and parenteral nutrition have been published by the American Society for Parenteral and Enteral Nutrition, and also serve as guidelines to health professionals for the implementation, administration, and termination of artificial feeding.[33] These guidelines specifically state that "if the procedures for supplying nutrition support impose burdens greater than the anticipated benefits; such procedures may be discontinued in accordance with the principles and practices governing the withholding and withdrawing of other forms of medical treatment."[33]

The standards of practice for the nutrition support dietitian and guidelines from the American Society for Parenteral and Enteral Nutrition are useful in conjunction with the above standards; these guidelines specifically address the professional responsibilities of the dietitian in the provision of specialized nutrition support therapy, including "the termination of enteral and parenteral therapies when appropriate."[34] King stated that the dietitian should be involved in decisions of withholding nutrition support, and she offers the following guidelines to be used in the decision-making process:

- Each case is unique and must be handled individually.
- The patient's expressed desire for extent of medical care is a primary guide for determining the level of nutrition intervention.
- The expected benefits, in contrast to the potential burdens, of nonoral feeding must be evaluated by the health care team and discussed with the patient. The focus of care should emphasize the patient's physical and psychological comfort.
- The decision to forgo hydration or nutrition support should be weighed carefully, because such a decision may be difficult or impossible to reverse within a period of days or weeks.
- The decision to forgo "heroic" medical treatment does not preclude baseline nutrition support.
- The physician's written diet order in the medical chart documents the decision to administer or forgo nutrition support. The dietitian should participate in this decision.
- The institution's ethics committee, if available, should assist in establishing and implementing defined, written guidelines for nutrition support protocol. The dietitian should be a required member of or consultant to such a committee.

The American Dietetic Association's position paper on issues in feeding the terminally ill adult[26] addresses the role of the dietitian in terms of ethical, legal, medical, and nutritional responsibilities that correspond with the content of this chapter.

CONCLUSIONS

The sophistication of modern medicine demands philosophic reflection on the appropriate and inappropriate use of today's medical miracles. Ethical analysis, legal precedents, and professional standards help clinicians to decide what they should do in an age when almost anything seems possible. Clinicians should be cautious in their approach to decisions regarding withholding or withdrawing nutrition support; they should know that do-not-feed does not mean do-not-care, do-not-pay-attention-to, as-good-as-dead, or worthless person. The decision to withhold or withdraw nutrition support means that caregivers should intensify their efforts to provide other forms of care. When the patient can no longer "rage against the dying of the light," it is time for the caregivers to do all that is in their power to provide comfort as the patient goes "gentle into that good night."[31]

REFERENCES

1. Dubler N. Health professions in the middle: legal and ethical dilemmas of medical technologies. Presented at Twelfth Clinical Congress of the American Society for Parenteral and Enteral Nutrition; January 18, 1988; Las Vegas, NV.

2. Office of Technology Assessment. Nutritional support and hydration. In: *Life Sustaining Technologies and the Elderly.* Washington, DC: Office of Technology Assessment; 1987:275–329.

3. Bresnahan JF, Drane JF. A challenge to examine the meaning of living and dying. *Health Prog.* December 1986:32–98.

4. Hiller MD. *Ethics and Health Administration: Ethical Decision Making in Health Management.* Arlington, VA: Association of University Programs in Health Administration; 1986:1–166.

5. Fahey C. Ethical issues in practice. Presented at 70th Annual Meeting of The American Dietetic Association; October 22, 1987; Atlanta, GA.

6. Maguire D. The meaning of morals. In: *The Moral Choice.* Minneapolis, MN: Winston Press; 1979:58–107.

7. Beauchamp TL, Walters L. *Contemporary Issues in Bioethics.* Belmont, CA: Wadsworth Publishing Co; 1982:1–41.

8. Francoeur RT. *Biomedical Ethics: A Guide to Decision Making.* New York: John Wiley & Sons Inc; 1983:5–198.

9. Maguire D. Love's strategy. In: *The Moral Choice.* Minneapolis, MN: Winston Press; 1979:108–127.

10. Harron F, Burnside J, Beauchamp T. *Health and Human Values: A Guide to Making Your Own Decisions.* New Haven, CT: Yale University Press; 1983.

11. Drane JF. A methodology for making ethical healthcare decisions. *Health Prog.* 67:36–64.

12. Paris JJ, McCormick RA. The Catholic tradition on the use of nutrition and fluids. *America.* May 2, 1987:356–361.

13. McCormick RA. To save or let die. *JAMA.* 1974;229:172–176.

14. McCartney JJ. Catholic positions on withholding sustenance for the terminally ill. *Health Prog.* October 1986:38–40.

15. Larue GA. *The Vatican's Declaration on Euthanasia, 1980.* Los Angeles, CA: Hemlock Society; 1980:35–44.

16. O'Rourke K. The AMA statement on tube feeding: an ethical analysis. *America.* November 22, 1986:321–324.

17. Paris JJ. Withholding or withdrawing nutrition and fluids: what are the real issues? *Health Prog.* December 1985:22–25.

18. Nelson LJ. Forgoing nutrition and hydration. *Clin Ethics Rep.* 1987;1:1–7.

19. American Health Consultants, Inc. AMA council issues controversial new life support rule. *Med Ethics Advis.* 1986;2:41–48.

20. Dresser R. Court cases on nutritional support. Presented at Tenth Clinical Congress of the American Society for Parenteral and Enteral Nutrition; February 9–12, 1986; Dallas, TX.

21. American Health Consultants, Inc. Massachusetts Supreme Court ruling: tube feeding is extraordinary measure. *Med Ethics Advis.* 1986;2:129–131.

22. Dresser RD. Discontinuing nutrition support: a review of the case law. *J Am Diet Assoc.* 1985;85:1289–1292.

23. Mishkin B. Withholding and withdrawing nutritional support. *Nutr Clin Pract.* 1986;1:50–52.

24. Rothenberg LS. The dissenting opinions: biting the hands that won't feed. *Health Prog.* December 1986:38–45.

25. Bayley C. The case of Elizabeth Bouvia: a strain on our ethical reasoning. *Health Prog.* July–August 1986:40–47.

26. Position of The American Dietetic Association: issues in feeding the terminally ill adult. *J Am Diet Assoc.* 1992;92:996–1005.

27. National Conference of Commissioners on Uniform State Laws. Uniform rights of the terminally ill act. Presented at Annual Conference; August 2–9, 1985; Minneapolis, MN.

28. Center for Bioethics. The need for hospital policies before a case arises. *Ethical Curr.* May 1987:1–2.

29. Brodeur D. Feeding policy protects patients' rights, decisions. *Health Prog.* June 1985:38–40.

30. Halligan M, Hamel RP. Ethics committee develops supportive care guidelines. *Health Prog.* December 1985:26–60.

31. Center for Bioethics. Forgoing food: symbol and reality. *Ethical Curr.* May 1987:2–8.

32. "Anon." Code of ethics for the profession of dietetics. *J Am Diet Assoc.* 1988;88:1592–1596.

33. A.S.P.E.N. Board of Directors Guidelines for the use of parenteral and enteral nutrition in adult and pediatric patients. *J Parenter Enter Nutr.* 1993;17:1SA–26SA.

34. American Society for Parenteral and Enteral Nutrition. Standards of practice: nutritional support dietitian. *Nutr Clin Pract.* August 1986:216–220.

CHAPTER 4

Macronutrient Requirements

Wanda Hain Howell

INTRODUCTION

The macronutrients carbohydrate, protein, and fat are the primary energy substrates in the diets of healthy individuals. During illness, carbohydrate and fat ideally should serve as the principal energy substrates, with protein reserved for anabolic processes. Although absolute requirements for carbohydrate and fat have not been established for states of health or disease, minimum levels have been suggested. In contrast, protein requirements have been defined by the National Research Council (NRC) for healthy individuals. Increases beyond these levels are estimated for individuals in states of disease.

Although quantitative considerations have traditionally been emphasized, new evidence suggests that qualitative aspects of the macronutrients merit close scrutiny. Specifically, the type of carbohydrate, protein, and fat in the diet may be of equal importance to the amount. Therefore, this review includes both quantitative and qualitative considerations in the estimation of macronutrient requirements.

MACRONUTRIENT REQUIREMENTS IN HEALTH

Carbohydrate Requirements

Dietary carbohydrate consists primarily of sugars (mono- and disaccharides) and complex carbohydrates (polysaccharides). Starches are polymers of glucose. Dietary fibers are indigestible and include insoluble complex carbohydrates in plant cell walls (cellulose, hemicellulose) and soluble pectin, gums, and mucilages.

Although humans do not exhibit carbohydrate-deficiency symptoms, disturbances in metabolism and intestinal function can appear when intake is very low. Carbohydrate-free diets promote gluconeogenesis from stored triglycerides and lean tissue mass, resulting in the accumulation of ketone bodies, dehydration, and loss of tissue proteins. The amount of dietary carbohydrate necessary to prevent these effects and "spare protein" is estimated to be 50 to 100 grams daily.[1] The NRC, however, recommends that more than 50% of total energy be provided by carbohydrate in order to reduce energy requirements from fat to about 30%.[2] Thus, for healthy adults consuming 2500 kcal/day, the recommended intake would be at least 310 g/day primarily from complex carbohydrate.

Interest in dietary fiber as a potentially important factor in reducing the risk of developing chronic disorders such as cardiovascular disease and colon cancer has led to recommendations for increased intake.[3] Current average intake of dietary fiber in the United States is estimated to be about 12 to 15 g/day.[4] The recommended level of 10 g/1000 kcals/day is associated with protective effects while avoiding potential detrimental effects.[3]

The protective effects of fiber have been attributed to its physical properties. The water-holding capacity of wheat bran fiber is associated with increased stool weight and decreased transit time, both of which are important for maintaining large bowel function.[5] Although these effects are specific to insoluble fiber, soluble fiber sources such as pectin may protect against colon cancer by producing short-chain fatty acids on fermentation.[6] Some animal studies, however, have reported that highly fermentable fibers promote tumor formation.[7] The significance of this effect in humans is poorly understood and requires further investigation.

Although insoluble fibers have a protective effect on large bowel function, these dietary fibers have no reported effect on plasma lipids. Water-soluble fiber intake, however, is positively associated with reduction in plasma total and low-density lipoprotein cholesterol with little change in high-density lipoprotein cholesterol. The soluble fiber physical properties of differential bile acid binding and increased viscosity of intestinal fluids are hypothesized to interfere with cholesterol absorption resulting in decreased plasma cholesterol levels.[8]

A very high intake of dietary fiber can decrease the availability of some nutrients. Both water-soluble and insoluble fiber sources have been reported to inhibit pancreatic enzyme activity, although the significance of this effect in healthy individuals is difficult to determine because of the excess of these enzymes produced in response to a meal.[9] Insoluble fiber, specifically the plant cell wall matrix in some foods, also provides a physical barrier to digestion and can result in decreased availability of nutrients in these foods.[10] Reduced mineral absorption (particularly iron, calcium, zinc, and copper) associated with the intake of cereal and some fruits is more likely to be due to the presence in these foods of phytic acid rather than fiber. Likewise, fiber *per se* has little if any effect on vitamin absorption.[10]

Lipid Requirements

Triglycerides are the primary lipid component in foods and nutrient products and provide the most concentrated source of energy among the macronutrients.

They are nonpolar (insoluble) but release polar (soluble) fatty acids on digestion. Fatty acids are classified as short-chain, medium-chain, or long-chain; and as saturated, monounsaturated, and polyunsaturated. Polyunsaturated fatty acids are subdivided into omega-3 (ω-3) or omega-6 (ω-6) fatty acids. The parent members of the ω-3 and ω-6 fatty acids are alpha-linolenic and linoleic acids, respectively. Saturated and monounsaturated fatty acids can be synthesized from acetyl coenzyme A and thus are not essential dietary components. Polyunsaturated fatty acids (linoleic and alpha-linolenic) are essential in the diet because they cannot be synthesized. They are precursors of cell membrane lipids (phospholipids) and eicosanoids (prostaglandins, thromboxanes, and leukotrienes).

Essential fatty acid (EFA) deficiency was first recognized in infants who were fed formulas deficient in linoleic acid.[11] Much later, this deficiency syndrome was identified in adults who were fed exclusively with fat-free intravenous solutions.[12] Clinical signs of EFA deficiency include scaly skin, hair loss, and impaired wound healing. Biochemical confirmation of EFA deficiency is an increased triene/tetraene ratio (greater than 0.1).[13] In the absence of sufficient linoleic acid (a tetraene), the metabolism of oleic acid produces elevated levels of eicosatrienoic acid.

EFA deficiency is seen almost exclusively in patients with medical problems affecting fat intake or absorption of fat. For this reason, there is currently no Recommended Dietary Allowance (RDA) for either linoleic or alpha-linolenic acid. The average American intake of polyunsaturated fatty acids is about 7% of total energy, which is well above the 1% to 2% sufficient to prevent EFA deficiency in adults.[2] The American Academy of Pediatrics recommends that infant formulas provide at least 2.7% of energy as linoleic acid.[14] This level is below the approximately 6% provided by human milk. The Food and Agriculture Organization and the World Health Organization recommend a minimum intake of 3% to 5% for adults.[15] To compensate for EFA losses in the placenta and milk during pregnancy and lactation, these organizations recommend intakes during these conditions of 4.5% and 7% of total energy, respectively.[15]

The ω-3 fatty acid, docosahexanoic acid (DHA), is an essential component of brain and retinal cell membrane phospholipids.[16] DHA deficiency in animals results in impaired vision and behavior alterations, including learning defects. One suspected case in a human has been described.[17] DHA and eicosapentenoic acid (EPA) can be synthesized in small amounts from dietary plant sources (linseed, canola, rapeseed, and soybean oils) of alpha-linolenic acid or obtained in much larger amounts directly from oily fish (tuna, trout, salmon, mackerel, herring, and sardines) that consume phytoplankton and algae. Evidence from animal studies suggests that a dietary intake of 0.5% to 1.0% of total energy from alpha-linolenic acid will provide optimal tissue levels and prevent deficiency symptoms.[18]

The interactions between the ω-6 and ω-3 fatty acids in eicosanoid metabolism are depicted in Figure 4–1. The ratio of ω-6 to ω-3 fatty acids can affect platelet aggregation and immune function.[19] The platelet aggregating and thrombogenic

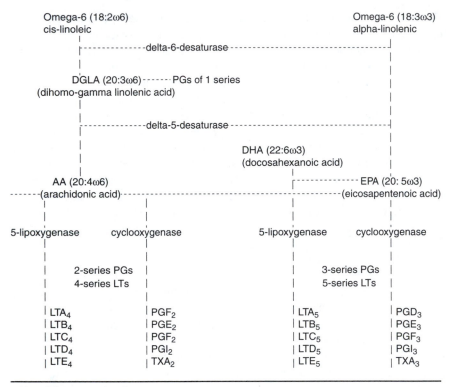

Figure 4–1 Interactions between Linoleic and Alpha-Linolenic Fatty Acids in Eicosanoid Metabolism.

prostaglandin TXA_2 and the inflammation mediator PGE_2 are derived from arachidonic acid, a product of linoleic acid, in response to injury. In the absence of injury, prostaglandins of the 1 series (from dihomo-gamma linolenic acid, also produced from linoleic acid) predominate and control platelet aggregation and inflammation. This control can also be enhanced by increasing ω-3 fatty acids relative to ω-6 fatty acids. Both classes of fatty acids compete for the enzyme delta-5-desaturase. With higher intakes of alpha-linolenic acid, EPA, and DHA, competitive inhibition of the conversion of arachidonic acid to 2-series prostaglandins occurs. This results in increased production of 3-series prostaglandins, which are inhibitors of platelet aggregation and inflammation. This suppression of platelet aggregation is the basis for the reported protective effect of ω-3 fatty acids in reducing cardiovascular disease risk.[19] Control of pathologic immune responses in diseases such as rheumatoid arthritis has also been reported with very high intakes of fish oil.[20] Fish oil supplementation, however, should be used cautiously due to the potential side effects of bleeding, vitamin E deficiency, and vitamin A and D toxicity.[20]

Protein and Amino Acid Requirements

The NRC has defined allowances for protein, although the requirement in biological systems is for amino acids. For this reason, a discussion of both protein and amino acid requirements is appropriate. The NRC followed three steps in establishing the 1989 RDA for protein[2]: (1) estimates of the average requirement for reference proteins (ie, highly digestible, high-quality protein such as egg, meat, milk, or fish) were made according to gender, age, and reproductive status; (2) the average requirement for reference protein for each group was increased by two standard deviations (estimated to meet the needs of 97.5% of the U.S. population) to derive the recommended allowance for reference protein; and (3) amino acid scoring patterns were calculated to determine if adjustment of the reference protein allowance would be necessary based on the quality of proteins consumed in the average American diet.

Methods used by the NRC to determine requirements for reference protein varied with age, gender, and reproductive status. Data from nitrogen balance studies are considered the most valid; however, adequate data are not available for elderly persons and women (this is true for women in general and for women who are pregnant or lactating). Nitrogen balance data for young men indicate an average daily requirement for reference protein of 0.6g/kg/day. After increasing this level by two standard deviations, the requirement becomes 0.75g/kg/day, or rounded off to 0.8g/kg/day. No protein quality adjustment was necessary. Although limited data for women are available, there is some evidence that the requirement, when adjusted for body weight, is not substantially different from that of adult men.[2] The protein RDA for elderly adults is also set at 0.8g/kg/day. Because of the changes in body composition with aging, this level is higher per unit of lean body mass in older adults and is considered to compensate for age-related decreases in protein utilization.

During pregnancy, the RDA for women is increased to provide additional protein for maternal, fetal, and placental tissues. Using the factorial method of estimating requirements, the amount of protein deposited in these tissues is quantified and adjustments are made for increases in nitrogen retention and the efficiency of the conversion of dietary protein to the added tissue burden during each of the three trimesters of pregnancy. The same method is used to estimate the average additional protein requirement during lactation based on the amount (750 mL) and composition (0.011 g protein/mL) of milk produced during the first and second 6 months of lactation. The specific additional requirements during pregnancy and lactation are presented in Table 4–1.

Infant protein requirements are based on human milk as the reference protein in amounts necessary for satisfactory growth. This level is estimated at 1.68 g/kg/day and increased by two standard deviations to the RDA of 2.2 g/kg/day. A modified factorial method is used to define the RDA for protein in older infants and children. These levels represent additional requirements for growth and nitrogen maintenance throughout childhood and adolescence plus adjustments for growth variability and efficiency of protein utilization. Specific values for each age group are presented in Table 4–1.

Table 4–1 Recommended Dietary Allowances for Protein

Category	Age (Years) or Condition	Weight	Recommended Dietary Allowance (g/kg)	Recommended Dietary Allowance (g/day)
Both sexes	0–0.5	6	2.2	13
	0.5–1	9	1.6	14
	1–3	13	1.2	16
	4–6	20	1.1	24
	7–10	28	1.0	28
Males	11–14	45	1.0	45
	15–18	66	0.9	59
	19–24	72	0.8	58
	25–50	79	0.8	63
	51+	77	0.8	63
Females	11–14	46	1.0	46
	15–18	55	0.8	44
	19–24	58	0.8	46
	25–50	63	0.8	50
	51+	65	0.8	50
Pregnancy	1st trimester			+10
	2nd trimester			+10
	3rd trimester			+10
Lactation	1st 6 months			+15
	2nd 6 months			+12

Source: Adapted with permission from Recommended Dietary Allowances: 10th Edition. Copyright 1989 by the National Academy of Sciences. Courtesty of the National Academy Press, Washington, D.C.

The importance of protein in the diet is primarily as a source of amino acids. All food proteins, with the exception of gelatin, contain some of each of the 20 amino acids used for protein synthesis. Nine of these are considered essential or indispensable because they cannot be synthesized via transamination. In humans, the essential amino acids are histidine, isoleucine, leucine, lysine, methionine, phenylalanine, threonine, tryptophan, and valine. Arginine may be provisionally essential in patients with liver dysfunction or when it is present in small amounts relative to other amino acids as in parenteral nutrient solutions.[21]

Short-term nitrogen balance studies in adults, infants, and children have provided data used to estimate essential amino acid requirements for adults and children (see Table 4–2). The limited data reported for the elderly suggest no difference in requirements from those of young adults.[22] No information is available on amino acid requirements for pregnant and lactating women.[2]

Table 4–2 Estimates of Amino Acid Requirements

	Requirements, mg/kg/day, by Age Group			
Amino Acid	Infants Age 3–4 mo[a]	Children, Age ~2 yr[b]	Children, Age 10–12 yr[c]	Adults[d]
Histidine	28	?	?	8–12
Isoleucine	70	31	28	10
Leucine	161	73	42	14
Lysine	103	64	44	12
Methionine plus cystine	58	27	22	13
Phenylalanine plus tyrosine	125	69	22	14
Threonine	87	37	28	7
Tryptophan	17	12.5	3.3	3.5
Valine	93	38	25	10
Total without histidine	714	352	214	84

[a]Based on amounts of amino acids in human milk or cow's milk formulas fed at levels that supported good growth.

[b]Based on achievement of nitrogen balance sufficient to support adequate lean tissue gain (16 mg N/kg/day).

[c]Based on upper range of requirement for positive nitrogen balance.

[d]Based on highest estimate of requirement to achieve nitrogen balance.

Source: Adapted with permission from Recommended Dietary Allowances: 10th Edition. Copyright 1989 by the National Academy of Sciences. Courtesy of the National Academy Press, Washington, D.C.

The NRC also developed methods to evaluate the protein quality of average diets and specific foods. Amino acid requirement patterns compare the essential amino acid profiles in the average diets of each age group to that of reference proteins. These requirement patterns are calculated by dividing each essential amino acid requirement by the recommended allowance of reference protein for each age group. Amino acid requirement patterns are expressed as milligrams of each essential amino acid per gram of reference protein. When requirement patterns were compared to amino acid patterns in average American diets, no substantial differences were found and no adjustments for protein quality were necessary. The RDAs for protein are, therefore, essentially the same as the desired allowance for reference proteins in each age group.

The method used by the NRC to evaluate and adjust for the protein quality of specific foods is the amino acid score. This score is calculated according to the most limiting amino acid (the one with the greatest deficit for the age group involved) by dividing its value in the food source by the value of the same amino acid in a reference protein source. A high score indicates that a particular food is a good source of a given amino acid. This methodology to evaluate protein quality is also important in the design and formulation of products used for specialized nutrition support. Amino acid scores can be and are used to develop nutrition products that meet specific needs during illness.

MACRONUTRIENT REQUIREMENTS IN STRESS

Metabolic Adaptation to Stress

The metabolic response to the stress of injury or trauma has been described by Cuthbertson as having two distinct phases: the ebb phase and the flow phase.[23] The initial phase, or *ebb phase,* is commonly referred to as shock. The system's protective response results in depression of metabolism with a corresponding decrease in oxygen consumption and heat production. Hypovolemia and hypotension occur and will compromise organ function unless corrected in the short term. Correction of these responses necessitates advancement to the *flow phase* of injury, characterized by increased resting energy expenditure (REE) and oxygen consumption. This catabolic phase is mediated by neuroendocrine responses and the production of immunoregulatory polypeptides known collectively as cytokines. The most important cytokines involved in the metabolic response to injury and infection are interleukin-1 (IL-1) and tumor necrosis factor (TNF) or cachectin.[24] IL-1 stimulates the induction of fever, granulopoeisis, synthesis of acute-phase proteins, and hyperinsulinemia. It also acts directly on lymphocytes, macrophages, granulocytes, bone marrow, the reticuloendothelial system, liver, muscles, and endocrine organs. The action of IL-1 is at least partially mediated by PGE_2. The effects of

TNF overlap with those of IL-1 and can stimulate the production of IL-1. The cytokines augment and supplement the neuroendocrine responses to stress.

The neuroendocrine changes with stress are depicted in Figure 4–2. The metabolic response to stress is initiated by the sympathetic nervous system and triggers the release of antidiuretic hormone (ADH), adrenocorticotropic hormone (ACTH), catecholamines, and glucagon. The secretion of ADH results in water and sodium retention and potassium excretion in response to acute volume depletion. ACTH prompts the release of the mineralocorticoid aldosterone and the glucocorticoid cortisol. Aldosterone works via the renin-angiotensin-aldosterone system and in conjunction with ADH to promote water and sodium retention and potassium loss in the presence of hypovolemia. Cortisol stimulates liver enzyme activity and, thus, gluconeogenesis from the catabolism of protein (proteolysis) and fatty acids (lipolysis) for energy substrate. Catecholamines, particularly epinephrine, promote lipolysis and glycolysis for the same purpose. In addition, both epinephrine and ACTH are associated with the release of glucagon. These effects, combined with peripheral insulin resistance, lead to the characteristic hyperglycemia and hyperinsulinemia of stress.

In the absence of insulin resistance, increases in both hepatic glucose production from glycolysis and gluconeogenesis and peripheral glucose uptake and oxidation may lead to the near normal serum glucose levels seen in some patients with injury or sepsis who are not receiving high-glucose feedings.[25] The distinc-

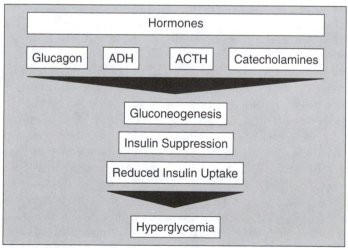

ACTH = adrenocorticotropic hormone; ADH = antidiuretic hormone

Figure 4–2 Neuroendocrine Changes with Stress.

tion between insulin resistance and glucose intolerance is important in this regard. Most patients who are injured or septic are relatively glucose intolerant in that exogenous glucose does not suppress the obligatory increase in hepatic glucose production. This has implications for determining acceptable serum glucose levels. Glucose concentrations from 160 to 200 mg/dL are recommended to maximize glucose uptake without causing hyperosmolarity.[26]

Carbohydrate Requirements

Glucose is the preferred substrate of many vital tissues, including the central nervous system, erythrocytes, immune cells, and injured tissue. Maintenance of glucose oxidation in these tissues as well as the sparing of protein via gluconeogenesis (although limited) can be achieved at a glucose infusion rate of approximately 4 mg/kg/ minute.[27] Higher rates of glucose infusion are likely to result in lipogenesis in both liver and adipose tissue as evidenced by respiratory quotient values greater than 1.0.[28] Furthermore, the catabolic effects of stress cannot be eliminated with higher rates of glucose infusion "covered" by high doses of insulin.[29]

It is necessary to consider carbohydrate requirements relative to total and non-protein energy requirements. To derive energy requirements, clinicians commonly use the Harris-Benedict equation to estimate basal energy expenditure and multiply by activity and stress factors. This method has been shown, however, to overestimate energy requirements for critically ill patients.[30] Measurement of oxygen consumption and carbon dioxide production by indirect calorimetry is generally considered a more accurate method to determine energy requirements and substrate utilization, thus reducing the incidence of overfeeding.[31] In addition to lipogenesis, consequences of overfeeding include hypertriglyceridemia; hyperglycemia with osmotic diuresis and dehydration and potentially azotemia; respiratory complications of increased carbon dioxide production, increased minute ventilation, and possible prolonged ventilator support; and hepatic dysfunction characterized by fat deposition, cholestasis, steatosis, and hepatomegaly.[25]

Specific recommendations for total energy and carbohydrate requirements depend on the method used to estimate these requirements. Requirements for total energy in nonstressed, malnourished patients can generally be estimated at 25% above REE (50% above REE in ambulatory patients); and in patients with injury or infection at 30% to 50% above REE. Alternatively, in the absence of REE data, total energy requirements can be estimated at 25 to 35 kcal/kg/day—with the lower end of the range for nonstressed, ventilated, or sedated patients and the upper end for severely injured or septic patients. The ultimate goal is to obtain positive nitrogen balance or, if not feasible, to minimize nitrogen loss. Frequent adjustments in estimates of total energy requirements should be made accordingly. Carbohydrate should routinely supply 50% to 60% of total kilocalories or 60% to

70% of nonprotein kilocalories.[25] In cases of extreme insulin resistance, characterized by very high serum glucose concentrations (>300 mg/dL), or in pulmonary compromise, carbohydrate intake should be reduced as necessary.

Lipid Requirements

Glucose is never recommended as the sole source of energy substrate in injured or septic patients. Exogenous lipids can be oxidized for energy and are necessary as a source of essential fatty acids in these patients. Exogenous lipids are particularly useful in volume-restricted and insulin-resistant or glucose-intolerant patients. The optimal carbohydrate/lipid mix is unknown, although several considerations are important. Under moderately stressful conditions, fat and glucose have comparable effects on nitrogen balance, whereas in severely stressed patients urea nitrogen excretion is decreased by carbohydrate and unchanged by lipid.[25] This results in fat sparing rather than protein sparing in these critically ill patients. Fat clearance is also impaired as a result of the reduced lipoprotein lipase activity associated with stress-induced cytokine production.[27] Excessive rates of lipid infusion have also been shown to stimulate the reticuloendothelial system, thereby possibly altering the response of this system to subsequent bacterial challenge.[32] Furthermore, high concentrations of linoleic acid in both enteral and parenteral feedings are associated with high PGE_2 levels (see Figure 4–1), which can result in immunosuppression and undesirable inflammatory response.[33,34] Due to these potential adverse effects of excessive lipid provision, protocols generally stipulate that lipids represent 25% to 35% of total kilocalories or 30% to 40% of nonprotein kilocalories.

Nontraditional lipid sources for enteral and parenteral support are currently being investigated. Results of these investigations indicate that some of the adverse effects associated with the provision of linoleic acid as the primary lipid source can be controlled by the use of mixed and structured triglycerides. Mixtures of long-chain triglycerides (LCT) and medium-chain triglycerides (MCT) may reduce the incidence of liver dysfunction (particularly steatosis) associated with long-term nutritional support providing primarily linoleic acid.[35] Combinations of MCTs and LCTs have been used with success in the enteral support of patients with fat maldigestion and malabsorption. In contrast to LCTs, MCTs may also offer a unique nitrogen-sparing effect.[36] Structured triglycerides have been developed to optimize fat-substrate mixtures. Fatty acids from a variety of triglycerides are liberated, followed by reesterification in combinations that produce desired metabolic effects.[37] For example, triglycerides have been structured to include MCTs as well as a high ratio of ω-3 to ω-6 fatty acids. When compared to physical mixtures of these fatty acids and linoleic acid-based enteral formulas, the structured triglyceride diet resulted in enhanced inhibition of tumor growth, weight gain, and nitrogen retention in tumor-bearing animals.[38] Similar results plus a re-duction in energy expenditure have been reported in animals with burn injury fed this type of structured lipid both enterally[39] and parenterally.[40] The extent to which these results apply to humans is unknown, although these studies are currently under way.

Protein and Amino Acid Requirements

Protein requirements in stress associated with injury and infection are com-monly expressed in g/kg actual dry body weight in nonobese patients and desir-able dry body weight in those who are obese (>25% above desirable weight). Al-though specific recommended levels vary somewhat by institution, most research supports a range of 1.5 to 2.0 g/kg/day during stress. This generally translates to between 15% and 20% of total energy expenditure. Requirements for protein, car-bohydrate, lipid, and kilocalories in stress are summarized in Table 4–3.

Risks of excessive protein intake include the metabolic load placed on the body in disposing of the byproducts of protein metabolism. The clearance of urea from excessive protein intake may even require dialysis in critically ill patients. In addi-tion, the production of excess heat from very high protein intakes may increase respiratory load and elevate body temperature. These symptoms may be inter-preted as infection and treated inappropriately with antibiotics, potentially with adverse side effects. There is some evidence that levels of protein intake higher than 1 g/kg/day do not significantly improve nitrogen balance of patients with major trauma.[41]

Table 4–3 Macronutrient Requirements in Stress

Macronutrient	Requirement
Calories	REE × 1.30 to 1.50 25–35 kcals/kg/day
Carbohydrate	≤4 mg/kg/minute or 6 g/kg/day 50%–60% of total calories 60%–70% of nonprotein calories
Lipid	~0.5 mg/kg/minute or 0.7 g/kg/day 25%–30% of total calories 30%–40% of nonprotein calories
Protein	1.5–2.0 g/kg/day 15%–20% of total calories

Standard enteral and parenteral formulations are designed to provide an amino acid profile similar to that of tissue protein rather than a reference food protein.[42] Based on recent research, requirements for specific amino acids may be increased in metabolic stress. Interest in the branched-chain amino acids (BCAA), isoleucine, leucine, and valine, has continued since early *in vitro* animal studies indicated that leucine supplementation was capable of stimulating protein synthesis and reducing protein degradation.[43] Although BCAA-enriched enteral and parenteral formulas are frequently used in the management of critically ill patients, little human data are available to support this practice.[44,45] The efficacy of BCAA supplementation has also been investigated in patients with hepatic failure and impending encephalopathy. The goal of this therapy is reversal of the abnormal BCAA to aromatic amino acid ratio seen in liver failure. In healthy individuals this ratio is 3.5 to 4.0. In liver failure, the ratio falls below 2.5; and in hepatic coma it drops below 1.2 to levels less than 0.8.[46] Increases in brain aromatic amino acids are associated with increases in false neurotransmitters derived from them. A meta-analysis of data in this area indicates slight improvements in encephalopathic patients given parenteral BCAA-enriched solutions, allowing larger amounts of protein to be administered.[47] Effects on mortality, however, are discrepant among the trials included in this analysis. For these reasons, clinical guidelines published by the American Society for Parenteral and Enteral Nutrition stipulate that BCAA-enriched enteral or parenteral formulas should be used in patients with hepatic encephalopathy only when, despite standard medical care, the encephalopathy makes it impossible to provide adequate protein to the patient.[48] These guidelines also state that due to the lack of supportive clinical data, the use of BCAA-supplemented formulas in other critically ill patients cannot be routinely advocated.

Glutamine has received recent attention as a potentially beneficial amino acid for patients in states of metabolic stress. Considerable evidence indicates that glutamine concentrations in skeletal muscle may decrease markedly in patients after undergoing surgery; receiving bone marrow transplantation; or suffering from sepsis, burns, or trauma.[49] Glutamine is derived primarily from the oxidation of BCAAs in skeletal muscle during stress. It is then transported to the gut as an oxidative fuel source for enterocytes and immune cells. Lack of adequate glutamine or its conditional deficiency during stress may result in altered structure and function of these cells. Supplementation of feedings with glutamine has been reported to improve nitrogen balance, control intestinal atrophy, reduce bacterial translocation, and enhance the absorptive capacity of the gut.[50,51] The development of glutamine dipeptides and cold sterilization techniques have made it possible to provide glutamine supplementation in the delivery of nutrition support.[49] Although standard parenteral formulations do not currently contain glutamine, and only a few enteral products are L-glutamine enriched, this situation is likely to change with further study of the safety and clinical efficacy of glutamine supplementation.

Arginine may be a conditionally essential amino acid in a wide range of clinical conditions. It is synthesized in the kidney from citrulline, which originates from the metabolism of glutamine in the gut.[52] The metabolism of arginine results in the production of ornithine, a necessary precursor for polyamine synthesis. Arginine is also the sole precursor for nitric oxide, which is thought to be important in the regulation of macrophage and lymphocyte activity.[53] Supplementation of arginine has been shown to have potentially beneficial effects including stimulation of the immune system, enhancement of wound healing, improvement in postoperative recovery, and prevention or inhibition of tumor growth in animals.[54] However, in one study of dietary arginine supplementation in human breast cancer patients, tumor growth was stimulated.[55] Mechanisms for the beneficial effects of arginine supplementation in humans are not well defined, but it has been reported to stimulate secretion of growth hormone and insulin-like growth factor-1.[56] Arginine-enriched formulas are available; however, more research is needed on the effects of arginine supplementation—particularly on its ability to enhance tumor growth—before widespread use is recommended.

CONCLUSIONS

The amount of carbohydrate, lipid, and protein required during states of health and metabolic stress are reasonably well defined. Each of these broad categories of macronutrients, however, is comprised of qualitatively very different types of nutrient compounds. All carbohydrates, lipids, and amino acids are not alike in their biological effects. For the critically ill patient, the focus of research has moved toward alternative lipid sources (such as the ω-3 fatty acids and structured lipids) and the conditionally essential amino acids (such as glutamine and arginine). Although there is no clear consensus as to their value, there is reason for optimism that further research on the clinical efficacy of these nutritional factors will lead to improvements in recovery and survival.

REFERENCES

1. Calloway S. Dietary components that yield energy. *Environ Biol Med.* 1971;1:175–186.
2. National Research Council, Food and Nutrition Board. *Recommended Dietary Allowances.* 10th ed. Washington, DC: National Academy Press; 1989.
3. National Research Council. *Diet and Health: Implications for Reducing Chronic Disease Risk. Report of the Committee on Diet and Health, Food and Nutrition Board.* Washington, DC: National Academy Press; 1989.
4. Lanza E, Jones DY, Block G, Kessler L. Dietary fiber intake in the U.S. population. *Am J Clin Nutr.* 1987;46:790–797.

5. Cummings JH, Bingham SA, Heaton KW, Eastwood MA. Fecal weight colon cancer risk and dietary intake of non-starch polysaccharides (dietary fiber). *Gastroenterology.* 1992;103:1783–1789.

6. McIntyre A, Gibson PR, Young GP. Butyrate production from dietary fiber and protection against large bowel cancer in a rat model. *Gut.* 1993;34:386–391.

7. Jacobs LR, Lupton JR. Effect of dietary fibers on rat large bowel mucosal growth and cell proliferation. *Am J Physiol.* 1984;246:G378–G385.

8. Eastwood MA, Morris ER. Physical properties of dietary fiber that influence physiological function: a model for polymers along the gastrointestinal tract. *Am J Clin Nutr.* 1992;55:436–442.

9. Schneeman BO, Gallagher DD. Effects of dietary fiber on digestive enzymes. In: Spiller GA, ed. *Dietary Fiber in Human Nutrition.* 2nd ed. Boca Raton, FL: CRC Press; 1993:377–385.

10. Snow P, Odea K. Factors affecting the rate of hydrolysis of starch in food. *Am J Clin Nutr.* 1981;34:2721–2727.

11. Weise HF, Hansen AE, Adam DJD. Essential fatty acids in infant nutrition. *J Nutr.* 58:345–360.

12. Richardson TJ, Sgoutas D. Essential fatty acid deficiency in four adult patients during total parenteral nutrition. *Am J Clin Nutr.* 1975;28:258–263.

13. Holman RT. Essential fatty acid deficiency. In: Holman RT, ed. *Progress in the Chemistry of Fats and Other Lipids.* New York: Pergamon Press; 1971;9:275–348.

14. American Academy of Pediatrics. Composition of human milk: normative data. In: Forbes GB, ed. *Pediatric Nutrition Handbook.* Elk Grove Village, IL: American Academy of Pediatrics. 1985:363–368.

15. Food and Agriculture Organization/World Health Organization. *Fat in Human Nutrition: Report of an Expert Consultation.* Rome: Publications Division, Food and Agriculture Organization; 1993.

16. Neuringer MD, Connor WE. ω-3 fatty acids in the brain and retina: evidence of their essentiality. *Nutr Rev.* 1986;44:285–294.

17. Holman RT, Johnson SB, Hatch TF. A case of human linolenic acid deficiency involving neurological abnormalities. *Am J Clin Nutr.* 1982;35:617–623.

18. Innis SM, Nelson CM, Rioux FM, King DJ. Development of visual acuity in relation to plasma and erythrocyte ω-6 and ω-3 fatty acids in healthy term gestation infants. *Am J Clin Nutr.* 1994;60:347–352.

19. Leaf A, Weber PC. Cardiovascular effects of ω-3 fatty acids. *N Engl J Med.* 1988;318:549–557.

20. Hansen HS. New biological and clinical roles for the ω-6 and ω-3 fatty acids. *Nutr Rev.* 1994;52:162–167.

21. Heird WC, Nicholson JF, Driscoll JM Jr, et al. Hyperammonemia resulting from intravenous alimentation using a mixture of synthetic L-amino acids: a preliminary report. *J Pediatr.* 1972;81:162–165.

22. Watts JH, Mann AN, Bradley L, Thompson DJ. Nitrogen balances of men over 65 fed the FAO milk patterns of essential amino acids. *J Gerontol.* 1964;19:370–374.

23. Cuthbertson DP. The physiology of convalescence after injury. *Br Med Bull.* 1945;3:96–106.

24. Elwyn DE, Bursztein S. Carbohydrate metabolism and requirements for nutritional support: part III. *J Nutr.* 1993;9:255–267.

25. Wojnar MM, Hawkins WG, Lang CH. Nutritional support of the septic patient. *Crit Care Clin.* 1995;11:717–733.

26. Moore RS, Cerra FB. Sepsis. In: Fischer JE, ed. *Total Parenteral Nutrition.* 2nd ed. Boston: Little, Brown & Co; 1991:347–365.

27. Wolfe RR, Shaw JHF. Glucose and FFA kinetics in sepsis: role of glucagon and sympathetic nervous system activity. *Am J Physiol.* 1985;248:E236–E242.

28. Askanazi J, Carpentier YA, Elwyn DH, et al. Influence of total parenteral nutrition on fuel utilization in injury and sepsis. *Ann Surg.* 1980;191:40–46.

29. Lang CH. Mechanism of insulin resistance in infection. In: Schlag G, Redl H, eds. *Pathophysiology of Shock, Sepsis, and Organ Failure.* New York: Springer-Verlag; 1993:609–625.

30. Cortes V, Nelson LD. Errors in estimating energy expenditure in critically ill surgical patients. *Arch Surg.* 1989;124:287–290.

31. Westenskow DR, Schipe CA, Raymond JL, et al. Calculation of metabolic expenditure and substrate utilization from gas exchange measurements. *J Parenter Enter Nutr.* 1988;12:20–24.

32. Seidner DL, Mascioli EA, Istfan NW, et al. Effects of long-chain triglyceride emulsions on reticuloendothelial system function in humans. *J Parenter Enter Nutr.* 1989;13:614–619.

33. Gottschlich MM, Jenkins M, Warden GD, et al. Differential effects of three enteral dietary regimens on selected outcome variables in burn patients. *J Parenter Enter Nutr.* 1990;14:225–236.

34. Yetiv JZ. Clinical applications of fish oil. *JAMA.* 1988;260:665–670.

35. Bach AC, Frey A, Lutz O. Clinical and experimental effects of medium-chain triglyceride-based fat emulsions: a review. *Clin Nutr.* 1989;8:223–235.

36. Seaton TB, Welle SL, Warenko MK, et al. Thermic effect of medium chain and long chain triglycerides in man. *Am J Clin Nutr.* 1986;44:630–634.

37. Babayan VK. Medium chain triglycerides and structured lipids. *Lipids.* 1987;22:417–420.

38. Ling PR, Istfan NW, Lopes SM, et al. Structured lipid made from fish oil and medium-chain triglycerides alters tumor and host metabolism in Yoshida-sarcoma-bearing rats. *Am J Clin Nutr.* 1991;53:1177–1184.

39. Two TC, DeMichele SJ, Selleck KM, et al. Administration of structured lipid composed of MCT and fish oil reduces net protein catabolism in enterally fed burned rats. *Ann Surg.* 1989;210:100–107.

40. Mok KT, Maiz A, Yamazaki K, et al. Structured medium-chain and long-chain triglyceride emulsions are superior to physical mixtures in sparing body protein in the burned rat. *Metabolism.* 1984;33:910–915.

41. Larsson J, Lennmarken C, Martensson J, et al. Nitrogen requirements in severely injured patients. *Br J Surg.* 1990;77:413–418.

42. McNurlan MA, Garlick PJ. Protein and amino acids in nutritional support. *Crit Care Clin.* 1995;11:635–650.

43. Buse MJ, Reid SS. Leucine: a possible regulator of protein turnover in muscle. *J Clin Invest.* 1975;56:1250–1255.

44. Heyland DK, Cook DJ, Guyatt GH. Does the formulation of enteral feeding products influence infectious morbidity and mortality rates in the critically ill patient? A critical review of the evidence. *Crit Care Med.* 1994;22:1192–1202.

45. Jimenez FJJ, Leyba CO, Mendez SM, et al. Prospective study of the efficacy of branched-chain amino acids in septic patients. *J Parenter Enter Nutr.* 1991;15:252–261.

46. Fischer JE, Funovics JM, Aguirre A, et al. The role of plasma amino acids in hepatic encephalopathy. *Surgery.* 1975;78:276–290.

47. Naylor CD, O'Rourke K, Detsky AS, et al. Parenteral nutrition with branched-chain amino acids in hepatic encephalopathy: a meta-analysis. *Gastroenterology.* 1989;97:1033–1042.

48. American Society for Parenteral and Enteral Nutrition. Guidelines for the use of parenteral and enteral nutrition in adult and pediatric patients. *J Parenter Enter Nutr.* 1993;14(suppl 4):1SA–52SA.

49. Zeigler TR, Smith RJ, Byrne TA, Wilmore DW. Potential role of glutamine supplementation in nutrition support. *Clin Nutr.* 1993;12(suppl 1):S82–S90.

50. Hammarqvist F, Wernerman J, Ali R, et al. Addition of glutamine to total parenteral nutrition after elective abdominal surgery spares free glutamine in muscle, counteracts the fall in muscle protein synthesis, and improves nitrogen balance. *Ann Surg.* 1989;209:455–461.

51. Van Der Hulst RRW, Van Kreel BK, Von Meyenfeldt MF, et al. Glutamine and the preservation of gut integrity. *Lancet.* 1993;341:1363–1365.

52. Windmueller HG, Spaeth AE. Source and fate of circulating citrulline. *Am J Physiol.* 1981; 241:E473–E479.

53. Hibbs JB Jr, Taintor RR, Vavrin Z. Macrophage cytotoxicity: role for L-arginine deaminase and amino nitrogen oxidation to nitrate. *Science.* 1987;235:473–478.

54. Barbul A. Arginine: biochemistry, physiology, and therapeutic implications. *J Parenter Enter Nutr.* 1986;10:227–236.

55. Park KGM, Heys SD, Blessing K, et al. Stimulation of human breast cancers by dietary L-arginine. *Clin Sci.* 1992;82:413–419.

56. Kirk SJ, Hurson M, Regan MC, et al. Arginine stimulates wound healing and immune function in elderly human beings. *Surgery.* 1993;114:155–160.

CHAPTER 5

Micronutrients

Michele M. Gottschlich and Theresa Mayes

INTRODUCTION

Micronutrients have long been regarded as being of minor importance compared to carbohydrate, protein, and fat; however, recently there has been a surge of interest in micronutrients in terms of their significance as components of enteral and parenteral nutrition support. It is now recognized that micronutrients not only prevent classic deficiency syndromes but also can cause derangements in metabolic processes. The effects of a deficiency state may not be immediately obvious, but can ultimately impact recovery and wellness. This chapter reviews the specific functions of the individual micronutrients. Emphasis is directed toward the assessment of micronutrient status and deficiency signs. Recommendations for allowances are detailed, with consideration given to the route of micronutrient delivery. It should be emphasized that such guidelines are somewhat empiric, and major gaps in the scientific literature currently remain. Implications regarding therapeutic intake are also explored.

VITAMIN A (RETINOL)

Vitamin A (retinol) influences vision, adrenal hormone biosynthesis, and mucopolysaccharide and glycoprotein synthesis. In addition, vitamin A maintains epithelial integrity and has a positive impact on wound healing.[1–5] Vitamin A also has a beneficial effect on certain neoplasms,[6,7] infections,[8–10] and many aspects of the immune system.[11–16] One of the ways vitamin A mediates immunocompetence is through its influence on the thymus gland[17] and its role (specifically beta-carotene [β-carotene], the major dietary vitamin A precursor) in the antioxidant defense systems.[18]

The most dramatic signs of vitamin A inadequacy are ocular. Xerophthalmia—a syndrome that includes night blindness, conjunctival xerosis, and Bitot's spots—is a classic characterization of vitamin A deficiency. It often occurs in malnourished children in underdeveloped countries in association with diarrheal disease,[19–21] parasitic infestation,[22] or infection.[19,20,23] Xerophthalmia is uncommon in the United States. However, subclinical hypovitaminosis A is prevalent in preterm infants[24–26]; in patients with gastrointestinal tract dysfunction (ie, hepatic disease and defective absorption[19–21,27,28]) and impaired vitamin A transport (ie, protein deficiency[29–31] and zinc deficiency[27,32]); and in conditions that augment vitamin A needs, such as burns, trauma, and major surgery.[33,34] Other characteristics of vitamin A deficiency include loss of appetite and hyperkeratosis.

There is a high incidence of respiratory ailments (such as pneumonia and bronchopulmonary dysplasia) in vitamin A–deficient humans,[19,35,36] probably due to the keratinization and drying of epithelial cells in the trachea and bronchi. Mucous secretions and cilial motion cease, allowing foreign material to remain. The dryness also causes breaks in the integrity of membranes, allowing the entry of infective agents into normally well-protected areas. Vitamin A supplementation appears to promote regenerative healing from lung injury.[35]

Suboptimal vitamin A nutriture results in a decrease of the vitamin in tissues. Since the liver is the major storage organ, hepatic concentration of retinol is a direct measure of vitamin A reserves. This information can be obtained from liver biopsy, but such a procedure can be justified only in special clinical cases. Serum measurement of vitamin A remains the only practical test, although care must be taken to avoid using hemolyzed blood samples (hemolysis results in inappropriately high levels of vitamin A). Low serum levels of vitamin A reflect not only suboptimal intake of the nutrient but also depleted liver stores, because these reserves are drawn upon during inadequate intake of the vitamin. Also, the status of its carrier proteins must be considered for proper interpretation.

Retinol-binding protein (RBP) can be used as an indirect indicator of vitamin A nutriture.[37,38] Vitamin A–deficient animals sequester RBP in the liver. When these animals are provided vitamin A, hepatic mobilization of RBP occurs.[39] On the other hand, decreased levels of RBP (such as that which occurs in protein malnutrition) affect vitamin A status because RBP is the only known carrier of vitamin A.[40,41]

Critically ill patients often demonstrate depressed serum RBP and vitamin A levels.[23,33,34,42] Stephenson et al recently reported that patients experiencing acute episodes of infection sustain increased urinary excretion of vitamin A.[23] Critically ill patients also frequently experience diarrhea. A relationship between vitamin A deficiency and diarrhea has been suggested.[19–21,43–45] The association of diarrhea with vitamin A status is understandable, since vitamin A deficiency profoundly affects the metabolism and differentiation of epithelial tissues, causing a thinning of the gut epithelium, decreased goblet cell numbers, diminished production of glycoprotein, loss of mucous secretion, and decreased formation of glycocalyx, which promotes bacterial adherence to small intestinal mucosal cells.[46,47]

Vitamin A dietary allowances are expressed in retinol equivalents, with one retinol equivalent equal to 3.33 international units (IU), or 0.6 μg of β-carotene (see Table 5–1). The decreased biologic activity of carotene is due to a low efficiency in converting carotene to vitamin A. Vitamin A deficiency is preventable if intake is individualized according to the patient's condition. The seriously malnourished patient with gastrointestinal tract dysfunction should receive supplemental vitamin A. Attention should likewise be given to vitamin A status in patients with diseases in which absorption is defective. It is also recommended that a daily supplement approximating five times the Recommended Dietary Allowance (RDA) be administered to all patients with severe injury.[1,8,48] The American Medical Association's (AMA's) parenteral allowances[49] for vitamin A are 3300 IU, although recommendations in the literature have ranged between 1500 and 4200 IU.[49–54] Lowry et al[50] studied vitamin A levels in 40 hospitalized patients receiving total parenteral nutrition (TPN). They found that normal serum vitamin A levels could be maintained by providing 1500 to 2000 IU/day, whereas Labadarios et al[55] demonstrated a 43% incidence of low plasma vitamin A levels when delivering a minimum of 2500 IU/day. Provision of 3300 IU in home parenteral nutrition programs yielded plasma levels within the normal or high-normal range.[52,53] Recommended intake of vitamin A during critical illness far exceeds the RDA and AMA allowance. Trauma, burn, and septic adults require 10,000 to 25,000 IU of vitamin A daily to account for increased demands.

Of equal concern is that hypervitaminosis A is becoming a clinical problem of increasing frequency in the United States. An intake of 25,000 IU/day is considered excessive and is associated with a toxicity risk.[56] Publicity regarding the value of vitamin A–related compounds as treatment of acne[57] and aging[6] or in the possible prevention of cancer,[6,7] along with a heightened trend toward self-medication, can lead to excessive consumption. There have also been reports of vitamin A toxicity in patients with renal failure[58,59]; increased teratogenic effects are evident among babies born to women who consume more than 10,000 IU vitamin A per day[60]; and liver damage may be caused by excessive vitamin A consumption.[61] Signs of toxicity include headaches, nausea, vomiting, hair loss, hyperkeratosis, skeletal pain, hepatomegaly, and hypercalcemia.[62,63] However, most symptoms are reversible upon cessation of overdosing.

VITAMIN D

More than 10 substances have vitamin D activity. Two of the most important are vitamin D$_2$ (ergocalciferol) and vitamin D$_3$ (cholecalciferol). Cholecalciferol is synthesized in the skin from endogenous or dietary cholesterol upon exposure to

Table 5–1 A Guide to Enteral Vitamin/Mineral Preparations

Vitamin/Mineral	Units	RDA, Adult Males	RDA, Children (1–10 years)	Berocca (Roche)	Berocca Plus (Roche)	Centrum (Lederle)	Clusivol Liquid (Whitehall Robins)	One-A-Day Essential (Bayer)	PolyViSol (Mead Johnson)	Theragran (Mead Johnson)	ViDaylin (Ross)
Vitamin A	IU RE	3300 1000	1332–2331	—	5000	5000	2500	5000	1500	5500	1500
Vitamin D	IU	200 10	400	—	—	400	400	400	400	400	400
Vitamin E	IU mg	10 10	6–7	—	30	30	—	30	5	30	5
Vitamin K	µg	80	15–30	—	—	25	—	—	—	—	—
Thiamine	mg	1.5	0.7–1.0	15	20	2.25	1.0	1.5	0.5	3	0.5
Riboflavin	mg	1.7	0.8–1.2	15	20	2.60	1.0	1.7	0.6	3.4	0.6
Niacin	mg	19	9–13	100	100	20	5	20	8	20	8
Vitamin B6	mg	2.0	1.0–1.4	4	25	3	0.6	2	0.4	3	0.4
Vitamin B12	µg	2.0	0.7–1.4	5	50	9	2	6	2.0	9	1.5
Ascorbic acid	mg	60	40–45	500	500	90	15	60	35	90	35
Folic acid	µg	200	50–100	500	800	400	—	400	—	400	—
Biotin	µg	*	*	—	—	45	—	—	—	30	—
Pantothenic acid	mg	*	*	18	25	10	3	10	—	10	—
Calcium	mg	800	800	—	—	162	—	—	—	—	—
Phosphorus	mg	800	800	—	—	125	—	—	—	—	—
Iodine	µg	150	70–120	—	—	150	—	—	—	—	—
Iron	mg	10	10	—	27	27	—	—	10	—	12
Magnesium	mg	350	80–170	—	50	100	3	—	—	—	—
Zinc	mg	15	10	—	22.5	15	0.5	—	—	—	—
Copper	mg	*	*	—	3	2	—	—	—	—	—
Manganese	mg	*	*	—	5	5	0.5	—	—	—	—
Chromium	µg	*	*	—	0.1	25	—	—	—	—	—

continues

Table 5–1 continued

Vitamin/Mineral	Units	RDA, Adult Males	RDA, Children (1–10 years)	Berocca (Roche)	Berocca Plus (Roche)	Centrum (Lederle)	Clusivol Liquid (Whitehall Robins)	One-A-Day Essential (Bayer)	PolyViSol (Mead Johnson)	Theragran (Mead Johnson)	ViDaylin (Ross)
Potassium	mg	*	*	—	—	30	—	—	—	—	—
Fluoride	mg	*	*	—	—	—	—	—	—	—	—
Selenium	µg	70	20–30	—	—	25	—	—	—	—	—
Molybdenum	µg	*	*	—	—	25	—	—	—	—	—
Sodium	µg	*	*	—	—	27.2	—	—	—	—	—
Chloride	mg	*	*	—	—	—	—	—	—	—	—

Note: RDA, Recommended Dietary Allowance; IU, International Unit; RE, Retinol Equivalent.
*Recognized as essential, but guidelines currently are not established.

Source: Physician's Desk Reference, Edition 51. Medical Economics, Inc. 1997.

ultraviolet light. Ergocalciferol is the plant form of vitamin D. Both are hydroxy-lated in the liver to produce 25-hydroxy (OH) vitamin D. The kidney further metabolizes it into 1,25-dihydroxy (OH)$_2$ vitamin D. Five micrograms of vitamin D are equivalent to the RDA of 200 IU for adult males.

Vitamin D promotes intestinal absorption of calcium and phosphorus, calcium reabsorption from the kidney, and mobilization of calcium and phosphorus from bone.[64,65] Vitamin D is therefore important for maintenance of skeletal integrity. More recent evidence indicates that vitamin D plays a wider biologic role than previously thought. It is now appreciated that vitamin D has immunoregulatory functions[66–69] in addition to modulating cellular proliferation and differentiation.[70]

The best specific laboratory indicator of vitamin D status is plasma 25-hydroxy (OH) vitamin D or plasma 1,25-dihydroxy (OH)$_2$ vitamin D; however, these measures are not routinely available.[71,72] Consequently, indirect measures are used more frequently. Vitamin D deficiency is indirectly manifested through an abnormality of serum levels of calcium, phosphorus, and parathyroid hormone. Serum calcium and phosphorus decrease as a result of vitamin D deficiency, while serum parathyroid hormone increases, potentiating secondary hyperparathyroidism. Additional signs of vitamin D deficiency include bone pain and tenderness, and demineralization of bone. Radiographic changes are also evident during chronic deficiency or toxicity and can be used in diagnosis. Serum parameters and radiographic data must be interpreted with caution, because alterations are not entirely specific to vitamin D deficiency.

The significance of vitamin D as a nutritional factor in the prevention of rickets in children and osteomalacia in adults was initially described nearly a century ago. Today, because of fortification efforts in the United States, vitamin D deficiency is rare during childhood. However, the elderly are at continued increased risk for skeletal fractures due to a diet potentially deficient in vitamin D, decreased absorption, and lack of exposure to sunlight.[73]

Many disease states can have a negative impact on vitamin D status. Patients suffering such disorders as tropical sprue, regional enteritis, and pancreatic insufficiency often develop osteomalacia because of malabsorption of vitamin D. Surgery such as gastric resection and jejunoileal bypass for obesity may impair absorption. Malfunction of the liver can interfere with absorption, transport, and utilization of vitamin D.[74] The observation of skeletal abnormalities and hypocalcemia in patients with renal compromise and the failure of these patients to respond to vitamin D supplementation can be explained by lowered kidney hydroxylation activity. Vitamin D deficiency is also common in patients with hip fractures[75] and hypoparathyroidism[76]; it is also common with the long-term use of certain drugs such as anticonvulsants, cimetidine, and isoniazid.[77]

Guidelines for enteral and parenteral intake are outlined in Tables 5–1 and 5–2.[78,79] The parenteral infusion of 200 IU/day has been shown to maintain 25-

Table 5–2 A Guide to Parenteral Vitamin/Mineral Preparations

Vitamin/Mineral	Units	AMA, Adult Recommendation	AAP, Children's Recommendation	Berocca Parenteral (Roche)	M.V.I. Pediatric (Astra)	M.V.I.-12 (Astra)	M.T.E.-5 (Lyphomed)
Vitamin A	IU RE	3300 1000	2300	3300	2300	3300	—
Vitamin D	IU µg	200 5	400	200	400	200	—
Vitamin E	IU mg	10 10	7	10	7	10	—
Vitamin K	µg	*	*	—	200	—	—
Thiamine	mg	3	1.2	3	1.2	3	—
Riboflavin	mg	3.6	1.4	3.6	1.4	3.6	—
Niacin	mg	40	17	40	17	40	—
Vitamin B$_6$	mg	4	1.0	4	1.0	4	—
Vitamin B$_{12}$	µg	5	1.0	5	1.0	5	—
Ascorbic acid	mg	100	80	100	80	100	—
Folic acid	µg	400	140	400	140	400	—
Biotin	µg	60	20	60	20	60	—
Pantothenic acid	mg	15	5	15	—	15	—
Calcium	mg	*	*	—	—	—	—
Phosphorus	mg	*	*	—	—	—	—
Iodine	µg	*	*	—	—	—	—
Iron	mg	*	*	—	—	—	—
Magnesium	mg	*	*	—	—	—	—
Zinc	mg	2.5–4.0					5
Copper	mg	0.5–1.5					1
Manganese	mg	0.15–0.8					0.5

Table 5-2 continued

Vitamin/Mineral	Units	AMA, Adult Recommendation	AAP, Children's Recommendation	Berocca Parenteral (Roche)	M.V.I. Pediatric (Astra)	M.V.I.-12 (Astra)	M.T.E.-5 (Lyphomed)
Chromium	μg	10–15	*	—	—	—	10
Potassium	mg	*	*	—	—	—	—
Fluoride	mg	*	*	—	—	—	—
Selenium	μg	*	*	—	—	—	60
Molybdenum	μg	*	*	—	—	—	—
Sodium	μg	*	*	—	—	—	—
Chloride	mg	*	*	—	—	—	—

Note: AMA, American Medical Association[49,78]; AAP, American Academy of Pediatrics[79]; IU, International Unit; RE, Retinol Equivalent.
*Recognized as essential, but guidelines currently are not established.

Source: Physician's Desk Reference, Edition 51. Medical Economics, Inc. 1997.

hydroxy (OH) vitamin D and 1,25-dihydroxy (OH)$_2$ vitamin D within the normal range in some patients,[53] but this is not always a consistent finding.[54,80] Many high-risk groups respond well to vitamin D supplementation. However, the administration of pharmacologic doses over a prolonged period potentiates vitamin D toxicity. The signs and symptoms of hypervitaminosis D are those associated with hypercalcemia (ie, weakness, nausea and vomiting, fatigue, anorexia, headache, diarrhea, confusion, psychosis, and tremors). Chronic hypercalcemia causes calcification of soft tissues with particularly serious injury to the kidneys. Shike et al[81] described a metabolic bone disease in patients on long-term parenteral nutrition that was characterized by hypercalciuria, intermittent hypercalcemia, decreased parathyroid hormone, and osteomalacia. These symptoms improved after withdrawal of vitamin D from the hyperalimentation solution. Others have reported similar findings.[82,83] The explanation of TPN-associated bone disease is not yet clear. At present, the clinician is cautioned to avoid overzealous use of supplemental vitamin D.

VITAMIN E

There are eight biologically active forms of vitamin E, commonly referred to as tocopherols. Alpha tocopherol (α-tocopherol) is the most active in the series. One milligram of dl-α-tocopherol has been designated as 1 IU. The major activity of vitamin E may be as an antioxidant,[18,84] inhibiting oxidation of unsaturated fatty acids by free radicals. It thereby functions in the maintenance of cell wall integrity, protecting vital membranes from peroxidative damage caused by free radicals. Vitamin E has been shown to be an effective inhibitor of prostaglandin and thromboxane synthesis,[85-88] thereby lessening the effects of inflammation and circulatory irregularities such as leg cramps and blood platelet adhesion.[89] It also has been found to enhance immune function[85,90-93] and inhibit the conversion of nitrates to nitrosamines, which are cancer-promoting substances.[89]

Clinical manifestations of vitamin E deficiency—such as increased platelet aggregation,[94] decreased red blood cell survival, and hemolytic anemia—have been well described.[95-97] Tocopherol deficiency has been associated with neurologic abnormalities,[98-100] decreased serum creatinine levels, excessive creatinuria,[97,101] and most recently, heart disease.[102-105] Prolonged depletion results in lesions in skeletal muscle resembling muscular dystrophy.[96] Measurement of plasma (or serum) tocopherol levels is the traditional laboratory means of evaluating vitamin E status, because a reasonably good correlation has been shown between serum and tissue levels of vitamin E.[106] Because the majority of plasma vitamin E is carried by lipoproteins, conditions that lower blood lipoproteins cause decreased circulatory vitamin E levels.[53,107] The erythrocyte peroxide hemolysis test, the red blood cell fragility test, and breath pentane[108] and ethane[109] analysis can also be used to assess vitamin E status.

Subjects at risk of developing vitamin E deficiency include infants[96,110,111]; patients with severe protein-calorie malnutrition;[97] and patients with prolonged steatorrhea, such as those with pancreatitis,[96,112] cystic fibrosis,[97,99,110] or short-bowel syndrome.[96,100] Patients with inhalation injury[113] and diseases related to the delivery of high concentrations of oxygen by mechanical ventilation have also been correlated with subnormal levels of plasma vitamin E.

The RDA for vitamin E is 3 to 10 mg α-tocopherol equivalents. However, the need for vitamin E can be influenced by a number of dietary factors. Requirements for vitamin E greatly increase with increasing polyunsaturated fatty acids in the diet,[114] and it is difficult to set guidelines for vitamin E intake unless the dietary level of polyunsaturated fatty acids is also specified. Interestingly, the U.S. diet has increased in polyunsaturated fatty acid content in recent years, and the plant sources responsible for the enhanced intake are rich in tocopherol. The vitamin E requirement is partially spared by dietary selenium[115] and sulfur amino acid intake.

Vitamin E intake during prolonged TPN has been studied by many, with variable results. Shils et al[53] and Dempsey et al[80] reported vitamin E levels in the lower end of the normal range, whereas Davis et al[52] found no apparent impairment in tocopherol status during the parenteral infusion of approximately 10 IU of vitamin E (plus that contained in fat emulsion). The current recommended parenteral intake according to the Nutrition Advisory Group of the AMA is 7 IU for children under 11 years of age and 10 IU for patients above 11 years.

Vitamin E supplementation is recommended for patients who were severely malnourished prior to the initiation of hyperalimentation. Therapeutic roles for augmented vitamin E intake in fibrocystic breast disease[116] and in the prevention of cancer have been suggested, although no definitive conclusions can be made. Vitamin E supplements are recommended for patients with cystic fibrosis and in the treatment of deficiencies caused by the malabsorption of fat. Various therapeutic doses of vitamin E have been proposed in diseases thought to be related to oxygen toxicity, such as retrolental fibroplasia[117–119] and bronchopulmonary dysplasia.[120] Multiple studies support the immunostimulatory effects of vitamin E[121–124]; therefore, supplementation of patients with acquired immune deficiency syndrome (AIDS) has been suggested.[125]

Most acute and chronic studies show that vitamin E is relatively nontoxic.[126] However, megadoses may inhibit immune function[127] and lead to prolongation of the clotting time.[128] Persons who require anticoagulation medication should avoid megadoses of vitamin E because the vitamin can exacerbate the blood coagulation defect of vitamin K deficiency caused by anticoagulant therapy.[129]

VITAMIN K

Vitamin K promotes hepatic biosynthesis of several factors necessary for normal blood clotting.[130] It also may serve a special role in bone metabolism.[8,131–135]

The requirement of the adult human for vitamin K is extremely low. There is little probability for developing a primary dietary deficiency of vitamin K. One reason is the ubiquity of vitamin K_1 (phylloquinone) in the diet. Another significant source is microflora-synthesized vitamin K_2 (menaquinone). Hence, there is no need for vitamin K supplements except in specific disease states or when dietary vitamin K is restricted due to impaired health.

The latest guidelines produced by the Food and Nutrition Board of the National Research Council establish an RDA for vitamin K at 80 μg/day.[136] Patients receiving long-term TPN are at risk for deficiency, given alterations in the flora due to nonactive gut hypertrophy. Vitamin K is therefore an important component of long-term intravenous feeding programs. Vitamin K is not included in regular parenteral multivitamin products to allow flexibility for the administration of anticoagulants. If vitamin K is not contraindicated by the use of anticoagulants, it should be given intramuscularly or subcutaneously on a weekly basis to prevent deficiency. The AMA's recommended weekly dose is 0.2 to 1.5 mg.[49] Others have suggested intramuscular or subcutaneous injections of 5 to 10 mg/wk.[53,137]

Occasionally vitamin K inadequacy occurs; it is characterized as a hemorrhagic disease because of the increased time required for blood to clot. A vitamin K deficiency may be encountered in newborns,[138,139] as neonates have a relatively sterile gut and consequently synthesize little vitamin K. The risk of vitamin K deficiency is at its peak a few days after birth and during breastfeeding.[140] The American Academy of Pediatrics therefore recommends routine intramuscular administration of prophylactic phylloquinone at birth.[141] Others in danger of suboptimal vitamin K status include the elderly[135,142] and patients with renal failure.[143,144] The absorption of vitamin K requires the presence of bile in the small intestine; therefore, subjects with malabsorption syndromes such as sprue, ulcerative colitis, chronic pancreatitis, biliary dysfunction, or bowel resection are at risk for deficiency. In addition, vitamin K deficiency is encountered in patients receiving certain drugs such as antibiotics, which can interfere with the intestinal synthesis of vitamin K[143,144]; anticoagulants (such as coumadin derivatives), which antagonize the action of vitamin K[145,146]; and cholestyramine therapy.[147] Furthermore, liver disease results in the failure of vitamin K to biosynthesize clotting factors resulting in hypoprothrombinemia[148]; however, vitamin K administration in patients with severe liver disease will not improve prothrombin time. Recently, vitamin K deficiency has been suggested as a contributing factor to coagulopathies observed in burn patients.[149] Burn patients appear at increased risk for vitamin K deficiency, due to increased blood loss, periodic episodes of diarrhea, and widespread antibiotic use.

A number of diagnostic tests are available to rule out whether a bleeding disorder is due to vitamin K deficiency.[150] Historically, the speed of conversion of prothrombin to thrombin in a plasma sample (prothrombin time) has been used to assess vitamin K status. However, prothrombin time has recently been scrutinized as an insensitive measure of vitamin K nutriture.[151] Although expensive, plasma phylloquinone concentration is the best indicator of vitamin K status. In addition, recent evidence correlates serum undercarboxylated osteocalcin to vitamin K depletion[151,152] and may prove useful in the measurement of vitamin K status. When the diagnosis of vitamin K deficiency exists, administration of the vitamin should result in prompt correction of an abnormal clotting time.

VITAMIN B₁ (THIAMINE)

Thiamine (vitamin B₁) has important biochemical functions. It is a precursor of thiamine pyrophosphate, a coenzyme in the oxidative decarboxylation of alpha-keto (α-keto) acids and transketolase reactions. In addition, thiamine is an essential cofactor for aerobic metabolism facilitating the entry of pyruvate into the Krebs cycle.[153] Decreased availability of thiamine results in impaired pyruvate metabolism. Hence, vitamin B₁ is essential for the efficient metabolism of energy and carbohydrate. Thiamine is also believed to be a structural component of nervous system membranes.[154]

Beriberi is the classic pathologic vitamin B₁ deficiency syndrome.[155] The condition is prevalent in the Orient, where unfortified, polished rice is a dietary staple. Beriberi can be subclassified by severity. Individuals who subsist on a diet containing slightly less than the thiamine requirement gradually develop the fairly subtle, dry form. Dry beriberi is chiefly a neurologic disease. Paresthesia, hypesthesia, anesthesia, and weakness are experienced in the lower extremities. Peripheral neuritis results from a degeneration of the myelin sheath. The more severe form of beriberi is wet beriberi, characterized by edema and cardiac involvement. Carbohydrate metabolism is blocked to a significant degree.

The most frequently encountered cause of primary thiamine deficiency in the United States is chronic alcoholism and may result in Wernicke's encephalopathy.[155,156] Factors associated with increased risk of secondary thiamine deficiency include conditions causing increased losses (such as diuresis, malabsorption, and dialysis) and increased requirements (such as fever, infection, hyperthyroidism, trauma, and burns).[157] Prolonged antacid therapy may lead to thiamine deficiency by alkaline destruction of the ingested vitamin.[158] Thiamine inadequacy has also been reported during TPN.[159-162] Deficiency symptoms occur within 2 to 3 weeks in malnourished patients.[163]

Clinical signs of thiamine deficiency include anorexia, fatigue, peripheral neuropathy, foot and wristdrop, cardiomegaly, and hyperlactemia[153,163] from impaired pyruvate utilization. Right ventricular heart failure was reversed in two thiamine-depleted patients who were provided thiamine supplementation.[164] Various biochemical procedures are useful in confirming a diagnosis based on clinical symptoms. One of the most commonly employed indexes of deficiency is a depressed

24-hour urinary thiamine.[155,165] The erythrocyte transketolase test represents a functional check of thiamine status.[155,166] It appears to be a more reliable indicator of vitamin B1 insufficiency than urinary measurements. The evaluation of blood thiamine levels has not found wide acceptance as a tool for assessing thiamine nutriture. Vitamin B1 deficiency may also cause elevated levels of pyruvate, since thiamine is required for pyruvate metabolism; however, this effect lacks sensitivity and specificity.[167]

The requirement for thiamine in human nutrition is related to caloric intake. Oral ingestion of approximately 0.6 mg/1000 kcal (or 1.7 mg/day) is recommended for the normal adult.[136,168] Important targets for pharmacologic doses of thiamine are alcoholics[155,160] and those with neurologic disorders.[169]

The parenteral recommendation for vitamin B1 is currently 3 mg/day.[49] Long-term follow-up of adult home TPN patients indicates that this amount is adequate to sustain normal transketolase activity,[55,170] but blood thiamine levels were slightly below normal.[53,170] Since functional tests remained within normal limits, the fall in blood thiamine levels probably has no clinical significance. Nevertheless, several centers recommend higher doses in the range of 10 to 50 mg of vitamin B1 for TPN patients.[51,171–173]

VITAMIN B2 (RIBOFLAVIN)

To be metabolically active, riboflavin (vitamin B2) must first be converted to its coenzyme derivatives: flavin mononucleotide and flavin-adenine dinucleotide (FAD), which act as intermediaries in the transfer of electrons in biologic oxidation-reduction reactions. These reactions include oxidative phosphorylation, beta-oxidation of fatty acids, purine degradation, and amino acid oxidation.

Populations at risk of riboflavin deficiency include those with diseases such as thyroid dysfunction,[174] diabetes, and alcoholism[175]; those who follow a strict vegan diet; and individuals with chronic malabsorption. In addition, periods of physiologic stress—such as during rapid cellular growth in childhood or during pregnancy, lactation, or wound healing—predispose subjects to vitamin B2 deficiency. Ariboflavinosis may also arise from pathologic stress, including burns, surgical procedures, fractures, and other forms of trauma. Chronic intake of certain drugs may increase the requirement for vitamin B2 by decreasing absorption, increasing its excretion, or antagonizing its action. For example, certain medications used to treat patients with psychiatric disorders (such as psychotropic drugs and tricyclic antidepressants) have been shown to affect riboflavin metabolism.[176] Some biochemical evidence also suggests depletion of riboflavin with use of oral contraceptives,[177] although this finding is controversial.[178,179]

Lipid metabolism is disturbed during riboflavin deficiency, marked by a decrease in fatty acid oxidation and by changes in phospholipid and fat cell membrane composition.[180,181] Glucose and amino acid metabolism is also affected by vitamin B_2 inadequacy.

Clinical manifestations of riboflavin deficiency include cheilosis, angular stomatitis, and glossitis. Seborrheic dermatitis often involves the nose. Other clinical symptoms include dermatitis over the joints and genital region, cessation of growth, and photophobia. Sydenstricker et al[182] suggest that riboflavin deficiency can be diagnosed by observing an increase in corneal vascularization.

Biochemical methods are more quantitative and can detect riboflavin deficiency before clinical signs appear. Urinary excretion of riboflavin has been used to assess nutritional adequacy. It correlates well with dietary intake and urine volume but not necessarily with riboflavin stores. Furthermore, a number of factors, such as age, physical activity, body temperature, and stress, can influence excretion of vitamin B_2. Serum riboflavin levels are also thought to reflect recent intake of the vitamin, and not tissue or total body status. A more sensitive and specific indicator of riboflavin involves the measurement of erythrocyte glutathione reductase. The activity of this FAD-containing enzyme is a long-term indicator of vitamin B_2 status and does not fluctuate dramatically on a day-to-day basis.

The current daily riboflavin allowances for oral intake[136] have been suggested as 0.6 mg/1000 kcal. The differences in RDAs among various age groups are primarily related to variances in calorie intake recommendations.[136] Several studies reveal that an increase in physical activity augments the requirement for riboflavin.[183,184] The AMA recommends the daily parenteral infusion of 3.6 mg of riboflavin in adults,[49] a level somewhat higher than oral allowances. Doses ranging from 1.8 to 4.2 mg of riboflavin have maintained normal red blood cell glutathione reductase activity levels in adult TPN patients.[51,55,162] At present, the only therapeutic application of riboflavin is to prevent or treat ariboflavinosis. No cases of toxicity from ingestion of riboflavin have been reported.

VITAMIN B_3 (NIACIN)

Niacin (vitamin B_3) is a component of nicotinamide adenine dinucleotide (NAD) and nicotinamide adenine dinucleotide phosphate, two coenzymes involved in many oxidation-reduction reactions such as the tricarboxylic acid cycle, electron transport, glycolysis, deamination, fat synthesis, beta-oxidation, and steroid biosynthesis. In the absence of niacin, metabolism is severely handicapped and most cells suffer. Therefore, it is not surprising that vitamin B_3 deficiency (pellagra) leads to many clinical changes. Because of the involvement of niacin in the energy system, early symptoms include weakness and fatigue. Niacin deficiency affects the digestive tract (diarrhea), the nervous system (dementia), and the skin (dermatitis); for this reason, it is recognized as the disease of the three Ds. The mucous membranes that line the gastrointestinal tract become inflamed and have atrophic lesions. This causes maldigestion and severe watery, and occasionally heme-occult-positive, stools. Steatorrhea can occur without the presence of diarrhea. Achlorhydria may be present. Early lesions of the nervous system are nonspecific and include dizziness, headaches, insomnia, irritability, and depression. Motor and sensory functions of peripheral nerves may also be impaired. In advanced pellagra, irreversible psychosis with delirium and catatonia may occur. The skin changes most often involve parts of the body exposed to sunlight; the skin becomes dry, thickened, and inflamed.

Biochemical procedures for evaluating vitamin B3 status are not entirely reliable, although measurement of urinary niacin metabolites[185] and whole-blood NAD[167] can be used to substantiate a niacin deficiency. To date, a functional biochemical test has not been developed for assessing vitamin B3 coenzyme status. A noted improvement in clinical symptoms in response to niacin supplementation may be adequate evidence for diagnosis of a deficiency state. A positive response to niacin therapy is usually noted within 24 hours.[186]

The high incidence and serious consequences of acute vitamin B3 deficiency have prompted enrichment programs. Pellagra has become relatively rare in the United States, since fortification of grains was instituted. Nevertheless, secondary niacin deficiency still persists. Patients at risk include those with a history of alcohol abuse, thyroid disorders, neoplasia,[187] isoniazid treatment for tuberculosis, anticancer drug mercaptopurine (6-MP) use, malabsorption, or burns.[157,188,189]

Niacin requirements for humans are expressed in terms of niacin equivalents, because niacin needs can be satisfied not only by vitamin B3 but also by synthesis from dietary tryptophan. Hence, the dietary requirement is influenced by the quantity and quality of ingested protein. For estimating dietary requirements, 60 mg of tryptophan is considered equivalent to 1 mg of niacin.[190] The daily allowance for niacin is also influenced by total caloric intake. The RDA for adults is 6.6 niacin equivalents/1000 kcal and not less than 13 niacin equivalents at a caloric intake less than 2000 kcal.[136] The current RDA for niacin is further supported by the work of Jacobs and colleagues.[191]

The AMA recommends 40 mg daily for adults on TPN.[49] Therapeutic dosage of niacin during a deficiency state is suggested at 50 to 150 mg/day.[192] However, when 100 mg/day is added to the TPN infusate, urinary excretion of niacin is noted to be excessive.[170] Daily parenteral delivery of only 10 mg results in whole-blood nicotinic acid levels in the lower or below normal range.[55]

Proposed benefits derived from pharmacologic doses of niacin include the healing of broken vessels, vasodilatation, and decreased plasma free fatty acids. Nicotinic acid in large amounts may have prophylactic value in preventing coronary heart disease.[193,194] However, when nicotinic acid is used in megadoses (ranging from 3 to 250 g/day), particularly when parenterally administered, transient symptoms of vasodilatation or "flushing" and sensation of heat, itching, nausea, vomiting, abdominal cramping, and headaches may occur. Oral administration of thera-peutic doses of nicotinic acid may reduce the adverse side effects. In addition, slow-release forms of the medication are available.[186] Due to gastrointestinal tract symptoms, high doses of niacin are contraindicated in patients with gastritis or peptic ulcer.

VITAMIN B6 (PYRIDOXINE)

Pyridoxal-5-phosphate (PLP) represents the coenzyme form of vitamin B6 for well over 60 different enzyme systems. It is involved in many reactions, including transamination, deamination, decarboxylation, and desulfhydration of amino ac-ids. The essential role of vitamin B6 in the maintenance of the functional integrity of the brain is illustrated by the fact that most of the neurotransmitters are formed by the decarboxylation of amino acid derivatives with the aid of pyridoxine-de-pendent enzymatic reactions. These neurotransmitters include dopamine, norepi-nephrine, serotonin, tyramine, taurine, and histamine. Vitamin B6 is also required for the synthesis of niacin from tryptophan and the formation of porphyrin. It is essential for glycogen phosphorylase activity. PLP is important for normal nucleic acid synthesis, carbohydrate and lipid metabolism, and maintenance of normal immune function[195,196] and is closely related to endocrine metabolism.

A clinical syndrome associated with pyridoxine deficiency in humans has been described. Initially, subjects develop personality changes, manifested by irritabil-ity and depression. Patients demonstrate stomatitis, glossitis, cheilosis, and sebor-rhea of the nasal folds, characteristics frequently indistinguishable from the le-sions of riboflavin and niacin deficiency. Because of pyridoxine's close association with neurotransmitters, it is not surprising that vitamin B6 deficiency results in disorders of the central nervous system. Normochromic, microcytic, or sideroblastic anemia may occur after prolonged pyridoxine deficiency because PLP is required for heme synthesis.[197,198]

Biochemical techniques used to substantiate clinical signs of vitamin B6 defi-ciency have been reviewed by Sauberlich et al.[199] Until about 1965, the acceptable method for determining pyridoxine status was the urinary measurement of xanthu-renic acid, a tryptophan metabolite. A test load of approximately 5 g of L-tryp-tophan leads to a marked increase in urinary excretion of xanthurenic acid in the vitamin B6–deficient subject.[200,201] Although the tryptophan load test is relatively easy to perform and has been widely used, test results need to be interpreted with care in view of the interrelated metabolic and hormonal factors involved in tryp-tophan metabolism.[202] Consequently, additional biochemical indexes should be employed whenever possible. A decreased urinary excretion of 4-pyridoxic acid can be used to assess immediate dietary intake,[201,203] but it is probably not indica-tive of body reserves. Measurement of the blood concentration of vitamin B6 may have promise as an index of pyridoxine status. Determination of transaminase activities, a functional test of B_6 reserves, appears to be the most useful test to date. Human pyridoxine depletion studies have demonstrated that glutamic-oxaloacetic transaminase (GOT) and glutamic-pyruvic transaminase (GPT) activities decrease erythrocytes (EGOT and EGPT) and serum (SGOT and SGPT).[201,203–205] Normal serum transaminase has a wide range. Therefore, SGOT and SGPT are less valuable than measurement of these enzymes in erythrocytes.[203,205]

The RDA for vitamin B_6 for an adult male is 2.0 mg.[136] Pregnant women may have lower-than-desirable levels of serum B_6; when this condition is not rectified, their newborns are also short of this vitamin.[206] Individuals have increased needs for vitamin B_6 during pregnancy and lactation, and during the consumption of high-protein diets.[136] High-protein intake hastens the onset of deficiency because of the active role the vitamin plays in protein metabolism. Pyridoxine deficiency also occurs frequently in uremic patients[207]; in patients with burns,[208] advanced age,[209] malignancies,[210] and asthma[211]; and in patients with malabsorption, alcoholism, and liver disease.[212] Certain drugs, such as isoniazid,[213] hydralazine, and penicillamine are vitamin B_6 antagonists and may produce a deficiency. Some researchers assert that women taking oral contraceptives may require additional pyridoxine,[214] but this is a controversial issue.

The Nutrition Advisory Group of the AMA recommends 4.0 mg of vitamin B_6 for children over 11 years old and for adults.[49] Hence, intravenous recommendations for pyridoxine are currently twice the RDA. Augmented parenteral intake is indicated. Jeejeebhoy et al[172] administered 5.5 mg of vitamin B_6 daily to patients on long-term hyperalimentation and found plasma pyridoxine levels to be slightly below normal in two of six patients.

FOLIC ACID

Folate coenzymes are principally involved in 1-carbon transfer reactions necessary for maintenance or restoration of red blood cells, nucleotide metabolism, and protein synthesis.[215] Folic acid is also involved in the production of S-adenosylmethionines (SAM) when dietary methionine is restricted. Vitamin B_{12} is necessary for metabolism and recycling of folic acid; therefore, cobalamin (vitamin B_{12}) deficiency can precede folate deficiency.

Folic acid deficiency is a widespread disorder. It has been referred to as the most common hypovitaminosis of humans. The indigent[216,217] and the elderly[218] often display signs of folic acid deficiency due to insufficient intake. Considerable loss of folic acid through dialysis[207,219,220] has led to deficiency states. Ileal disease, inflammatory bowel disease, sprue, celiac disease, and gastrectomies may produce megaloblastic anemia by reducing absorption of folate from food.[221–223]

Folic acid deficiency has been associated with anticonvulsant therapy. It is usually manifested by reduced serum and erythrocyte folate levels, but occasionally megaloblastic anemia appears.[224,225] Interference with conjugases,[224] malabsorption,[226] and coincidence of inadequate dietary intake are poorly understood theories of folic acid deficiency commonly seen with anticonvulsants.

Folic acid deficiency is a frequent complication of alcoholism, due in part to dietary deprivation of folic acid.[227–229] Other factors include malabsorption of folate[230–232] and alcohol's interference with folate utilization.[233] In addition to alcohol, a large array of folic acid–antagonist drugs inhibit the utilization of folic acid. These include chemotherapeutic agents (such as methotrexate and aminopterin)[234,235] and certain potassium-sparing diuretics (such as triamterene.)[236] Some investigators have proposed impaired absorption of pteroylglutamic acid, the major constituent of food folate, in patients taking oral contraceptives[230,237,238]; however, others have not found oral contraceptive–induced malabsorption of folic acid.[239]

An increased requirement for folic acid may occur in any condition that increases the metabolic and cell division rate, such as infection, hyperthyroidism, trauma, and burns.[240,241] Similarly, augmented cell turnover—as seen in pregnancy, lactation, early infancy, chronic hemolytic anemias, and malignant tumors—enhances folate needs.[136,242] Patients receiving chronic hemodialysis typically receive routine supplementation with folate, although the rationale has been scrutinized.[243] Due to increased red blood cell hemolysis, folate needs are postulated as higher among those with thalassemia and sickle cell anemia.[244] Folic acid deficiency has been implicated in the predisposition to neural tube defects such as spina bifida and anencephaly.[245,246] A growing body of experimental evidence correlates low dietary folate and carcinogenesis.[246–251] This observation is related to the intricate role of folic acid in DNA and RNA synthesis and cell division.

Classic folic acid deficiency in humans results in a smooth, sore tongue and gastrointestinal disturbances. Symptoms of nervous instability, dementia, depression, diarrhea, and weight loss are often revealed. Cell-mediated immunity is depressed during folic acid deficiency. The most striking feature of folic acid inadequacy is an anemia indistinguishable from the anemia of vitamin B_{12} deficiency.[252,253] This blood disturbance, termed macrocytic anemia, exhibits mature red blood cells fewer in number and larger than normally seen. The younger erythrocytes in the bone marrow fail to mature during dietary folate deprivation. In addition, a lack of SAM directly reduces the activity of the enzyme cystathionine beta-synthase, thus elevating plasma homocysteine. Hyperhomocysteinemia has been implicated in coronary heart disease.[254]

To distinguish between vitamin B_{12} and folic acid deficiency, a number of biochemical measurements are available.[252,255,256] Such procedures include the assay of serum folate and red blood cell folate, and the measurement of urinary excretion of formiminoglutamic acid (FIGLU). Of these procedures, quantitation of serum folic acid level is most commonly performed. It is an early sign of folate deficiency.[252,255,256] Low serum levels provide little information regarding tissue reserves. However, chronically low levels of serum folic acid eventually are accompanied by advanced deficiency signs such as megaloblastic anemia.

The assay of folate concentration in red blood cells is generally more helpful than serum measurement of folate status since red blood cell folate is reported to parallel tissue stores.[257] However, red blood cell folate determinations do not differentiate between the megaloblastic anemias of vitamin B_{12} deficiency versus folic acid deficiency. The functional test for evaluating folate coenzyme function (based on the increased urinary excretion of FIGLU) is an additional index of folate deficiency.

Ample evidence exists demonstrating that pteroylglutamic acid in a dose of 50 μg/day will correct a state of pure folic acid deficiency and prevent biochemical lesions from developing in healthy adults.[255] The current RDA of 180 to 200 μg for the nonpregnant, nonlactating adult is obviously above the minimal daily requirement of 50 μg, even though approximately 50% less than recommended prior to 1989. This RDA provides a margin of safety for such factors as possible losses from cooking and bioavailability in foods.[255] In addition, the recommended folate allowance provides for liver storage of the vitamin to prevent deficiency during brief episodes of decreased dietary intake.

Given the relationship between adequate folic acid nutriture and the prevention of several disease states (atherosclerosis, malignancies, tubular defects), widespread fortification of foodstuff has been suggested. However, Campbell[258] suggests that before folic acid consumption is increased in the general public, concerns such as increased difficulty diagnosing vitamin B_{12} deficiency, folate neurotoxicity, drug interactions, and altered zinc metabolism should be addressed.

Until recently, folic acid was not a component of parenteral multivitamin preparations. Instead, folic acid was administered in weekly intramuscular doses or not at all. Numerous reports of folic acid deficiency during TPN[229,241,256] make it clear that it is necessary in parenteral feeding regimens, even for those patients undergoing brief periods of TPN. Stromberg et al[162] administered 200 μg daily to patients on TPN and found this amount to be adequate for maintenance but inadequate for correcting deficiencies. Nichoalds et al[51] have shown that a parenteral protocol containing a daily dose of 300 μg is insufficient to maintain serum folate levels, whereas a dose of 600 μg normalizes serum folate. The AMA Nutrition Advisory Group recommends the intravenous daily delivery of 400 μg to adults receiving TPN.[49]

VITAMIN B_{12}

Vitamin B_{12} is a coenzyme required for the transfer of methyl groups in the synthesis of nucleic acids and choline. It is necessary for normal carbohydrate, protein, and fat metabolism because it is involved in the formation of succinate from methylmalonate and in the synthesis of the amino acid methionine. It is essential for cellular reproduction, including red blood cell and myelin formation, and is crucial for folic acid regeneration. This explains why the hematologic picture of folate and cobalamin (vitamin B_{12}) deficiency are indistinguishable. In addition to megaloblastic anemia, the most prominent signs and symptoms of B_{12} deficiency are loss of appetite, weight loss, fatigue, glossitis, leukopenia, thrombocytopenia, and achlorhydria. Inadequate myelin synthesis with irreversible nerve damage results from vitamin B_{12} inadequacy but not folic acid deficiency. Additional neurologic symptoms of vitamin B_{12} deficiency include paresthesia, poor muscular coordination, confusion, hallucinations, and possibly psychosis, most notably in the elderly.

Enterohepatic cycling and liver stores conserve vitamin B_{12}, and therefore a deficiency state may not develop for as long as 3 years. Clinical deficiency due to dietary insufficiency is relatively rare and occurs almost exclusively in vegetarians.[259,260] In the United States, most cases of cobalamin deficiency are due to failure of absorption of the vitamin resulting from a lack of intrinsic factor in gastric juice (pernicious anemia), not dietary restriction.[260] Total gastrectomy produces vitamin B_{12} deficiency, since this procedure removes the source of intrinsic factor. Malabsorption of cobalamin may also result from tropical and nontropical sprue, ileal resection, gastric bypass surgery, stagnant bowel syndrome, and intestinal parasite infestations. The development of deficiency in this manner may occur rapidly because enterohepatic cycling is interrupted. Lifelong treatment with injectable vitamin B_{12} is necessary therapy for persons with pernicious anemia and permanent gastric or ileal compromise.[225,256,261] Vitamin B_{12} deficiency has also been associated with drugs that damage cobalamin absorption, such as neomycin, colchicine, potassium chloride, para-aminosalicylic acid, and ethanol.[225] An increased requirement for vitamin B_{12} exists during pregnancy, lactation, infancy, and hyperthyroidism.

The most common procedure for diagnosing deficiency has been the determination of serum vitamin B_{12} levels. Low serum cobalamin has been associated with low body content of the vitamin.[262] Elevated urinary excretion of FIGLU, as described in folic acid deficiency, may also occur in subjects with vitamin B_{12} inadequacy.[252,255,257] When the causative factor is vitamin B_{12} deficiency, this abnormality is corrected by the administration of cobalamin.[252,255]

Once biochemical tests have established that a vitamin B_{12} deficiency exists, the etiology should be evaluated to determine whether the condition is due to lack of intrinsic factor, other malabsorptive disorders, or inadequate nutrient intake. Pernicious anemia can be diagnosed by using the urinary excretion (Schilling) test. This involves measuring the absorption of oral vitamin B_{12} administered with and without intrinsic factor.[260] If vitamin B_{12} deficiency is of the pernicious anemia type, the Schilling test would indicate improved cobalamin absorption when vitamin B_{12} is administered with intrinsic factor. As previously noted, vitamin B_{12} is necessary to catalyze the conversion of methylmalonate to succinate. Inadequate cobalamin inhibits this reaction, causing an increase in the urinary excretion of methylmalonic acid. This characteristic test can also be used to confirm a vitamin B_{12} deficiency state.[136]

The RDA for adults is 2.0 µg, which maintains adequate vitamin B_{12} nutriture and a substantial body pool.[136] Little information is available regarding parenteral needs. Investigators have administered 2 to 12.5 µg of vitamin B_{12} per day, and all studies failed to detect any abnormalities of vitamin B_{12} status.[50,51,162,172] The AMA Nutrition Advisory Group recommends 5.0 µg for adults as a daily maintenance dose for intravenous use.[49]

VITAMIN C (ASCORBIC ACID)

Vitamin C has several important biochemical functions. It is involved in numerous enzyme systems, such as the hydroxylation of proline and lysine during collagen formation.[263,264] Ascorbic acid is needed for normal matrices of cartilage and bone, as well. It also plays a metabolic role in the synthesis of carnitine, steroids, and catecholamines. Vitamin C participates in tyrosine metabolism and the conversion of folic acid to tetrahydrofolic acid. Furthermore, it participates in biologic oxidation and reduction reactions, in which it is oxidized to dehydroascorbic acid. Through this function, vitamin C enhances the absorption of iron[265] by reducing the ferric form of iron to ferrous. It promotes the elimination of toxic transition metal ions by reducing them. Other roles include its ability to destroy free radicals derived from oxygen.[18] Ascorbic acid is involved in the immunologic and antibacterial function of white blood cells[266] and the metabolism of nucleotides, prostaglandins, and histamine. Finally, it may act to regulate cholesterol metabolism, as a deficiency is associated with depressed synthesis of bile acids from cholesterol.

Mild deficiencies of vitamin C can occur from inadequate intake or under stressful situations that lead to enhanced metabolism or poor utilization. It presents as fatigue, anorexia, muscular pain, and increased susceptibility to infection and stress. More severe deficiency is termed scurvy and is characterized by anemia; hemorrhagic disorders; weakening of collagenous structures in bone cartilage, teeth, and connective tissue; degeneration of muscles; gingivitis; capillary weakness; and rheumatic leg pain. In the United States, scurvy is primarily present in infants relying on cow's milk as a staple[136] and speaks to the significance of continuing breast milk or infant formula until a child is at least 12 months of age. Clinical symptoms of vitamin C inadequacy are accompanied by a reduction of vitamin C concentration in plasma, leukocytes, and urine. A summary of the investigative evidence supporting the role of vitamin C in multiple forms of cancer was recently published.[267] It appears that vitamin C has a protective function in preventing cancers of the following type: oral, esophageal, gastric, pancreatic, cervical, rectal, lung, and breast.

Ascorbic acid is detected in the urine when the body pool exceeds 1500 mg. Urinary excretion declines dramatically with depletion.[136,268] Measurement of urinary ascorbic acid is not as sensitive as blood plasma and leukocyte assay for assessing nutritional adequacy.[269] Measurement of plasma (or serum) ascorbic acid is currently the most commonly used and practical procedure.[268,270] However, plasma and serum levels do not represent optimal measures of vitamin C status; these measures tend to reflect recent dietary intake,[269] and levels fall to negligible values long before tissue is depleted.

Without the availability of a functional biochemical procedure, leukocyte ascorbate levels represent the most reliable index of vitamin C content of tissue stores.[269,271] Because leukocyte ascorbate levels do not fall as rapidly with dietary depletion as do plasma levels, they are representative of long-term vitamin C nutriture. Changes in concentration of the vitamin in white blood cells are more pronounced with the onset of scurvy. Unfortunately, the determination of ascorbic acid in white blood cells is difficult and currently requires relatively large amounts of blood. Therefore, leukocyte assay is not practical for routine use in the assessment of vitamin C status; however, these difficulties are expected to be resolved with modern technology.

The optimal dietary intake of vitamin C is debatable, and a wide range of recommended levels of intake exist.[50,51,54,55,136,170] A daily oral intake of 60 mg has been recommended for healthy, nonpregnant, nonlactating adults.[136] Individuals who probably require increased intake of vitamin C include pregnant or lactating women, cigarette smokers,[272] alcoholics, the elderly,[273] and oral contraceptive users.[274] Patients frequently reported to have ascorbate deficiency include surgical,[275,276] cancer,[277] and burn patients.[157] In addition, plasma ascorbate is reportedly low in critically ill patients, which is not necessarily a result of decreased intake. Schorah et al[278] postulate that vitamin C acts much like a negative acute-phase reactant. However, it is not clear whether decreased levels are the result of redistribution, increased utilization, enhanced oxidation as a result of free radicals produced during the inflammatory response, or augmented losses. Further studies are needed to clarify possible beneficial effects of vitamin C supplementation in asthma, atherosclerosis, and common cold prophylaxis. However, it is doubtful that more than a small percentage of the population will gain any advantage from the use of more than 100 to 500 mg/day.

A wide spectrum of parenteral guidelines exists. The provision of 34 mg of vitamin C per day has been associated with an 83% incidence of low plasma ascorbate levels,[55] whereas 100 to 140 mg daily results in normal blood concentrations.[51,170] Experience with the parenteral administration of much higher levels (700 to 3500 mg) has been reported.[50,54] The AMA recommends supplementation of parenteral nutrition programs with 100 mg of vitamin C.

Generally, pharmacologic intakes (both enteral and parenteral) are well tolerated, since excesses are rapidly cleared by the kidneys. It is not apparent that adults are harmed by the ingestion of several grams daily. There is evidence that higher doses of vitamin C (in the range of 5 to 15 g/day) may be associated with nausea and diarrhea. Some ascorbic acid is converted to oxalate, and large doses may lead to urinary stone formation. Megadoses may also interfere with tests for glycosuria.

BIOTIN

Biotin serves as a coenzyme in a number of carboxylation reactions. In this capacity, biotin has essential roles in gluconeogenesis, lipogenesis, propionate and pyruvate metabolism, and branched-chain amino acid catabolism. Biotin deficiency has been induced experimentally[278] and can be precipitated by the ingestion of large quantities of raw egg whites (which contains avidin, a biotin-binding protein).[279–281] Subjects at risk include alcoholics, patients with partial gastrectomies[282] and burns,[283] and women during pregnancy and lactation.[284] Deficiencies secondary to antibiotic therapy and in association with long-term TPN[285–287] have been reported. Clinical manifestations of biotin deficiency include anorexia, nausea, vomiting, weight loss, glossitis, pallor, depression, lassitude, myalgia, scaly dermatitis, anergy, desquamation of the lips, arthralgia, anemia, and alopecia. Measurement of biotin levels in the blood and urine can help determine status[280]; however, biotin deficiency can exist despite a plasma level within normal limits. Additional means of determining biotin deficiency include persistent lactic acidosis[286,288]; reduced plasma nonesterified fatty acid concentration[287]; and urinary accumulation of 30H-isovaleric acid, 30H-propionic acid, and 30H-butyric acid.[286] The skewed detection of any combination of the recommended tests along with clinical signs warrants scrutiny of the nutrition regimen for biotin adequacy.

Much of the daily requirement for biotin can be produced by intestinal bacteria. Unless the gut flora is disturbed by antibiotics, this can be a significant source. No dietary standards for oral biotin intake have been established, but the safe and adequate level for adults is estimated as 30 to 100 µg.[136]

Biotin typically had been omitted from parenteral vitamin preparations until the AMA published guidelines. Currently, the AMA-recommended level of intravenous supplementation is 60 µg.[49] Nichoalds et al[289] and McClain et al[285] have found this amount to satisfy requirements in adult TPN patients, whereas Dempsey et al[80] reported a 50% incidence of suboptimal biotin status when 60 µg was infused daily.

PANTOTHENIC ACID

Pantothenic acid is present in all living cells, primarily as a constituent of coenzyme A (CoA).[290] A second known coenzyme-like substance containing a pantothenic acid prosthetic group is acyl-carrier protein (ACP).[291] At least 70 enzymes are known to require CoA or ACP. CoA serves as a carrier of acyl groups and participates in enzymatic reactions concerned with energy release from fat, carbohydrate, and ketogenic amino acids. It is also involved in the synthesis of sterols (such as cholesterol and steroid hormones), the acetylation of amines (such as choline to form acetylcholine), the acetylation of sulfonamide drugs prior to excretion, and the synthesis of heme. ACP functions with a multienzyme system known as the fatty acid synthetase complex, which is necessary for fat synthesis. There is also evidence to suggest that pantothenic acid has a role in the maintenance of normal immune function.[292,293]

Deficiency in animals manifests as symptoms of tissue failure; poor growth; weight loss abnormalities of skin, hair, and feathers; fatty liver; gastrointestinal ulceration; adrenal gland necrosis; neuromuscular disorders; decreased leukocyte formation; and inhibition of antibody formation.[290] Spontaneous pantothenic acid deficiency is very uncommon in humans and is thought to occur only in chronically malnourished individuals presenting with other B-vitamin deficiencies[294] or in association with the administration of pantothenic acid antagonists.[295] Alcoholics may also be at risk of suboptimal pantothenic acid status. Symptoms of deficiency in humans include diarrhea, insomnia, mental depression, fatigue, malaise, numbness and tingling of the hands and feet, increased susceptibility to infection, inhibition of antibody formation,[292,293] poor wound healing and graft take,[292] growth impairment, neuromuscular disturbances, and lesions of the adrenal gland.

Pantothenic acid deficiency is difficult to diagnose because symptoms mask multiple other vitamin and/or mineral deficiencies. Techniques for evaluating pantothenic acid nutriture are limited. Present assessment relies mainly on urinary excretion of the vitamin. In studies that control the dietary intake of pantothenic acid, urinary excretion is related to ingestion.[296] Serum pantothenic acid appears to be less sensitive than urinary excretion to dietary pantothenic acid intake; however, serum levels do respond to extreme differences in intake.[297] The activity of CoA in red blood cells may represent a functional method of assessing pantothenic acid status.[298]

The essentiality of pantothenic acid is well established, but there is no clear indication as to the daily requirement. Deficiency states are rare because of widespread distribution in foods. No RDA has been proposed, but the Food and Nutrition Board of the National Research Council estimates a safe and adequate intake for pantothenic acid to be 4 to 7 mg/day in adults.[136] Stress situations elevate needs, so requirements are likely to be high during pregnancy and lactation.[299,300] Pantothenic acid supplementation has been suggested as having beneficial effects in wound healing,[301] arthritis, and the treatment of postoperative ileus, but its efficacy remains to be proven. The AMA currently recommends a parenteral dose of 15 mg/day for adults.[49] This guideline has been derived empirically since pantothenate nutriture in parenterally nourished subjects has not been well studied. Pantothenic acid is present in intravenous multivitamin preparations in the form of dexpanthenol, which is more stable than the free vitamin or its salt. In addition, pantothenic acid is frequently incorporated into oral multivitamin preparations.

ZINC

Zinc acts as a cofactor in more than 100 different enzyme systems, including alkaline phosphatase, alcohol dehydrogenase, DNA and RNA polymerase, carbonic anhydrase, and carboxypeptidase. It also has a role as a ligand that helps maintain the structural integrity of certain nonenzymatic substances such as albumin, nucleotides, histidine, and cysteine. Zinc promotes protein synthesis, cellular replication, and collagen formation.[302,303] It plays an important function in immune and antioxidant defense systems.[18,304–308] Zinc is necessary for normal taste acuity.[309–311] Finally, an important interaction exists between zinc and vitamin A.[312–314]

Zinc deficiency handicaps metabolism extensively, and the resulting symptoms are diverse. The most commonly recognized findings are hair loss and dermatitis.[315–319] The skin may become scaly and inflamed, and wound repair is impeded.[303,320–322] One of the most important consequences of zinc deficiency is growth failure.[311,323,324] Zinc deficiency is associated with low circulating levels of insulin-like growth factor-1 (IGF-1)[325–327] and, therefore, zinc supplementation has been studied as a means to mediate growth by improving serum IGF-1.[328] Delayed sexual maturation and testicular atrophy are observed with advanced zinc deficiency. Smell and taste acuity often decline[309–311]; loss of appetite is common[316]; and depression,[310,315] diarrhea,[315,316] decreased dark adaptation,[312,314] and immune dysfunction[304–308] are all symptomatic of zinc deficiency.

A prodigious number of laboratory tests, both biochemical and functional, have been used in the evaluation of zinc status; yet assessment remains highly problematic. Approaches have included the measurement of plasma, serum, sweat, saliva, red blood cells, white blood cells, platelets, skin, hair, nails, urine, and alkaline phosphatase. The mainstay for the assessment of zinc nutriture has been the determination of plasma or serum zinc concentration. However, levels of zinc in the blood can be depressed to less than 50% of the premorbid level during the acute-phase response to injury,[329,330] probably mediated by corticotropin, interleukin-1, or other stress hormones.[330,331] As a consequence, zinc is redistributed in tissues; however, total body zinc content is believed to remain the same. Therefore, blood levels of zinc may not always be an accurate reflection of total body zinc and should not be relied on alone in critical care. It is also important to recognize that hemolysis alters concentrations of zinc, since red blood cells contain 75% of whole blood zinc whereas plasma contains about 22%.[332] Extreme caution must be exercised to avoid pitfalls in the quantitation or interpretation of serum or plasma zinc. Naber and colleagues[333] suggest a method of distinguishing zinc deficiency in animals due to the inflammatory response and a true zinc deficiency using in-vitro uptake of [65]Zn by the blood. Although the methodology requires validation in humans, preliminary work is promising.

Urinary excretion of zinc is decreased as a result of zinc deficiency.[315,321,334–336] However, it is not a reliable diagnostic aid—particularly in stress situations such as surgery, trauma, and burns, which cause hyperexcretion of zinc. Other tests include the measurement of zinc levels in hair and nails. Because hair and nail tissue turns over slowly, zinc levels do not reflect recent changes in body zinc stores. There are potential problems with contamination of this tissue by shampoos, nail treatments, and other preparations.

Functional indexes of zinc include the assessment of wound healing and nitrogen retention, which can be cumbersome to measure. Some researchers have reported that a decrease in serum alkaline phosphatase activity is associated with the onset of zinc deficiency manifestations.[318,319,337] Other functional procedures include dark adaptometry and taste acuity. Due to the lack of precision in the biochemical measurements used to diagnose zinc deficiency, several authors suggest studying the effect of zinc supplementation on linear growth to verify zinc status in children.[338–340]

The RDA is set at 15 mg for adults,[136] and the AMA has established guidelines for parenteral zinc infusion in stable adults at 2.5 to 4.0 mg/day.[78] Primary zinc deficiency is most commonly seen in patients on TPN when inadequate zinc is supplied intravenously.[315,318,341–343] Only 10% to 40% of the zinc supplied to the gastrointestinal tract is absorbed; therefore enteral administration of 220 mg of zinc sulfate (approximately 50 mg of elemental zinc) supplies 5 to 20 mg of zinc. Decreased intake is a potential cause of zinc depletion, as are decreased absorption (such as seen in inflammatory bowel disease,[344] short-bowel syndrome,[342] and high phytate intake[345]), decreased utilization (such as that occurring with cirrhosis of the liver), and increased loss (such as occurs in gastrointestinal fistula, decubitus ulcer, diarrhea, thermal burn exudation, and drug ingestion).[307,346] Increased zinc is required during pregnancy and lactation,[347] by neonates,[348] after trauma,[336] and during postburn reepithelialization.[309,321,335,336,349] Zinc supplementation has also been shown to reduce the duration of the common cold.[350,351] Iron supplementation is known to decrease zinc absorption; however, if these minerals are consumed in foodstuff, the interaction is less pronounced.[352] Zinc toxicity has been reported in humans, although the emetic effect that ensues consumption of large doses aids to minimize hazardous effects. Other signs of zinc toxicity include dehydration, lack of muscle coordination, abdominal pain, dizziness, hypocupremia, microcytosis and neutropenia, decreased high-density lipoproteins,[353] and compromised immunity.[354]

COPPER

Another essential trace element in humans is copper. Its primary role is as a component of copper metalloenzymes.[355] The cross-linking reactions of collagen and elastin synthesis require various copper-containing amine oxidases.[356] Copper is an essential component of superoxide dismutase, which scavenges potentially damaging free radicals.[18,357] Copper is notable as a cofactor in the formation of skin and hair pigment (tyrosinase)[358] and in the release of energy by the respiratory chain (cytochrome *c* oxidase). Copper is also incorporated into dopamine β-hydroxylase, a cuproenzyme involved in the synthesis of norepinephrine and epinephrine. Copper is necessary to catalyze the oxidation of Fe^{2+} to Fe^{3+} during hemoglobin and transferrin formation.[359] Moreover, copper plays an essential role in cholesterol metabolism, phospholipid production, and prostaglandin synthesis.[360] It is important for an effective immunologic response to a variety of pathogenic challenges. Furthermore, copper is required for red and white blood cell maturation, myocardial contractility, and brain development.[361] Other physiologic functions include its involvement in taste sensation[362] and glucose metabolism.

Important symptoms of copper deficiency include skeletal demineralization,[363,364] poor wound healing,[365] immune defects,[366,367] hypotonia, cholesterol abnormalities, impaired glucose tolerance, and central nervous system and cardiovascular disorders. Another expression of copper deficiency is defective iron metabolism. Anemia,[364,365,369] neutropenia,[363,365,368–370] and leukopenia develop.[363,365,369] Multiple metabolic alterations observed in copper deficiency may also contribute to atherogenesis.[371] Less devastating are the changes observed in hair and skin pigmentation.

Copper status is usually assessed by the serum copper or ceruloplasmin concentration. Low circulating levels may suggest suboptimal copper nutriture. However, blood levels are frequently elevated during an infection[372,373] because ceruloplasmin, the copper-carrier protein, acts as an acute-phase reactant. Hypercupremia is also observed in subjects taking steroid contraceptives as well as in pregnancy,[373,374] leukemia, and neoplasia. Because circulating values do not always reliably reflect whole-body copper status, copper has also been measured in the urine, hair, and nails; however, these measures remain problematic.[375] Differential blood counts may be useful in conjunction with other tests. Functional indexes include glucose intolerance and impaired immunocompetence. More recently, some investigators have recommended serum assay of various cuproenzymes (such as superoxide dismutase and lysyl oxidase) in the assessment of copper status,[376] but such analyses are not yet routinely available in the average clinical laboratory. Milne and Johnson[377] report that during copper deficiency, the enzymatic activity of ceruloplasmin is decreased and circulating ceruloplasmin is increased; these authors suggest using the ratio of enzymatic activity to the concentration of ceruloplasmin as an indicator of copper nutriture.

Primary deficiency of copper is rare, although failure to supply sufficient parenteral copper during the early years of TPN was documented.[363,368–370] A variety of malabsorptive syndromes (such as short-bowel syndrome, sprue, jejunoileal bypass, chronic diarrhea, Crohn's disease, and celiac disease) may contribute to secondary copper deficiency. Antacids and high-dose oral zinc therapy can have a depressive effect on copper absorption. The hypocupremia observed in nephrotic syndrome, protein-calorie malnutrition,[378] and perhaps burns is postulated to be the result of decreased circulating protein and, thus, an inability to provide sufficient protein for the protein-copper complex, ceruloplasmin. Decreased serum copper[365,379] and high urinary copper output[335,379] have been reported after burns, although these findings have not always been confirmed by others.[309,336]

Wilson's disease is an inborn error of metabolism related to copper. This disorder causes an accumulation of copper due to the inability to excrete the mineral properly. Acute copper toxicity is characterized by nausea, vomiting, diarrhea, hemolysis, convulsions, and gastrointestinal bleeding. Drug therapy (penicillamine) is available to treat this disease.

There are, as yet, no RDAs for copper.[136] Safe and adequate enteral intake has been estimated to be 1.5 to 3 mg/day. The AMA has established guidelines for parenteral copper infusion in the adult at 0.5 to 1.5 mg/day.[78] This amount may be excessive, as studies by Shike et al[376] have demonstrated that normal copper status could be achieved by lower doses of 0.2 to 0.3 mg/day in stable TPN patients.

SELENIUM

A well-characterized selenoenzyme is glutathione peroxidase,[380] which reduces intracellular hydroperoxides. In this manner, selenium, along with vitamin E, protects membrane lipids from oxidant damage.[18] This function of selenium metabolism suggests a role in cancer prevention.[381] Other functions of this trace mineral are largely speculative. It plays a poorly understood role in growth and in the preservation of normal anatomy and physiology of cardiac and skeletal muscle.

Selenium deficiency has been described in protein-calorie malnutrition,[382] burns,[383,384] and in patients receiving TPN.[385–389] Others at greater risk for possible selenium deficiency include patients with small-bowel resection,[390] malabsorption,[391] pancreaticointestinal insufficiency,[392] AIDS,[393] cancer[394,395]; preterm infants[396]; and patients with cystic fibrosis.[389,395] Clinical signs of selenium deficiency in humans include growth retardation, muscle pain and weakness,[388] myopathy,[389] and cardiomyopathy.[385,386,397] Excess selenium is correlated with growth retardation, muscular weakness, infertility, hepatic necrosis, dysphagia, dysphonia, bronchopneumonia, and respiratory compromise. Selenium toxicity can also produce symptoms such as nausea, diarrhea, abdominal pain, nail and hair changes, fatigue, irritability, and peripheral neuropathy.[398]

A number of methods for the biochemical assessment of selenium status have been described.[399] One of the most widely used tests is the assay of erythrocyte selenium concentration, which has the advantage of requiring minimal processing and is not subject to error from hemolysis. Erythrocyte selenium levels are usually characteristic of selenium nutriture in patients not requiring blood transfusions whose dietary intake is relatively constant over time.

The diagnosis of selenium deficiency is also suggested by low levels of selenium in serum or plasma. Such determinations may be more appropriate measures because they are less influenced by transfusions and are more acutely responsive to changes in selenium intake than are erythrocyte levels.[400] Depressed selenium concentrations in urine, hair, and nails represent additional evidence suggestive of deficiency,[399,401] but these results are less conclusive. The functional activity of glutathione peroxidase in erythrocytes or platelets has been proposed to be responsive to changes in selenium intake, although questions of sensitivity and specificity exist.[402,403] Selenoprotein P, a selenium carrier protein, has recently been isolated and appears promising as an indicator of selenium status.[404] At present, the accurate assessment of selenium status requires the measurement of several of these biochemical parameters in addition to considering several interacting nutrients, such as vitamin E and polyunsaturated fatty acids.

On the basis of available information, the National Research Council has established the RDA for selenium for adults at 70 µg.[136] The AMA does not currently have guidelines for selenium supplementation during TPN.[78] A reasonable amount of intravenous selenium for the maintenance of selenium balance in nondepleted patients is probably in the range of 20 to 40 µg/day.[405] Therapeutic dose of intravenous selenium during deficiency is suggested at 80 to 160 µg/day.[406] Monitoring of serum selenium levels approximately every 10 days is recommended until normal levels are achieved.[392]

IRON

Iron regulates two important oxidative processes. First, it has a central role in the transportation of oxygen in the body via hemoglobin in red blood cells and myoglobin in the muscle. Second, iron functions in the respiratory chain, influencing the oxidative processing of energy nutrients. Iron is a cofactor in some enzyme systems, including catalase, peroxidase, and xanthine oxidase. It is also necessary for the hydroxylation of lysine and proline, cell replication, and DNA synthesis. Considerable evidence also suggests that iron has a role in host resistance.[12,407,408]

Iron deficiency is the most common nutrient inadequacy. A suboptimal iron status is usually the result of insufficient intake, especially among those whose needs are unusually high (such as in infants, adolescents, and pregnant women),[409] individuals with impaired absorption (for example, postgastrectomy and in gastrointestinal diseases),[410] or individuals with extensive iron losses (which can be caused by blood loss from acute hemorrhage, or long-term losses from hiatal hernia, peptic ulcer, gastrointestinal bleeding, diverticulitis, ulcerative colitis, cancer, and esophageal varices). Hypoferremia has also been documented following surgery and during septic episodes.[411]

Early stages of iron deficiency can be detected by diminished serum ferritin concentrations, as ferritin decreases in parallel with depletion of body iron stores. The only cause of low serum ferritin levels is exhausted iron stores.[412] However, certain conditions (such as rheumatoid arthritis, cancer, inflammatory disease, or surgery)[413] may mask deficiency by elevating circulating ferritin levels. In any event, during uncomplicated cases of iron depletion, a low serum ferritin level is followed by a decrease in serum iron level, an increase in total iron-binding capacity, and therefore a low transferrin saturation index. When iron levels become sufficiently reduced, impairment of hemoglobin synthesis occurs, and anemia develops that is characterized by hypochromic, microcytotic erythrocytes. Hemoglobin, hematocrit, mean corpuscular volume, and mean corpuscular hemoglobin concentration fall below normal levels.

Iron deficiency affects many other tissues in the body as well. Epithelial disturbances include cheilosis, glossitis, atrophy of the tongue, hair loss, brittle fingernails, and koilonychia (spoon-shaped nails). Pallor, tissue hypoxia, exertional dyspnea, and coldness in extremities have been associated with iron deficiency. Heart enlargement is common, but after treatment the heart usually returns to its normal size. Less specific are changes affecting behavior and cognition.[414,415] Controversy continues to surround the role of iron deficiency in producing eating disorders (such as pica), menorrhagia, and immune defects.

Suboptimal iron nutriture has been associated with increased susceptibility to infection, reduced lymphocyte counts, decreased secretory immunoglobulin A, impaired interleukin-1 production, and depressed neutrophil bactericidal activity.[12,407,408,416–420] However, these findings must be balanced by reports that iron excess may likewise be a critical determinant of infectious outcome. Unbound iron seems to encourage bacterial and fungal growth.[421,422] Weinberg[423] has presented conditions in which hosts stressed by excessive iron demonstrated enhanced susceptibility to infection. Host response to bacterial invasion is characterized by a reduction in plasma iron, brought about by depressed intestinal assimilation and increased liver storage of iron. Hence, routine iron supplementation should probably be avoided when associated with infection and hypotransferrinemia.

The adult RDA is 15 mg for women and teenage boys, and 10 mg for men.[136] Small-dose enteral supplements (around 15 mg) may be indicated if iron-rich foods are unavailable, if absorption-enhancing factors are missing in the diet, or if a person is on a calorie-restricted diet. Patients with severe iron deficiencies are instructed to consume a minimum of three 320-mg hydrated ferrous sulfate tablets per day. Each tablet contains 60 mg of elemental iron; however, only an approximate 20% of the elemental iron is absorbed. Therefore, 36 mg of elemental iron may be absorbed from the three recommended ferrous sulfate tablets. In order to replace iron stores, 36 to 48 mg of elemental iron is suggested, so this recommendation is not excessive. Normalization of hemoglobin and replenishment of iron stores are usually observed following 3 months of iron-replacement therapy. Whether from foodstuff or supplement, nonheme iron absorption is enhanced by simultaneous ingestion of ascorbic acid.

Routine parenteral administration of iron is controversial, and the AMA makes no recommendations for iron intake.[382] TPN patients are in a dubious predicament in that they are likely to have experienced blood loss and therefore are predisposed to the development of iron deficiency. On the other hand, TPN patients are also prone to infectious sequelae; hence judicious iron supplementation is warranted to avoid excessive circulating free iron, which is a risk factor for infection. Iron supplementation is a standard component of TPN protocols at some institutions,[424,425] either as a part of the hyperalimentation solution or as an intramuscular supplement. Others recommend more conservative treatment[426] using blood transfusions as a means of administering iron.

CONCLUSIONS AND FUTURE DIRECTIONS

It is clear that providing adequate intake of many vitamins and trace minerals involves more than simply preventing clinical deficiency signs. Accumulating scientific evidence indicates that micronutrients are critical in terms of promoting well-being, minimizing the risk or severity of acute and chronic disorders, and maximizing outcome potential during recovery from disease and critical illness. Exciting new information will improve our understanding and hence facilitate the construction of improved micronutrient practice guidelines during enteral and parenteral support.

REFERENCES

1. Levenson SM, Gruber CA, Rettura G, Gruber DK, et al. Supplemental vitamin A prevents the acute radiation induced defect in wound healing. *Ann Surg.* 1984;200:494–511.

2. Winsey K, Simon RJ, Levenson SM, Seifter E, et al. Effect of supplemental vitamin A on colon anastomotic healing in rats given preoperative irradiation. *Am J Surg.* 1987;153:153–156.

3. Ehrlich HP, Tarver H. Effect of beta-carotene, vitamin A and glucocorticoids on collagen synthesis in wounds. *Proc Soc Exp Biol.* 1971;137:936–938.

4. Ortonne JP, Schmidt D, Bennet G, Thivolet J. Influences of retinoic acid on epidermal wound healing in man. In: Orfanos CE, ed. *Retinoids.* New York: Springer-Verlag; 1981:497–500.

5. Seifter E, Crowley LV, Returra G, Nakav K, et al. Influence of vitamin A on wound healing in rats with femoral fracture. *Ann Surg.* 1975;181:836–841.

6. Weiss JS. Topical tretinoin improves photoaged skin: a double blind vehicle controlled study. *JAMA.* 1988;259:527–532.

7. Bollag W. Vitamin A and retinoids: from nutrition to pharmacotherapy in dermatology and oncology. *Lancet.* 1983;1:860–863.

8. Levenson SM, Seifter E. Dysnutrition, wound healing and resistance to infection. *Clin Plast Surg.* 1977;4:375–388.

9. Cohen BE, Elin RJ. Vitamin A-induced nonspecific resistance to infection. *J Infect Dis.* 1974;129:597–600.

10. Cohen BE, Elin RJ. Enhanced resistance to certain infections in vitamin A-treated mice. *Plast Reconstr Surg.* 1974;54:192–195.

11. Cohen BE, Gill G, Cullen PR, Morris PJ. Reversal of postoperative immunosuppression in man by vitamin A. *Surg Gynecol Obstet.* 1979;149:658–662.

12. Beisel WR. Single nutrients and immunity. *Am J Clin Nutr.* 1982;35:417–468.

13. Fusi S, Kupper TS, Green DR, Ariyan S. Reversal of postoperative immunosuppression in man by vitamin A. *Surgery.* 1984;96:330–335.

14. Parent G, Rouseaux-Prevost R, Carlier Y. Influence of vitamin A on the immune response of Schistosoma monsoni-infected rats. *Trans R Soc Trop Med Hyg.* 1984;78:380–383.

15. Santos MS, Meydani SN, Leka L, Wu D, et al. Natural killer cell activity in elderly men is enhanced by β-carotene supplementation. *Am J Clin Nutr.* 1996;64:772–777.

16. Pasatiempo AMG, Bowman TA, Taylor CE, Ross AC. Vitamin A depletion and repletion: effects on antibody response to the capsular polysaccharide of streptococcus pneumonia, type III (SSS-III). *Am J Clin Nutr.* 1989;49:501–510.

17. Seifter E, Rettura G, Swifter J, Davidson H, et al. Thymotropic action of vitamin A. *Fed Proc.* 1973;32:947A.

18. Rock CL, Jacob RA, Bowen PE. Biological characteristics of the antioxidant micronutrients, vitamin C, vitamin E and the carotenoids: an update. *J Am Diet Assoc.* 1996;96:693–702.

19. Sommer A, Katz J, Tarwotje I. Increased risk of respiratory disease and diarrhea in children with preexisting mild vitamin A deficiency. *Am J Clin Nutr.* 1984;40:1090–1095.

20. Sivakumar B, Reddy V. Absorption of labelled vitamin A in children during infection. *Br J Nutr.* 1972;27:299–304.

21. Stoll BJ, Banu H, Kabir I, Molla A. Nightblindness and vitamin A deficiency in children attending a diarrhea disease hospital in Bangladesh. *J Trop Pediatr.* 1985;31:36–39.

22. Mahalanabis D, Simpson TW, Chakraborty ML, Ganguli C, et al. Malabsorption of water miscible vitamin A in children with giardiasis and ascariasis. *Am J Clin Nutr.* 1979;32:313–318.

23. Stephenson CB, Alvarez JO, Kohatsu J, Hardmeier R, et al. Vitamin A is excreted in the urine during acute infection. *Am J Clin Nutr.* 1994;60:388–392.

24. Hustead VA, Gutcher GR, Anderson SA, Zachman RD. Relationship of vitamin A (retinol) status to lung disease in the preterm infant. *J Pediatr.* 1984;105:610–615.

25. Woodruff CW, Latham CB, Mactier H, Hewett JE. Vitamin A status of preterm infants: correlation between plasma retinol concentration and retinol dose response. *Am J Clin Nutr.* 1987;46:985–988.

26. Zachman RD. Retinol (vitamin A) and the neonate: special problems of the human premature infant. *Am J Clin Nutr.* 1989;50:413–424.

27. Jacob RA, Sandstead HH, Solomons NW, Rieger C, et al. Zinc status and vitamin A transport in cystic fibrosis. *Am J Clin Nutr.* 1978;31:638–644.

28. Howard L, Chu R, Feman S, Mintz H, et al. Vitamin A deficiency from long term parenteral nutrition. *Ann Intern Med.* 1980;93:576–577.

29. Arroyave G, Wilson D, Mendez J, Behar M, et al. Serum and liver vitamin A and lipids in children with severe protein malnutrition. *Am J Clin Nutr.* 1961;9:180–185.

30. Rechcigel M, Berger S, Loosli JK, Williams HH. Dietary protein and utilization of vitamin A. *J Nutr.* 1962;76:435–440.

31. Smith FR, Suskind R, Thanangkul O, Leitzman C, et al. Plasma vitamin A, retinol-binding protein and prealbumin concentrations in protein calorie malnutrition, II: response to varying dietary treatments. *Am J Clin Nutr.* 1975;28:732–738.

32. Smith JC, McDaniel EG, Fan FF, Halsted JA. Zinc: a trace element essential in vitamin A metabolism. *Science.* 1973;181:954–955.

33. Szebeni A, Negyesi G, Feuer L. Vitamin A levels in the serum of burned patients. *Burns.* 1980;7:313–318.

34. Rai K, Courtemanch AD. Vitamin A assay in burned patients. *J Trauma.* 1975;15:419–424.

35. Shenai JP, Kennedy KA, Chytil F, Stahlman MT. Clinical trial of vitamin A supplementation in infants susceptible to bronchopulmonary dysplasia. *J Pediatr.* 1987;111:269–277.

36. Hussey GD, Klein M. A randomized, controlled trial of vitamin A in children with severe measles. *N Engl J Med.* 1990;323:160–164.

37. Goodman DS. Vitamin A and retinoids in health and disease. *N Engl J Med.* 1984;310:1023–1037.

38. Winston WK, Krug-Wispe S, Succop P, Tsang RC, et al. Effect of different vitamin A intakes on very-low-birth-weight-infants 1-3. *Am J Clin Nutr.* 1995;62:1216–1220.

39. Muto Y, Smith JF, Milch PO, Goodman DS. Regulation of retinol-binding protein metabolism by vitamin A status in the rat. *J Biol Chem.* 1972;247:2542–2551.

40. Moody BJ. Changes in the serum concentrations of thyroxine-binding prealbumin and retinol-binding protein following burn injury. *Clin Chim Acta.* 1982;188:87–92.

41. Smith FR, Goodman DS, Zaklama MS, Gabr MK, et al. Serum vitamin A, retinol-binding protein, and prealbumin concentrations in protein-calorie malnutrition: a functional defect in hepatic retinol release. *Am J Clin Nutr.* 1973;26:973–981.

42. Kasper H, Brodersen M, Schedel R. Concentration of vitamin A, retinol-binding protein and prealbumin in serum in response to stress. *Acta Hepatogastroenterol.* 1975;22:403–408.

43. Sommer A, Djunaedi E, Loeden AA, Taruretjo I, et al. Impact of vitamin A supplementation on childhood mortality. *Lancet.* 1986;1:1169–1173.

44. Skogh M, Sundquist T, Tagesson C. Vitamin A in Crohn. *Lancet.* 1980;1:766.

45. Gottschlich MM, Warden GD, Michel M, Havens P, et al. Diarrhea in tube-fed burn patients: incidence, etiology, nutritional impact and prevention. *J Parenter Enter Nutr.* 1988;12: 338–345.

46. Gabriel EP, Lindquist BL, Lee PC. Vitamin A deficiency promotes bacterial adherence to rat small intestinal mucosal cells. *Am J Clin Nutr.* 1987;45:846.

47. DeLuca L, Wolf G. Vitamin A and mucous secretion. *Int J Vitam Nutr Res.* 1970;40:284–290.

48. Barbul A, Thysen B, Rettura G, Levenson SM, et al. White cell involvement in the inflammatory wound healing and immune actions of vitamin A. *J Parenter Enter Nutr.* 1978;2:129–138.

49. American Medical Association. Multivitamin preparations for parenteral use: a statement by the Nutrition Advisory Group. *J Parenter Enter Nutr.* 1979;3:258–262.

50. Lowry SF, Goodgame JT, Maher MM, Brennan MF. Parenteral vitamin requirements during intravenous feeding. *Am J Clin Nutr.* 1978;31:2149–2158.

51. Nichoalds GE, Meng HC, Caldwell MD. Vitamin requirements in patients receiving total parenteral nutrition. *Arch Surg.* 1977;112:1061–1064.

52. Davis AT, Franz FP, Courtnay DA, Ullrey DE, et al. Plasma vitamin and mineral status in home parenteral nutrition patients. *J Parenter Enter Nutr.* 1987;11:480–485.

53. Shils ME, Baker H, Frank O. Blood vitamin levels of long-term adult home total parenteral nutrition patients: the efficacy of the AMA-FDA parenteral multivitamin formulation. *J Parenter Enter Nutr.* 1985;9:179–188.

54. Kirkimo AK, Burt ME, Brennan MF. Serum vitamin level maintenance in cancer patients on total parenteral nutrition. *Am J Clin Nutr.* 1982;35:1003–1009.

55. Labadarios D, O'Keefe SJ, Dicker J, Stuijvenberg LV, et al. Plasma vitamin levels in patients on prolonged total parenteral nutrition. *J Parenter Enter Nutr.* 1988;12:205–211.

56. Hathcock JN, Hattan DG, Jenkins MY, McDonald JT, et al. Evaluation of vitamin A toxicity. *Am J Clin Nutr.* 1990;52:183–202.

57. Plewig G, Nikolowski J, Wolff HH. Action of isotretinoin in acne rosacea and gram-negative folliculitis. *J Am Acad Dermatol.* 1982;6:766–785.

58. Gotloib L, Sklan D, Mines M. Hemodialysis: effect on plasma levels of vitamin A and carotenoid. *JAMA.* 1978;239:751.

59. Yatzidis H, Digenis P, Koutsicos D. Hypervitaminosis A accompanying advanced chronic renal failure. *Br Med J.* 1975;3:352–353.

60. Rothman KJ, Moore LL, Singer MR, Nguyen US, et al. Teratogenicity of high vitamin A intake. *N Engl J Med.* 1995;333:1369–1373.

61. Geubel AP, DeGalocsy C, Alves N, Rahier J, et al. Liver damage caused by therapeutic vitamin A administration: estimate of dose-related toxicity in 41 cases. *Gastroenterology.* 1991;100:1701–1709.

62. Gamble JG, Ip SC. Hypervitaminosis A in a child from megadosing. *J Pediatr Orthop.* 1985;5:219–221.

63. Smith FR, Goodman DS. Vitamin A transport in human vitamin A toxicity. *N Engl J Med.* 1976;294:805–808.

64. Wilz DR, Gray RW, Dominguez JH, Lemann J. 1,25-(OH)$_2$-vitamin D concentrations and net intestinal calcium, phosphate, and magnesium absorption in humans. *Am J Clin Nutr.* 1979;32:2052–2060.

65. Harrison E, Harrison HC. Intestinal transport of phosphate: action of vitamin D, calcium and potassium. *Am J Physiol.* 1961;201:1007–1012.

66. Monolagas SC, Provvedini DM, Tsoukas CD. Interactions of 1,25-dihydroxyvitamin D$_3$ and the immune system. *Mol Cell Endocrinol.* 1985;43:113–122.

67. Adams JS, Sharama OP, Gacod MA, Singer FR. Metabolism of 25 hydroxyvitamin D$_3$ by cultured pulmonary alveolar macrophages in sarcoidosis. *J Clin Invest.* 1983;72:1856–1860.

68. Tsoukas CD, Provvedini DM, Manolagas SC. 1,25-dihydroxyvitamin D$_3$: A novel immuno-regulatory hormone. *Science.* 1984;224:1438–1439.

69. Toss G, Symreng T. Delayed hypersensitivity response and vitamin D deficiency. *Int J Vitam Nutr Res.* 1983;53:27–31.

70. Simpson RV, Arnold AJ. Calcium antagonizes 1,25-dihydroxyvitamin D$_3$ inhibition of breast cancer cell proliferation. *Endocrinology.* 1986;119:2284–2289.

71. Avioli LV, Haddad JG. Vitamin D's: more and more measured better and better. *N Engl J Med.* 1977;297:1006–1007.

72. Shepard RM, Horst RL, Hamstra AJ, DeLuca HF. Determination of vitamin D and its metabolites in plasma from normal and anephric man. *Biochem J.* 1979;182:55–69.

73. Mowe M, Bohmer T, Haug E. Serum calcidiol and calcitriol concentrations in elderly people: variations with age, sex, season and disease. *Clin Nutr.* 1996;15:201.

74. Avioli LV, Lee SW, McDonald JK, Lund J, et al. Metabolism of vitamin D$_3$-3H in human subjects: distribution in blood, bile, feces, and urine. *J Clin Invest.* 1967;46:983–992.

75. Lips P, van Ginkel FC, Jongen MJ, Rubertus F, et al. Determinants of vitamin D status in patients with hip fracture and in elderly control subjects. *Am J Clin Nutr.* 1987;46:1005–1010.

76. Ireland AW, Clubb JS, Neale FC, Posen S, et al. The calciferol requirements of patients with surgical hypoparathyroidism. *Ann Intern Med.* 1968;69:81–89.

77. Bengoa JM, Bolt MJ, Rosenberg IH. Hepatic vitamin D 25-hydroxylase inhibition by cimetidine and isoniazid. *J Lab Clin Med.* 1984;104:546–552.

78. American Medical Association. Guidelines for essential trace element preparations for parenteral use. *JAMA.* 1979;241:2051–2054.

79. Greene HL, Hambidge KM, Schanler R, Tsang RC. Guidelines for the use of vitamins, trace elements, calcium, magnesium, and phosphorus in infants and children receiving total parenteral nutrition. *Am J Clin Nutr.* 1988;48:1324.

80. Dempsey DT, Mullen JL, Rombeau JL, Crosby LD, et al. Treatment effects of parenteral vitamins in total parenteral nutrition patients. *J Parenter Enter Nutr.* 1987;11:229–237.

81. Shike M, Harrison JE, Sturtridge WC, Tam CS, et al. Metabolic bone disease in patients receiving long term parenteral nutrition. *Ann Intern Med.* 1980;92:343–350.

82. Klein FL, Horst RL, Norman AW, Ament ME, et al. Reduced serum levels in 11-25-dihydroxyvitamin D during long-term parenteral nutrition. *Ann Intern Med.* 1981;94:638–643.

83. Seligman JV, Basi SS, Deitel M, Bayley TA, et al. Metabolic bone disease in a patient on long-term total parenteral nutrition: a case report with review of literature. *J Parenter Enter Nutr.* 1984;8:722–727.

84. Jacob RA, Burri BJ. Oxidative damage and defense. *Am J Clin Nutr.* 1996;63:1855.

85. Likoff RO, Guptill DR, Lawrence LM, McKay CC, et al. Vitamin E and aspirin depress prostaglandins in protection of chickens against *Escherichia coli* infection. *Am J Clin Nutr.* 1981;34:245–251.

86. Hamelin S, Chan AC. Modulation of platelet thromboxane and malonaldehyde by dietary vitamin E and linoleate. *Lipids.* 1983;18:267–269.

87. Panganamala RV, Cornwell DG. The effects of vitamin E on arachidonic acid metabolism. *Ann N Y Acad Sci.* 1982;393:376–391.

88. Pentland AP, Morrison AR, Jacobs SC, Hruza LL, et al. Tocopherol analogs suppress arachidonic and metabolism via phospholipase inhibition. *J Biol Chem.* 1992;267:15578–15584.

89. Vitamin E Research and Information Service (VERIS). *The Vitamin E Fact Book.* LaGrange, IL: VERIS; 1994.

90. Bendich A, Gabriel E, Machlin LJ. Effect of dietary level of vitamin E on the immune system of the spontaneously hypotensive and normotensive Wistar Kyota rat. *J Nutr.* 1983;113:1920–1926.

91. Tanaka J, Fujiwara H, Torisu M. Vitamin E and immune response, I: enhancement of helper T cell activity by dietary supplementation of vitamin E in mice. *Immunology.* 1979;38:727–734.

92. Rundas C, Peterson VM, Zapata-Sirvent R, Hansbrough J, et al. Vitamin E improves cell-mediated immunity in the burned mouse: a preliminary study. *Burns.* 1984;11:11–15.

93. Meydani SN, Barkland MP, Liu S, Meydani M, et al. Vitamin E supplementation enhances cell-mediated immunity in healthy elderly subjects. *Am J Clin Nutr.* 1990;52:557.

94. Lake AM, Stuart MJ, Osku FA. Vitamin E deficiency and enhanced platelet function: reversal following E supplementation. *J Pediatr.* 1977;90:722–725.

95. Horwitt MK, Century B, Zeman AA. Erythrocyte survival time and reticulocyte levels after tocopherol depletion in man. *Am J Clin Nutr.* 1963;12:99–106.

96. Binder HJ, Herting DC, Hurst V, Finch SC, et al. Tocopherol deficiency in man. *N Engl J Med.* 1965;273:1289–1297.

97. Majaj AS, Dinning JS, Azzam SA, Darby WJ. Vitamin E responsive megaloblastic anemia in infants with protein calorie malnutrition. *Am J Clin Nutr.* 1963;12:374–379.

98. Sitrin MD, Lieberman F, Jensen WE, Noronha A, et al. Vitamin E deficiency and neurologic disease in adults with cystic fibrosis. *Ann Intern Med.* 1987;107:51–54.

99. Bye AM, Muller DP, Wilson J, Wright VM, et al. Symptomatic vitamin E deficiency in cystic fibrosis. *Arch Dis Child.* 1985;60:162–164.

100. Howard L, Ovesen L, Satya-Murti S, Chu R. Reversible neurological symptoms caused by vitamin E deficiency in patients with short bowel syndrome. *Am J Clin Nutr.* 1982;36:1243–1249.

101. Nitowsky HM, Tildon JT, Levin S, Gordon HH. Studies of tocopherol deficiency in infants and children, VII: the effect of tocopherol on urinary, plasma and muscle creatine. *Am J Clin Nutr.* 1962;10:368–378.

102. Gey KF, Puska P, Jordon P, Moser UK, et al. Inverse correlation between plasma vitamin E and mortality from ischemic heart disease in cross-cultural epidemiology. *Am J Clin Nutr.* 1991;53:326S–334S.

103. Stampler MJ, Hennekens CH, Manson JE, Calditz GA, et al. Vitamin E consumption and the risk of coronary disease in women. *New Engl J Med.* 1993;328:1444.

104. Rimm EB, Stampfer MJ, Ascherio A, Giorannucci E, et al. Vitamin E consumption and the risk of coronary heart disease in men. *New Engl J Med.* 1993;328:1450.

105. Verlangieri AJ, Bush MJ. Prevention and regression of primate induced atherosclerosis by d-alpha tocopherol. *J Am Coll Nutr.* 1992;11:131.

106. Thurlow PM, Grant JP. Vitamin E and total parenteral nutrition. *Ann N Y Acad Sci.* 1982;393:121–132.

107. Vanderwoude MG, Van Gaal LF, Vanderwoude MF, DeLeeuw IH. Vitamin E status in normocholesterolemic and hypercholesterolemic diabetic patients. *Acta Diabetol Lat.* 1987;24:133–139.

108. Lemoyne M, Van Gossum A, Kurian R, Ostro M, et al. Breath pentane analysis as an index of lipid peroxidation: a functional test of vitamin E status. *Am J Clin Nutr.* 1987;46:267–272.

109. Riley CA, Cohen G, Lieberman M. Ethane evolution: a new index of lipid peroxidation. *Science.* 1974;183:208–210.

110. Gordon HH, Nitowsky HM, Cornblath M. Studies in tocopherol deficiency in infants and children. *Am J Dis Child.* 1955;90:669–681.

111. Phelps DL. Current perspectives on vitamin E in infant nutrition. *Am J Clin Nutr.* 1987;46:187–191.

112. Braunstein H. Tocopherol deficiency in adults with chronic pancreatitis. *Gastroentrology.* 1961;40:224–231.

113. Gottschlich MM, Jenkins M, Washam M, Warden GD, et al. The relationship between vitamin E status and inhalation injury in burn patients. *Proc Am Burn Assoc.* 1988;20:76.

114. Horwitt MK. Status of human requirements for vitamin E. *Am J Clin Nutr.* 1974;27:1182–1193.

115. Scott ML. Advances in our understanding of vitamin E. *Fed Proc.* 1980;39:2736–2739.

116. London RS, Sundaram GS, Schultz M, Nair PP, et al. Endocrine parameters and alpha tocopherol therapy of patients with mammary dysplasia. *Cancer Res.* 1981;41:3811–3813.

117. Johnson L, Schaffer D, Boggs T, Quinn G, et al. Vitamin E treatment of retrolental fibroplasia grade III or worse. *Pediatr Res.* 1980;14:601.

118. Johnson L, Schaffer D, Boggs TR. The premature infant, vitamin E deficiency and retrolental fibroplasia. *Am J Clin Nutr.* 1974;27:1158–1173.

119. Johnson L, Schaffer D, Quinn G, Goldstein D, et al. Vitamin E supplementation and the retinopathy of prematurity. *Ann N Y Acad Sci.* 1982;393:473–495.

120. Ehrenkranz RA, Bonta BW, Ablow RC, Warshaw JB. Amelioration of bronchopulmonary dysplasia after vitamin E administration: a preliminary report. *N Engl J Med.* 1978;299:564–569.

121. Kline K, Rao A, Romach Eh, Kidao S, et al. Vitamin E modulation of disease resistance and immune responses. *Ann N Y Acad Sci.* 1990;587:294.

122. Wang Y, Huang DS, Liang B, Watson RR. Nutritional status and immune responses in mice with murine AIDS are normalized by vitamin E supplementation. *J Nutr.* 1994;124:2024.

123. Wang Y, Liang B, Watson RR. Normalization of nutritional status by various levels of vitamin E supplementation during retrovirus infection causing murine AIDS. *Nutr Res.* 1994;14:1375.

124. Meydani SN, Meydani M, Verdon CP, Shapiro AA, et al. Vitamin E supplementation suppresses prostaglandin E_2 synthesis and enhances the immune response in aged mice. *Mech Aging Dev.* 1986;34:191.

125. Liang B, Chung S, Araghiniknam M, Lane LC, et al. Vitamins and immunomodulation in AIDS. *Nutr.* 1996;12:1.

126. Farrell PM, Bieri JG. Megavitamin and supplementation in man. *Am J Clin Nutr.* 1975;28:1381–1386.

127. Prasad JS. Effect of vitamin E supplementation on leukocyte function. *Am J Clin Nutr.* 1980;33:606–608.

128. Corrigan JJ, Marcus FI. Coagulopathy associated with vitamin E ingestion. *JAMA.* 1974;230:1300–1301.

129. Diplock AT. Safety of antioxidant vitamins and β-carotene. *Am J Clin Nutr.* 1995;62:1510S–1516S.

130. Suttie JW. The metabolic role of vitamin K. *Fed Proc.* 1980;39:2730–2735.

131. Hauschka PV, Reid ML. Vitamin K dependence of a calcium binding protein containing gamma-carboxyglutamic acid in chicken bone. *J Biol Chem.* 1978;253:9063–9068.

132. Lian JB. Osteocalcin: functional studies and postulated role in bone resorption. In: Suttie JW, ed. *Current Advances in Vitamin K Research.* New York: Elsevier Science Publishers; 1988:245.

133. Price PA. Vitamin K-dependent formation of bone Gla protein (osteocalcin) and its function. *Vitam Horm.* 1985;42:65–108.

134. Binkley NC, Suttie JW. Vitamin K nutrition and osteoporosis. *J Nutr.* 1995;125:1812–1821.

135. Roberts NB, Holding JD, Walsh JPJ, Klenerman L, et al. Serial changes in serum vitamin K, triglyceride, cholesterol, osteocalcin, and 25-hydroxyvitamin D_3 in patients after hip replacement for fractured neck of femur or osteoarthritis. *Eur J Clin Invest.* 1996;26:24–29.

136. Food and Nutrition Board, National Research Council. *Recommended Dietary Allowances.* 10th ed. Washington, DC: National Academy Press, 1989.

137. Jeppson B, Gimmon Z. Vitamins. In: Fischer JE, ed. *Surgical Nutrition.* Boston: Little, Brown & Co; 1983:241–281.

138. American Academy of Pediatrics Committee on Nutrition. Vitamin K supplementation for infants receiving milk substitute infant formulas and for those with fat malabsorption. *Pediatrics.* 1971;48:483–487.

139. Shearer MJ, Barkhan P, Rahim S, Stimmler L. Plasma vitamin K in mothers and their newborn babies. *Lancet.* 1982;2:460–463.

140. Keenan WJ, Jewett T, Glueck HI. Role of feeding and vitamin K in hypoprothrombinemia of the newborn. *Am J Dis Child.* 1971;121:271–277.

141. American Academy of Pediatrics Committee on Nutrition. Vitamin K supplementation for infants receiving milk substitute infant formulas and for those with fat malabsorption. *Pediatrics.* 1971;48:483–487.

142. Hazell K, Baloch KH. Vitamin K deficiency in the elderly. *Gerontol Clin.* 1970;12:10–15.

143. Pineo GF, Gallus AS, Hirsh J. Unexpected vitamin K deficiency in hospitalized patients. *Can Med Assoc J.* 1973;109:880–883.

144. Ansell JE, Kumar R, Deykin D. The spectrum of vitamin K deficiency. *JAMA.* 1977;238:40–42.

145. Hall JG, Pauli RM, Wilson KM. Maternal and fetal sequelae of anticoagulation during pregnancy. *Am J Med.* 1980;68:122–140.

146. O'Reilly RA, Rytand DA. Resistance to warfarin due to unrecognized vitamin K supplementation. *N Engl J Med.* 1980;303:160–161.

147. Gross L, Brotman M. Hypoprothrombinemia and hemorrhage associated with cholestyramine therapy. *Ann Intern Med.* 1970;72:95–96.

148. Blanchard RA, Furie BC, Jorgenson M, Kruger SF, et al. Acquired vitamin K-dependent carboxylation deficiency in liver disease. *N Engl J Med.* 1981;305:242–248.

149. Jenkins M, Gottschlich MM, Khoury J, Warden GD. A prospective analysis of serum vitamin K in severely burned pediatric patients. *J Burn Care Rehabil.* In press.

150. Didisheim P. Screening tests for bleeding disorders. *Am J Clin Pathol.* 1967;47:622–630.

151. Sokoll LJ, Sadowski JA. Comparison of biochemical indexes for assessing vitamin K nutritional status in a healthy adult population. *Am J Clin Nutr.* 1996;63:566–573.

152. Sokoll LJ, O'Brien ME, Camilo ME, Sadowski J. Undercarboxylated osteocalcin and development of a method to determine vitamin K status. *Clin Chem.* 1995;41:1128.

153. Stryer L. *Biochemistry.* New York: WH Freeman & Co; 1988.

154. Itokaiva Y, Schulz RA, Cooper JR. Thiamine in nerve membranes. *Biochim Biophys Acta.* 1972;266:293–299.

155. Sauberlich HE. Biochemical alterations in thiamine deficiency: their interpretation. *Am J Clin Nutr.* 1967;20:528–542.

156. Victor M, Adams RD. On the etiology of the alcoholic neurologic diseases, with special reference to the role of nutrition. *Am J Clin Nutr.* 1961;9:379–397.

157. Lund CC, Levenson SM, Green RW, Grueber FS, et al. Ascorbic acid, thiamine, riboflavin and nicotinic acid in relation to acute burns in man. *Arch Surg.* 1947;55:557–583.

158. Christakis G, Miridjanian A. Diets, drugs and their interrelationships. *J Am Diet Assoc.* 1968;52:21–24.

159. Kramer J, Goodwin JA. Wernicke's encephalopathy: complication of intravenous hyperalimentation. *JAMA.* 1977;238:2176–2177.

160. Nadel AM, Burger PC. Wernicke encephalopathy following prolonged intravenous therapy. *JAMA.* 1976;235:2403–2405.

161. Blennow G. Wernicke encephalopathy following prolonged artificial nutrition. *Am J Dis Child.* 1976;129:1456.

162. Stromberg P, Shenkin A, Campbell RA, Spooner RJ, et al. Vitamin status during total parenteral nutrition. *J Parenter Enter Nutr.* 1981;5:295–299.

163. Campbell C. The severe lactic acidosis of thiamine deficiency: acute pernicious or fulminating beriberi. *Lancet.* 1984;2:446.

164. Mad LC, Kranz A, Liebisch B, Traindl O, et al. Lactic acidosis in thiamine deficiency. *Clin Nutr.* 1993;12:108.

165. Leveille GA. Modified thiochrome procedure for the determination of urinary thiamin. *Am J Clin Nutr.* 1972;25:273–274.

166. Warnock LG. A new approach to erythrocyte transketolase measurement. *J Nutr.* 1970; 100:1057–1062.

167. Shibata K, Murata K. Blood NAD as an index of niacin nutrition. *Nutr Int.* 1986;2:177–181.

168. Sauberlich HE, Herman YF, Stevens CO, Herman RH. Thiamin requirements of the adult human. *Am J Clin Nutr.* 1979;32:2237–2248.

169. Zbinden G. Therapeutic use of vitamin B1 diseases other than beriberi. *Ann N Y Acad Sci.* 1962;98:550–561.

170. Howard L, Bigaouette J, Chu R, Krenzer BE, et al. Water soluble vitamin requirements in home parenteral nutrition patients. *Am J Clin Nutr.* 1983;37:421–428.

171. Broviac JW, Scriber BH. Prolonged parenteral nutrition in the home. *Surg Gynecol Obstet.* 1974;139:24–28.

172. Jeejeebhoy KN, Langer B, Tsallas G, Chu RC, et al. Total parenteral nutrition at home: studies in patients surviving four months to five years. *Gastroenterology.* 1976;71:943–953.

173. Dudrick SJ, MacFayden BV, Souches EA, Englert DM, et al. Parenteral nutrition techniques in cancer patients. *Cancer Res.* 1977;37:2440–2450.

174. Rivlin RS. Riboflavin metabolism. *N Engl J Med.* 1970;283:463–472.

175. Rosenthal WS, Adham NF, Lopez R, et al. Riboflavin deficiency in complicated chronic alcoholism. *Am J Clin Nutr.* 1973;26:858–860.

176. Pinto J, Huang YP, Rivlin RS. Inhibition of riboflavin metabolism in rat tissues by chlorpromazine, imipramine and amitriptyline. *J Clin Invest.* 1981;67:1500–1506.

177. Newman LR, Lopez R, Cole HS, Boria MC, et al. Riboflavin deficiency in women taking oral contraceptive agents. *Am J Clin Nutr.* 1978;31:247–249.

178. Roe DA, Bogusz S, Sheu J, McCormick DB. Factors affecting riboflavin requirements of oral contraceptive users and nonusers. *Am J Clin Nutr.* 1982;35:495–501.

179. Lewis CM, King JC. Effect of oral contraceptive agents on thiamin, riboflavin, and pantothenic acid status in young women. *Am J Clin Nutr.* 1980;33:832–838.

180. Olpin SE, Bates CJ. Lipid metabolism in riboflavin status deficient rats: effect of dietary lipids on riboflavin status and fatty acid profiles. *Br J Nutr.* 1982;47:577–588.

181. Pinto J, Dutta P, Rivlin R. Alterations in age-related decline of β-adrenergic receptor binding in adipocytes during riboflavin deficiency. *Clin Res.* 1985;33:526A.

182. Sydenstricker VP, Sebrell WH, Cleckley HM, Kruse SE. The ocular manifestations of ariboflavinosis. *JAMA.* 1940;114:2437–2445.

183. Belko AZ, Obarznak E, Kalkway HJ, Rotter BS, et al. Effects of exercise on riboflavin requirements of young women. *Am J Clin Nutr.* 1983;37:509.

184. Trebler-Winters LR, Yoon J-S, Kalkway HJ, Chalfin-Davies J, et al. Riboflavin requirements and exercise adaptation in older women. *Am J Clin Nutr.* 1992;56:526.

185. Carter EGA. Quantitation of urinary niacin metabolites by reversed phase liquid chromatography. *Am J Clin Nutr.* 1982;36:926–930.

186. Sriram K, Suchitra VJ. Acute niacin deficiency. *J Nutr.* 1996;12:355.

187. Basu TK, Raven RW, Bates C, Williams DC. Excretion of 5-hydroxyindole acetic acid and N'-methylnicotinamide in advanced cancer patients. *Eur J Cancer.* 1973;9:527–528.

188. Barlow GB, Sutton JL, Wilkinson AW. Metabolism of nicotinic acid in children with burns and scalds. *Clin Chim Acta.* 1977;75:337–342.

189. Hilton JG, Wells CH. Nicotinic acid reduction of plasma volume after thermal trauma. *Science.* 1976;191:861–862.

190. Horwitt MK, Harper AE, Henderson LM. Niacin-tryptophan relationships for evaluating niacin equivalents. *Am J Clin Nutr.* 1981;34:423–427.

191. Jacobs RA, Swendseid ME, McKee RW, Fu CS, et al. Biochemical markers for assessment of niacin status in young men: urinary and blood levels of niacin metabolites *J Nutr.* 1989;119:591.

192. Rombeau JL, Rolandelli RH, Wilmore DW. Nutritional support. In: Wilmore DW, et al, eds. *Scientific American Surgery, Perioperative Management and Surgical Technique.* New York: Scientific American Inc; 1994;1.

193. Shepherd J, Packard CJ, Potseh JR, Grotto AM, et al. Effects of nicotinic acid therapy on plasma high density lipoprotein subfraction distribution and composition and on apolipoprotein A metabolism. *J Clin Invest.* 1979;63:858–867.

194. Levy RI, Fredrickson DS, Shulmon R, Bilheimer DW, et al. Dietary and drug treatment of primary hyperlipoproteinemia. *Ann Intern Med.* 1972;77:267–294.

195. Chandra RK, Au B, Heresi G. Single nutrient deficiency and cell-mediated immune responses, II: pyridoxine. *Nutr Res.* 1981;1:101–106.

196. Axelrod AE, Trakatellis AC. Relationship of pyridoxine to immunological phenomena. *Vitam Horm.* 1964;22:591–607.

197. Weintraub LR, Conrad ME, Crosby WH. Iron-loading anemia treatment with repeated phlebotomies and pyridoxine. *N Engl J Med.* 1966;275:169–176.

198. Hines JD, Harris JW. Pyridoxine-responsive anemia: description of three patients with megaloblastic erythropoiesis. *Am J Clin Nutr.* 1964;14:137–146.

199. Sauberlich HE, Canham JE, Baker EM, Raica N, et al. Biochemical assessment of the nutritional status of vitamin B6 in the human. *Am J Clin Nutr.* 1972;25:629–642.

200. Greenberg LD, Bohr DF, McGrath H, Rinehart JF. Xanthurenic acid excretion in the human subject on a pyridoxine-deficient diet. *Arch Biochem.* 1949;21:237–239.

201. Linkswiler H. Biochemical and physiological changes in vitamin B6 deficiency. *Am J Clin Nutr.* 1967;20:547–557.

202. Coursin DB. Recommendations for standardization of the tryptophan load test. *Am J Clin Nutr.* 1964;14:56–61.

203. Baysal A, Johnson BA, Linkswiler H. Vitamin B6 depletion in man: blood vitamin B6, plasma pyridoxal-phosphate, serum cholesterol, serum transaminases and urinary vitamin B6 and 4-pyridoxic acid. *J Nutr.* 1966;89:19–23.

204. Cinnamon AD, Beaton JR. Biochemical assessment of vitamin B6 status in man. *Am J Clin Nutr.* 1970;23:696–702.

205. Cheney M, Sabry ZI, Beaton GH. Erythrocyte glutamic-pyruvic transaminase activity in man. *Am J Clin Nutr.* 1965;16:337–338.

206. Roepke J, Kirksey A. Vitamin B₆ nutriture during pregnancy and lactation, I: vitamin B₆ intake levels of the vitamin in biological fluids and condition of the infant at birth. *Am J Clin Nutr.* 1979;32:2249–2256.

207. Kopple JD, Swendseid ME. Vitamin nutrition in patients undergoing maintenance hemodialysis. *Kidney Int.* 1975;7(suppl):79–84.

208. Barlow GB, Wilkinson AW. Plasma pyridoxal phosphate levels and tryptophan metabolism in children with burns and scalds. *Clin Chim Acta.* 1975;64:79–82.

209. Rose CS, Gyorgy P, Butler M, Andres R, et al. Age differences in vitamin B₆ status of 617 men. *Am J Clin Nutr.* 1976;29:847–853.

210. Potera C, Rose DP, Brown RR. Vitamin B₆ deficiency in cancer patients. *Am J Clin Nutr.* 1977;30:1677–1679.

211. Reynolds RD, Natta CL. Depressed plasma pyridoxal phosphate concentrations in adult asthmatics. *Am J Clin Nutr.* 1985;41:684–688.

212. Baker H, Frank O, Zetterman RK, Rajan KS, et al. Inability of chronic alcoholics with liver disease to use food as a source of folates, thiamin and vitamin B₆. *Am J Clin Nutr.* 1975;28:1377–1380.

213. Bender DA, Russell-Jones R. Isoniazid induced pellagra despite vitamin B₆ supplementation. *Lancet.* 1979;2:1125–1126.

214. Roepke J, Kirksey A. Vitamin B₆ nutriture during pregnancy and lactation, II: the effect of long-term use of oral contraceptives. *Am J Clin Nutr.* 1979;32:2257–2264.

215. Menzies R, Crossen PE, Fitzgerald PH, Gunz FW. Cytogenic and cytochemical studies on marrow cells in folate deficiency. *Blood.* 1966;28:581–594.

216. Leevy CM, Cardi L, Frank O, Gellene R, et al. Incidence and significance of hypovitaminosis in a randomly selected hospital population. *Am J Clin Nutr.* 1965;17:259–271.

217. Herbert V. Megaloblastic anemia as a problem in world health. *Am J Clin Nutr.* 1968;21:1115–1120.

218. Girwood RH. Folate depletion in old age. *Am J Clin Nutr.* 1969;22:234–237.

219. Hampers CL, Streiff R, Nathan DG, Merrill JP. Megaloblastic hematopoiesis in uremia and in patients on long term hemodialysis. *N Engl J Med.* 1967;276:551–554.

220. Whitehead VM, Comty CH, Posen GA, Kaye M. Homeostasis of folic acid in patients undergoing hemodialysis. *N Engl J Med.* 1968;279:970–974.

221. Markkanen T. Absorption tests with natural folate material in controls and in gastrectomized patients. *Am J Clin Nutr.* 1968;21:473–481.

222. Mollin DL, Hines JD. Observations on the nature and pathogenesis of anemia following partial gastrectomy. *Proc R Soc Med.* 1964;57:575–580.

223. Hoffbrand AV, Necheles TF, Maldonado N, Horta E, et al. Malabsorption of folate polyglutamate in tropical sprue. *Br Med J.* 1969;2:543–547.

224. Druskins MS, Wallen MH, Bonagura L. Anticonvulsant associated megaloblastic anemia. *N Engl J Med.* 1962;267:483–485.

225. Waxman S, Corcino JJ, Herbert V. Drugs, toxins and dietary amino acids affecting folic acid absorption on utilization. *Am J Med.* 1970;48:599–608.

226. Gerson CD, Hepner GW, Cohen N, Butterworth CE, et al. Inhibition of diphenylhydration on folic acid absorption in man. *J Clin Invest.* 1970;49:33. Abstract.

227. Halstead CH, Robles EA, Mezey E. Decreased jejunal uptake of labeled folic acid in alcoholic patients: roles of alcohol and nutrition. *N Engl J Med.* 1971;285:701–706.

228. Herbert V, Zalusk R, Davidson CS. Correlating folate deficiency with alcoholism and associated macrocytosis, anemia and liver disease. *Ann Intern Med.* 1963;58:977–988.

229. Shah PC, Zafar M, Patel AR. Folate deficiency during intravenous hyperalimentation. *J Med Clin Exp Theor.* 1977;8:383–392.

230. Hartshorn EA. Food and drug interactions. *J Am Diet Assoc.* 1977;70:15–19.

231. Halstead CH, Harris JW. The effect of alcoholism on the absorption of folic acid evaluated by plasma levels and urine excretion. *J Lab Clin Med.* 1967;69:116–131.

232. Halsted CH, Robles EA, Mezey E. Intestinal malabsorption in folate deficient alcoholics. *Gastroenterology.* 1973;64:526–532.

233. Sullivan LW, Herbert V. Suppression of hematopoiesis by ethanol. *J Clin Invest.* 1964;43:2048–2062.

234. Hellman S, Iannitti AT, Bertino JR. Determinations of the levels of serum folate in patients with carcinoma of the head and neck treated with methotrexate. *Cancer Res.* 1964;24:105–113.

235. Werkheiser WC. The biochemical, cellular and pharmacological action of folic acid antagonists. *Cancer Res.* 1963;23:1277–1285.

236. Lieberman FL, Bateman JR. Megaloblastic anemia posssibly induced by triamterene in patients with alcoholic cirrhosis. *Ann Intern Med.* 1976;68:168–173.

237. Necheles TF, Snyder LM. Malabsorption of folate polyglutamates associated with oral contraceptive therapy. *N Engl J Med.* 1970;282:858–859.

238. Streiff R. Folate deficiency and oral contraceptives. *JAMA.* 1970;214:105–108.

239. Stephens ME. Oral contraceptives and folate metabolism. *Clin Sci.* 1972;42:405–414.

240. Barlow GB, Wilkinson AW. 4"-amino-imidazole-5-carboxamide excretion and folate status with burns and scalds. *Clin Chim Acta.* 1970;29:355–358.

241. Steinberg D. Folic acid deficiency: early onset of megaloblastosis. *JAMA.* 1972;222:490.

242. Alperin JB, Hutchinson HI, Levin WC. Studies of folic acid requirements in megaloblastic anemia of pregnancy. *Arch Intern Med.* 1966;117:681–688.

243. Reid DJ, Barr SL, Leichter J. Effects of folate and zinc supplementation on patients undergoing chronic hemodialysis. *J Am Diet Assoc.* 1992;92:574.

244. Hine RJ. Folic acid: contemporary clinical perspective. *Perspect Appl Nutr.* 1993;1:3–14.

245. Milunsky A, Jick H, Jick SS, Bruell CL, et al. Multivitamin/folic acid supplementation in early pregnancy reduces the risk of neural type defects. *JAMA.* 1989;262:2847.

246. Czeizel AE, Dudas I. Prevention of the first occurrence of neural tube defects by periconceptional vitamin supplementation. *N Engl J Med.* 1992;327:1832.

247. Butterworth CE. Effect of folate on cervical cancer: synergism among risk factors. *Ann N Y Acad Sci.* 1992;669:293–313.

248. Giovannucci E, Stampfer MJ, Colditz GA, Rimm EB, et al. Folate, methionine and alcohol intake and risk of colorectal cancer. *J Natl Cancer Inst.* 1993;85:875.

249. Frevdenheim JL, Graham S, Marshall JR, Haughey BP, et al. Folate intake and carcinogenesis of the colon and rectum. *Int J Epidemiol.* 1991;20:368.

250. Jaskiewicz K, Marasas WFO, Lazarus C, Campbell NRC, et al. Association of esophageal cytological abnormalities with vitamin and lipotrope deficiencies in populations at risk for esophageal cancer. *Anticancer Res.* 1988;8:871.

251. Butterworth CE, Hatch K, Macaluso M, Cole P, et al. Folate deficiency and cervical dysplasia. *JAMA.* 1992;267:528.

252. Herbert V. Biochemical and hematologic lesions in folic acid deficiency. *Am J Clin Nutr.* 1967;20:562–569.

253. Varadi S, Abbot D, Elwis A. Correlation of peripheral white cell and bone marrow changes with folate levels in pregnancy and their clinical significance. *J Clin Pathol.* 1966;19:33–36.

254. Clark R, Daly L, Robinson, CP Suel NM, et al. Hyperhomocysteinemia: an independent risk factor for vascular diseases. *N Engl J Med.* 1991;349:1149.

255. Herbert V. Nutritional requirements for vitamins B_{12} and folic acid. *Am J Clin Nutr.* 1968;21:743–752.

256. Kahn SB. Recent advances in the nutritional anemias. *Med Clin North Am.* 1970;54:631–645.

257. Hoffbrand AV, Newcombe BF, Mollin DL. Method of assay of red cell folate activity and the value of the assay as a test for folate deficiency. *J Clin Pathol.* 1966;19:17–28.

258. Campbell NRC. How safe are folic acid supplements. *Arch Intern Med.* 1996;156:1638.

259. Winawer SJ, Steiff R, Zamchek N. Gastric and hematological abnormalities in a vegan with nutritional vitamin B_{12} deficiency: effect of oral vitamin B_{12}. *Gastroenterology.* 1967;53:130–135.

260. Baker SJ. Human vitamin B_{12} deficiency. *World Rev Nutr Diet.* 1967;8:52–69.

261. Boylan LM, Sugerman HJ, Driskell JA. Vitamin E, vitamin B_6, vitamin B_{12} and folate status of gastric bypass surgery patients. *J Am Diet Assoc.* 1988;88:579–585.

262. Boddy K, Adams JF. The long-term relationship between serum vitamin B_{12} and total body vitamin B_{12}. *Am J Clin Nutr.* 1972;25:395–400.

263. Kramer GM, Dillios LC, Bowler EC. Ascorbic acid treatment on early collagen production and wound healing in the guinea pig. *J Periodontol.* 1979;50:189.

264. Sengupta KP, Deb SK. Role of vitamin C in collagen synthesis. *Indian J Exp Biol.* 1978;16:1061.

265. Cook JD, Monsen ER. Vitamin C, the common cold and iron absorption. *Am J Clin Nutr.* 1977;30:235–241.

266. Thomas WR, Holt PG. Vitamin C and immunity: an assessment of the evidence. *Clin Exp Immunol.* 1978;32:370–379.

267. Block G. Vitamin C and cancer prevention: the epidemiologic evidence. *Am J Clin Nutr.* 1991;53:270S.

268. Hodges RE, Hood J, Canham JE, Sauberlich HE, et al. Clinical manifestation of ascorbic acid deficiency in man. *Am J Clin Nutr.* 1971;24:432–443.

269. Jacob RA, Skala JH, Omaye ST. Biochemical indices of human vitamin C status. *Am J Clin Nutr.* 1987;46:818–826.

270. Pearson WN. Biochemical appraisal of the vitamin nutritional status in man. *JAMA.* 1962;180:49–55.

271. Denson KW, Bowers EF. The determination of ascorbic acid in white blood cells. *Clin Sci.* 1961;21:157–162.

272. Pelletier O. Vitamin C status of cigarette smokers and nonsmokers. *Am J Clin Nutr.* 1970;23:520–524.

273. Bates CJ, Rutishauser I, Black AE, Paul AA. Long-term vitamin status and dietary intake of healthy elderly subjects. *Br J Nutr.* 1977;42:43–55.

274. Rivers JM, Devine MM. Plasma ascorbic acid concentrations and oral contraceptives. *Am J Clin Nutr.* 1972;25:684–689.

275. Crandon JH, Lennihan R, Mikal S, Reif AE. Ascorbic acid economy in surgical patients. *Ann N Y Acad Sci.* 1961;92:246–267.

276. Irvin TT, Chattopadhyay DK, Smythe A. Ascorbic acid requirements in postoperative patients. *Surg Gynecol Obstet.* 1978;147:49–55.

277. Cameron E, Pauling L, Leibowitz B. Ascorbic acid and cancer: a review. *Cancer Res.* 1979;39:663–681.

278. Schorah CJ, Downing C, Piripitsi A, Gallivan L, et al. Total vitamin C, ascorbic acid, and dehydroascorbic acid concentrations in plasma of critically ill patients. *Am J Clin Nutr.* 1996;63:760–765.

279. Sydenstricker VP, Singl SA, Briggs AP, DeVaughn NM, et al. Observations on the egg white injury in man and its cure with a biotin concentrate. *JAMA.* 1942;118:1199–1200.

280. Baugh CM, Malone JH, Butterworth CE. Human biotin deficiency: a case history of biotin deficiency induced by raw egg consumption in a cirrhotic patient. *Am J Clin Nutr.* 1968;21:173–182.

281. Sweetman L, Suhr L, Baker H, Peterson RM, et al. Clinical and metabolic abnormalities in a boy with dietary deficiency of biotin. *Pediatrics.* 1981;68:553–558.

282. Markkanen T. Studies on the urinary excretion of thiamine, riboflavin, nicotinic acid, pantothenic acid and biotin in achlorhydria and after partial gastrectomy. *Acta Med Scand.* 1960;360 (suppl):1–56.

283. Barlow GB, Dickerson JA, Wilkinson AW. Plasma biotin levels in children with burns and scalds. *J Clin Pathol.* 1976;29:58–59.

284. Bhagavan HN, Coursin DB. Biotin content of blood in normal infants and adults. *Am J Clin Nutr.* 1967;20:903–906.

285. McClain GJ, Baker H, Onstad GR. Biotin deficiency in an adult during home parenteral nutrition. *JAMA.* 1962;247:3116–3117.

286. Carlson GL, Williams N, Barber D, Shaffer JL, et al. Biotin deficiency complicating long-term total parenteral nutrition in an adult patient. *Clin Nutr.* 1995;14:186.

287. Matsuse S, Kashihara S, Takeda H, Koizumi S. Biotin deficiency during total parenteral nutrition: its clinical manifestation and plasma nonesterified fatty acid level. *J Parenter Enter Nutr.* 1985;9:760–763.

288. Thoene J, Baker H, Yoshino M, Sweetman L. Biotin-responsive carboxylase deficiency associated with subnormal plasma and urinary biotin. *N Engl J Med.* 1981;304:817.

289. Nichoalds GE, Luther RW, Sykes TR, Kinney JM, et al. Biotin status of adult TPN patients. *J Parenter Enter Nutr.* 1982;6:577.

290. Novelli GD. Metabolic functions of pantothenic acid. *Physiol Rev.* 1953;33:525–543.

291. Pugh EL, Wakil SJ. Studies on the mechanism of fatty acid synthesis, XIV: the prosthetic group of acyl carrier protein and its mode of attachment of the protein. *J Biol Chem.* 1965;240:4727–4733.

292. Hodges RE, Beam WB, Ohlson MA, Bleiler RE. Factors affecting human antibody response, III: immunologic responses of men deficient in pantothenic acid. *Am J Clin Nutr.* 1962;11:85–93.

293. Axelrod AE, Hopper S. Effects of pantothenic acid, pyridoxine and thiamine deficiencies upon antibody formation to influenza virus PR-8 in rats. *J Nutr.* 1960;72:325–330.

294. Kerry E, Crispin S, Fox HM, Kies C. Nutritional status of preschool children, I: dietary and biochemical finding. *Am J Clin Nutr.* 1968;21:1274–1279.

295. Lubin R, Daum KA, Beam WB. Studies of pantothenic acid metabolism. *Am J Clin Nutr.* 1956;4:420–433.

296. Fox HM, Linkswiler H, Geschwender D. Effect of altering the pantothenic acid intake on the urinary excretion of this vitamin. *Fed Proc.* 1959;18:525.

297. Kies C, Wishart C, McGee M, Foss Z, et al. Pantothenic acid levels in urine, blood serum and whole blood of adult humans fed graded levels of pantothenic acid. *Fed Proc.* 1982;41:276.

298. Ellestad JJ, Nelson RA, Adson MA, Palmer WM. Pantothenic acid and coenzyme A activity in blood and colonic mucosa from patients with chronic ulcerative colitis. *Fed Proc.* 1970;29:820.

299. Song WO, Wyse BW, Hansen RG. Pantothenic acid status of pregnant and lactating women. *J Am Diet Assoc.* 1985;85:192–198.

300. Cohenour SH, Calloway DH. Blood, urine and dietary pantothenic acid levels of pregnant teenagers. *Am J Clin Nutr.* 1972;25:512–517.

301. Aprahamian M, Dentinger A, Stock-Damge C, Kouassi J, et al. Effects of supplemental pantothenic acid on wound healing: experimental study in rabbits. *Am J Clin Nutr.* 1985;41:578–589.

302. Eckhert CD, Hurley LS. Reduced DNA synthesis in zinc deficiency: regional differences in embryonic rats. *J Nutr.* 1977;107:855–861.

303. Rahmat A, Norman JN, Smith G. The effect of zinc deficiency on wound healing. *Br J Surg.* 1974;61:271–273.

304. Lennard ES, Bjornson AB, Petering HG, Alexander JW. An immunologic and nutritional evaluation of burn neutrophil function. *J Surg Res.* 1974;16:286–298.

305. Chandra RK, Au B. Single nutrient deficiency and cell-mediated immune responses, I: zinc. *Am J Clin Nutr.* 1980;33:736–738.

306. Fernandes G, Nair M, Onoe K, Tanaka T, et al. Impairment of cell-mediated immunity functions by dietary zinc deficiency in mice. *Proc Natl Acad Sci.* 1979;76:457–461.

307. Pekarek RS, Sandstead HH, Jacob RA, Barcome DF. Abnormal cellular immune response during acquired zinc deficiency. *Am J Clin Nutr.* 1979;32:1466–1471.

308. Briggs WA, Pederson MM, Mahajan SK, Dale HS, et al. Lymphocyte and granulocyte function in zinc-treated and zinc deficient hemodialysis patients. *Kidney Int.* 1982;21:827–832.

309. Cohen IK, Schechter PJ, Henkin RI. Hypogeusia, anorexia and altered zinc metabolism following thermal burn. *JAMA.* 1973;223:914–916.

310. Henkin RI, Schechter PJ, Hoye R, Mattern CFT. Idiopathic hypogeusia, with dysgeusia, hyposmia, and dysomia. *JAMA.* 1971;217:434–440.

311. Hambidge KM, Hambidge C, Jacobs M, Baum JD. Low levels of zinc in hair, anorexia, poor growth and hypogeusia in children. *Pediatr Res.* 1972;6:868–874.

312. Huber AM, Gershoff SN. Effects of zinc deficiency on the oxidation of retinol and ethanol in rats. *J Nutr.* 1975;105:1486–1490.

313. Halsted JA, Smith JC, Irwin MI. A conspectus of research on zinc requirements of man. *J Nutr.* 1974;104:345–378.

314. Solomons NW, Russell RM. The interaction of vitamin A and zinc: implications for human nutrition. *Am J Clin Nutr.* 1980;33:2031–2040.

315. Kay RG, Tasman-Jones C, Pybus J, Whiting R, et al. A syndrome of acute zinc deficiency during total parenteral alimentation in man. *Ann Surg.* 1976;183:331–340.

316. Weber TR, Sears N, Davis B, Grosfeld JL. Clinical spectrum of zinc deficiency in pediatric patients receiving total parenteral nutrition (TPN). *J Pediatr Surg.* 1981;16:236–240.

317. Tucker SB, Schroeter AL, Brown PW, McCall JT. Acquired zinc deficiency. *JAMA.* 1976;235:2399–2402.

318. Arakawa T, Tamura T, Igaraski Y, Suzuki H, et al. Zinc deficiency in two infants during total parenteral alimentation for diarrhea. *Am J Clin Nutr.* 1976;29:197–204.

319. Strobel CT, Byrne WJ, Abramavits W, Newcomer VJ, et al. A zinc deficiency dermatitis in patients on total parenteral nutrition. *Int J Dermatol.* 1978;17:575–581.

320. Gang RK. Adhesive zinc tape in burns: results of a clinical trial. *Burns.* 1981;7:322–325.

321. Hanzel JW, DeWeese MS, Lichti EL. Zinc concentrations within healing wounds. *Arch Surg.* 1970;100:349–357.

322. Pories WJ, Henzel JH, Robb CG, Strain WH. Acceleration of wound healing in man with zinc sulfate given by mouth. *Lancet.* 1967;1:121–124.

323. Solomons N, Rosenfield RL, Jacob RA, Sandstead HH. Growth retardation and zinc nutrition. *Pediatr Res.* 1976;10:923–927.

324. Butrimovitz GP, Purdy WC. Zinc nutrition and growth in a childhood population. *Am J Clin Nutr.* 1978;31:1409–1412.

325. Cossack ZT. Decline in somatomedin-C (insulin like growth factor-1) with experimentally induced zinc deficiency in human subjects. *Clin Nutr.* 1991;10:284.

326. Dorup I, Flyvbrjerg A, Everts ME, Clausen T. Role of insulin-like growth factor-1 and growth hormone in growth inhibition induced by magnesium and zinc deficiencies. *Br Med J.* 1991;66:505.

327. Ninh NX, Thissen JP, Maiter D, Adam E, et al. Reduced liver insulin-like growth factor-1 gene expression in young zinc deprived rats is associated with a decrease in liver growth hormone (GH) receptors and serum GH-binding protein. *J Endocrinol.* 1995;144:449.

328. Ninh NX, Thissen JP, Collette L, Gerard G, et al. Zinc supplementation increases growth and circulating insulin-like growth factor-1 (IGF-1) in growth retarded Vietnamese children. *Am J Clin Nutr.* 1996;63:514.

329. Pekarek RS, Wannemacher RW, Chapple FE, Powanda MC, et al. Further characterization and species specificity of leukocyte endogenous mediator (LEM). *Proc Soc Exp Biol Med.* 1972;141:643–648.

330. Falchuk HH. Effect of acute disease and ACTH on serum zinc proteins. *N Engl J Med.* 1977;296:1129–1134.

331. Dinarello CA. Interleukin-1. *Rev Infect Dis.* 1984;6:51–93.

332. Vallee BL, Gibson JG. The zinc content of normal human whole blood, plasma, leukocytes and erythrocytes. *J Biol Chem.* 1948;176:445–457.

333. Naber THJ, Heymer F, Van Der Hamer CJA, Van Der Broek WJM, et al. The in-vitro uptake of zinc by blood cells in rats with long term inflammatory stress. *Clin Nutr.* 1994;13:247.

334. Nielson SP, Jemec B. Zinc metabolism in patients with severe burns. *Scand J Plast Reconstr Surg.* 1968;2:47–52.

335. Carr G, Wilkinson AW. Zinc and copper urinary excretions in children with burns and scalds. *Clin Chim Acta.* 1975;61:199–204.

336. Shakespeare PG. Studies on the serum levels of iron, copper and zinc and the urinary excretion of zinc after burn injury. *Burns.* 1982;8:358–364.

337. Moser PB, Borel J, Majerus T, Anderson RA. Serum zinc and urinary zinc excretion of trauma patients. *Nutr Res.* 1985;5:253–261.

338. Castilo-Duran C, Gardia H, Venegas P, Torreal BAI, et al. Zinc supplementation increases growth velocity of male children and adolescents with short stature. *Acta Paediatr.* 1994;83:833.

339. Gibson RS, Heywood A, Yaman C, Sohlstrom A, et al. Growth in children from the Wosera subdistrict, Papua New Guinea, in relation to energy and protein intake and zinc status. *Am J Clin Nutr.* 1991;53:782.

340. Cavan KR, Gibson RS, Grazioso CF, Isalgue AM, et al. Growth and body composition of periurban Guatemalan children in relation to zinc status: a cross-sectional study. *Am J Clin Nutr.* 1993;57:334.

341. Okada A, Takagi Y, Itakura T, Satani M, et al. Skin lesions during intravenous hyperalimentation: zinc deficiency. *Surgery.* 1976;80:629–635.

342. Latimer JS, McClain CJ, Sharp HL. Clinical zinc deficiency during zinc-supplemented parenteral nutrition. *J Pediatr.* 1980;97:434–437.

343. Younaszi HD. Clinical zinc deficiency in total parenteral nutrition: zinc supplementation. *J Parenter Enter Nutr.* 1983;7:72–74.

344. McClain CJ, Le-Chu S, Gilbert H, Cameron P. Zinc deficiency induced retinal dysfunction in chronic disease. *Dig Dis Sci.* 1983;28:85–87.

345. Oberleas D, Harland BF. Phytate content of foods: effect on dietary zinc bioavailability. *J Am Diet Assoc.* 1981;79:433–436.

346. Lyle WH. Penicillamine and zinc. *Lancet.* 1974;2:1140.

347. Hunt IF, Murphy NJ, Cleaver AE, Faraji B, et al. Zinc supplementation during pregnancy: zinc concentration of serum and hair from low-income women of Mexican descent. *Am J Clin Nutr.* 1983;37:572–582.

348. Krieger I, Alpern BE, Cunnane SC. Transient neonatal zinc deficiency. *Am J Clin Nutr.* 1986;43:955–958.

349. Pochon JP, Kloeti J. Zinc and copper replacement therapy in children with deep burns. *Burns.* 1978;5:123–126.

350. Mossad SB, Macknin ML, Medendorp SV, Mason P. Zinc gluconate lozenges for treating the common cold: a randomized, double-blind, placebo-controlled study. *Ann Intern Med.* 1996;125:81–88.

351. Godfrey JC, Conant-Sloane B, Smith DS, Turco JH, et al. Zinc gluconate and the common cold: a controlled clinical study. *J Int Med Res.* 1992;20:234–246.

352. Pennington JAT. Nutritional elements in U.S. diets: results from the total diet study, 1982 to 1986. *J Am Diet Assoc.* 1989;89:659–664.

353. Hooper PL, Visconti L, Garry PJ, Johnson GE. Zinc lowers high density lipoprotein-cholesterol levels. *JAMA.* 1980;244:1960–1961.

354. Chandra RK. Excessive intake of zinc impairs immune responses. *JAMA.* 1984;252:1443–1446.

355. Evans GW. Copper homeostasis in the mammalian system. *Physiol Rev.* 1973;53:535–570.

356. Carnes WH. Role of copper in connective tissue metabolism. *Fed Proc.* 1971;30:995–1000.

357. McCord JM, Fridovich I. Superoxide dismutase: an enzymatic function for erythrocuprein. *J Biol Chem.* 1969;244:6049–6055.

358. Pomerantz SH. Separation, purification and properties of two tyrominases from hamster melanoma. *J Biol Chem.* 1963;238:2351–2357.

359. Osaki S, Johnson DA, Frieden E. The possible significance of the ferrous oxidase activity of ceruloplasmin in normal human serum. *J Biol Chem.* 1966;241:2746–2751.

360. Maddox IS. The role of copper in prostaglandin synthesis. *Biochim Biophys Acta.* 1973;306: 74–81.

361. Danks DM. Copper deficiency in humans. *Ann Rev Nutr.* 1988;8:235–237.

362. Henkin RI, Keiser HR, Jaffe IA. Decreased taste sensitivity after D-penicillamine reversed by copper administration. *Lancet.* 1967;2:1268–1271.

363. Karpel JT, Peden VH. Copper deficiency in long-term parenteral nutrition. *J Pediatr.* 1972;80:32–36.

364. Heller RM, Kirchner SG, O'Neill JA, Hough AJ, et al. Skeletal changes of copper deficiency in infants receiving prolonged total parenteral nutrition. *J Pediatr.* 1978;92:947–949.

365. Brian JE, Caldwell FT, Woody RC, Bowser-Wallace BH. Hypocupremia in a major burn. *J Trauma.* 1987;27:335–336.

366. Koller LD, Mulhern SA, Frankel NC, Steven MG, et al. Immune dysfunction in rats fed a diet deficient in copper. *Am J Clin Nutr.* 1987;45:997–1006.

367. Prohaska JR, Lukasewycz OA. Copper deficiency suppresses the immune response of mice. *Science.* 1981;213:559–561.

368. Dunlop WM, James GW III, Hume DM. Anemia and neutropenia caused by copper deficiency. *Ann Intern Med.* 1974;80:470–476.

369. Vilter RW, Bozian RC, Hess EV, Zellner DC, et al. Manifestations of copper deficiency in a patient with systemic sclerosis on intravenous hyperalimentation. *N Engl J Med.* 1974;291:188–191.

370. Sriram K, O'Gara JA, Strunk JR, Peterson JK. Neutropenia due to copper deficiency in total parenteral nutrition. *J Parenter Enter Nutr.* 1986;10:530–532.

371. Lynch SM, Frei B. Mechanisms of copper and iron dependent oxidative modification of human low density lipoprotein. *J Lipid Res.* 1993;34:1745–1753.

372. Pekarek RS, Powanda MC, Wannemacher RW. The effect of leukocytic endogenous mediator (LEM) on serum copper and ceruloplasmin concentrations in the rat. *Proc Soc Exp Biol Med.* 1972;141:1029–1031.

373. Markowitz H, Gubler CJ, Mahoney JP, Cartwright GE, et al. Studies on copper metabolism, XIV: copper, ceruloplasmin and oxidase activity in sera of normal human subjects, pregnant women, and patients with infection, hepatolenticular degeneration and the nephrotic syndrome. *J Clin Invest.* 1955;34:1498–1508.

374. Vir SC, Love AHG, Thompson W. Serum and hair concentrations of copper during pregnancy. *Am J Clin Nutr.* 1981;34:2382–2388.

375. Hambidge KM. Increase in hair copper concentration with increasing distance from the scalp. *Am J Clin Nutr.* 1973;26:1212–1215.

376. Shike M, Roulet M, Kurian R, Whitwell J, et al. Copper metabolism and requirements in total parenteral nutrition. *Gastroenterology.* 1981;81:290–297.

377. Milne DB, Johnson PE. Assessment of copper status: effect of age and gender on reference ranges in healthy adults. *Clin Chem.* 1993;39:883–887.

378. Mason KE. A conspectus of research on copper metabolism and requirements of man. *J Nutr.* 1979;109:1979–2006.

379. Boosalis MG, McCall JT, Solem LD, Ahrenholz DH, et al. Serum copper and ceruloplasmin levels and urinary copper excretion in thermal injury. *Am J Clin Nutr.* 1986;44:899–906.

380. Rotruck JT, Hoekstra WG, Pape AL, Ganther H, et al. Relationship of selenium to glutathione peroxidase. *Fed Proc.* 1972;31:691.

381. Willett WC, MacMahon B. Diet and cancer: an overview. *N Engl J Med.* 1984;310:697–703.

382. Burk RF, Pearson NN, Wood RP II, Vietri F. Blood selenium levels and *in vitro* red blood cell uptake of 75 Se in kwashiorkor. *Am J Clin Nutr.* 1967;20:723–733.

383. Boosalis MG, Solem LD, Ahrendholz DH, McCall JT, et al. Serum and urinary selenium levels in thermal injury. *Burns.* 1986;12:236–240.

384. Hunt DR, Lane HW, Beesinger D, Gallagher K, et al. Selenium depletion in burn patients. *J Parenter Enter Nutr.* 1984;8:695–699.

385. Johnson RA, Baker SS, Fallow JT, Maynard EP, et al. An accidental case of cardiomyopathy and selenium deficiency. *N Engl J Med.* 1981;304:1210–1212.

386. Fleming CR, Lie JT, McCall JT, O'Brien JF, et al. Selenium deficiency and fatal cardiomyopathy in a patient on home parenteral nutrition. *Gastroenterology.* 1982;83:689–693.

387. Fleming CR, McCall JT, O'Brien JF, Forsman RW, et al. Selenium status in patients receiving home parenteral nutrition. *J Parenter Enter Nutr.* 1984;8:258–262.

388. Baptista RJ, Bistrian BR, Blackburn GL, Miller DG, et al. Suboptimal selenium status in home parenteral nutrition patients with small bowel resections. *J Parenter Enter Nutr.* 1984;8:542–545.

389. Watson RD, Cannon RA, Kurland GS, Cox KL, et al. Selenium responsive mytositis during prolonged home parenteral nutrition in cystic fibrosis. *J Parenter Enter Nutr.* 1985;9:58–60.

390. Rannem T, Hylander E, Ladefoged K, Stawn M, et al. The metabolism of [^{75}Se] selenite in patients with short bowel syndrome. *J Parenter Enter Nutr.* 1996;20:412–416.

391. Kearns PJ, Kagawa FT. Selenium deficiency in patients receiving oral and enteral nutrition. *J Parenter Enter Nutr.* 1986;10(suppl):7.

392. Yagi M, Tani T, Hashimoto T, Shimizu K, et al. Four cases of selenium-deficiency in postoperative long-term enteral nutrition. *Nutrition.* 1996;12:40–43.

393. Dworkin BM, Rosenthal WS, Wormser GP, Weiss L. Selenium deficiency in the acquired immunodeficiency syndrome. *J Parenter Enter Nutr.* 1986;10:405–407.

394. Broghamer WL, McConnell KP, Blotcky AL. Relationship between serum selenium levels in patients with carcinoma. *Cancer.* 1976;37:1384–1388.

395. Stead RJ, Hinks LJ, Hodson ME, Redington AN, et al. Selenium deficiency and possible increased risk of carcinoma in adults with cystic fibrosis. *Lancet.* 1985;2:862–863.

396. Tyrala EE, Borschel MW, Jacobs JR. Selenate fortification of infant formulas improves the selenium status of preterm infants. *Am J Clin Nutr.* 1996;64:860–865.

397. Rannem T, Ladefoged K, Hylander E, Christiansen J, et al. The effect of selenium supplementation on skeletal and cardiac muscle in selenium-depleted patients. *J Parenter Enter Nutr.* 1995;19:351–355.

398. Helzlsouer K, Jacobs R, Morris S. Acute selenium intoxication in the United States. *Fed Proc.* 1985;44:1610.

399. Levander OA. Considerations on the assessment of selenium status. *Fed Proc.* 1985;44:2579–2583.

400. Thompson CD, Robinson MF. Selenium in human health and disease with emphasis on those aspects peculiar to New Zealand. *Am J Clin Nutr.* 1980;33:303–323.

401. Robberecht HJ, Deelstra HA. Selenium in human urine: concentration levels and medical implications. *Clin Chim Acta.* 1984;136:107–120.

402. Beilstein MA, Whangu PP. Distribution of selenium and glutathione peroxidase in blood fractions from humans, rhesus and squirrel monkeys, rats and sheep. *J Nutr.* 1983;113:2138–2147.

403. Levander OA, Alfthan G, Arvilommi H, Gref CG, et al. Bioavailability of selenium to Finnish men as assessed by platelet glutathione peroxidase activity and other blood parameters. *Am J Clin Nutr.* 1983;37:887–897.

404. Rannem T, Persson-Moschos M, Huang W, Stawn M, et al. Selenoprotein P in patients on home parenteral nutrition. *J Parenter Enter Nutr.* 1996;20:287–291.

405. Lipkin EW. Selenium in the parenterally nourished patient. *Nutr Int.* 1986;2:12–18.

406. Van Rij AM, Thompson CD, McKenzie JM. Selenium deficiency in total parenteral nutrition. *Am J Clin Nutr.* 1989;32:2076.

407. Chandra RK, Saraya AK. Impaired immunocompetence associated with iron deficiency. *J Pediatr.* 1975;86:899–902.

408. Krantman HJ, Young SR, Ank BJ, O'Donnell CM, et al. Immune function in pure iron-deficiency. *Am J Dis Child.* 1982;136:840–844.

409. Scott DE, Pritchard JA. Iron deficiency in healthy young college women. *JAMA.* 1967;199:897–900.

410. Harju E, Lindberg H. Lack of iron stores is common in patients with gastrointestinal diseases. *Surg Gynecol Obstet.* 1985;161:362–366.

411. Shanbhogue LK, Paterson N. Effect of sepsis and surgery on trace minerals. *J Parenter Enter Nutr.* 1990;14:287–289.

412. Jacobs A, Worwood M. Ferritin in serum. *N Engl J Med.* 1975;292:951–959.

413. Mohammed R, McCall KE, Veitch D. Changes in iron metabolism following surgery. *Br J Surg.* 1983;70:161–162.

414. Lozoff B, Brittenham GM, Viteri FE, Wolf AWC, et al. Developmental deficits in iron-deficient infants: effects of age and severity of iron lack. *J Pediatr.* 1982;101:948–952.

415. Oski FA, Honig AS, Helw B, Howanitz P. Effect of iron therapy on behavioral performance in nonanemic, iron-deficient infants. *Pediatrics.* 1983;71:877–880.

416. Koutras AK, Vigorita VJ, Quiroz E. Effect of iron-fortified formula on SIgA of gastrointestinal tract in early infancy. *J Pediatr Gastroenterol Nutr.* 1986;5:926–930.

417. Joynson DHM, Jacobs A, Walker DM, Dolby AE. Defect of cell-mediated immunity in patients with iron-deficiency anemia. *Lancet.* 1972;2:1058–1059.

418. Bagchi K, Mohanram M, Reddy V. Humoral responses in children with iron-deficiency anemia. *Br Med J.* 1980;2:1249–1251.

419. Helyar L, Sherman AR. Iron deficiency and interleukin-1 production by rat leukocytes. *Am J Clin Nutr.* 1987;46:346–352.

420. Dallman PR. Iron deficiency and the immune response. *Am J Clin Nutr.* 1987;46:329–334.

421. Weinberg ED. Infection and iron metabolism. *Am J Clin Nutr.* 1977;30:1485–1490.

422. Fletcher J. The effect of iron and transferrin on the killing of *Escherichia coli* in fresh serum. *Immunology.* 1971;20:493–500.

423. Weinberg ED. Iron and susceptibility to infectious disease. *Science.* 1974;184:952–956.

424. Shenkin A, Fraser WD, McLelland AJD, Fell GS, et al. Maintenance of vitamin and trace element status in intravenous nutrition using a complete nutritive mixture. *J Parenter Enter Nutr.* 1987;11:238–242.

425. Hull RE. Trace element requirements in hyperalimentation. *Am J Hosp Pharm.* 1974;31:1035–1039.

426. Bothe A, Benotti P, Bistrian BR, Blackburn GL. Use of iron with total parenteral nutrition. *N Engl J Med.* 1975;293:1153.

CHAPTER 6

Fluid, Electrolyte, and Acid-Base Balance

David L. Paskin

INTRODUCTION

The management of fluid and electrolyte balance, to those unfamiliar with it, seems to be a mystery with no solution. Because of this, medical and paramedical staffs turn away without trying to spend a little extra time to understand the basic, uncomplicated pathophysiology of disease states and their constant, profound effects on fluid balance. With an understanding of body composition and its alterations by hormone mediators (antidiuretic hormone [ADH], epinephrine, glucocorticoids, glucagon, and aldosterone), clinicians can understand the concept of fluid management.

BODY COMPOSITION

The body is composed of adipose tissue and lean body mass (LBM). The LBM is further subdivided into extracellular mass (ECM) and body cell mass (BCM).[1]

Adipose tissue is a relatively anhydrous mass: its water content is only about 20% by weight, whereas the water content of skeletal muscle is 80% by weight.

The ECM consists of extracellular fluid (ECF) and supporting structures. The ECF is composed of plasma, interstitial water, and transcellular water (cerebrospinal fluid, pericardial fluid, and fluid that is in the joint spaces). The supporting structures—skeleton, tendons, and cartilage—are stable and do not vary in fluid, electrolyte, or acid-base balance.

The BCM is the metabolically active portion of the LBM. It consists of skeletal muscle (60%), viscera (30%), and the cells of the supporting structures of the ECM (10%), such as red blood cells and the cells of adipose tissue. A 70-kg man contains about 20 kg of adipose tissue and about 50 kg of LBM, the LBM being equally divided by weight as ECM and BCM.

Increased Total Body Water

With starvation, protein and fat are the endogenous sources of calories. There is a resulting change in body composition with an increasing ECM to BCM ratio, secondary to an absolute decrease in BCM and an absolute increase in ECM. This change occurs secondary to decreased insulin levels and increased levels of glucagon, catecholamines, ADH, glucocorticoids, and aldosterone.

As the ECM to BCM ratio increases, the normal 1:1 ratio of exchangeable sodium (ECM) to exchangeable potassium (BCM) increases.[2] This is secondary to potassium loss due to decreased BCM, sodium retention secondary to elevated levels of aldosterone, and an excess of intracellular sodium possibly secondary to alterations in the sodium pump. As starvation progresses, body fat and BCM continue to erode and ECM continues to increase.

With sepsis and trauma, sustained elevated levels of glucagon, glucocorticoids, epinephrine, ADH, aldosterone, and insulin cause an extremely catabolic state. Protein losses are much greater than in simple starvation and can equal 150 g of protein per day, or about 24 g of nitrogen. This hormonal milieu prevents adaptation that results in the decreased protein loss seen in simple starvation. A rapid and devastating erosion of BCM with an even more intense increase in the ratio of ECM to BCM—and thus an even more marked increase in total body water—ensues.

Relationship of Body Composition to Fluid Balance

The correlation between body composition and fluid balance is obvious. In a 70-kg man, 60% of total body weight is water (42 L). Of the total body weight, 40% is intracellular fluid (ICF) (28 L) and 20% is ECF (14 L [11 L of interstitial fluid and 3 L of plasma]). This 14 L of ECF is the labile portion of the ECM. Therefore, any condition that allows for an increase in ECM will increase the amount of ECF.

With simple fluid loss, there is a rapid refill of plasma volume from the interstitial fluid space. At the same time, increased levels of ADH and aldosterone cause a decreased loss of fluid and a decrease in sodium at the renal level. When fluid repletion is planned, both plasma volume and interstitial fluid should be repleted.

The hormonal environment for fluid conservation increases the ECM to BCM ratio as evidenced by increased interstitial fluid, increased total body sodium, and decreased total body potassium secondary to loss of BCM and the effects of aldosterone.

As fluid repletion occurs, there is always overfill of the interstitial fluid space. This occurs whether crystalloids or colloids are used. The exact mechanism is unknown. As fluid leaves the plasma volume, it is sequestered in the interstitial space. In sepsis and trauma, this sequestration is even greater than when it is secondary to mere hypovolemia, and there is a proportionally greater reexpansion of the ECF than of the ICF. With hypovolemia, there is an equal repletion of both ICF and ECF.[3]

Decreased Total Body Water (Dehydration, Underhydration)

The diagnosis of dehydration is made by history, physical examination, and clinical and laboratory tests. The keys to diagnosis are the history and physical examination. Clinical and laboratory tests are useful as corroborating evidence.

History

Thirst is an early symptom of dehydration. In hospitalized patients, thirst may also be caused by a dry mouth secondary to drug therapy or by nasal obstruction (eg, nasogastric tubes) that results in mouth breathing. Diarrhea, vomiting, and nasogastric or nasoenteral suction result in loss of body water. Therefore, when these tubes are present, volume loss must be anticipated.

Physical Examination

Physical examination is extremely important in evaluating fluid status. Loss of sweat in the axillary area usually means some degree of dehydration, as does a loss of tissue turgor. An increased pulse rate may reflect dehydration. Lethargy and unconsciousness may be present with severe dehydration. Blood pressure may be normal or decreased. The patient may have a positive "tilt test," which is a fall in blood pressure and/or an increased pulse rate when the patient goes from a flat position to an erect or semierect position.

Clinical Tests

Urinary Output. Urinary output is one of the most accurate indicators of the state of hydration if renal function is normal. An adequate urinary output usually connotes no evidence of moderate or severe dehydration.

Weight. The simple measure of body weight, while difficult to obtain on a hospitalized patient, accurately reflects acute fluid changes. As water weighs 1 kg/L; a 24-hour weight gain of 2 kg means that 2 L of fluid have accumulated for that period of time. BCM can be gained only at a rate of 200 g/day; thus any acute weight change (either increase or decrease) usually indicates a gain or loss of ECF.

Laboratory Tests

Patients with dehydration may have an elevated blood urea nitrogen level, an elevated blood urea nitrogen-creatinine ratio (normal is usually 10:1), and an increased serum sodium level.

Treatment

The amount of fluid to be given depends on the degree of loss, the etiology of the loss, and the response to therapy. Clinical estimates of dehydration allow for repletion guides. Severe dehydration or severe hypovolemia correlates with a 10% loss of body weight. Therefore, this is the amount of fluid that should be replaced. For moderate or mild losses, the estimates are 6% and 3% of total body weight, respectively. Maintenance fluid needs of about 30 to 40 mL/kg/day must also be administered. Repletion is achieved by administering half the calculated deficit in the first 8 hours and the remaining half over the next 16 hours. With severe dehydration in a 70-kg man, the loss would be 10% of 70 kg, or 7 L, and maintenance needs would be 2100 mL; thus, the total amount of fluid to be given for repletion would be 9100 mL over 24 hours.

Monitoring of pulse, blood pressure, urinary output, central venous pressure, and pulse pressure is essential during resuscitation. With sepsis, the amount of fluid repletion to effect adequate perfusion may be two or three times as great as it is with hypovolemia. Because interstitial fluid and plasma volume are being lost, the infusion of some type of balanced salt solution (saline or Ringer's lactate) is an appropriate form of therapy. If additional losses from gastric juice, diarrhea, or fistula drainage occur, repletion should be achieved with an electrolyte solution similar to the fluid lost. The electrolyte content of common intravenous fluids is presented in Table 6–1.

During resuscitation, decreased blood pressure, decreased urinary output, or other signs of decreased perfusion usually indicate an inadequate plasma volume and the need for additional fluid.[4] Once resuscitation is completed and perfusion problems occur, pulmonary artery wedge pressure should be monitored. Inotropic drugs and diuretic agents may be necessary. In the early postresuscitation period,

Table 6–1 Electrolyte Content of Common Intravenous Fluids

Intravenous Fluid	Na+ (mEq/L)	K+ (mEq/L)	Cl (mEq/L)	HCO₃ (mEq/L)	Glucose (g/L)
Normal Saline	154	—	154	—	—
D₅ Normal Saline	154	—	154	—	50
1/2 Normal Saline	77	—	77	—	—
D₅ 1/2 Normal Saline	77	—	77	—	50
D₅ 1/4 Normal Saline	38	—	38	—	50
D₅ Water	—	—	—	—	50
D₁₀ Water	—	—	—	—	100
Lactated Ringer's Solution	130	4	112	28	—

decreased urinary output and decreased tissue perfusion even with high-normal or normal pulmonary wedge pressure may be the only signs that fluid is still indicated, since critically ill patients seldom have early primary myocardial problems.

Summary

All of the above conditions alter ECM. As the ECM decreases, dehydration is evident; as the ECM increases, overhydration is the result. Chronic renal, cardiac, and hepatic diseases; sepsis; starvation; trauma with repletion; postresuscitative states; and postsurgical states exist to some degree with a hormonal milieu that causes or allows a relative or absolute increase in ECM and therefore a relative increase in total body water.

SODIUM

Sodium is the main extracellular cation and, under normal circumstances, the serum sodium level correlates with total body sodium. However, with an expanded ECM and an increase in intracellular sodium, the serum sodium level is normal or low despite an increase in total body sodium. This occurs because circumstances that increase the ECM always allow for slightly greater fluid retention than sodium retention. Also, the hormonal milieu is such that some sodium is intracellular. For every extra liter of ECF, about 135 mmol of sodium are added to the body economy. Therefore, any condition that increases ECF will increase total body sodium, even though in all of these states the serum sodium value will be low or low-normal. Thus, the serum sodium level correlates inversely with total body sodium.

Dilutional Hyponatremia

Dilutional hyponatremia is secondary to an increased ADH level and the administration of large amounts of hypotonic salt solution during resuscitation and thereafter. This condition occurs in almost all patients receiving intravenous fluids, whether they require resuscitation or not. Despite the fact that the serum sodium level is low, the patient has retained too much sodium and too much water; therefore, the treatment of choice is restriction of fluids and sodium with or without diuretics. When administering parenteral or enteral nutrition support, clinicians must remember that most hospitalized patients with chronic wasting diseases, chronic diseases, or acute diseases have an increased ECM. By definition, these patients have retained too much sodium and water, and treatment regimens must be directed at sodium and water restriction.

Hypernatremia

Paradoxically, hypernatremia usually reflects depleted total body sodium, depleted ECM, and ECF deficit. This condition usually occurs secondary to marked dehydration or desalting water losses. The treatment is repletion of the ECF space. The amount of fluid to be given is calculated according to the formula for fluid repletion.

Electrolyte concentration is calculated according to the type of fluid loss. If there is a 4-L deficit and the loss has been from the extracellular space, the fluid should contain electrolytes in the same relative concentration as that present normally in both plasma and interstitial fluid. The electrolyte content of body fluids is found in Table 6–2. Serum electrolyte concentrations are then monitored so that additions or subtractions may be made.

POTASSIUM

Because potassium is the main intracellular cation, serum potassium levels have no correlation at all with the total body content of or capacity for potassium. Star-

Table 6–2 Electrolyte Composition of Body Fluids

Type of Fluid	Volume (mL/24 h)	Na (mEq/L)	K (mEq/L)	Cl (mEq/L)	HCO$_3$ (mEq/L)	Mg (mEq/L)
Saliva	1500	60	20	15	50	0.9
Stomach	2500	60	10	90	0	0.1–3.4
		(30–90)	(4–12)	(50–150)*		
Pancreatic fistula	>1000	140	5	75	80	0.4
		(135–155)	(4–6)	(60–100)	(70–90)	(0.2–0.7)
Bile	600	145	5	100	45	0.2–3.0
			(135–155)	(4–6)	(80–110)	(35–50)
Mid-jejunum	3000	105	5	100	45	NA
		(70–125)	(3.5–6.5)	(70–125)	(10–20)	
Ileostomy	—	120	5	105	20	NA
		(90–140)	(4–10)	(60–125)	(15–50)	
Diarrhea	—	25–50	35–60	20–40	35–45	5.8
						0.9–13.9
Blood	—	132–145	3.7–5.1	98–108	22–30	1.2–1.9
Urine	—	30–80	30–80	50–100	NA	4–6

*Lower in achlorhydria

Source: Reprinted with permission from Cerra, ed., *Manual of Critical Care,* p. 189, © 1987, Mosby-Year Book.

vation, trauma, sepsis, diuretics, nasogastric drainage, and posttraumatic and post-surgical changes cause a decrease in total body potassium. However, the serum potassium level relates to the acid-base balance. A low serum potassium level may be either the cause or the effect of metabolic alkalosis. If the serum potassium level is high, the most common cause is metabolic acidosis, as in renal failure, congestive heart failure, or other poor perfusion syndromes.

Hypokalemia

Depletion of BCM, diuretics, the hormonal influence of aldosterone and ADH, and nasogastric drainage are etiologic factors in hypokalemia. Potassium, hydrogen ion, and chloride are lost at the renal level with reabsorption of sodium and bicarbonate, so metabolic alkalosis will be present. The treatment is repletion of potassium and chloride.

Hyperkalemia

Poor perfusion and metabolic acidosis result in hyperkalemia. There is a loss of bicarbonate with a decrease in the serum CO_2. Correction of the etiology of the poor perfusion will correct the acidosis and the hyperkalemia.

IATROGENIC FLUID AND ELECTROLYTE ABNORMALITIES

Many drugs are mixed with 5% dextrose and water and given as small volume parenteral fluids (intravenous riders or solusets). Inotropic and antiarrhythmic agents are diluted in water or saline. Antibiotics given as sodium salts also contribute to excess water and sodium administration. With multiple drug regimens, the amount of free water given may equal 2–3 L/24 hours. Care must be taken to monitor judiciously the type and amount of fluid the patient receives.

The administration of fluid and electrolytes in any setting requires careful monitoring and common sense. The greater majority of patients who are postresuscitative, postoperative, or postanesthetic have increased total body water and increased sodium; the presence of hyponatremia in these patients always means too much water and sodium and, therefore, restrictive measures should be applied. The presence of hypokalemia commonly connotes metabolic alkalosis, which is correctable by the addition of potassium chloride. However, once the potassium level becomes normal or even at the high end of the normal range, it is often omitted from parenteral fluids and the patient again experiences a total potassium deficit. Normalization of the serum potassium level does not mean that potassium should be withdrawn from intravenous solutions.

Once a careful history has been obtained to determine the etiology of the fluid and electrolyte loss, correction to a normal state should be slow and steady, except when signs of shock are present. Overcorrection is not well tolerated. Constant overhydration and then diuresis followed by overhydration are common in the intensive care setting. This roller-coaster method of fluid administration should be replaced by judicious, carefully planned fluid and electrolyte therapy.

ELEVATED BLOOD GLUCOSE LEVELS IN CRITICALLY ILL PATIENTS

The hormonal milieu in critically ill, hospitalized patients is such that there is an increased glucagon-to-insulin ratio. The clearance of glucose continues at an increased rate, but the utilization is decreased. There is insulin resistance. All of these factors lead to an elevated blood glucose level, even though the insulin level might be much higher than normal. The stage is set for hyperosmolar, nonketotic coma.

Normal serum osmolarity is 290 to 300 mOsm. Serum osmolarity can be measured directly or calculated by measuring the serum sodium concentration and blood glucose level. Serum osmolarity is equal to twice the serum sodium concentration in mmol/L plus the blood glucose level measured in mOsm/L. To determine blood glucose in mOsm/L, the concentration (mg/dL) of blood glucose is divided by 18. If the blood glucose level is 72 mg/dL, this would contribute 4 mOsm; if the serum sodium level is 145 mmol/L, this would contribute 290 mOsm. Therefore, the two values added together (290 + 4) equal 294 mOsm/L (within the normal range).

As the blood glucose level increases, the osmolarity also increases. If the blood glucose level is 900 mg/dL, there would be a 50-mOsm rise in serum osmolarity (900 mg ÷ 18 = 50 mOsm) attributable to blood glucose.

Because of the osmotic effect of glucose, renal diuresis occurs, resulting in large fluid and electrolyte losses in the urine. There is replenishment of the ECF loss by ICF. The ICF loss becomes greater in order to replete losses and maintain osmotic neutrality. A particle split occurs within the cell, which results in an increased number of osmotically active particles within the cell. This equalization of osmolarity slows the movement of water from the cells into the extracellular space and therefore maintains osmotic neutrality on both sides of the cell membrane without losing more ICF. However, by the time this occurs, there has already been a large loss of fluid and electrolytes. The patient becomes confused and comatose; if the condition is not corrected quickly, death ensues.

The treatment of hyperosmolar nonketotic coma requires judicious fluid and electrolyte repletion and careful correction of the elevated blood glucose levels. Both abnormalities are corrected concomitantly. Because osmotic neutrality occurs on both sides of the cell membrane, slow correction of the extracellular hyperosmolar state must be achieved. If the decrease in osmolarity in the ECF space occurs too rapidly, large amounts of fluid will be transferred to the intracellular space; intracellular edema will occur, leading to rapid cell destruction and death. Patients in nonketotic coma are particularly sensitive to insulin. If these patients were treated with the same doses used to treat patients in diabetic coma, they would become hypoglycemic rapidly and the osmolarity would drop too quickly. Treatment therefore should be directed at correcting the blood glucose level with insulin doses lower than those that would be used for a similar blood glucose level in true ketotic diabetic coma.

Repletion of the lost ECF is the most important treatment. The ECF should be replenished with normal saline. This seems paradoxical because the serum sodium level during hyperosmolar coma is high-normal or elevated; but despite this elevation in serum sodium, total body sodium is markedly depleted. During repletion, urinary output, pulse rate, and blood pressure should be monitored, as should serum electrolytes and blood glucose. As repletion occurs, alterations in fluid and electrolyte therapy may be undertaken. Normal saline is always used to replace fluid and electrolyte losses in patients with hyperosmolar nonketotic coma except when edema is present. The presence of edema means increased ECF and increased total body sodium; under these circumstances, fluid should be replaced with half-normal saline rather than normal saline. Fluid should never be replaced as free water. The infusion of free water during hyperosmolar nonketotic coma leads to severe dilutional hyponatremia, cerebral edema, and death. This sequence occurs because of rapid fluid shifts from the ECF space to the ICF space secondary to the presence of osmotically active particles within the cell. These particles are produced to compensate cellular fluid losses early in the pathophysiology of hyperosmolar coma.

ACID-BASE DISORDERS

The metabolic pathways are such that the products of glycolysis, whether anaerobic or aerobic, and the oxidative metabolism of fats result in the production of acids. These acids must be disposed of, which requires transport from the cells where they are produced to the two main disposal organs—the kidneys and the lungs. The transport must not effect a change in the acid-base balance (pH) of the transport medium (eg, both the interstitial and plasma components of ECF).

An acid is a proton donor. Hydrogen ion (H^+) is a proton. Therefore, any compound yielding a hydrogen ion is an acid. The normal concentration of H^+ is 0.00004 mmol/L (compared with sodium, which is 140 mmol/L or potassium, which is 4.5 mmol/L). Because this number is so small that clinical use would be cumbersome, pH is used instead.[5] The pH is the negative log of the H^+ concentration to the base 10. Although the mathematical concept is confusing, the practical application is such that simpler numbers are used to describe H^+ concentration (7.42 pH versus 0.00004 mmol/L). Because pH is the negative log, the relationship of pH to H^+ is inverse. Therefore, a decreasing pH means an increasing H^+ concentration (acidemia), and an increasing pH means a decreasing H^+ concentration (alkalemia).

Calculating H$^+$ Concentration from pH

The H$^+$ concentration in serum at a pH of 7.40 is 0.00004 mmol/L, or 40 nmol/L. The H$^+$ concentration can be approximated by knowing the pH change. For every measured increase of 0.1 pH unit above 7.4, 40 nmol/L is multiplied by 0.8. For every decrease of 0.1 pH unit below 7.4, 40 nmol/L is multiplied by 1.25.[6] For example, if the pH is 7.5, 40 is multiplied by 0.8, which equals 32 nmol/L of H$^+$ concentration. Therefore, a decreased amount of H$^+$ accompanies the increased pH. On the other hand, if the pH falls to 7.3, 40 nmol/L of H$^+$ is multiplied by 1.25, and the H$^+$ concentration is 50 nmol/L. If the pH falls to 7.2, then the nmol value must be multiplied by a factor for each tenth of a pH unit fall. In other words, if the pH falls from 7.4 to 7.2, the H$^+$ concentration goes from 40 nmol/L to 62.5 nmol/L (40 × 1.25 = 50; 50 × 1.25 = 62.5). If it then falls to 7.1, the H$^+$ concentration will rise to 78 nmol/L (62.5 × 1.25). Therefore, for each tenth of a pH unit drop, the relative amount of H$^+$ is greater (so that from pH 7.4 to 7.3 there is a 10-nmol increase in H$^+$ concentration; from pH 7.3 to 7.2 there is a 12.5-nmol increase in H$^+$ concentration; and from pH 7.2 to 7.1 the increased H$^+$ concentration is 16 nmol/L).

Dissociation Constant (pK)

The pH is the negative log of the acid's ability to dissociate. Therefore, the stronger the acid, the lower the pK; the weaker the acid, the higher the pK. Because the physiologic pH is 7.4, a good buffer will have a pK close to that pH value. The pH is directly proportional to the pK and the concentration of base and inversely proportional to the concentration of acid. The pH is equal to the pK plus the log of the ratio of the concentration of base to acid.

Equation 1

$$pH = pK + \frac{\log [base]}{\log [acid]}$$

Equation 1 represents the Henderson-Hasselbalch equation. Conceptually, the main point of the equation is that the relationship of base to acid is really what determines pH. Any rise in the numerator or base will increase pH, and any rise in the denominator or acid will decrease pH. The converse is also true. Any decrease in the numerator will decrease the pH, and any decrease in the denominator will increase the pH.

Buffers

A buffer is a substance that can donate or accept H$^+$ and thereby minimize pH changes. The best buffers are acids that do not totally dissociate or do not bind H$^+$

too tightly. The major ECF buffer is the carbonic acid system (equation 2), which is an excellent buffer at a physiologic pH. Because carbonic acid is so abundant, clinical measurement of this buffer system accounts for the main determination of acid-base balance. However, other buffer systems are available.

Equation 2

$$H_2O + CO_2 \rightleftharpoons H_2CO_3 \rightleftharpoons H^+ + HCO_3^-$$

Acid (H^+ donor)   Base (H^+ acceptor)
(Carbonic acid)   (Bicarbonate)

LABORATORY TESTS FOR DETERMINING ACID-BASE BALANCE

Blood gas determinations measure the partial pressure of oxygen (P_{O2}), the partial pressure of carbon dioxide (P_{CO2}), and the H^+ concentration (pH) in whole blood drawn from the arterial side of the circulation. The pH can be measured directly by a pH electrode that reflects H^+ concentration. The P_{CO2} is the amount of CO_2 dissolved in the blood. When CO_2 is combined with water, it yields carbonic acid (H_2CO_3); therefore, its determination (equation 3) accounts for the amount of acid representing the denominator of the pH equation.

Equation 3

$$pH \cong \frac{[\text{Base}]}{[\text{Acid}]}$$

$$pH \cong \frac{[\text{Base}]}{[P_{CO_2}]}$$

The normal value of P_{CO2} is 40 mm Hg. Because CO_2 is a volatile gas, it is eliminated from the system via the lungs. Any condition that causes decreased or impaired ventilation will cause CO_2 retention and an increased P_{CO2} (hypoventilation secondary to general anesthesia, chronic lung disease, narcolepsy, or airway obstruction). When the P_{CO2} increases, the ratio of base to acid decreases, the pH decreases, and the H^+ concentration increases; the result is acidosis (equation 4). When the acidosis is primarily due to an increase in P_{CO2}, it is primary respiratory acidosis.

Equation 4

$$\downarrow pH = \frac{[\text{Base}]}{[P_{CO_2}] \uparrow}$$

If the P_{CO2} is reduced, therefore decreasing the denominator, the pH will increase and the H^+ will decrease. This will cause alkalosis. If decreasing P_{CO2} is the initial event, the alkalosis is referred to as respiratory alkalosis. Any condition causing hyperventilation will precipitate respiratory alkalosis (equation 5). The most common etiologic factors in a hospital setting are early gram-negative septicemia, central nervous system disorders, hypoxemia, and increased CO_2 disposal secondary to mismanagement of ventilators.

Equation 5

$$\uparrow pH = \frac{[Base]}{[Pco_2]\downarrow}$$

Serum CO_2

The CO_2 content is measured in serum (Pco_2 is measured in whole blood). It is one of the four determinations made when serum electrolytes are measured, and yields the total CO_2 content of the serum; the average normal value is 25 mmol/L (range 22 to 28 mmol/L). Because the entire range of the equation is measured— that is, dissolved CO_2 (Pco_2), carbonic acid (H_2CO_3), and bicarbonate (HCO_3^-) (equation 6)—the value refers to the total CO_2 and should not be confused with Pco_2, which measures only the partial pressure of CO_2.

Equation 6

$$H_2O + CO_2 \rightleftharpoons H_2CO_3 \rightleftharpoons H^+ + HCO_3^-$$

$$\underbrace{\hspace{5cm}}_{CO_2 \text{ Content}}$$

The acid component must be subtracted from the total CO_2 content to get the true amount of base. The conversion of Pco_2 from mm Hg to mmol/L is done by assuming that 1 mm Hg of Pco_2 is equal to 0.03 mmol/L. Therefore, 40 mm Hg is equal to 1.2 mmol of CO_2 ($40 \times 0.03 = 1.2$).[7] If the CO_2 content by electrolyte determination is 25.2 mmol/L and the Pco_2 by blood gas measurement is 40 mm Hg (1.2 mmol/L), then the total base would equal the total CO_2 minus the acid, or 24 mmol/L 25.2 − 1.2 = 24). The difference between 25.2 and 24 is insignificant clinically; therefore, the CO_2 content is conveniently used as a measure of total base (HCO_3^-). The equation for the pH of serum is shown in equation 7.

Equation 7

$$pH = pK + \log \frac{[Base]\ (CO_2\ Content)}{[Acid]\ (Pco_2)}$$

$$pH = 6.1 + \log \frac{[24]}{[1.2]}$$

$$pH = 6.1 + \log 20$$

$$pH = 6.1 + 1.3$$

$$pH = 7.4$$

The pK of the carbonic acid system is always constant at 6.1; therefore, if any two of the three values (pH, CO_2 content, and P_{CO_2}) are known, the third value can always be calculated.

Metabolic Acidosis

If a process produces an increased amount of acid, therefore consuming bicarbonate (base) and decreasing the numerator of the equation, the pH will decrease, resulting in acidosis. If the primary change is a decrease in bicarbonate (CO_2 measured by serum electrolytes), the disorder is metabolic acidosis. Conditions commonly causing metabolic acidosis in a hospital setting are diarrhea, enteral diversion (ileal loop, sigmoid loop), renal failure, diabetic ketoacidosis, and any state where there is poor tissue perfusion with resulting lactic acidosis.

Metabolic Alkalosis

If the primary change is an increase in the bicarbonate or the numerator, the pH increases, resulting in primary metabolic alkalosis. Metabolic alkalosis usually occurs secondary to a loss of H^+ with an attempt to increase the production of H^+, thereby causing the equation to move toward the right.

Equation 8

$$H_2O + CO_2 \rightleftharpoons H_2CO_3 \rightleftharpoons H^+ + HCO_3^-$$

With the increase in generation of HCO_3^-, the numerator will increase and the pH will increase. If the primary change is an increase in HCO_3^-, the resulting abnormality is metabolic alkalosis.

METABOLIC ABNORMALITIES

Just as the variation in P_{CO_2} (acid) is controlled by the lungs, the changes in CO_2 content (base) are regulated by the kidneys. Renal function is complex but simple. The primary function of the kidney is to conserve water and sodium. The secondary function is to maintain acid-base balance. The kidneys are most efficient in accomplishing this: 180 L of glomerular filtrate per day results in only 1 L of urine. With this ability to conserve water, the kidneys are equally efficient in conserving sodium. To maintain electrical neutrality, the kidneys in retaining cation (sodium) must lose some cation; the two obvious choices are H^+ and K^+. This concept is important in metabolic acid-base disorders. As excess H^+ is lost in the urine, K^+ is retained, and serum potassium levels may increase. The major cause of increased serum potassium levels during metabolic acidosis, however, is an attempt to drive the H^+ intracellularly so that potassium comes out into the ECF. An opposite effect can occur during metabolic alkalosis: increased bicarbonate can cause potassium and sodium to enter the cell and H^+ to exit the cell. Therefore, the serum potassium level is an indicator of acid-base status. In alkalosis, the serum potassium level is low or normal; in acidosis, it is normal or high.

COMPENSATION

The regulatory ability of the lungs and kidneys is so efficient that, when a primary change in acid-base status occurs in one organ, the other organ corrects in a similar direction so that the acid-base ratio always stays as close to 20:1 as possible.

The lungs can blow off more CO_2 (P_{CO_2}—acid) by increasing the rate of respiration and conversely can retain CO_2 by decreasing the respiratory rate. In this way, the lungs can compensate for a metabolic (renal) change. A classic example of this phenomenon is diabetic ketoacidosis (equation 9). The large production of ketones (acetoacetic acid) overwhelms the system with acid (H^+ or proton donor). To buffer the effect of the ketones immediately, base (bicarbonate HCO_3^-) is consumed, and the amount of base decreases. The numerator of the pH equation therefore decreases, and the pH decreases also.

Equation 9

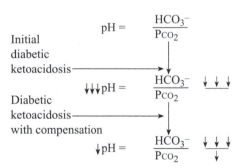

To compensate for this sequence and to try to return the pH toward but not to normal, the denominator of the equation (acid—P_{CO_2}) must decrease to maintain the ratio as close to 20:1 as possible. To decrease the P_{CO_2}, the lungs begin to blow off more CO_2, resulting in metabolic acidosis with compensatory respiratory alkalosis (primary decrease in bicarbonate followed by a secondary decrease in the P_{CO_2}).

Initially in metabolic alkalosis, there is a loss of H^+ and an increased production of bicarbonate, and therefore an increase in total CO_2 (base). The respiratory response is hypoventilation to retain P_{CO_2} (acid), and both the numerator (base) and the denominator (acid) change in the same direction in an attempt to keep the pH toward normal (20:1 ratio). The final correction for metabolic alkalosis is to decrease absolutely the base (bicarbonate) and retain H^+. At the renal level, bicarbonate is lost and chloride is retained. There is an attempt to retain H^+, and therefore potassium must be lost. Serum potassium levels decrease. If too much K^+ is lost and none is replaced, the kidney begins to conserve K^+ and lose H^+ in its place. This creates a paradox—the loss of H^+ (acid) at a time when bicarbonate (base) is overabundant. To help correct for this type of metabolic alkalosis, exogenous potassium should be given.

Clinically, metabolic alkalosis occurs in patients with large gastric losses secondary to nasogastric suction, obstructing duodenal ulcer, or gastric outlet obstruction. These patients classically have an increased CO_2 content with an increased pH and a compensatory increase in P_{CO_2}. The urine should have a basic pH (since the increased amount of alkali should be excreted by the kidney with retention of H^+). If the urine becomes acidic in the presence of metabolic alkalosis, K^+ must be given so that the H^+ will be retained to help decrease the bicarbonate excess and return the pH toward normal. The compensation for all acid-base disturbances is always toward but not to a normal pH.

Metabolic disorders (bicarbonate) require eventual metabolic correction, even though respiratory mechanisms can help compensate. Primary problems of P_{CO_2} or CO_2 disposal via the lungs require a primary correction of the respiratory mechanism even though metabolic compensation can help stabilize the pH. Complete correction of the pH by compensatory mechanisms does not occur. If the compensation were complete, the stimulus for the primary problem to correct itself would be diminished. Compensatory mechanisms are just that—they compensate, but they do not completely correct a problem. If there is an acid-base disturbance with a normal pH, two or more problems with both metabolic and respiratory components must be occurring simultaneously. These components are primary rather than compensatory. This mixed disturbance is diagnosed by the presence of a normal pH with an abnormally elevated CO_2 content and P_{CO_2}, or conversely with an abnormally low CO_2 content accompanied by an abnormally low P_{CO_2}.

Table 6–3 shows the values for a patient with metabolic alkalosis (vomiting secondary to obstructing duodenal ulcer) and respiratory acidosis (chronic lung disease). Metabolic alkalosis is demonstrated by a CO_2 combining power of 36

Table 6–3 Mixed Acid-Base Disturbance with Normal pH

Acid-Base Balance	pH	CO_2 (mmol/L)	P_{CO_2} (mm H)	Ratio
No disturbance	7.4	24	40	20:1
Mixed disturbance	7.4	36 ↑↑	60 ↑↑	20:1

Exhibit 6–1 Clinical Relevance of Each Laboratory Parameter

pH	
Decreased	Primary metabolic acidosis
	Primary respiratory acidosis
Increased	Primary metabolic alkalosis
	Primary respiratory alkalosis
CO₂ (Serum CO₂ or Base)	
Increased	Primary metabolic alkalosis
	Compensation for respiratory acidosis
Decreased	Primary metabolic acidosis
	Compensation for respiratory alkalosis
Pco₂ (Blood Gas or Acid)	
Increased	Primary respiratory acidosis
	Compensation for metabolic alkalosis
Decreased	Primary respiratory alkalosis
	Compensation for metabolic acidosis

mmol/L; respiratory acidosis by a P_{CO_2} of 60 mm Hg. The ratio of base to acid is normal, and therefore the pH is normal. However, both the CO_2 combining power and the P_{CO_2} are elevated. This is a classic mixed disturbance: the pH is normal, but two primary problems are occurring in the opposite acid-base direction.

INTERPRETING LABORATORY RESULTS

To assess acid-base status clinically, blood gases (pH, P_{CO_2}) and serum electrolytes (K^+, CO_2, NaCl) are determined. The clinical relevance of the laboratory results is shown in Exhibit 6–1. Serum CO_2 is equivalent to $HCO_3^- = $ base $= $ numerator $= $ metabolic disturbance $= $ kidney. Blood P_{CO_2} is equivalent to $H^+ = $ acid $= $ denominator $= $ respiratory disturbance $= $ lung.

Simple Acid-Base Disturbances

Four primary disturbances are possible: (1) metabolic acidosis (primary decrease in base), (2) metabolic alkalosis (primary increase in base), (3) respiratory acidosis (primary increase in acid), and (4) respiratory alkalosis (primary decrease in acid) (see Table 6–4). Common causes for simple acid-base disorders are shown in Exhibit 6–2.

Each disturbance, metabolic or respiratory, is accompanied by a compensating change in the other in a similar direction (see Exhibit 6–3).

Exhibit 6–2 Common Causes for Acid-Base Disorders

Respiratory Acidosis
- acute and chronic lung disease
- central nervous system depression (sedatives, trauma)
- neuromuscular disorders (eg, Guillain-Barré syndrome)

Respiratory Alkalosis
- anxiety with hyperventilation
- central nervous system disorder (eg, cerebrovascular accident)
- early gram-negative sepsis
- ventilator mismanagement

Metabolic Acidosis
- renal failure
- diabetic ketoacidosis
- diarrhea
- ureteral diversion (ileal and sigmoid loops)
- lactic acidosis (poor perfusion, shock)

Metabolic Alkalosis
- vomiting (especially with duodenal obstruction)
- Cushing's syndrome

Table 6–4 Simple Acid-Base Disturbances with Altered pH

Acid-Base Balance	pH	P_{CO_2} (mm Hg)	CO_2 (mmol/L)	Base-Acid Ratio
Normal	7.4	40	24	N
Metabolic acidosis	↓	↓	↓↓	↓
Metabolic alkalosis	↑	↑	↑↑	↑
Respiratory acidosis	↓	↑↑	↑	↓
Respiratory alkalosis	↑	↓↓	↓	↑

Exhibit 6–3 Compensatory Changes in Acid-Base Disturbances

↓ Base (metabolic)	Compensatory ↓ acid (respiratory)
↑ Base (metabolic)	Compensatory ↑ acid (respiratory)
↑ Acid (respiratory)	Compensatory ↑ base (metabolic)
↓ Acid (respiratory)	Compensatory ↓ base (metabolic)

Note: Smaller arrows indicate that the compensating change is always smaller than the primary change.

REFERENCES

1. Moore FD. *The Body Cell Mass and Its Supportive Environment.* Philadelphia: WB Saunders Co; 1963.

2. Shizgal HM. Body composition and nutritional support. *Surg Clin North Am.* 1981;61:727–741.

3. Elwyn DH, Bryan-Brown CW, Shoemaker WC. Nutritional aspects of body water dislocations in postoperative and depleted patients. *Ann Surg.* 1975;182:76–85.

4. Lucas CE, Ledgerwood AM. The fluid problem in the clinically ill. *Surg Clin North Am.* 1983;63:439–454.

5. Sorensen SPH. Enzymstudien. II. Mitteilung. Über die Messung and die Bedetung der Wasserstoffionenkonzentration bei enzymatischen Prozessen. *Biochem Z.* 1909;21:131.

6. Fagen TJ. Estimation of hydrogen ion concentration. *N Engl J Med.* 1973;288:915.

7. Narins RG, Emmet M. Simple and mixed acid-base disorders: a practical approach. *Medicine (Baltimore).* 1980;59:161–187.

CHAPTER 7

Indirect Calorimetry

Carol S. Ireton-Jones

INTRODUCTION

Nutritional care of patients begins with the determination of calorie requirements. Careful attention to calorie requirements is important to prevent overfeeding and underfeeding, both of which may have deleterious effects on recovery. Energy requirements may be calculated or measured. This chapter focuses on the measurement of energy expenditure using indirect calorimetry. The methodology for indirect calorimetry and guidelines for interpretation of measured energy expenditure (MEE) are provided. Home care, outpatient, and research applications of indirect calorimetry are also included.

Estimation of energy requirements is not an exact science because of the many individual variations among people in size, stature, intake, output, and race. Energy expenditure and requirements may be estimated with simple balance studies that can ascertain the effectiveness of the nutrition regimen for a healthy person. In most cases, if weight loss occurs, too few calories are being consumed; if weight gain occurs, too many calories are being consumed. Adjustments to account for activity level may be made, but in the normal person this estimation is quite accurate. The application of the simple balance equation to sick, hospitalized patients is complicated by hydration status, disease status, nutrient regimen, nutritional status, and individual response to disease or injury. Energy expenditure formulas are often used to determine adequate nutrition support regimens; however, inaccuracy exists in each formula. Estimation of energy expenditure can be obviated using direct or indirect calorimetry to measure energy expenditure. To fully understand measurement of energy expenditure, the components of daily energy expenditure must be defined.

PHYSIOLOGY OF ENERGY EXPENDITURE

The maintenance of body functions is dependent upon a constant amount of voluntary and involuntary energy expenditure. Energy is expended in the human body for microprocesses such as active transport, macromolecule synthesis, and muscle contraction. The total daily energy expenditure of humans consists of several components, including basal energy expenditure (basal metabolic rate [BMR]), resting energy expenditure (REE), diet-induced thermogenesis (the "thermic effect of food"), shivering and nonshivering thermogenesis, and the energy expenditure for physical activity.[1] The extent of each of these components varies among individuals.

Basal metabolism is defined as the minimal heat production of an individual. The BMR is the approximate energy cost of maintaining basic physiologic activities including heartbeat, respiration, kidney function, osmotic balance, brain activity, and body temperature.[2] It is determined 12 to 14 hours after the ingestion of food and with the individual at complete rest.[3] The BMR varies with the size of an individual. REE includes the BMR and the increases in energy expenditure that occur following awakening but with minimal activity.[4] REE is the main component of the average daily metabolic rate.[5]

The *thermic effect of food,* or diet-induced thermogenesis, is said to account for a 5% to 10% increase above REE in daily energy expenditure.[1,6] Diet-induced thermogenesis is an obligatory process due to the inevitable energy costs of digestion, absorption, and processing or storage of substrates and a component that involves stimulation of the sympathetic nervous system.[6] Nicotine and caffeine are the most active thermogenic agents contributing to an increase in energy expenditure.[7] Shivering, or cold-induced thermogenesis, plays a minor role in everyday life. Nonshivering thermogenesis is difficult to demonstrate in adult individuals and therefore is considered to be of little or no consequence in overall daily energy expenditure.[8]

Physical activity is the most difficult component of energy expenditure to predict; however, it must be considered.[9] The energy costs of many activities have been measured, and researchers have found that the amount of energy expended is proportionate to the rate of sustained muscle contraction.[10] Energy expenditure varies with body size and composition, age, and gender.[5] It is also proportionate to the body surface area and to the percentage of lean body mass.[11] Males typically have higher metabolic rates than do females. Energy expenditure is generally depressed during starvation and in chronic dieters and anorexics.[12] It is normally increased in people who reside in cold climates, in the obese, in smokers, and under conditions of stress and disease.[11,13–15]

CALORIMETRY

The theory of calorimetry is not new. A review of the history of calorimetry by Feurer and Mullen[1] reported that in the late 1700s Black and Lavoisier used calorimeters to relate oxygen consumption to heat production in animal studies. Bidder and Schmidt described BMR using gas exchange, and Pettenkofer and Voit built a respiration chamber for human studies in the mid-1800s. Rubner performed calorimetric measurements on dogs using both indirect and direct methods, and he showed the correlation between the two methods.[3] Atwater, Rosa, and Benedict developed a respiration chamber large enough for adults and initiated some of the landmark studies in human energy expenditure in 1890. In 1903, Atwater and Benedict demonstrated the correlation between direct and indirect calorimetry in humans. It was during this same time that the classic equations of Harris and Benedict were published.[16] The work done by these pioneering researchers in metabolism remains useful and standard today.

Energy expenditure can be quantified in humans using either direct or indirect calorimetry. These two methods do not measure energy expenditure in the same fashion. Direct calorimetry is the measurement of energy expenditure in the form of heat lost by the body, whereas, indirect calorimetry allows for the assessment of energy expenditure by measuring respiratory gas exchange.[5]

Direct Calorimetry

Direct calorimetry is used to measure heat production or the total rate of heat loss by the body. Because all types of energy in the body are converted to heat, direct calorimetry can be measured to determine energy expenditure. Direct calorimetry can be used to measure metabolic rate provided that body thermal equilibrium is maintained and no external work is done.[5,17] To determine energy expenditure by direct calorimetry, the subject is placed in a sealed, insulated chamber with an oxygen supply. A known volume of water is circulated through a series of pipes located at the top of the chamber. Because the entire chamber is well insulated, the heat produced and radiated by the individual is absorbed by the circulating water. The change in water temperature reflects metabolic energy release.[9] Human energy expenditure was determined by direct calorimetry in classic studies done in the early twentieth century on young men who rested or worked in a sealed, insulated chamber.[18] These studies demonstrated that energy expenditure was almost directly related to the consumption of oxygen.

Bradham[19] used direct calorimetry to measure the energy expenditure of a burned patient. He did this to determine the quantity and individual variation of energy required during an illness; the procedure allowed him to predict the course of his patient's physical condition. Since direct calorimetry requires the use of a chamber or cumbersome equipment in which the subject is placed for the duration of the study, it is difficult to achieve in a clinical setting where continuous patient care is required. This technique is therefore of little use in the routine clinical care of hospitalized patients.

Indirect Calorimetry

Because the first law of thermodynamics can be applied to the human body, the energy released by oxidative processes and by anaerobic glycolysis is ultimately transformed into heat or external work.[5,20] Indirect calorimetry is based on the premise that all energy is derived from the oxidation of protein, carbohydrate, and fat and that the amount of oxygen consumed and carbon dioxide produced are characteristic and constant for each fuel.[5] When using indirect calorimetry, heat production (energy expenditure) is determined by measuring the oxygen consumption and carbon dioxide production during respiratory gas exchange.[21] From those values, energy expenditure can be calculated with the use of the Weir[22] or similar equations.

Indirect calorimetry is simpler to perform than direct calorimetry and permits individualized determination of energy expenditure.[23-26] A method for performing indirect calorimetry was described by Douglas[21] in 1911; today it is used predominantly in research settings.[27] With the advent of microprocessors that allow miniaturization and advancing computer technology, indirect calorimetry methodology has become portable in size and technique. Although the methodology of indirect calorimetry has been cumbersome in the past, reliable, automated, portable indirect calorimeters (called metabolic measurement carts) now allow for rapid and easy measurement of energy expenditure.[25,26,28]

Indirect calorimetry may be performed using either open- or closed-circuit methodology.[29] In the *open-circuit method,* the subject breathes air from the environment, while expired air is collected for volumetric measurement. The expired gas volume is then corrected for standard conditions and is analyzed for its oxygen and carbon dioxide content, with a subsequent calculation being done to determine oxygen consumption and carbon dioxide production. The *closed-circuit method* isolates the subject from outside air during the measurement by having the subject breathe entirely through a closed system. In the closed-circuit system, the subject often breathes from a reservoir containing pure oxygen; as the subject exhales, carbon dioxide is removed by a material such as soda lime. The decrease in the gas volume in the closed system is related to the rate of the oxygen consumption, from which the metabolic rate is then calculated.

Several instruments are commercially available to allow the clinician or researcher to measure oxygen consumption and carbon dioxide production at the bedside. Although systems are available that use both open- and closed-circuit methods of measurement, the most frequently used systems employ an open-circuit system for measuring energy expenditure. Examples of some of open-circuit, commercially available systems are the Vmax 29n Energy Measurement System and the DeltaTrac II Metabolic Cart (SensorMedics, Yorba Linda, California) and the CCM (Medical Graphics Corporation, St. Paul, Minnesota). In addition to performing indirect calorimetry, some instruments are capable of providing cardiopulmonary exercise testing and pulmonary function testing.

Some investigators have assembled indirect calorimetry systems from readily available components.[30] Although a laboratory-assembled system is accurate, it requires a research setting for validation of the system and for continuous maintenance.

Metabolic Cart Methodology

Indirect calorimetry performed using a portable metabolic measurement cart for measuring oxygen consumption and carbon dioxide production is applicable to the clinical setting for many reasons. The cart can be easily transported and used at the patient's bedside. Both ventilator-dependent and spontaneously breathing patients can be measured in a minimal amount of time.[23,31] Oxygen consumption (V_{O_2}) and carbon dioxide production (V_{CO_2}) are measured instantaneously. Spontaneously breathing patient measurements may be accomplished using a nose clip and mouthpiece or a mask that covers the nose and mouth; however, these measurements are done most comfortably by using an enclosed breathing chamber called a canopy. The canopy measurement technique used with the DeltaTrac II (Metabolic Cart) allows for the head of the patient to be covered with a transparent plastic canopy. A constant flow of air goes through the canopy and to the metabolic cart with the exact value of this flow calibrated by the instrument. All expired air is collected into this constant flow so that calculations of oxygen consumption and carbon dioxide production can be completed (see Exhibit 7–1).

When using a mask or a nose clip and mouthpiece, it is important to maintain an adequate seal because inspiratory or expiratory air leakage invalidates data. A non-rebreathing valve is connected to the mask or mouthpiece so that gas collection can be accomplished. Patients with tracheotomies can be measured as long as the non-rebreathing valve fits snugly over the cuffed endotracheal tube and the cuff is inflated.[32]

Patients supported by mechanical ventilators are measured using a single-piloted exhalation valve. A mechanical ventilator manufacturer has developed a system that is attached to the ventilator that allows the clinician to obtain both respiratory and metabolic data (7250 Metabolic Monitor, Nellcor Puritan Bennett, USA). Although this system allows for continuous measurement of oxygen consumption and carbon dioxide production, use is limited to patients who are being mechanically ventilated with the 7200 AE ventilator.

Exhibit 7–1 Sample Metabolic Cart Protocol

METHODOLOGY

- *Spontaneously breathing patients* are connected to the metabolic measurement cart using a mask and non-rebreathing valve or a canopy.
- *Ventilator-dependent patients* are connected to the metabolic measurement cart using a single-piloted exhalation valve to collect expired gas. Inspired gas is sampled on the "dry side" of the ventilator humidifier.

INTERPRETATION

Measurements of oxygen consumption, carbon dioxide production, and ventilatory volume are made in 1-minute intervals until a steady state is achieved. Measured energy expenditure (MEE) and respiratory quotient (RQ) are calculated. A steady state is achieved when three consecutive 1-minute measurements of MEE are within 10% of one another and the corresponding RQs are within 5% of one another.

Indirect calorimetry measurements include the following:

- V_{O_2} (oxygen consumption L/minute)
- V_{CO_2} (carbon dioxide production L/minute)
- RQ (respiratory quotient)
- v_T (tidal volume)
- v_E (minute ventilation)
- fr (frequency of ventilation breaths)
- VEQ_{O_2} (ventilatory equivalent of oxygen)

These measurements are used to determine the MEE and RQ, and as check points to validate the methodology.

EQUATION

The modified Weir equation, used to calculate energy expenditure from oxygen consumption (V_{O_2}) and carbon dioxide production (V_{CO_2}), is written as follows:

$$MEE = ([V_{O_2} \times 3.796] + [V_{CO_2} \times 1.214]) \times 1440, \text{ where}$$

MEE = measured energy expenditure (kcal/day)
V_{O_2} = oxygen consumption (L/min)
V_{CO_2} = carbon dioxide production (L/min)

Indirect calorimetry is a useful and accurate technique to determine MEE in acutely and chronically ill patients; however, certain conditions must be maintained to obtain reliable measurements.[20,31] The MEE can be accurately determined under the following conditions:

- Patients should be measured when they are awake but at rest and in a supine position.

- Patients should be measured 2 hours after a meal unless they are on continuous nutrition support.
- Measurements should be taken at least 1 hour following strenuous activity such as a dressing change, chest physiotherapy, or physical therapy.

When these conditions are met, MEEs are considered to be reliable, useful assessments of a patient's energy expenditure.[25,26,31-33] The best time to measure a patient is when the surroundings are less hectic and when vital signs such as heart rate and ventilatory status are most stable. There are some limitations to indirect calorimetry due to physiological and mechanical factors. The following situations may cause indirect calorimetry measurements of energy expenditure to be unreliable[34]:

- patients measured while receiving high-frequency mechanical ventilation
- patients with chest tubes that leak air
- patients receiving mechanical ventilation with fractional inspired oxygen concentrations >60% when open-circuit measurement systems are used
- patients in whom the tracheotomy tube has an incompetent or nonexistent tracheal cuff
- patients receiving inconsistent sources of inspired oxygen (variable levels of inspired oxygen)
- unskilled personnel conducting the metabolic measurement

MEASUREMENT DATA

Prior to initiating an indirect calorimetric measurement of energy expenditure, the metabolic cart should be calibrated according to instrument specifications. Measurement data are collected and analyzed by predetermined standards as to steady-state measurement data (that is, reproducible data). The length of time for a test depends on the testing standards set for the metabolic cart. Standards may be determined from data obtained at the institution or according to recommendations by the manufacturer. Swimnamer et al[33] analyzed measurement data over a continuous period of 24 hours and correlated data with individual measurements of energy expenditure; they found that the data obtained under standard conditions for 30 minutes were not significantly different from those obtained from a 24-hour measurement of energy expenditure.

Measured Energy Expenditure

The measurement of oxygen consumption and carbon dioxide production provides data required for the calculation of energy expenditure. These data are used to calculate MEE from the Weir equation. Some metabolic carts may use a modification of the Weir equation to obtain energy expenditure data from oxygen consumption and carbon dioxide production.[13] To obtain an energy expenditure assessment, oxygen consumption and carbon dioxide production are measured at 1- to 5-minute intervals. At the same time, respiratory quotient (the ratio of oxygen consumed to carbon dioxide produced) is determined.

A steady-state measurement of energy expenditure is determined by averaging a specified interval of consecutive MEE values that are reproducible. One technique used to determine a steady-state MEE is to obtain three consecutive minute measurements of MEE within 10% of each other that have corresponding respiratory quotients (RQs) that are within 5% of each other.[13,31] An average of the three values for the MEE and RQ is obtained to provide what is considered to be the patient's daily MEE and RQ. In patients where the MEE and RQ are not consecutively within ±10% and ±5%, respectively, the median of 10 consecutive MEE values may be used to determine the average daily MEE. In some metabolic carts, MEE, RQ, or V_{O_2} and V_{CO_2} are graphically displayed and a steady state measurement is determined by physiologic wave-form monitoring. A steady state measurement is obtained by selecting the most representative sample of data (Tech Notes, MedicalGraphics Corporation, St. Paul, Minnesota).

Respiratory Quotient

Metabolic measurement systems capable of measuring both oxygen consumption and carbon dioxide production also have the advantage of permitting calculation of the RQ. RQ is calculated from the ratio of carbon dioxide produced (V_{CO_2}) to oxygen consumed (V_{O_2}) and reflects net substrate utilization (V_{CO_2}/V_{O_2}).[35] Oxidation of each major nutrient class occurs at a known RQ, ranging from 0.7 for fat oxidation to 1.0 for glucose oxidation (see Table 7–1). Net fat synthesis is demonstrated by the occurrence of an RQ greater than 1.0.[35,36] RQs greater than 1.0 can occur when carbohydrate (glucose) intake or total caloric intake is excessive. The

Table 7–1 Respiratory Quotients (RQs)

Energy Source	RQ
Fat	0.70
Protein	0.80
Carbohydrate (glucose)	0.95–1.00
Mixed diet	0.85
Net fat synthesis	>1.01
Hyperventilation	>1.10
Ketosis	<0.60

effect is probably a function of high carbohydrate (glucose) intake. Excess caloric intake, especially in the form of carbohydrate, increases energy expenditure.[37] A very low RQ is often seen with inadequate nutrition support such as hypocaloric feeding or in patients who have had prolonged periods of inadequate nutrient intake. If nitrogen excretion is measured, the nonprotein RQ may be calculated.[1] Often urinary nitrogen excretions are not available from which to calculate the proportion of protein in the energy expenditure. Weir[22] analyzed this problem and showed that by employing a formula for calculating energy expenditure and taking into account estimated nitrogen excretion, the resulting error in calculation was no more than 2% for energy expenditure and RQ. With the inaccuracies found in urinary nitrogen excretion collection when it is not done under scrupulous conditions, deleting the nitrogen value in the MEE determination is probably more accurate than including available nitrogen excretion data if they are not absolutely accurate.

RQ has been used to determine the efficacy of nutrition support regimens for hospitalized patients.[35] Intensive nutrition support of hospitalized patients is often administered intravenously, using glucose as the major energy source. In a study comparing RQs of patients receiving glucose-based parenteral nutrition to RQs of patients receiving balanced proportions of carbohydrate, protein, and fat either enterally or parenterally, RQs greater than 1.0 were noted more frequently in patients who received the glucose-based parenteral nutrition.[35] The authors of this study suggested that fat added to nutrition support regimens containing carbohydrate and protein optimizes substrate utilization.[35]

CLINICAL APPLICATIONS OF INDIRECT CALORIMETRY

An understanding of the relationship between energy expenditure and energy requirements is fundamental in clinical nutritional assessment. An indirect calorimetric measurement of energy expenditure in the hospitalized patient contains the components of daily energy expenditure including the BMR; thermic effect of food; and the effect of disease state, stress, and/or trauma.[25,26] MEE should be done under controlled conditions mentioned previously so that reproducible results are obtained.

Guidelines for Interpretation of Measured Energy Expenditure

Indirect calorimetric measurements of energy expenditure are interpreted for adults (>14 years of age) using guidelines developed following intensive review of indirect calorimetry and energy expenditure, and from clinical expertise gained from experience with the methodology (see Exhibit 7–2).[26,38] These guidelines are presented as an example and must be assessed for their usefulness within each

Exhibit 7–2 Recommended Energy Intake (kcal/day)

Maintenance regimen (nonstressed patient):	$REI = MEE \times 1.0$
Maintenance regimen (stressed patient):	$REI = MEE \times 1.1$
Repletion regimen (stressed patient):	$REI = MEE \times 1.3$

MEE = measured energy expenditure in kcal/day

institution. Specialized guidelines may be necessary for neonates, infants, or children to account for anabolic processes such as growth and development.[39]

The MEE is used to determine a patient's recommended energy intake (REI). The REI provides for the daily energy expenditure plus any additional energy required to replete body cell mass such as with a repletion regimen. A maintenance regimen is used for the nonstressed, inactive outpatient who is in normal nutritional status. Any adjustments upward will be figured for activity only. The Harris-Benedict equations[16] for calculating REE may be used in place of the MEE for these individuals. A maintenance regimen that provides the MEE is used for a stressed inpatient who has a normal nutritional status and a normal or mildly catabolic level as determined by urinary urea nitrogen excretion and severity of illness. Some clinicians have reported adding a factor of 10% to the MEE for these patients.[40] A repletion regimen is employed for a stressed inpatient who is malnourished or severely catabolic. This may involve increasing the MEE by 30%.[25,26,39–41] Occasionally, a patient has mixed criteria such as an abnormal nutritional status but a normal catabolic level. In this case, clinical judgment must be used in deciding whether to increase the MEE.

Who Should Be Measured?

Anyone who has an illness or injury that may potentially affect metabolic rate or anyone who has a metabolism suspected to be altered from the normal state is a potential candidate for an energy expenditure assessment by indirect calorimetry. When clinicians follow a large group of patients, they should determine certain priorities so that patients who will benefit the most from an MEE will be measured first (see Exhibit 7–3). All patients receiving intensive nutrition support should have an MEE completed as a part of the nutritional assessment. Patients currently in the intensive care unit would be expected to have first priority. Energy expenditures of burn patients should be reassessed following each surgical procedure or weekly.[42] Other patients requiring intensive care should have their energy expenditures reassessed weekly. Patients receiving parenteral nutrition other than those

Exhibit 7–3 Sample Energy Expenditure Assessment Protocol

1. All patients who are being followed by the nutrition support team and who are receiving intensive nutrition support (enteral or parenteral) will have their energy expenditures measured by indirect calorimetry.
2. Due to the number of patients being followed, patients are prioritized according to location and diagnosis:
   - **First priority:** ICU patients on TPN
   - **Second priority:** ICU patients on enteral nutrition
   - **Third priority:** Ward patients on TPN
   - **Fourth priority:** Ward patients on enteral nutrition
   - **Fifth priority:** any other patient needing an energy expenditure assessment
3. Patients are measured initially and measurements are repeated according to the above priority list. All ICU patients are measured weekly; all patients receiving TPN on the ward are measured biweekly; and ward patients receiving enteral nutrition are remeasured at 2-week intervals if still in the hospital.
4. Other patients such as those on a research protocol or special patients will be worked into the priority schedule as needed.

Note: ICU—intensive care unit; TPN—total parenteral nutrition

in the intensive care unit should be the next priority. All other patients would then follow. Patients falling into the last two categories should have their energy expenditures reassessed biweekly unless otherwise indicated. All patients' energy expenditure should be reassessed when a significant change occurs such as a change in the route or type of nutrition support (eg, parenteral to enteral) or change in the method of ventilation from mechanical ventilation support to spontaneous breathing. Indirect calorimetry can be an important component of an initial nutritional assessment and useful for serial monitoring of energy requirements.

The accurate assessment of energy expenditure is important, since overfeeding of patients may be as harmful as underfeeding. Glucose infused in amounts in excess of 7 mg/kg/min is not oxidized. Rather, it is synthesized into fat, which may lead to hepatic steatosis.[35,43] Also, extra carbon dioxide and fluid loads produced as a result of excess nutrient intake exert deleterious effects in patients with impaired ventilatory function.

Other Applications of Indirect Calorimetry

Indirect calorimetry can be used for patients other than those receiving intensive nutrition support. It is difficult to estimate energy expenditure in obese patients, and indirect calorimetry may be used to guide a nutrition support regimen.[44–46] Inpatient and outpatient centers that deal with eating disorders find the assessment of energy expenditure a useful adjunct to therapy.[12] Study protocols may be devised to examine segments of the patient population in conjunction with specific diseases or injuries.[29,47–49] Indirect calorimetry may be integrated as a component of other hospital-based or outpatient-based programs such as wellness programs.

Because the type and complexity of patients seen at home is increasing, the use of indirect calorimetry in this setting can be an important part of initial and follow-up assessments for people receiving nutrition support. Patients on home total parenteral nutrition support may be inadequately nourished when the Harris-Benedict equations are used to estimate energy requirements.[50] In the past, most metabolic carts were too large and cumbersome and not portable enough to take into the patient's home. One metabolic cart has been successfully used in home care applications because it is small and, although heavy, can be carried into a patient's home.[50,51]

Because a metabolic measurement cart is a very specialized, expensive instrument, clinicians should consider the following points before acquiring one: the population the metabolic cart will be applied to (ventilator-dependent or spontaneously breathing adult or pediatric patients); the type of measuring technique the metabolic cart uses (mixing chamber or breath by breath); the type and ease of connections to ventilator-dependent patients; and the type and ease of connections to spontaneously breathing patients (mask, canopy). Special considerations such as ease of movement, warranty, training, and support services (both technical and scientific) should also be included.

Using a metabolic measurement cart in numerous patient care settings increases revenue sources. In addition, documenting the cost-effectiveness of individualizing nutrition support regimens and using dietitians/clinicians who can accurately interpret the measurement data add to the value of the measurement.

The virtues of indirect calorimetry have been presented. However, this technique has some limitations. Metabolic measurement carts to perform indirect calorimetry are expensive, and they require an experienced technician with a thorough understanding of patient airway management. Indirect calorimetry may not be available at all times or applicable in all patient care situations. Thus, at times it is necessary to use equations.

ENERGY EQUATIONS

Energy requirements in hospitalized patients cannot be accurately predicted from equations developed from healthy individuals.[23,28,52] There have been several formulas developed for estimating caloric requirements. Foster and colleagues[47] have identified 191 different published formulas for predicting energy expenditures. The predictive equations of Harris and Benedict, Fleish, Klieber, Cunningham, and others are generally good predictors for normal populations but are unpredictably inaccurate for individuals whose metabolic function is compromised by illness or injury.[32] Each formula is designed to estimate an individual's energy expenditure. Some of the formulas are appropriate for normal subjects, and some are attempts at estimating a hospitalized person's energy expenditure. All are estimations only; none are exact.

Long and colleagues[14] used indirect calorimetry to estimate energy needs of patients suffering from various types of trauma. Patients who had undergone elective surgery, had skeletal trauma, or were suffering from sepsis or burns had their energy expenditures measured by indirect calorimetry and expressed as "percent increases in metabolic rate above normal." All patients' energy expenditures were greater than normal as would be expected.[14] Measurements obtained by indirect calorimetry allowed for a more precise approximation of the patients' energy expenditures than did the Harris-Benedict equations. Turner and colleagues[13] compared MEE in burn patients to energy expenditures calculated using the Harris-Benedict equations and a standard burn formula. These authors concluded that neither the Harris-Benedict equations nor the burn formula accurately predicted the MEEs in the severely burned patients.[13]

Two equations have been developed that are useful in predicting the energy expenditure of hospitalized patients. These equations are used for estimating the energy expenditures of ventilator-dependent patients and spontaneously breathing patients.[31] The equations were developed using statistical analysis similar to that used by Harris and Benedict in the development of the REE. Easily measured variables were correlated with indirect calorimetric measurements of energy expenditure from hospitalized patients using multiple regression analysis. These equations are described in Exhibit 7–4.[31]

The energy equations in Exhibit 7–4—EEE(v) and EEE(s)—were developed using 200 patients and were validated using a separate, independent set of data from 100 patients. Validation showed no significant difference between the patients' actual (MEE) and predicted energy expenditures (EEE). The equations were found to be accurate in predicting the energy requirements of hospitalized patients when indirect calorimetry is not available.[31] The same guidelines for applying MEEs to the REIs of hospitalized patients are used for the energy equations, substituting EEE(v) or EEE(s) where MEE is mentioned.

These equations have been further validated by other researchers in a similar patient group; with a critically ill patient population; and in mechanically ventilated, obese patients.[54–56] In each study, the equations were found to be significantly correlated to MEE and useful for the clinical setting.

The use of indirect calorimetry to measure energy expenditures is efficacious.[14,16,20,23,25,26,29,32,46] It allows clinicians to tailor a patient's nutrition support

Exhibit 7–4 Equations To Predict Energy Expenditure of Hospitalized Patients

Ventilator-Dependent Patients

$$EEE(v) = 1784 - 11(A) + 5(W) + 244(S) + 239(T) + 804(B)$$

Spontaneously Breathing Patients

$$EEE(s) = 629 - 11(A) + 25(W) - 609(O)$$

Where:

EEE = kcal/day
s = spontaneously breathing
v = ventilator dependent
A = age (years)
W = body weight (kg)
S = sex (male = 1, female = 0)
T = diagnosis of trauma (present = 1, absent = 0)
B = diagnosis of burn (present = 1, absent = 0)
O = obesity >30% above ideal body weight from 1959 Metropolitan Life Insurance tables (present = 1, absent = 0)

Note: These equations have been statistically reevaluated, and the equation for ventilator-dependent patients is revised from the original reference.

Source: Data from Ireton-Jones, Turner, Liepa, Baxter, 1992 (31) and Ireton-Jones, Jones, 1997 (53).

regimen and to determine a patient's response to the regimen. Bedside, portable indirect calorimetry provides nutrition support clinicians with precise, individualized determinations of energy expenditures. It is applicable clinically, in research settings, and in various home care and outpatient settings. However, when indirect calorimetry is not available, the energy equations described above provide a statistically accurate and practically useful solution to the problem of predicting energy expenditures of hospitalized patients.

REFERENCES

1. Feurer ID, Mullen JL. Measurement of energy expenditure. In: Rombeau JL, Caldwell MD, eds. *Parenteral Nutrition.* Philadelphia: WB Saunders Co; 1986:224–236.
2. Nestle M. Nutrition. In: Martin DW, Mayes PA, Rodwell VW, Granner DK, eds. *Harper's Review of Biochemistry.* Los Altos, CA: Lange Medical Publications; 1985:350–378.
3. Kleiber M. *The Fire of Life.* New York: John Wiley & Sons; 1961:177–214.

4. Owen OE. Resting metabolic requirements of men and women. *Mayo Clin Proc.* 1988;63:503–510.

5. Westerterp KR. Energy expenditure. In: Westerterp MS, Fredrix EWHM, Steffens AB, eds. *Food Intake and Energy Expenditure.* Boca Raton, FL: CRC Press; 1994:237–257.

6. Reed GW, Hill JO. Measuring the thermic effect of food. *Am J Clin Nutr.* 1996;63:164–169.

7. Acheson KJ, Zahorska-Markiewiez B, Pittet P, Anantharaman K, et al. Caffeine and coffee: their influence on metabolic rate and substrate utilization in normal weight and obese individuals. *J Clin Nutr.* 1980; 33:989–997.

8. Jequeir E, Gygax PH, Pittet P, Vanotti A, et al. Increased thermal body insulation: relationship to the development of obesity. *J Appl Physiol.* 1974;36:674–678.

9. Katch F, McArdle W. *Nutrition, Weight Control and Exercise.* Philadelphia: Lea & Febiger; 1988:93–112.

10. Girandola R, Katch F. Effects of physical training on ventilatory equivalent and respiratory exchange ratio during weight supported, steady state exercise. *Eur J Appl Physiol.* 1976;35:119–123.

11. Jeevanandam M, Young DH, Schiller WR. Obesity and the metabolic response to severe multiple trauma in man. *J Clin Invest.* 1987;87:262–269.

12. Sedlet KL, Ireton-Jones CS. Energy expenditure and the abnormal eating pattern of a bulimic: a case study. *J Am Diet Assoc.* 1989;89:74–77.

13. Turner WW, Ireton CS, Hunt JL, Liepa GU, et al. Predicting energy expenditures in burned patients. *J Trauma.* 1985;25:11–17.

14. Long CL, Schaffel N, Geiger JW, Schiller WR, et al. Metabolic response to injury and illness: estimation of energy and protein needs from indirect calorimetry and nitrogen balance. *J Parenter Enter Nutr.* 1997;3:452–459.

15. Turner WW. Nutritional considerations in the patient with disabling brain disease. *Neurosurgery.* 1985;16:707–713.

16. Harris JA, Benedict FG. *Biometric Studies of Basal Metabolism in Man.* Washington, DC: Carnegie Institution of Washington; 1919. Publication no 270.

17. Jequier E. Studies with direct calorimetry in humans: thermal body insulation and thermoregulatory responses during exercise. In: *Assessment of Energy Metabolism in Health and Disease.* Columbus, OH: Ross Laboratories; 1980:15–20.

18. DuBois EF. *Basal Metabolism in Health and Disease.* Philadelphia: Lea & Febiger; 1924.

19. Bradham GB. Direct measurement of the total metabolism of a burned patient. *Arch Surg.* 1972;105:410–417.

20. Jequier E. Measurement of energy expenditure in clinical nutritional assessment. *J Parenter Enter Nutr.* 1987;11:86S–89S.

21. Douglas CG. A method for determining the total respiratory exchange in man. *J Physiol (London).* 1911;42:xvii–xxvi.

22. Weir JW. New methods for calculating metabolic rate with special reference to protein metabolism. *J Physiol.* 1949;109:1–9.

23. Ireton CS, Turner WW, Hunt JL, Liepa GU, et al. Evaluation of energy expenditures in burn patients. *J Am Diet Assoc.* 1986;86:331–333.

24. Thompson J, Manore MM. Predicted and measured resting metabolic rate of male and female endurance athletes. *J Am Diet Assoc.* 1996;96:30–34.

25. McClave SA, Snider HL. Use of indirect calorimetry in clinical nutrition. *Nutr Clin Pract.* 1992;7:208–221.

26. Porter C, Cohen N. Indirect calorimetry in critically ill patients: role of the clinical dietitian in interpreting results. *J Am Diet Assoc.* 1996;96:49–57.

27. Lane LD, Winslow EH. Oxygen consumption, cardiovascular response, and perceived exertion in healthy adults during rest, occupied bedmaking, and unoccupied bedmaking activity. *Cardiovasc Nurs.* 1987;23:31–35.

28. Osborne BJ, Saba AK, Wood SJ, Nyswonger GD, et al. Clinical comparisons of three methods to determine resting energy expenditure. *Nutr Clin Pract.* 1994;9:241–246.

29. Kinney JM. Indirect calorimetry in malnutrition: nutritional assessment or therapeutic reference? *J Parenter Enter Nutr.* 1987;11:90S–94S.

30. Head CA, McManus CB, Seitz S, Grossman GD, et al. A simple and accurate indirect calorimetry system for assessment of resting energy expenditure. *J Parenter Enter Nutr.* 1984;8:45–48.

31. Ireton-Jones CS, Turner WW, Liepa GU, Baxter CR, et al. Equations for estimation of energy expenditures in patients with burns with special reference to ventilatory status. *J Burn Care Rehab.* 1992;13:330–333.

32. Dietrich KA, Romero MD, Conrad SA. Effects of gas leak around endotracheal tubes on indirect calorimetry measurements. *J Parenter Enter Nutr.* 1990;14:408–413.

33. Swimnamer DL, Phang PT, Jones RL, Grace M, et al. Twenty-four hour energy expenditure in critically ill patients. *Crit Care Med.* 1987;15:637–643.

34. Shronts EP, Lacy JA. Metabolic support. In: Gottschlich MM, Matarese LE, Shronts EP, eds. *Nutrition Support Dietetics Core Curriculum.* Silver Spring, MD: A.S.P.E.N.; 1993:356.

35. Ireton-Jones CS, Turner WW. The use of respiratory quotient to determine the efficacy of nutritional support regimens. *J Am Diet Assoc.* 1987;87:180–183.

36. Elia M, Livesey G. Theory and validity of indirect calorimetry during net lipid synthesis. *Am J Clin Nutr.* 1988;47:591–607.

37. Askanazi J, Rosenbaum SH, Hyman AI, Silverberg PA, et al. Respiratory changes induced by the large glucose loads of total parenteral nutrition. *JAMA.* 1980;243:1444–1447.

38. Pursell TP, Turner WW, eds. *Handbook of Intensive Nutritional Support.* Dallas, TX: University of Texas Southwestern Medical Center; 1988.

39. Mayes T, Gottschlich MM, Khoury J, Warden GD, et al. Evaluation of predicted and measured energy requirements in burned children. *J Am Diet Assoc.* 1996;96:24–29.

40. McClave SA, Snider HL, Greene L, Lowen C, et al. Effective utilization of indirect calorimetry during critical care. *Intern Care World.* 1992;9:194–200.

41. Rutten P, Blackburn GL, Flatt JP, Hallowell E, et al. Determination of the optimal hyperalimentation infusion rate. *J Surg Res.* 1975;18:477–483.

42. Ireton-Jones C, Turner WW. The effect of burn wound excision on measured energy expenditure and urinary nitrogen excretion. *J Trauma.* 1987;27:217–220.

43. Wolfe RR, O'Donnell TF Jr, Stone MD, Richmond DA, et al. Investigation of factors determining the optimal glucose infusion rate in total parenteral nutrition. *Metabolism.* 1980;29:892–900.

44. Astrup A, Buemann B, Christensen NJ, Madsen J, et al. The contribution of body composition, substrates, and hormones to the variability in energy expenditure and substrate utilization in premenopausal women. *J Clin Endocrinol Metab.* 1992;74:279–286.

45. Ireton-Jones CS, Francis C. Obesity: nutrition support practice and application to critical care. *Nutr Clin Pract.* 1995;10:144–149.

46. Ireton-Jones CS, Turner WW. Actual or ideal body weights: which is more accurate to estimate energy expenditure? *J Am Diet Assoc.* 1990;90:193–195.

47. Foster GD, Knox LS, Dempsey DT, Mullen JL, et al. Caloric requirements in total parenteral nutrition. *J Am Coll Nutr.* 1987;6:231–253.

48. Szeluga DJ, Stuart RK, Brookmeyer R, Uternohlen V, et al. Energy requirements of parenterally fed bone marrow transplant recipients. *J Parenter Enter Nutr.* 1985;9:139–143.

49. Merrick HW, Long CL, Grecos GP, Dennis, et al. Energy requirements for cancer patients and the effect of total parenteral nutrition. *J Parenter Enter Nutr.* 1988;12:8–14.

50. Ireton-Jones CS, Garritson BK, Long A. The use of indirect calorimetry in the assessment of energy expenditures in patients receiving home nutritional support. *J Am Diet Assoc.* 1994;94(suppl):A24.

51. Ireton-Jones CS, Morris D, Barbaro D. Energy expenditures of symptomatic HIV+ individuals. Presented at American Society for Parenteral and Enteral Nutrition; January 29, 1992; Orlando, FL. Abstract.

52. Roza AM, Shizgal HM. The Harris Benedict equation reevaluated: resting energy requirements and the body cell mass. *Am J Clin Nutr.* 1984;40:168–182.

53. Ireton-Jones CS, Jones JD. Why use predictive equations for energy expenditure assessment? *J Am Diet Assoc.* 1997;97(suppl):A-44.

54. Wall JO, Wall PT, Ireton-Jones CS, et al. Accurate prediction of the energy expenditures of hospitalized patients. *J Am Diet Assoc.* 1995;95(suppl):A-24.

55. Gagliardi E, Brathwaite LEM, Ross SE. Predicting energy expenditure in trauma patients: validation of the Ireton-Jones equation. *J Parenter Enter Nutr.* 1995;19(suppl):22S.

56. Amato P, Keating KP, Quercia RA, et al. Formulaic methods of estimating calorie requirements in mechanically ventilated obese patients: a reappraisal. *Nutr Clin Pract.* 1995;10:229–232.

PART II

Impact of Organ Function and Disease Process on Nutrition Therapy

CHAPTER 8

Esophagus, Stomach, and Intestines

John M. Draganescu and William H. Lipshutz

INTRODUCTION

In patients for whom nutrition therapy is indicated, there is an obvious need for early determination of the safe and effective use of the gastrointestinal tract, as well as the optimal route of delivery of enteral feedings. This can be best accomplished through a complete assessment of the gastrointestinal system. Depending upon the situation, various diagnostic studies and the expertise of health care specialists may be required before this determination can be made. This chapter reviews the many processes and frank disease states involving the gastrointestinal system that may absolutely contraindicate enteral feeding, permit its use with concomitant therapeutic measures, or merely modify its route of delivery.

THE ESOPHAGUS

The esophagus is a hollow tube 25 to 35 cm long in the adult; it is composed of striated muscle in the upper one third and smooth muscle in the lower two thirds. The esophagus extends from the pharynx, where the cricopharyngeal muscle comprises the upper esophageal sphincter, to the stomach. The lower end is composed of a specialized arrangement of the muscle fibers that form the lower esophageal sphincter (LES). This is a high-pressure zone maintained by active tension that relaxes upon swallowing, thereby allowing solids and liquids that have been pushed down the length of the esophagus by a peristaltic wave to be propelled into the stomach. The function of the LES is affected by numerous hormones, drugs, and other exogenous agents, as shown in Exhibit 8–1.

Disorders involving the esophagus can be characterized by actual mechanical obstruction of the esophageal lumen, dysfunction of the esophageal sphincters or the peristaltic activity between them, or varying degrees of both mechanical obstruction and faulty motor function. These disorders may prevent consideration of the

Exhibit 8–1 Drugs and Other Agents That Affect Lower Esophageal Sphincter Pressure

Increase Sphincter Pressure
  alpha-adrenergic agonists
  antacids
  bethanechol
  gastrin
  histamine
  metoclopramide
  prostaglandin F_2
  protein in diet
Decrease Sphincter Pressure
  alpha-adrenergic antagonists
  anticholinergics
  beta-adrenergic agonists
  cholecystokinin
  ethanol
  fat in diet
  glucagon
  prostaglandins E, E_2
  secretin
  smoking

nasoenteric route for delivering enteral feedings and may also predispose toward various complications if feedings are initiated. Consequently, it is important to assess for the presence of these disorders in patients so that appropriate decisions regarding enteral alimentation and any indicated therapeutic measures can be made.

Gastroesophageal Reflux Disease

Gastroesophageal reflux disease (GERD) involves the symptomatic reflux of gastric contents—particularly acid, pepsin, and bile—into the esophagus with resultant damage to the esophageal mucosa, leading to esophagitis and heartburn. Although the prevalence of this frequently encountered problem is difficult to ascertain, one study of presumably normal hospital personnel revealed that 7% suffered heartburn daily, and 36% experienced it at least once each month.[1] In assessing the suitability of the gastrointestinal tract for enteral feeding, there are multiple reasons why GERD must be appreciated if present: (1) Already existing complications of GERD (eg, stricture) preclude nasoenteric tube feeding. (2) Heartburn and other related symptoms may be exacerbated after feedings are started. (3) Immediate and possibly life-threatening complications such as pulmonary aspiration may be elicited by enteral feedings. (4) Steady progression of GERD can be sustained by continued enteral feedings, with potential development of new complications. For all of these reasons, a review of various elements of this disease is warranted.

Clinical Presentation

The most common symptom of GERD is heartburn—a substernal burning sensation that rises toward the throat, often elicited by lying flat or bending over. If the reflux is severe enough, these same body positions may also evoke actual regurgitation of gastric fluid into the mouth—causing choking, coughing, and possible pulmonary aspiration, with symptoms of wheezing and dyspnea. Other symptoms include dysphagia—difficulty in swallowing usually involving solid foods—which may be experienced with or without development of an actual stricture; odynophagia—pain on swallowing—usually experienced after chronic, severe reflux has caused significant mucosal damage; and water brash, when the mouth suddenly fills with a large amount of fluid possibly secreted by the salivary glands. Gastroesophageal reflux may also result in hemorrhage that occasionally can be severe and readily apparent, resulting in the detection of bright red blood or "coffee grounds," but more often occult.

Pathogenesis

Multiple mechanisms of GERD have been established[2] that are operative in varying degrees in any given patient: (1) low LES pressure, resulting in inadequate protection against reflux, that may be persistently low or decreased periodically throughout the day; (2) increased abdominal pressure, seen with contraction of the diaphragm (coughing), abdominal musculature (straining, exercise, and stooping), or both; (3) mechanical predisposition toward reflux (when recumbent or bent over); (4) damaged mucosa because of refluxed acid, pepsin, and bile salts, with increased concentrations of these substances due to increased production, decreased gastric emptying, or reflux of duodenal contents; and (5) inefficient esophageal clearance mechanisms with a resultant increase in duration of mucosal exposure to damaging elements, eg, loss of gravity assist (recumbency) and decreased effective peristalsis (esophageal motor disorders). Varying combinations of these mechanisms may be present in any patient with GERD; the severity of the esophagitis is dependent upon the concentration of the damaging components in refluxed material and the duration of its contact with the esophageal mucosa.[2]

Diagnostic Evaluation

A number of studies can be employed to assess for the presence of GERD[3]:

Barium Swallow with Upper Gastrointestinal Series. Used as an initial study, the barium swallow with upper gastrointestinal series is more effective in ruling out other diagnoses (eg, peptic ulcer disease) and in assessing for gross lesions (eg, esophageal stricture, ulcer, or cancer) than in detecting esophageal mucosal damage or actual reflux.

Endoscopy. The most widely employed diagnostic modality, endoscopy allows direct examination of the entire mucosal surface and biopsy of the mucosa and any visualized lesions.

If the above studies are not definitive, the following may be employed to assess for gastroesophageal reflux.

Acid Perfusion (Bernstein) Test. A tube is placed in the upper third of the esophagus of a patient sitting upright, and normal saline is infused, followed by 0.1 N HCl for 30 minutes or until related symptoms are produced. The test is deemed positive if symptoms are reproduced twice during acid infusion and are relieved by saline infusion.

Esophageal Manometry. Using a multilumen water-perfused catheter assembly generally passed in nasogastric fashion, recordings of LES pressure and determination of the nature of peristaltic activity can be attained.

Prolonged pH Monitoring. After a pH electrode is placed 5 cm above the LES and the pH meter is connected to a recording device, the patient is given a normal diet (ensuring that no solids or liquids have a pH lower than 5.0). During the monitoring period, the patient records onset of symptoms and body position (supine or upright). The presence of reflux is indicated by a decrease in recorded pH to less than 4.0. After an overnight or 24-hour period of recording, assessments of the frequency and duration of episodes of reflux and the concomitant body position can be made.

In patients whose history and clinical pictures suggest gastroesophageal reflux, one can employ a number of studies of increasing complexity in attempting to diagnose it. The health care team can then consider various therapeutic measures, which are discussed later in this chapter, prior to initiating enteral feeding.

Complications of Reflux

Stricture. Long-term reflux can result in strictures that usually form in the lower esophagus; they are generally focal but can be long and extensive, a result of severe reflux. Patients complain of dysphagia when eating solid foods that worsens progressively, prompting them to reduce the size of the solid food swallowed, and gradually switch to soft foods and liquids as the stricture becomes increasingly narrow. When a bolus impacts completely at the stricture, the patient generally must regurgitate it. Diagnosis of an esophageal stricture is readily attained by barium swallow and endoscopy. Stricture is often the result of severe reflux, and its presence obviously contraindicates the nasoenteric route of enteral feeding and warrants instituting an effective antireflux regimen as well as considering jejunal instead of gastric feeding to minimize gastroesophageal reflux as much as possible. Strictures can be widened by using progressively larger-diameter, flexible dilators passed over guidewires under endoscopic and fluoroscopic guidance.

Ulcer. Gastroesophageal reflux can also produce esophageal ulcers. These are generally shallow, but some may deepen and on rare occasions can perforate the esophageal wall. Patients with esophageal ulcers may experience steady pain at rest as well as on swallowing. Hemorrhage, occasionally severe, may further complicate their clinical course. Barium swallow and endoscopy will detect these lesions, and the same considerations about enteral feeding apply with ulcers as with strictures.

Barrett's Esophagus. Chronic reflux can produce transformation of the typical squamous epithelium of the lower esophagus into columnar, or Barrett's, epithelium. The vertical extent of this process varies with each patient and is related to some degree to the severity of the reflux. The clinical importance of Barrett's esophagus stems from its potential to give rise to adenocarcinoma. Consequently, in addition to performing endoscopy and multiple biopsies to assess for adenocarcinoma, effective antireflux measures are warranted to control the formation of Barrett's esophagus and reduce the risk of malignancy. These measures should be well in place, and jejunal or continual gastric feeding should be considered before enteral feeding is deemed necessary for a patient with Barrett's esophagus.

Management

A number of factors contribute in varying degrees to the development of GERD. Effective therapy therefore simultaneously addresses these various components. A proposed therapeutic approach is summarized in Exhibit 8–2. Initially, one can employ simple maneuvers that are often very effective in reducing gastroesophageal reflux. The head of the bed should be elevated at least 6 inches; blocks may be placed under the legs of a nonhospital bed.[4] Patients should eat dinner or receive their last bolus feeding several hours before retiring, avoid late-night snacks, and refrain from lying flat after meals. Dietary modification entails avoiding alcohol, fatty foods, and chocolate (which can lower LES pressure), and coffee, tomato products, and orange juice (which can irritate esophageal mucosa).[5] Smoking, which also lowers LES pressure, should be eliminated.[6]

Drugs that lower LES pressure and thereby promote gastroesophageal reflux should be avoided, if possible,[3] including anticholinergics; α-adrenergic antagonists; β-adrenergic agonists; calcium-channel blockers; meperidine, morphine, and other opiates; progesterone; and theophylline. Calcium-channel blockers can

Exhibit 8–2 Therapeutic Approach to GERD

Phase 1
    Elevation of head of the bed
    Dietary modification
    Decrease or stop smoking
    Avoid potentially harmful medications
    Antacids or alginic acid
Phase 2
    Histamine H2 antagonists
        Cimetidine
        Ranitidine
    Bethanechol
    Metoclopramide
Phase 3
    Antireflux surgery

Source: Reprinted with permission from J.E. Richter, "A Critical Review of Current Medical Therapy for Gastroesophageal Reflux Disease," *Journal of Clinical Gastroenterology,* Vol. 8, Supp. 1, p. 78, © 1986, Lippincott-Raven Publishers.

---

predispose toward reflux by inhibiting esophageal contractions, thereby reducing the ability of the esophagus to clear refluxed acid.[7] Active therapeutic measures include the use of antacids—especially at bedtime—which not only neutralize acid but also increase LES pressure and reduce reflux.[8] Alginic acid, found in combination with antacids in Gaviscon (Marion Laboratories, Kansas City, MO), forms a viscous layer on top of the gastric contents that physically reduces the frequency and quantity of reflux.[9]

If a patient does not respond to the initial regimen above, more aggressive intervention can be undertaken. Histamine H2 receptor-blocking agents—cimetidine, ranitidine, and famotidine—assist by decreasing gastric acid production for hours after each administration. One of these agents should be used alone for at least 8 weeks before assessing the patient's response. Unrelieved symptoms can be addressed with the addition of metoclopramide; which is a dopamine antagonist that also increases LES pressure and in addition significantly enhances gastric emptying in reflux patients with either normal or delayed basal gastric emptying.[10] Through both of these mechanisms, metoclopramide can diminish the symptoms and mucosal damage of gastroesophageal reflux and accordingly reduce antacid use.[11] However, one must also be vigilant for its associated side effects, particularly neurologic ones such as drowsiness, lethargy, anxiety, and movement disorder. Cisapride, a prokinetic agent, has been used to relieve heartburn and regurgitation symptoms and is equally effective to histamine H2 blockers in healing esophagitis.[12] Omeprazole has also been effectively used to heal ulcers or erosions seen with GERD.[13]

Another agent that may be used at any point in the medical therapy of GERD is sucralfate (Carafate, Marion Laboratories). Given four times daily as a slurry made by dissolving a 1-g tablet in water, this aluminum hydroxide salt of sucrose octasulfate works locally by binding to inflamed esophageal mucosa and forming a protective barrier against acid and pepsin. Sucralfate also binds bile acids and therefore may significantly reduce their contribution to esophageal mucosal damage in patients with GERD.[14]

For the occasional patient who fails maximal medical therapy and has persistent severe symptoms, significant hemorrhage, progressive Barrett's esophagus, pulmonary complications, or strictures that cannot be dilated, antireflux surgery may be considered. Significant improvement is often seen postoperatively; however, recurrence of symptoms as well as histologic evidence of esophagitis as time progresses has been reported.[15] As the clinical situation permits, one must therefore ensure that an intensive therapeutic regimen has been employed fully before a refractory patient is referred for surgery.

In summary, one must assess for GERD in a patient whose clinical picture suggests its presence. When GERD is diagnosed, therapeutic measures should be implemented immediately. Clinical judgment regarding the severity of the disease and any of its complications should dictate the timing and delivery route of enteral feeding. In mild cases, nasogastric or gastrostomy tube feeding may be considered once antireflux measures are in place. More severe cases warrant consideration of continuous gastric or jejunal feeding in an attempt to minimize gastroesophageal reflux. Complications such as an esophageal stricture or severe ulceration preclude using nasoenteric tubes; however, the presence of these and other complications also mandates serious and thorough determination as to whether enteral feeding can be initiated safely and, if so, how long after therapeutic measures have been implemented. Careful clinical assessment increases the probability of safely delivering enteral feedings in appropriate patients without exacerbating existing GERD and risking serious and potentially life-threatening complications.

Mechanical Obstruction

Esophageal obstruction can result from a number of disorders and requires thorough assessment to rule out carcinoma and initiate appropriate therapy. Although the nasoenteric route of delivering enteral solutions is prohibited initially, occasionally a benign cause of obstruction (eg, a ring or web) can be resolved quickly, allowing for timely use of nasoenteric feeding if desired. Determination of the nature of the obstruction is therefore important in deciding upon the route and timing of enteral feedings.

Three of the most common causes of mechanical obstruction are (1) strictures, (2) tumors, and (3) Schatzki ring. Strictures can result from GERD, as previously discussed, and from caustic injury due to ingestion of alkali or acid. Tumors may be benign, such as leiomyomas and lipomas, or malignant, such as squamous cell carcinoma and adenocarcinoma. Schatzki ring is a thin, concentric narrowing in the lower esophagus without concomitant inflammation and fibrosis.

The clinical picture associated with mechanical obstruction includes dysphagia, which may be gradual or sudden in onset and generally is progressive in severity. Dysphagia is generally experienced with solid foods, although high-grade obstructing lesions can result in dysphagia with liquids also. Complete impaction of a solid-food bolus, generally meat, can be a presenting complaint, as is sometimes seen with Schatzki ring, or it may characterize a patient's course at any point because of progressive narrowing of the esophagus. Substernal or back pain may result from gastroesophageal reflux that produces strictures, or from carcinoma that can bore through the esophageal wall. Anorexia and weight loss are usually seen in patients with carcinoma. Iron-deficiency anemia due to slow, chronic blood loss—and, rarely, brisk acute hemorrhage—can mark the course of patients with reflux esophagitis and strictures, and cancer of the esophagus.

The diagnosis of mechanical obstruction can be accomplished by obtaining a barium swallow, which generally is definitive in revealing an obstructing lesion. Further assessment of the exact nature of the lesion is achieved through endoscopy, which allows direct visualization, and biopsy and cytology if indicated. If a tumor is discovered, a computed tomography scan can demonstrate any invasion through the esophageal wall, further extension into the mediastinum, and lymph node involvement. Management of strictures and Schatzki ring includes dilatation with tapered dilators, using endoscopic guidance as warranted. Antireflux measures are always needed for peptic strictures. Benign tumors generally require surgical therapy; esophageal carcinoma is treated by surgery, radiation therapy, or a combination of these, or by palliative measures depending upon the location and extent of the tumor and the patient's overall clinical status.

Although mechanical obstruction contraindicates nasoenteric feeding at the outset, quick resolution of Schatzki ring by dilatation allows early use of this route of delivering enteral feedings. This is not the case with peptic strictures or tumors, whose treatment extends over longer periods of time, thereby necessitating use of an enterostomy. Peptic strictures represent severe GERD, and continuous gastric or jejunal feeding to minimize gastroesophageal reflux is indicated.

Motor Disorders

Disorders of esophageal motility and LES function can result in dysphagia and other complications that may affect enteral feedings. These disorders may be primary (ie, when they occur in the absence of gastric carcinoma, esophagitis, systemic illness, or neuromuscular disease). An example of a primary esophageal motility disorder is achalasia. Alternatively, a systemic disease that involves the esophagus produces a similar clinical picture, as can be seen in scleroderma. A review of these two processes follows.

Achalasia

Achalasia is characterized by incomplete relaxation of the LES after swallowing, thereby producing an impediment to the movement of ingested material from the esophagus to the stomach. Resting LES pressure is usually increased, and the LES is supersensitive to cholinergic drugs.[16] Accompanying these abnormalities of the LES is the absence of normal peristalsis of the esophagus, which also contributes to ineffective delivery of solids and liquids into the stomach. Adequate oral feeding of enteral solutions and even nasoenteric tube placement obviously are difficult to achieve in this setting. Detection and treatment of achalasia, therefore, are crucial prior to instituting these two methods of enteral alimentation.

Clinically, patients experience dysphagia that is usually gradual in onset, not progressive, and noted with solids and liquids. Cold liquids or rapid eating may exacerbate symptoms, and impaction of a food bolus can usually be relieved by drinking large amounts of fluids. Odynophagia is occasionally present. Regurgitation of material from the esophagus is a common manifestation, especially at night, when patients may experience paroxysms of coughing or find food contents on the pillow upon awakening. Pulmonary aspiration of regurgitated material can also produce wheezing, dyspnea, or actual pneumonia. Weight loss may be seen in severe cases.

The diagnosis of achalasia begins with radiographic assessment. Occasionally a plain, upright chest X-ray reveals a widened esophagus with an air-fluid level due to retained food, and lack of a gastric air bubble. Barium swallow provides a more definitive assessment. Classic findings include lack of normal peristalsis, dilatation of the esophagus, and a "beak" appearance of the terminal esophagus (see Figure 8–1). Not all of these findings may be present. In all cases, the definitive diagnosis is made by esophageal manometry, which reveals the aforementioned findings of LES dysfunction and aperistalsis. Endoscopy should be performed to ensure that no tumor of the gastroesophageal junction or cardia of the stomach is causing secondary achalasia.

Complications of achalasia include the pulmonary manifestations of recurrent aspiration from regurgitation, and an increased incidence of squamous cell carcinoma of the esophagus. Treatment with pharmacologic agents has been studied. Nifedipine,[17] isosorbide dinitrate,[18] β-adrenergic agonist,[19] terbutaline sulfate, and nitroglycerin[20] have been shown to lower LES pressure significantly; however, the duration of this benefit and correlated relief of dysphagia are variable, and effec-

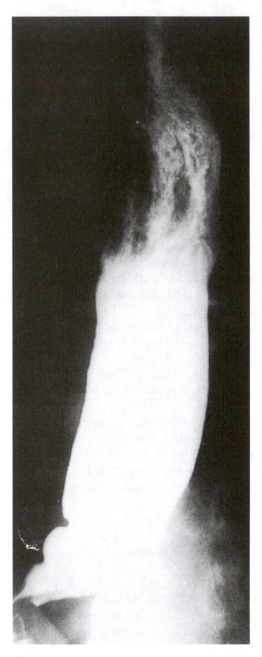

Figure 8–1 Barium Swallow from Patient with Achalasia. Note typical findings of a dilated esophagus that narrows distally, producing a beak appearance.

tive clinical use over a long period of time remains to be proven. Definitive treatment consists of actual destruction of the muscle fibers at the LES. In most patients, this can be safely accomplished by pneumatic dilatation. After evacuation of the esophagus, a bag dilator is passed orally into the esophagus; with fluoroscopic guidance, the unit's bag is positioned at the LES and then inflated to 15 psi for approximately 15 to 20 seconds. Most patients are markedly improved within hours, and this procedure can be repeated at a later time if the patient's dysphagia recurs or worsens. If contraindications to bag dilatation exist, or if a patient fails multiple sessions, myotomy and an antireflux procedure should be performed.

Recognition of achalasia prior to institution of oral or nasoenteric feeding is important to prevent significant regurgitation and pulmonary aspiration with its adverse sequelae. Because pneumatic dilatation can be accomplished shortly after diagnosis of achalasia, oral or nasoenteric feeding should be delayed until it is performed, if the patient's clinical picture permits. Otherwise, parenteral alimentation may be employed around the time of pneumatic dilatation or myotomy.

Scleroderma

Achalasia is a primary esophageal motor disorder, but a systemic disease that involves the esophagus may also produce abnormal motility and LES function. Scleroderma is such an example. This disease is marked by a proliferation of connective tissue with fibrosis of multiple organs. Although any segment of the gastrointestinal tract can be involved, the esophagus is the most common site, as manometric abnormalities can be detected in three fourths of patients.[21] Less commonly involved are the small bowel, colon, and stomach, in decreasing order of frequency.[22] Esophageal manometry reveals decreased amplitude or absent peristaltic waves at the distal two thirds, and an incompetent LES; LES pressure is usually low but may be normal in some patients. This LES dysfunction predisposes to an increased frequency of gastroesophageal reflux, and the lack of effective peristalsis results in impaired clearance of refluxed acid, pepsin, and bile. These elements consequently attack the esophageal mucosa for extended periods, and severe esophagitis ensues.

Expectedly, the clinical manifestations of this disorder include heartburn, due to development of GERD. Dysphagia with solids and/or liquids may be experienced, secondary to the characteristic abnormal peristalsis or to the development of a peptic stricture—seen in about 40% of patients—which represents a complication of GERD.[23]

Diagnosis of esophageal involvement in scleroderma begins with a barium swallow. Esophageal dilatation, diminished peristalsis, and frank gastroesophageal reflux can be seen. Large, wide-necked diverticula of the esophagus may be present, like those reported in the small bowel and colon of patients with scleroderma.[24] Esophageal manometry generally demonstrates the aforementioned findings of diminished, if not absent, peristalsis and LES incompetency.

Adverse sequelae of the esophageal motor disorder in scleroderma include the known complications of GERD. Not only are peptic strictures seen, but Barrett's metaplasia may occur, as was detected endoscopically in one study in 37% of patients reviewed.[25] Adenocarcinoma therefore remains a potential consequence in such patients.

No treatment exists to reverse the motor disorder seen in patients with scleroderma with esophageal involvement. Aggressive antireflux measures are clearly indicated, as many of these patients suffer severe GERD and may develop multiple complications.

Enteral feedings may be used in patients who do not have extensive small-bowel involvement and significant malabsorption. Patients with scleroderma with evidence of esophageal involvement, however, are most likely to benefit from continuous gastric or jejunal feeding implemented only after a vigorous antireflux regimen is already in place. Effective enteral alimentation can then take place without exacerbating gastroesophageal reflux and predisposing toward development of its complications.

THE STOMACH

Evaluation of the stomach and its rate of emptying is an important element in the assessment of a patient for whom enteral feeding is being considered. Adequate gastric emptying is crucial for safe and effective administration of both oral and gastric feeding. Where oral feeding is not possible, gastric feeding has a number of advantages over small bowel feeding, including (1) greater reservoir capacity, permitting the use of bolus feedings where no contraindications exist; (2) greater tolerance of osmotic loads without abdominal cramping, distention, vomiting, and fluid and electrolyte shifts; (3) resultant larger variety of enteral feeding formulas; and (4) easier maintenance of enteral access with nasogastric or percutaneous endoscopic gastrostomy tubes. These advantages relate directly to both the reservoir function of the stomach and its regulation of the emptying of liquids into the small bowel. The main disadvantage of gastric feeding is its potential to evoke a new onset of gastroesophageal reflux or exacerbate already ongoing reflux. A number of esophageal disorders predispose toward the development of gastroesophageal reflux. Gastric feeding places these patients at even greater risk; and, in addition, delayed gastric emptying potentiates further reflux not only in these patients but in every patient receiving oral or gastric feeding. Therefore, identification of delayed gastric emptying is necessary to prevent progressive gastroesophageal reflux and life-threatening complications such as pulmonary aspiration.

Delayed Gastric Emptying

Clinical manifestations of delayed gastric emptying may be mild or severe and include abdominal fullness and distention, nausea and vomiting (especially after meals), and anorexia and weight loss. On physical examination, a succussion splash may be detected occasionally: with the stethoscope placed at the epigastrium, the patient is rocked from side to side. If a splash of intragastric contents is heard, especially if hours have passed since the last feeding, delayed gastric emptying is probably operative. Gross abdominal distention may also be seen on examination, but its occurrence is variable. More definitive means of diagnosis generally are required.

Diagnosis

A simple, noninvasive means of assessing for delayed gastric emptying is the upper gastrointestinal barium series. A dilated stomach, retained gastric contents, and slow or absent passage of barium into the duodenum may be seen. Lesions such as ulcers and neoplasms that can cause mechanical obstruction, discussed later in this chapter, may also be detected. However, radiographic assessment of patients without complete obstruction is gross and qualitative; the rate of emptying cannot be quantitated on plain radiographs, since no measurement of the volume of residual barium is possible. Nevertheless, the upper gastrointestinal series is a useful initial study in evaluating the patient for decreased gastric emptying.

If the upper gastrointestinal series is not definitive, further assessment can consist of radionuclide scanning, which attempts to quantitate physiologically gastric motility and emptying. Radioisotopes that emit low levels of γ-radiation are used to label solids and liquids, which the patient ingests. A counter placed over the stomach determines the amount of radioisotope remaining in the stomach at different times, determining the rate of emptying. Several factors may affect the accuracy of the test, depending on the methodology used (eg, the concomitant volume of gastric secretion diluting the labeled meal cannot be quantitated). Nevertheless, the results of radionuclide scanning may provide strong evidence of delayed gastric emptying in a given patient. Endoscopy can also be used as a diagnostic tool. It provides for direct visualization of the gastric, pyloric, and duodenal mucosa to ascertain any possible causes of mechanical obstruction, and for biopsy of any lesions such as neoplasms or gastric ulcers. The diagnosis of delayed gastric emptying generally can be established through evaluation of the patient's clinical picture and use of one or more of the above diagnostic methods.

Pathogenesis

Delayed gastric emptying can result from mechanical obstruction by structural lesions located at critical sites. Many factors that do not involve a mechanical process can also produce diminished motility of the stomach. Both possibilities need to be considered in the evaluation of a patient with evidence of delayed gastric emptying.

Mechanical Gastric Outlet Obstruction. Any lesions located between the antrum and the duodenum inclusively can produce partial or complete gastric outlet obstruction. The severity of the obstruction can increase with time as the particular lesion progresses. Some causal factors are (1) prepyloric, pyloric, or duodenal ulcers with resultant inflammation and edema; (2) gastric carcinoma; (3) hypertrophic pyloric stenosis; and (4) prolapsing gastric polyps.

Nonmechanical Gastric Retention. Significantly delayed gastric emptying can also be seen in several scenarios in the absence of any structural lesions causing obstruction, as shown in Exhibit 8–3. Diabetic gastroparesis is a known complication of insulin-dependent diabetes mellitus, and the correlating symptoms may range from none to very severe. Complaints in any affected patient vary significantly with time, as completely asymptomatic periods may be experienced. Manometric assessment of the stomachs of these patients has revealed reduced gastric motor activity that is likely due to gastric neuropathy and not to any myopathy.[26,27] Delayed emptying of solids is most commonly seen, but with progression of the gastroparesis, emptying of liquids can also be diminished.[28] Hyperglycemia itself may also contribute to reduced gastric activity. One study of normal subjects demonstrated that induced hyperglycemia significantly reduced emptying of liquid meals containing protein with or without fat, but generally did not affect emptying of saline.[29] This finding suggests that hyperglycemia may enhance separate inhibitory mechanisms that diminish gastric motor function rather than cause this directly. The variable intensity of gastroparesis that marks the course of many patients with long-term diabetes can make control of their diabetes more difficult with oral or gastric feeding. Inconsistent rates of passage of enteral feeding solutions into the duodenum produce greater swings in serum glucose levels even with the same insulin regimen and schedule. Clinicians must keep this phenomenon in mind when attempting to achieve better glucose control through manipulations of the enteral hyperalimentation and insulin therapies.

Vagotomy and gastric surgery occasionally may produce delayed gastric emptying, although often transient. Truncal vagotomy and pyloroplasty have been shown to delay emptying of solids shortly after surgery, but improvement is noted 1 to 4 months after surgery and normal emptying is demonstrated within 3 years.[30] Liquid emptying in these patients is quicker as measured 3 months after surgery.[31] Selective (total gastric) vagotomy in humans results in a more rapid initial gastric emptying of liquids but an increased time for complete emptying.[32] When pyloroplasty is also performed, the time required for complete emptying is normal. A study using dogs demonstrated delayed emptying of solids after selective vagot-

Exhibit 8–3 Delayed Gastric Emptying States

Mechanical factors
  Gastric carcinoma
  Duodenal, pyloric, or prepyloric ulcers
  Idiopathic hypertrophic pyloric stenosis
Acid-peptic diseases
  Gastroesophageal reflux
  Gastric ulcer disease
Gastritis
  Atrophic gastritis ± pernicious anemia
  Viral gastroenteritis (acute—? chronic)
Metabolic and endocrine
  Diabetic ketoacidosis (acute)
  Diabetic gastroparesis (chronic)
  Hypothyroidism
  Pregnancy?
  Uremia?
Collagen vascular diseases—scleroderma
Pseudoobstruction
  Idiopathic
  Secondary (eg, amyloidosis, muscular dystrophies)
Postgastric surgery
  Postvagotomy and/or postgastric resections
Medications
  Anticholinergics, narcotic analgesics, L-dopa
Hormones (pharmacologic studies)
  Gastrin, cholecystokinin, somatostatin
Anorexia nervosa—? bulimia
Idiopathic
  Gastric dysrhythmias—tachygastria
  Gastroduodenal dyssynchrony
  ? Role of central nervous system (eg, depression)

Source: Reprinted with permission from H. Minami and R.W. McCallum, "The Physiology and Pathophysiology of Gastric Emptying in Humans," *Gastroenterology,* Vol. 86, pp. 1592–1610, © 1984, W.B. Saunders Company.

omy, but normal emptying occurred when the vagotomy was combined with pyloroplasty.[33] Superselective (proximal gastric) vagotomy also results in rapid initial emptying of liquids, but the time required for complete emptying is normal.[32] When both truncal vagotomy and antrectomy are performed, delayed emptying of solids is noted after surgery, but this resolves by 6 months.[34] Delayed gastric emptying of solids and/or liquids can thus be seen in varying degrees postoperatively depending on the type of vagotomy and gastric surgery performed, as well as the time interval between surgery and evaluation. The longer this interval, the less likely it is that significantly delayed emptying is due to such surgery, and other causes need to be considered.

A number of drugs are known to diminish gastric emptying. Opiate analgesics have been shown in dogs to decrease the frequency of gastric contractions.[35] Anticholinergics and tricyclic antidepressants may also produce delayed gastric emptying. L-Dopa has been shown to delay gastric emptying, potentially through stimulation of inhibiting dopamine receptors in the stomach.[36] β-Adrenergic agonists such as isoproterenol and salbutamol can decrease gastric emptying.[37] Aluminum hydroxide gel has also been shown to delay gastric emptying.[38]

Other notable causes of decreased gastric motor activity include elemental diets whose high osmolality and amino acid concentration may be responsible for a longer emptying time than found with blenderized foods with a similar caloric content.[39] Total parenteral nutrition (TPN) has also been shown to decrease gastric emptying through an unknown mechanism, although the effect of amino acids on gastric acid secretion and the effect of hyperglycemia on gastric emptying may be contributory.[40] This phenomenon may explain the nausea and anorexia experienced by some patients on TPN who are started on enteral feeding supplements. Consequently, discontinuation of TPN may be required to determine whether it is responsible for the patient's intolerance of enteral feeding.

Various metabolic and endocrine abnormalities can result in diminished gastric emptying. Hypokalemia, hypomagnesemia, hypocalcemia, hypercalcemia, uremia, and hypothyroidism have been implicated. Viral gastroenteritis can be linked to abnormal gastric motor function.[41] A systemic disease such as scleroderma can also involve the stomach and produce gastric stasis.

Therapy

Before oral or gastric feeding of a patient with delayed gastric emptying is initiated, the cause of the problem must be determined so that specific and directed therapy can be undertaken. The many different causes warrant many different approaches. Prokinetic agents can supplement directed therapy of delayed emptying. Metoclopramide significantly improves gastric emptying through its antagonism of dopamine, which is an inhibitory neurotransmitter in the gastrointestinal tract.[42] This agent also has cholinergic properties that are mediated by local intramural cholinergic neurons. The typical oral dosage of metoclopramide is 10 mg given one-half hour before each meal and at bedtime. A maximum dose of 80 mg each day can be tried, but side effects are more frequent above 40 mg. The agent is also available in parenteral form. Because impaired renal function prolongs the drug's half-life, patients with chronic renal failure should receive a reduced dosage. Side effects are seen in up to 20% of patients, and include drowsiness, lassitude, anxiety, agitation, and, uncommonly, extrapyramidal dystonic reactions. These side effects are generally reversible after withdrawal of the agent. Two other prokinetic agents that are currently used in clinical trials are domperidone and cisapride. Both promise to be effective alternatives in treating decreased gastric motility in a number of clinical situations. Successful resolution of gastric stasis prior to oral or gastric feeding minimizes the exacerbation of associated symptoms such as upper abdominal pain, distention, early satiety, bloating, nausea, and vomiting, and reduces the risk of gastroesophageal reflux. Prior to resolution of delayed emptying, continuous jejunal feeding can be used.

Rapid Gastric Emptying

A number of clinical situations are marked by rapid gastric emptying. Some have already been described: vagotomy with pyloroplasty or antrectomy, and superselective (proximal gastric) vagotomy. Patients with a gastroenterostomy may also have rapid emptying. The clinical significance of rapid gastric emptying relates to the possible onset of the *dumping syndrome,* which can be quite distressing. Early symptoms seen within 30 minutes of a feeding include bloating, epigastric discomfort, flushing, dizziness, tachycardia, nausea, and vomiting. Late symptoms that occur 1 to 2 hours after a meal are those of hypoglycemia: sweating, palpitations, and weakness. While the mechanism of the dumping syndrome is not fully understood, humoral factors may mediate the symptoms.

Therapy directed toward rapid gastric emptying should be attempted if the dumping syndrome is seen. Dietary manipulations such as frequent, small feedings with a low-carbohydrate content, and small volumes of liquids—especially those without simple sugars—may be helpful. If enteral solutions are to be used, one should select a formula containing complex carbohydrates such as dextrins, cornstarch, and corn syrups, as opposed to sucrose, fructose, maltose, lactose, and glucose oligosaccharides. A formula with a high percentage of carbohydrate comprising the caloric content should be avoided; continuous feeding or the delivery of small boluses is potentially beneficial. If oral feeding is possible, pectin, a dietary fiber, can be added to reduce the rate of gastric emptying and assist in minimizing related symptoms of the dumping syndrome.[43] An opiate may help to diminish gastric motility. Surgical procedures attempting to resolve severe rapid gastric emptying have inconsistent outcomes, and the above measures should be maximized before a surgical remedy is considered.

While there are known advantages to utilizing gastric feeding for enteral hyperalimentation, a thorough assessment of each patient must be made to ensure that it can be used safely. Delayed gastric emptying, particularly involving complete mechanical obstruction, speaks against immediate oral or gastric feeding. A history or clinical picture of GERD warrants determination as to whether gastric feeding can even be considered, and what antireflux measures should be instituted to avoid the serious and debilitating complications that can be evoked by enteral feeding.

THE INTESTINES

A functioning, patent, small intestine is essential for adequate digestion and absorption of required nutrients. A fundamental component of the absorptive capacity of the small intestine is adequate length. Surgical resection or bypass of segments of the small intestine produces a variable picture of malabsorption depending upon the site and length of bowel involved. Resection of the jejunum may result in minimal fat malabsorption but no carbohydrate malabsorption because the ileum undergoes hyperplasia to compensate for the decreased absorptive capacity. The ileum is the site of selective absorption of bile salts and vitamin B_{12}, which cannot be performed by the jejunum; therefore, significant resection of the ileum results in maldigestion and more severe malabsorption of fat, and diarrhea and steatorrhea ensue. Without parenteral supplementation, Vitamin B_{12} deficiency may eventually develop. Carbohydrate absorption is generally adequate in these patients. As iron is absorbed most quickly in the duodenum, removal or bypass of this segment may result in significantly decreased iron absorption, especially if dietary intake of iron is limited. Microcytic anemia, atrophy of the papillae of the tongue, and angular stomatitis may develop as a result of iron deficiency. In addition, a large number of diseases that involve these segments of the small intestine may produce malabsorption because of the reduction of functioning small intestine. (For an expanded discussion of maldigestion and malabsorption, see Chapter 19.)

The patient's surgical history and any known history of diseases involving the small intestine provide important information in determining the suitability of enteral feeding. One must inquire about and investigate clinical manifestations of fat or carbohydrate malabsorption, including diarrhea and steatorrhea. Enteral hyperalimentation with formulas selected to provide a high number of calories, vitamins, and minerals can be utilized if malabsorption is not severe. For patients who have just undergone extensive small-bowel resection and are being maintained on TPN, initial enteral feedings should consist of elemental components. Small volumes and diluted formulas are required at the start in order to minimize the osmotic load and prevent the dumping syndrome and severe diarrhea. Tolerance of these elemental diets can be followed by more complex formulas. For patients who have persistent severe malabsorption due to inadequate length of functioning small intestine, either permanently or temporarily, enteral feeding may not provide adequate nutrient uptake. Parenteral nutrition is required until this condition is resolved.

Mechanical Obstruction

An important element in assessing the gastrointestinal tract is determining whether there is any hindrance to the flow of intestinal contents. Enteral feedings should not be initiated if such intestinal obstruction can be documented. Causes of mechanical obstruction are listed in Exhibit 8–4; they include intrinsic and extrinsic bowel lesions and various obturating, or occluding, processes. Adhesions that

Exhibit 8–4 Mechanical Intestinal Obstruction

I. **Obturation (obstruction)**
   A. Polypoid tumors
   B. Intussusception
   C. Gallstones
   D. Foreign bodies
   E. Bezoars
   F. Feces
II. **Intrinsic bowel lesions**
   A. Atresia
   B. Stenosis
   C. Strictures
      1. Neoplastic
      2. Inflammatory
      3. Chemical
      4. Anastomotic
   D. Vascular abnormality
      1. Arterial occlusion
      2. Venous occlusion
III. **Extrinsic bowel lesions**
   A. Adhesions
      1. Previous surgery
      2. Previous peritonitis
   B. Hernias
      1. Internal
      2. External
   C. Neoplasm
   D. Abscesses
   E. Volvulus
   F. Congenital bands

Source: Reprinted with permission from M.H. Sleisenger and J.S. Fordtran, *Gastrointestinal Disease*, p. 312, © 1983, W.B. Saunders Company.

create extrinsic compression are the most common cause of small-bowel obstruction. Neoplasms most commonly cause obstruction of the colon, with its larger diameter.

Clinical Picture

Signs and symptoms related to mechanical intestinal obstruction include crampy abdominal discomfort and recurrent vomiting, and their frequency is often higher in patients with proximal small-bowel obstruction. Abdominal distention resulting from accumulating secretions and gas in the bowel may occur, especially with distal small-bowel or colonic obstruction. Fever, rigors, hypotension, and tachycardia suggesting sepsis and shock can occur if unrelieved obstruction results in ischemia and necrosis of the bowel.

Physical examination may reveal scars from previous abdominal surgery and abdominal distention. Bowel sounds are often high-pitched, and rushes and tinkling are heard. Diffuse abdominal tenderness can be detected on palpation, and frank masses may be noted when neoplasms are responsible for the obstruction.

Diagnosis

The history and physical examination provide the greatest contribution in establishing the diagnosis of mechanical intestinal obstruction. Confirmation of the diagnosis can be attained radiographically. Abdominal plain films generally reveal dilated, gas-filled segments of bowel proximal to the site of obstruction, but little gas in the bowel distal to the obstruction. Small-bowel obstruction therefore generates multiple loops of distended small bowel on supine films but little or no gas in the colon. Upright films may demonstrate air-fluid levels and hairpin loops of small intestine. The frequency and degree of these findings depend on the location of small-bowel involvement. Distal obstruction produces more extensive abnormalities than does proximal obstruction. In addition, a complete obstruction will produce a greater number of abnormal plain findings than will a partial obstruction. Colonic obstruction produces distention of the colon, but small bowel dilatation usually is seen only if the ileocecal valve is incompetent. Patients with a competent ileocecal valve often have a severely dilated cecum. Discrimination between dilated segments of small intestine and colon usually can be made by evaluation of plain X-ray films. Should doubt exist as to the location of distended bowel, a single-contrast barium enema can safely provide useful information.

Treatment

Initial management of a patient with diagnosed mechanical intestinal obstruction consists of stabilizing measures. Intravenous fluid and electrolyte repletion is essential. Enteral alimentation should not be utilized. Plasma or other volume expanders and antibiotics are warranted if signs of shock and sepsis are present.

Decompression of the dilated bowel can be achieved with suction through a nasoenteric tube placed in the stomach or preferably the small intestine. Occasionally an uncomplicated, partial small-bowel obstruction due to adhesions, for example, will resolve with these measures alone, because the degree of extrinsic compression can vary with time. Most cases, however, require surgery to relieve the obstruction.

Successful treatment depends largely on prompt institution of stabilizing therapy and optimal timing of indicated surgery, depending on the cause of the obstruction and the clinical status of the patient.[44] Enteral alimentation should be avoided in patients with intestinal obstruction.

Adynamic Ileus

Adynamic ileus is most commonly seen after abdominal surgery and involves the diffuse loss of adequate gastrointestinal motility. Other causes of adynamic ileus include sepsis, electrolyte imbalance, intestinal perforation, and peritonitis. Clinically, patients have varying degrees of abdominal distention and usually do not pass stools or flatus. Bowel sounds are absent or decreased. Signs of sepsis, shock, or peritonitis may be present if one of these processes is responsible for the ileus. Abdominal X-ray films demonstrate intestinal dilatation and air-fluid levels that may be difficult to distinguish from those present in mechanical obstruction. A feature often seen with ileus, however, is extensive intestinal distention that can involve the stomach, small intestine, colon, and rectum. Treatment of adynamic ileus consists of the administration of intravenous fluids and correction of any electrolyte imbalance. Nasogastric suction is usually effective; if not, a long Cantor tube may be placed into the small intestine to provide continuous suction.

In the postoperative setting, adynamic ileus usually resolves within 3 days, although some patients may have slightly longer courses. An extended period of ileus warrants an assessment of other possible causes, including mechanical intestinal obstruction. Oral or enteral feeding can be started when the patient reports passage of flatus or stools and the abdomen is soft and nondistended with normal, active bowel sounds. Progressive advancement of the diet can continue as long as the patient does not have signs or symptoms of mechanical obstruction or ileus.

CONCLUSIONS

The utility of employing enteral feeding in meeting a patient's nutritional goals is well known. A number of advantages over parenteral hyperalimentation have been described. Before enteral alimentation is initiated, a thorough assessment of the gastrointestinal system is always required to ensure that the nutrition therapy will be safe and effective. A systematic review starting with the esophagus and moving aborally increases the chances of both detecting previously unrecognized pathologic conditions and acknowledging already documented disease states. Various diagnostic studies and therapeutic measures may then be warranted to ascertain whether enteral feeding can be used. If it can be used, one must determine (1) the optimal time for initiating enteral alimentation; (2) the therapeutic regimen, if indicated, to be used concomitantly; and (3) the optimal method of delivery of the enteral feeding solutions. In this manner, the probability of successfully meeting established nutritional goals without serious complications and further morbidity is greatly enhanced.

REFERENCES

1. Nebel OT, Fornces MF, Castell DO. Symptomatic gastroesophageal reflux: incidence and precipitating factors. *Am J Dig Dis.* 1976;21:953–956.

2. Dodds WJ, Hogan WJ, Helm JF, et al. Pathogenesis of reflux esophagitis. *Gastroenterology.* 1981;81:376–394.

3. Richter JE, Castell DO. Gastroesophageal reflux: pathogenesis, diagnosis, and therapy. *Ann Intern Med.* 1982;97:93–103.

4. Johnson LF, DeMeester TR. Evaluation of elevation of head of the bed, bethanechol, and antacid foam tablets on gastroesophageal reflux. *Dig Dis Sci.* 1981;26:673–680.

5. Price SF, Smithson KW, Castell DO. Food sensitivity in reflux esophagitis. *Gastroenterology.* 1978;75:240–243.

6. Dennish GW, Castell DO. Inhibitory effect of smoking on the lower esophageal sphincter. *N Engl J Med.* 1971;284:1136–1137.

7. Richter JE, Dalton CB, Brice RG, et al. Nifedipine: a potent inhibitor of contractions in the body of the human esophagus. *Gastroenterology.* 1974;89:549–554.

8. Higgs RH, Smyth RD, Castell DO. Gastric alkalinization: effect on lower esophageal sphincter pressure and serum gastrin. *N Engl J Med.* 1974;291:486–490.

9. Malmud LS, Fisher RS. Quantitation of gastroesophageal reflux before and after therapy using the gastroesophageal scintiscan. *South Med J.* 1978;71(suppl 1):10–15.

10. Fink SM, Lange RC, McCallum RW. Effect of metoclopramide on normal and delayed gastric emptying in gastroesophageal reflux patients. *Dig Dis Sci.* 1983;28:1057–1061.

11. Bright-Asare P, El-Bassorrasi M. Cimetidine, metoclopramide, or placebo in the treatment of symptomatic gastroesophageal reflux. *J Clin Gastroenterol.* 1980;2:149–156.

12. Wiseman LR, Faulds D. Cisapride: an updated review of its pharmacology and therapeutic efficacy as a prokinetic agent in gastrointestinal motility disorders. *Drugs.* 1994;47:116–152.

13. Skoutakis VA, Joe RH, Hard DS. Comparative role of omeprazide in the treatment of gastroesophageal reflux disease. *Ann Pharmacother.* 1995;29:1252–1262.

14. Hameeteman W, Boomgaard DM, Dekker W, et al. Sucralfate versus cimetidine in reflux esophagitis. *J Clin Gastroenterol.* 1987;9:390–394.

15. Brand DL, Eastwood IR, Martin D, et al. Esophageal symptoms, manometry, and histology before and after anti-reflux surgery. *Surgery.* 1979;76:1393–1401.

16. Cohen S, Fisher R, Fuch A. The site of denervation in achalasia. *Gut.* 1972;13:556–558.

17. Bortolotti M, Labo G. Clinical and manometric effects of nifedipine in patients with esophageal achalasia. *Gastroenterology.* 1981;80:39–44.

18. Gelfond M, Rozen P, Gilat T. Isosorbide dinitrate and nifedipine treatment of achalasia: a clinical, manometric and radionuclide evaluation. *Gastroenterology.* 1982;83:963–969.

19. Dimarino AJ, Cohen S. Effect of an oral beta₂-adrenergic agonist on lower esophageal sphincter pressure in normals and in patients with achalasia. *Dig Dis Sci.* 1982;27:1063–1066.

20. Wong RKH, Maydonovich C, Garcia JE, et al. The effect of terbutaline sulfate, nitroglycerin, and aminophylline on lower esophageal sphincter pressure and radionuclide esophageal emptying in patients with achalasia. *J Clin Gastroenterol.* 1987;9:386–387.

21. Turner R, Lipshutz W, Miller W, et al. Esophageal dysfunction in collagen disease. *Am J Med Sci.* 1973;265:191–199.

22. Olmsted WW, Madewell JE. The esophageal and small bowel manifestations of progressive systemic sclerosis. *Gastrointest Radiol.* 1976;1:33–36.

23. Cohen S. Motor disorders of the esophagus. *N Engl J Med.* 1979;301:184–192.

24. Clements JL, Abernathy J, Weens HS. Atypical esophageal diverticula associated with progressive systemic sclerosis. *Gastrointest Radiol.* 1978;3:383–386.

25. Katzka DA, Reynolds JC, Saul SH, et al. Barrett's metaplasia and adenocarcinoma of the esophagus in scleroderma. *Am J Med.* 1987;82:46–52.

26. Fox S, Behar J. Pathogenesis of diabetic gastroparesis: a pharmacologic study. *Gastroenterology.* 1980;78:757–763.

27. Malagelada J, Rees WDW, Mazolta LJ, et al. Gastric motor abnormalities in diabetic and postvagotomy gastroparesis: effect of metoclopramide and bethanechol. *Gastroenterology.* 1980;78:286–293.

28. McCallum RW, Meyer CT, Marignani P, et al. A multicenter placebo-controlled clinical trial of oral metoclopramide in diabetic gastroparesis. *Diabetes Care.* 1983;6:463–467.

29. MacGregor IL, Gueller R, Watts H, et al. The effect of hyperglycemia on gastric emptying in man. *Gastroenterology.* 1976;70:190–196.

30. Cowley DJ, Vernon P, Jones T, et al. Gastric emptying of solid meals after truncal vagotomy and pyloroplasty in human subjects. *Gut.* 1972;13:176–181.

31. Cobb JS, Banks S, Marks IN, et al. Gastric emptying after vagotomy and pyloroplasty. *Am J Dig Dis.* 1971;16:207–215.

32. Clarke RJ, Alexander-Williams J. The effect of preserving antral innervation and of a pyloroplasty on gastric emptying after vagotomy in man. *Gut.* 1973;14:300–307.

33. Interone VC, DelFinado JE, Miller B, et al. Parietal cell vagotomy. *Arch Surg.* 1971;102:43–44.

34. Kalbasi H, Hudson FR, Herring A, et al. Gastric emptying following vagotomy and antrectomy and proximal gastric vagotomy. *Gut.* 1975;16:509–513.

35. Konturek SJ. Opiates and the gastrointestinal tract. *Am J Gastroenterol.* 1980;74:285–291.

36. Berkowitz DM, McCallum RW. Interaction of levodopa and metoclopramide on gastric emptying. *Clin Pharmacol Ther.* 1980;27:414–420.

37. Rees MR, Clark RA, Holdsworth CD, et al. The effect of beta-adrenoreceptor agonists and antagonists on gastric emptying in man. *Br J Clin Pharmacol.* 1980;10:551–554.

38. Hurewitz A, Robinson RG, Vats TS. Effects of antacids on gastric emptying. *Gastroenterology.* 1976;71:268–273.

39. Bury KD, Jambunathan G. Effects of elemental diets on gastric emptying and gastric secretion in man. *Am J Surg.* 1974;127:59–64.

40. MacGregor IL, Wiley CD, Lavigne ME, et al. Total parenteral nutrition slows gastric emptying of solid food. *Gastroenterology.* 1978;74:1059. Abstract.

41. Meeroff JC, Schreiber DS, Trier JS. Abnormal gastric motor function in viral gastroenteritis. *Ann Intern Med.* 1980;92:370–373.

42. Albibi R, McCallum RW. Metoclopramide: pharmacology and clinical application. *Ann Intern Med.* 1983;98:86–95.

43. Leeds AR, Raephs DN, Ebied F, et al. Pectin in the dumping syndrome: reduction of symptoms and plasma volume changes. *Lancet.* 1981;1:1075–1078.

44. Stewardson RH, Bombeck CT, Nyhus LM. Clinical operative management of small bowel obstruction. *Ann Surg.* 1978;187:189.

CHAPTER 9

Pancreatic Function

Janet A. Furman

INTRODUCTION

The pancreas plays a vital role in the digestion and absorption of nutrients, and pancreatic dysfunction can result in malabsorption, weight loss, and malnutrition. Pancreatic diseases often result in the need for nutrition support. Diabetes, pancreatitis, and pancreatic adenocarcinoma can significantly affect patient tolerance to nutrition support. Pancreatic disease can also result in considerable hypermetabolic stress, and adequate nutrient delivery can be a challenge.

PANCREATIC FUNCTIONS

Exocrine Function

The pancreas consists of acinar cells and duct cells, which are responsible for its exocrine function. Digestive enzymes, zymogens, and bicarbonate are secreted from the acini. Pancreatic exocrine secretions drain into small ducts that terminate into the main pancreatic duct, and eventually drain into the duodenum. When released into the intestine, pancreatic zymogens begin an important cascade that activates a host of other enzymes needed for digestion. The primary proteolytic enzyme in pancreatic secretions is trypsin. Carbohydrate digestion is facilitated by pancreatic amylase. Dietary fats are hydrolyzed by pancreatic lipase. Pancreatic duct cells secrete large amounts of bicarbonate to neutralize gastric acid and protect the duodenum from acid erosion.

Pancreatic stimulation occurs in three phases—the cephalic phase, the gastric phase, and the intestinal phase.[1] The *cephalic phase* involves the central nervous system, particularly the vagus nerve. Vagal stimulation by the act of smelling, seeing, or thinking about food stimulates the release of enzymes from the pancreas. Cephalic stimulation also plays a role in basal pancreatic secretion and pancreatic response to cholecystokinin (CCK). The *gastric phase* is mediated by the stomach, and gastrin release results in stimulation of the acinar cells, thus promoting secretin release.[1] Gastric distention with feeding also stimulates the pancreas. The *intestinal phase* occurs with CCK and secretin release, which is facilitated by the presence of chyme in the small intestine. CCK provokes the pancreas to release enzymes and zymogens into the duodenum, and secretin induces the release of large amounts of fluid and bicarbonate from the pancreas into the duodenum.[2,3] It appears that these hormones act in tandem. The presence of CCK is required for secretin to affect the pancreas.[2] The delicate interplay of neurologic and hormonal mechanisms is important in the control of pancreatic exocrine function, which leads to the proper digestion and absorption of nutrients.

Endocrine Function

The pancreas secrets insulin and glucagon, and therefore plays a pivotal role in energy metabolism, utilization, and storage. The endocrine cells of the pancreas are clustered in groups called the islets of Langerhans, which account for only 2% of the total cells of the pancreas. With feeding, insulin is released into the bloodstream from the beta cells. Insulin is an anabolic hormone, and its primary purpose is to counteract the effects of glucagon-mediated fuel oxidation, which results in storage of nutrients in the body. Insulin also increases glucose transport into cells and adipose tissues for glycogen and fatty acid synthesis, respectively.[2] This lowers serum glucose levels during the fed state. Glucagon is a catabolic hormone that induces the mobilization of stored energy in the absence of adequate energy intake or during times of fasting. This keeps the level of blood glucose from dropping excessively between meals and provides a constant supply of glucose to the brain. Using both catabolic and anabolic hormone release, the pancreas strives to achieve glucose homeostasis.

NUTRITION MANAGEMENT IN PANCREATIC DISEASE

Two major diseases of the pancreas that may require specialized nutrition support are diabetes and pancreatitis. Diabetes is a relatively common endocrine disorder, and occurs in 2% to 4% of the U.S. population.[3] Pancreatitis, in its acute form, can be fatal. Chronic pancreatitis may occur in 4% to 5% of the U.S. population and is often associated with alcoholism.[4]

Diabetes

Diagnosis of diabetes includes one or more of the following: elevated glucose levels in the presence of classic symptoms (weight loss, polyurea, polydipsia, and ketonuria), elevated fasting glucose on more than one occasion, or prolonged elevation of serum glucose (greater than 200 mg/dL) during an oral glucose tolerance test. Elevated fasting glucose is defined as serum measurement greater than 140 mg/dL.[3] The presence of excess serum glucose may cause the glycosylation of proteins such as hemoglobin. Glycosylation is dependent on the extent of hyperglycemia and may cause cellular damage and functional defects.[5] Glycosylated hemoglobin (HgB A1C) is used to measure glycemic control over approximately 6 to 8 weeks. A glycosylated hemoglobin concentration of greater than 6% is abnormal and indicates prolonged hyperglycemia. Many people have impaired glucose tolerance that does not progress to diabetes. In the face of stress and illness, these patients may exhibit significant glucose intolerance during nutrition support.

Type I and Type II Diabetes

The two types of diabetes are type I (insulin dependent) and type II (non–insulin dependent). Type I diabetes is characterized by little or no insulin secretion. Its precise etiology is unknown; however, antibodies have been detected in some diabetics suggesting an autoimmune process rendering the insulin-producing cells of the pancreas ineffective.[3,5] Type II diabetes is characterized by decreased insulin secretion. Individuals with type II diabetes commonly exhibit resistance to the effects of insulin when it is exogenously administered.

Nutrition Support in Diabetes

Diabetic patients frequently experience hyperglycemia. It has been reported that leukocyte function, phagocytosis, and host defense are impaired in uncontrolled diabetes.[6–8] Decreased immune function has been found in people with glucose levels greater than 250 mg/dL, and it is prudent to keep glucose levels in the 200 to 250 mg/dL range.[6–9] During nutrition support, care should be taken not to exceed the maximal glucose oxidation capacity of the liver (5 mg/kg/min), as this may precipitate hyperglycemia. The main goal of nutrition support is to provide adequate energy while maintaining glucose control.

Elevations in blood glucose levels may necessitate the addition of insulin to parenteral nutrition solutions. A careful and conservative approach to adding insulin to the solution is safe, effective, and time saving. A common guideline for initiating therapy is to add 0.1 unit of regular insulin to the solution for each gram of dextrose provided.[9] Another approach is to limit carbohydrate in the initial parenteral nutrition infusion to less than 150 grams of carbohydrate and add one half of the usual daily insulin requirement to the solution.[10] Subcutaneous insulin should be used to maintain serum glucose levels less than 200, using the algorithm provided in Table 9–1. Once the patient is stable, the insulin in the total parenteral nutrition (TPN) solution can then be increased daily as needed by adding two thirds of subcutaneously injected insulin to the previous insulin dose.[9] For example, if a patient requires an extra 15 units of insulin overnight, then two thirds of

Table 9–1 Recommendations for Insulin Dosage

Capillary Glucose (mg/dL)	IDDM* (Dose in Units)	NIDDM** (Dose in Units)	Stress (Dose in Units)
200–250	3	5	5
251–300	6	10	10
301–350	9	15	15
351–400	12	20	20

*IDDM—insulin-dependent diabetes mellitus (type I)
**NIDDM—non–insulin-dependent diabetes mellitus (type II)

Source: Data from R.A. DeFronzo et al., Influence of Basal Insulin and Glucagon Secretion on Potassium and Sodium Metabolism, *J Clin Invest,* Vol. 61, pp. 472–479, © 1978, and L.D. Wagman et al., The Effect of Acute Discontinuation of Total Parenteral Nutrition, *Ann Surg,* Vol. 204, pp. 524–529, © 1986.

this amount (10 units) should be added to the next bag of TPN solution, provided that blood sugars remain above 100. Another approach involves increasing the insulin in increments of 0.5 unit per gram of dextrose delivered in the next bag of TPN solution if insulin is administered beyond the dose contained in the previous TPN.[9] These approaches are conservative and safe. Dextrose should be increased in the solution only when glycemic control is acceptable (ie, 200 mg/dL or below).

Although glucose control is paramount in the diabetic patient, insulin should be added sparingly to parenteral nutrition solutions to avoid the possibility of hypoglycemia, which may result in discontinuation and wasting of the TPN solution. Serum glucose levels should be monitored at least three times daily and insulin carefully adjusted in the TPN solution to ensure adequate glucose control. Patients who are unstable or experiencing wide fluctuations in blood sugars may need more frequent monitoring. Even in patients who have achieved an acceptable level of glucose control, careful monitoring is appropriate. During the course of parenteral nutrition, many changes can affect serum glucose levels. Patients may experience infection, which can result in hyperglycemia. Medications may be modified, many of which can cause aberrations in blood glucose. Renal function should also be closely monitored. A decline in renal function may increase the half-life of insulin in the body and exaggerate its effects. It is also important to note that subcutaneous insulin injection may be less effective in patients with marked edema, hypoalbuminemia, or peripheral vascular disease. These patients often respond more appropriately to intravenously supplied insulin.[11]

Recovery of regular insulin from TPN solutions has been researched, and results are conflicting. Some researchers believe that a decreased availability is related to adherence of the insulin molecule to the administration set, in-line filters, and macronutrient concentrations in the solution. Factors that may affect insulin availability include insulin concentration, amino acid concentration, and container type and size.[12] Studies have shown as little as 50% of regular insulin is available from TPN solution; however, more recent reports suggest that 90% to 95% of total insulin is recovered from TPN solution.[12,13] The introduction of TPN bags that do not contain polyvinyl chloride, as well as changes in amino acid solutions and insulin manufacturing, may account for this increase in insulin recovery.[8] There is no widely accepted factor on which to base dosing adjustment for insulin adherence. However, clinicians should be aware that a decrease in the availability of insulin may occur, and that patients receiving TPN may need more than their usual insulin dose to maintain glucose control.

Aberrations in serum glucose levels along with insulin infusion may also affect serum electrolyte levels. Hyperglycemia may precipitate a pseudohyponatremia and osmotic diuresis of water and electrolytes, which may result in the need for electrolyte supplementation. According to McMahon and Rizza, for every 62 mg/dL increase in plasma glucose above normal, plasma sodium concentration is reduced by 1 mEq/L.[9] Insulin administration may enhance potassium and phosphorus uptake by the cells and decrease serum levels. Insulin infusion may also affect renal sodium handling and increase sodium resorption.[9,14] Careful monitoring and assessment of serum electrolytes, as well as an understanding of the physiologic effects of insulin, are necessary to ensure safe and appropriate use of parenteral nutrition in diabetic patients.

During the transition from parenteral nutrition to enteral feeding or oral diet, glucose control can be complicated by inconsistent oral or enteral intake. Insulin in the TPN solution should be dosed conservatively, because sporadic oral intake may cause blood glucose to fluctuate. Once the patient is receiving 1000 enteral calories, insulin should be decreased or discontinued from the TPN solution and ordered via standing daily dose (with appropriate use of intermediate- and/or long-acting insulin). Elevated blood sugars resulting from increasing enteral intake should be covered with subcutaneous insulin administration, and every effort should be made to keep carbohydrate intake stable until glucose is well controlled. Macronutrients in the TPN solution may also be adjusted to account for enteral intake.

Sudden cessation in TPN administration has been reported to cause hypoglycemia in diabetic patients. However, recent investigation suggests that this outcome is somewhat variable and patient specific.[15] Unless the TPN contains large amounts of insulin, tapering of the solution over several hours is probably not necessary. If the patient is receiving no other significant source of carbohydrate, it may be prudent to decrease the infusion rate by half for the last hour of administration,[9] and monitor glucose levels at appropriate intervals after discontinuation of the TPN.

In the diabetic patient receiving enteral feeding, gastrointestinal complications as well as alterations in serum glucose levels may be present. Diabetic gastroparesis may affect as many as 20% to 30% of all diabetics. The rate of gastric emptying is further slowed by hyperglycemia.[16,17] Gastroparesis appears to occur more commonly in patients with prolonged presence of diabetes or those with diabetic neuropathies.[18,19] As many as 76% of diabetic patients may experience gastrointestinal symptoms related to diabetes.[20–21] Patients may experience either slowed or rapid gastric emptying with solid or liquid meals.[21–22] Alterations in intestinal transit time may manifest as nausea, vomiting, diarrhea, constipation, early satiety, or fecal incontinence.[22] Patients may also exhibit radiographic evidence of altered gastric emptying with no outward clinical signs. Altered intestinal transit may affect enteral intake and result in widely fluctuating serum glucose levels.

Prokinetic agents such as metoclopromide, erythromycin, and cisapride have been used successfully in the treatment of gastroparesis.[20–23] Table 9–2 outlines methods of action and side effects of these treatments. In the patient with severe gastroporesis, jejunostomy feedings have also been used with success.[24]

Enteral Feeding Formulas Used in Diabetes

Composition of enteral feeding formulas appropriate for the diabetic patient has been the subject of considerable debate. Specialized formulas have been developed to improve glucose tolerance in patients receiving enteral feeding. While low-carbohydrate formulas *do* blunt the glycemic response to feeding, the macronutrient composition of these formulas does not meet currently accepted dietary

---

Table 9–2 Methods of Action and Side Effects in Treatment of Gastroparesis

Medication	Class	Method of Action	Side Effects
Metoclopromide	Dopamine antagonist	Increases antral contractions; enhances lower esophageal sphincter (LES)	Parkinsonian symptoms, tardive dyskinesia, restlessness, drowsiness
Erythromycin	Macrolide (antibiotic)	Motilin receptor agonist	Hepatitis, nausea, vomiting, diarrhea, abdominal cramping
Cisapride	Benzamide	Enhances acetylcholine release in the gut, increases antral contractions, enhances LES tone, increases colonic motility	Abdominal cramping, diarrhea, dizziness, headache

DeFronzo et al. 1978 (ref. 15) and Wagman et al. 1986 (ref. 15)

guidelines for those with diabetes.[25] The American Diabetes Association states that while the total grams of carbohydrate do have an impact on blood glucose levels, the evidence for using higher-fat formulas or fiber-containing formulas is not completely convincing. American Diabetes Association guidelines for the diabetic patient recommend a diet that is less than 30% fat and less than 10% of saturated fat to avoid the cardiovascular complications of diabetes. The specialized formulas available for diabetes tend to be greater than 40% fat and may not be appropriate for long-term use. Gastric emptying may also be slowed by the presence of fat or insoluble fiber in the digestive tract,[26] and it is important to avoid high-fat enteral feedings as well as those containing large amounts of fiber in the patient with gastroparesis. Further research is needed on the long-term effects of a low-carbohydrate feeding on glucose and lipid levels.[27,28]

It has been suggested that the addition of fiber to enteral feeding formulas may decrease serum glucose levels. Although the addition of wheat bran and guar gum to feedings has been successful in blunting glycemic response and reducing insulin requirements,[26,29,30] the addition of these substances to feeding formulas is impractical because they are gel-forming and affect the viscosity of the feeding formula. The fiber routinely added to enteral formulas is soy polysaccharide. Results of studies on glucose response to soy polysaccharide have been inconsistent. Many researchers report no significant difference or only mild positive effects in glucose absorption in patients receiving fiber-containing formulas.[31-34] Arguments against the use of fiber-supplemented formulas include reduction of vitamin and mineral absorption, slowed gastric emptying, and untoward gastrointestinal side effects, but these may not occur often.[34] Although the fiber-containing formulas are readily employed, research has not justified their routine use in diabetic patients.[25,28]

Insulin administration during enteral feeding warrants discussion. For continuous feedings, regular insulin should be given three to four times daily, depending on serum glucose levels. Hyperglycemia during intermittent feedings is also best treated with regular insulin so its effects occur while the feeding is administered and not postprandially. Bolus feedings, which more closely resemble "meals," may be managed with NPH insulin and regular insulin; however, glucose levels should be monitored daily.

Pancreatitis

Acute or chronic inflammation of the pancreas can lead to malabsorption, maldigestion, weight loss, and malnutrition. The spectrum of pancreatic disease can range from mild, self-limiting inflammation to chronic pancreatic degeneration with eventual loss of endocrine and exocrine functions. In acute pancreatitis, attacks may be isolated, and complete return of pancreatic function is possible. Patients with chronic disease usually have pancreatic abnormalities such as inflammation, scarring, calcification, and necrosis prior to their attack. These abnormalities do not resolve after symptoms have subsided.[4,35]

Acute Pancreatitis

The two most common causes of acute pancreatitis in the United States are alcohol abuse and cholelithiasis. Other possible causes of acute pancreatitis are listed in Table 9–3. The etiology of pancreatitis in alcoholism is poorly understood. One hypothesis suggests a change in consistency of the proteins secreted in the pancreas, which results in blockage of the pancreatic ducts.[3] Biliary stones may cause pancreatic obstruction that can lead to pancreatic inflammation.

Acute pancreatitis commonly presents with nausea, vomiting, and severe abdominal pain. Additional symptoms may include ileus, fever, leukocytosis, tachycardia, and ascites. Systemic aberrations that may arise from the release of pancreatic enzymes into circulation include respiratory distress, renal failure, and subcutaneous fat necrosis. Progression of acute pancreatitis can lead to critical illness. Of all cases, 10% are fatal.[3]

The diagnosis of pancreatitis involves thorough clinical evaluation of the patient,as well as biochemical and radiographic assessment. One of the most common biochemical abnormalities in pancreatitis is elevation of serum amylase.

Table 9–3 Conditions Associated with Acute Pancreatitis

*Ethanol abuse
Cholelithiasis
*Abdominal trauma
Hypercalcemia
Hyperlipidemia
Drugs—anticonvulsant (valproic acid), antibiotics (tetracycline, sulfonamides), antimetabolite (6-mercaptopurine), diuretics (hydrochlorothiazide, furosemide)
Viral infections—mumps, Coxsackie, hepatitis, others
Scorpion bite
Pancreatic cancer
*Pancreas divisum
Peptic ulcer with posterior penetration
*Hereditary pancreatitis
Endoscopic retrograde cholangiopancreatography
Hypoperfusion
Abdominal surgery

*associated with chronic pancreatitis

Source: Reprinted with permission from T.E. Andreoli et al., *Cecil Essentials of Medicine,* © 1993, W.B. Saunders Company.

However, this phenomenon does not occur in all cases. Hyperamylasemia can occur in many other pathological conditions such as intestinal ileus, liver disease, renal failure, gallstones, malignancies, and ketoacidosis.[36] Other criteria, such as C-reactive protein and methemalbumin levels may also predict severity of pancreatic disease, but are not routinely used.[37] Therefore, radiographic studies such as computed tomography (CT) scans are used to confirm diagnosis. A CT scan may aid in determining the size of the pancreas and the extent of necrosis and inflammation.

Local pancreatic abnormalities and complications are often seen in pancreatitis. Necrotic tissue and debris may collect in a pancreatic pocket known as a pseudocyst. Pseudocysts can occur in acute or chronic pancreatitis, and they may spontaneously resolve depending on the severity of the disease. Pseudocysts can rupture into the peritoneum, causing severe infection and pancreatic ascites. Pancreatic fistulas may develop with pancreatic trauma or injury. The amount of pancreatic fistula output depends on its location and whether ductal abnormalities are present. High-output pancreatic fistulas can result in fluid and electrolyte losses. Treatment includes replacement therapy, adequate drainage, and prevention of infection at the site of the fistula.[37] Complete bowel rest and TPN may also be necessary.

Treatment of acute pancreatitis usually consists of supportive measures, and may include complete bowel rest and parenteral nutrition support, fluid resuscitation, pain management, and treatment of concurrent side effects. Prognosis can be evaluated using Ranson criteria (see Table 9–4) upon admission and 48 hours later.[37,39] Fewer than three positive Ranson criteria indicate less than 1% mortality risk, five or six positive criteria predict a 40% mortality risk, and more than seven positive criteria indicate 100% mortality risk. Cause of death related to acute pancreatitis is usually secondary to systemic effects compromising other organ function.

Chronic Pancreatitis

Chronic pancreatitis results from a gradual destruction of pancreatic tissue, resulting in varying degrees of calcification and fibrosis. The most common cause of chronic pancreatitis is alcoholism, which may account for 60% of all cases.[40] It is hypothesized that calcification results from decreased overall pancreatic secretion with hypersecretion of protein in pancreatic juice. Deficiencies in proteins that maintain calcium balance in the pancreatic duct may occur, resulting in disordered calcium balance in the pancreatic ducts.[40,41]

The patient with chronic pancreatic disease usually experiences intermittent exacerbation of abdominal pain. Over time, other symptoms such as steatorrhea, malabsorption, weight loss, gastrointestinal bleeding, and diabetes may appear. Fever or significant elevations in serum amylase and glucose may not be detected, making diagnosis difficult to confirm in the early stages of the disease.[40] Radiographic studies and pancreatic function tests can be used to determine the extent of the disease.[3,40]

Table 9–4 Ranson Criteria for Evaluation of Pancreatitis

Ranson Criteria	Non-Gallstone Pancreatitis	Gallstone Pancreatitis
On admission		
Age (years)	>55	>70
WBC/mL	>16000	>18000
Glucose (mg/mL)	>200	>220
LDH (IU/L)	>350	>400
AST (IU/L)	>250	>250
Within 48 hours		
Hct decreases (points)	>10	
BUN increases (mg/dL)	>5	>2
Calcium (mg/dL)	<8	<8
P_{O_2} (mm Hg)	<60	—
Base deficit (mEq/L)	>4	>5
Fluid (L) (I-O)	>6	>4

Notes: AST—aspartate aminotransferase; BUN—blood urea nitrogen; hct—hematocrit; I-O—intake-output; P_{O_2}—arterial partial pressure of oxygen; LDH—lactate dehydrogenase; WBC—white blood cells

Source: Reprinted with permission from W.M. Steinberg, Predictors of severity of acute pancreatitis, *Gastroenteral Clinics of North America,* Vol. 19, No. 4, 849–860, © 1990, W.B. Saunders Company.

Insufficient insulin production and secretion may result in glucose intolerance, depending on the severity of pancreatic disease. Decreased glucagon reserve may enhance response to insulin therapy and precipitate hypoglycemia.[40] Careful blood sugar monitoring is necessary, because hypoglycemia may further be complicated by alcoholism and malnutrition.

Steatorrhea occurs once 90% to 95% of acinar function is lost.[40] Stools are commonly oily, bulky, and foul smelling. Patients may exhibit malabsorption of all macronutrients and fat-soluble vitamins. The weight loss and physical stress that follows malabsorption may decrease the body's ability to launch immune defense, and many patients with chronic pancreatitis succumb to recurrent infections. Malabsorption of vitamin B_{12} in pancreatitis has been suggested, based on the role of pancreatic enzymes in the transfer of cobalamin to intrinsic factor. However, this concept warrants further study.[42] Treatment of chronic pancreatic disease is geared toward replacement of insufficient pancreatic enzymes, pain management, and prevention of further pancreatic injury. Pancreatic enzyme therapy and treatment of hyperglycemia is usually instituted. Vitamin and mineral replacement may also be necessary. Complications such as ascites, pseudocysts, and gastrointestinal bleeding may necessitate surgery. Prognosis in chronic pancreatitis is usually related to complications, because the majority of patients do not die directly from an acute exacerbation.[40] Appropriate medical follow-up and patient compliance with treatment are important to avoid life-threatening complications.

Nutrition Support in Pancreatitis

Nutrition support in acute and chronic pancreatitis can be challenging. Patients with acute pancreatitis may have depressed ventricular function and defective oxygen transport consistent with sepsis.[43] Metabolic rate may vary, depending on the severity of diseases and complications; one investigation reported a variance in metabolic rate ranging between 77% and 139% of expenditure rates.[44] Predictive equations to determine energy and protein needs may not be accurate. Patient-specific metabolic testing is appropriate to determine energy needs accurately.

Protein requirements should be determined with concurrent complications, level of stress, and nutritional status in mind. Patients with severe and acute pancreatitis are often hypermetabolic and in negative nitrogen balance; parenteral nutrition may promote nitrogen retention in these patients and improve visceral protein indicators.[45,46] Monitoring nitrogen balance and prealbumin will aid in assessing the adequacy of the nutrition support regimen.

The goal of nutrition support in pancreatitis is to minimize the stimulation of pancreatic secretions, thereby avoiding the associated pain and life-threatening complications. Complete bowel rest is often indicated, and parenteral nutrition may be used if a prolonged period (greater than 5 to 7 days) without oral intake is anticipated. There has been considerable investigation into the appropriateness and efficacy of parenteral nutrition in pancreatitis. One study reported that parenteral nutrition support has no positive effect on length of stay, incidence of complications, or outcome[47]; other researchers suggest that parenteral nutrition may play an important role in the nutrition management of patients with pancreatitis—especially those with severe, acute disease.[45,46] In acute pancreatitis, TPN may be the most appropriate route of nutrition support until symptoms subside.

Long-term parenteral nutrition may be associated with gut atrophy and bacterial translocation, which may only complicate the hospital course of a patient with pancreatitis. Because of the increased expense and possibly higher rate of infection associated with parenteral nutrition, enteral nutrition has also been employed in pancreatitis. Again, this regimen should be designed with the goal of minimizing pancreatic stimulation. Investigators have reported that elemental and polymeric formulas stimulate pancreatic secretion when infused into the duodenum.[48-50] Elemental diets infused into the jejunum have been successful in providing nutrition and minimizing pancreatic secretion in some cases[51-53]; although conflicting evidence has been reported, it has not been reproduced.[54] The appropriateness of routine use of enteral feedings in pancreatitis remains in question, and further investigation is certainly warranted.

Macronutrient Tolerance in Pancreatitis

The patient with pancreatitis may exhibit carbohydrate intolerance due to endocrine dysfunction. With diabetic patients, care should be taken not to exceed the maximal glucose oxidation rate of the liver (3–5 mg dextrose/kg/min). Insulin therapy may be indicated and may be used as described in the section on diabetes.

There is a well-known association between pancreatitis and hyperlipidemia, and elevated blood lipids have been reported in 12% to 38% of patients with pancreatitis, independent of alcohol intake.[55,56] Serum triglyceride levels greater than 1000 mg/dL may precipitate acute pancreatitis.[56–58] The mechanism by which this occurs remains unclear. Lipid clearance may remain impaired after the pancreatitis has resolved.[57]

The use of intravenous lipids in pancreatitis has been controversial. Case reports have related lipid infusion to the development of acute pancreatitis.[59–61] However, two out of three of these reports involved patients treated with steroids, which also have been implicated in pancreatitis.[62] These patients were also receiving lipid doses exceeding current maximum lipid recommendations (30% of total kcal or 3 g/kg in pediatrics).[63] Lipids provided 42% of total calories in one case[59] and 4 g/kg in another involving pediatric patients.[61] The first case involved a 17-year-old boy who tolerated 20% lipid infusion for 6 weeks before recurrence of pancreatitis following a small meal; the patient was noncompliant with strict NPO recommendations. Upon reinitiation of the same lipid regimen, the patient again had pancreatitis symptoms. It would be difficult, however, to attribute the sole cause of the patient's recurrence to the concentrated lipid infusion. Therefore, no conclusive evidence can be extrapolated from these case reports.

Infusion of parenteral lipids in pancreatitis may be associated with hyperlipidemia, which can precipitate and complicate pancreatitis. Studies have produced conflicting results regarding the effect of intravenous lipid on pancreatic secretion.[64–67] However, researchers have found evidence that parenteral macronutrients as well as mixed substrate solutions do *not* significantly increase pancreatic secretion, and routine use of lipids is accepted as safe.[46,48,67] It is generally accepted that appropriate dosages of intravenous lipids (not exceeding 1 g lipid per kg of body weight) are safe in patients with or without preexisting pancreatic disease, and may be a useful source of calories in glucose-intolerant and malnourished patients.

It is prudent to monitor serum triglyceride levels regularly to avoid hyperlipidemia. Intravenous lipids may be used if triglyceride levels are maintained at 400 mg/dL during lipid infusion, and less than 250 mg/dL 4 hours after lipid infusion is complete.[63] Elevated triglyceride levels may also occur in glucose intolerance, renal disease, and alcoholism; therefore, it may be difficult to discern the exact etiology of the hyperlipidemia. If hyperlipidemia appears to be directly related to lipid infusion, it is wise to decrease the provision of intravenous fat and continue to monitor serum triglycerides. In the patient with preexisting dyslipidemia unrelated to pancreatitis, parenteral lipids should be provided in doses only sufficient to avoid essential fatty acid deficiency.

OTHER ISSUES

Electrolytes

Monitoring serum electrolytes and minerals is important in patients receiving nutrition support. Acidosis related to sepsis, vomiting, and diarrhea may cause fluctuations in serum potassium levels. Sodium and chloride losses may also be present due to nasogastric suctioning during bowel rest. Hypomagnesemia often occurs in pancreatitis and may be related to diarrhea and alcohol abuse. Magnesium should be supplemented as needed to avoid concurrent fluctuations of potassium, calcium, and phosphorus.

Pancreatitis itself may cause hypocalcemia, and the mechanism of calcium depletion in pancreatitis is unclear. Theories include calcium soap formation upon exposure to pancreatic enzymes, increased calcium deposition in the pancreas, and reduced parathyroid hormone secretion.[68] Investigators have also identified a relationship between elevated free fatty acids in serum and hypocalcemia.[69] Ionized calcium levels should be monitored carefully. Interestingly, hypercalcemia in patients receiving TPN has been implicated as a cause of pancreatitis. This may be related to blockage of the pancreatic duct due to deposition of excess calcium in the duct.[68,70]

Surgical Procedures

Surgical management is most often utilized in cases of pancreatic carcinoma or unrelenting, chronic pancreatitis.[71] Common procedures include subtotal pancreatectomy, total pancreatectomy, and pancreaticoduodenectomy (Whipple procedure). These procedures are increasingly well tolerated, and surgical management is becoming more common in pancreatic cancer and pancreatitis. The 5-year survival rate of pancreatic cancer has increased from 5% to 20%,[72] and surgery appears to provide significant improvement in pancreatitis, as well.[72,73] The most common side effect associated with pancreatic resection (especially Whipple procedure) appears to be delayed gastric emptying; however, pylorus-preserving procedures may decrease the incidence of this symptom.[74,75] Other reported side effects include early satiety, dumping syndrome, and diarrhea.[75] In the severely malnourished patient who requires surgery, parenteral nutrition may be initiated preoperatively. Postoperatively, enteral feedings should be initiated and advanced as quickly as possible.

Pancreatic Enzyme Replacement

Pancreatic enzyme replacement remains the mainstay of treatment for exocrine insufficiency due to pancreatic surgery or chronic pancreatitis. Enzyme replacement may aid the absorption of enteral nutrients and also appears to have an analgesic effect that may reduce mild pain associated with pancreatic insufficiency in some patients. Better control of fat malabsorption and diarrhea has been achieved using pH-sensitive, enteric-coated enzyme preparations that resist inactivation in the presence of gastric acid and are soluble in the small intestine.[76,77] It has been suggested that pancreatic enzyme therapy may affect folate status by forming a complex with the vitamin.[78] Long-term follow-up should include screening for folate deficiency.

CONCLUSIONS

Pancreatitis and pancreatic disease often result in the need for nutrition support. Parenteral nutrition is often the route of choice for providing nutrients, but investigations are beginning to relay the practicality and tolerability of enteral nutrition support. Acute pancreatic disease may result in considerable stress and catabolism. Chronic pancreatitis may cause malabsorption and significant malnutrition. It is important for nutrition practitioners to be aware of the effects of pancreatic disease on metabolism, serum electrolytes, and vitamin and mineral status. Knowledge of treatment options such as surgery and enzyme replacement may also be helpful in providing safe and effective nutrition support.

REFERENCES

1. Havala T, Shronts E, Cerra F. Nutritional support in pancreatitis. *Gastroenterol Clin North Am.* 1989;18:525–540.
2. Brody T. *Nutritional Biochemistry.* San Diego, CA: Academic Press Inc; 1994:50–63.
3. Andreoli TE, Bennet JC, Carpenter CC, Plum F, et al. *Cecil Essentials of Medicine.* Philadelphia: WB Saunders Co; 1993:311–318.
4. Steer ML, Waxman I, Freedman S. Chronic pancreatitis. *N Engl J Med.* 1995;332:1482–1490.
5. Shils ME, Olsos JA, Shike M, eds. *Modern Nutrition in Health and Disease.* 8th ed. Philadelphia: Lea & Febiger; 1994;2:1259–1266.
6. Bagdade JD, Nielson KL, Bulger RJ. Reversible abnormalities in phagocytic function in poorly controlled diabetic subjects. *Am J Med Sci.* 1972;263:451–456.
7. Bagdade JD, Root RK, Bulger RJ. Impaired leukocyte function in patients with poorly controlled diabetes. *Diabetes.* 1974;23:9–15.
8. Repine JE, Clawson CC, Goetz FC. Bactericidal function of neutrophils from patients with acute bacterial infections and from diabetics. *J Infect Dis.* 1980;142:869–874.

9. McMahon MM, Rizza RA. Diabetes mellitus. In: Zaloga GP, ed. *Nutrition in Critical Care.* St. Louis, MO: Mosby-Year Book; 1994:801–813.

10. McMahon MM, Manji N, Driscoll DF, Bistrian BR. Parenteral nutrition in patients with diabetes mellitus: theoretical and practical considerations. *J Parenter Enter Nutr.* 1989;13:545–553.

11. Pitts DM, Kilo KA, Pontious SL. Nutritional support for the patient with diabetes. *Crit Care Nurs Clin North Am.* 1993;5:47–56.

12. Seres DS. Insulin absorption to parenteral infusion systems: case report and review of the literature. *Nutr Clin Pract.* 1990;5:111–117.

13. Marcuard SP, Dunham B, Hobbs A, Caro JF. Availability of insulin from total parenteral nutrition solutions. *J Parenter Enter Nutr.* 1990;14:262–264.

14. DeFronzo RA, Sherwin RS, Dillingham M, Hendler R, et al. Influence of basal insulin and glucagon secretion on potassium and sodium metabolism. *J Clin Invest.* 1978;61:472–479.

15. Wagman LD, Newsome HH, Miller KB, Thomas RB, et al. The effect of acute discontinuation of total parenteral nutrition. *Ann Surg.* 1986;204:524–529.

16. Peters AL. Enteral and parenteral nutrition in patients with diabetes. *Diab Prof.* 1990;spring:1–16.

17. Nompleggi D, Bell SJ, Blackburn GL, Bistrian BR, et al. Overview of gastrointestinal disorders due to diabetes mellitus: emphasis on nutritional support. *J Parenter Enter Nutr.* 1989;13:84–91.

18. Kanatsuka A, Osegawa T, An T, Suziki T, et al. Augmented gastrin responses in diabetes patients with vagal neuropathy. *Diabetologia.* 1984;26:449–452.

19. Tougas G, Hunt RH, Fitzpatrick D, Upton AR. Evidence of impaired afferent vagal function in patients with diabetes gastroparesis. *Pace.* 1992;15:1597–1602.

20. Clark DW, Nowak TV. Diabetic gastroparesis: what to do when gastric emptying is delayed. *Postgrad Med.* 1994;95:195–204.

21. Feldman M, Schiller LR. Disorders of gastrointestinal motility associated with diabetes mellitus. *Ann Intern Med.* 1983;98:378–384.

22. Loo FD, Palmer DW, Soergel KH, Kalbfleisch JH, et al. Gastric emptying in patients with diabetes mellitus. *Gastroenterology.* 1984;86:485–494.

23. Gilman AG, Rall AW, Nies AS, Taylor P, eds. *The Pharmacological Basis of Therapeutics.* 8th ed. New York: Pergamon Press; 1990:927–928, 1134.

24. Jacober SJ, Narayan A, Strodel WE, Vinik AI. Jejunostomy feeding in the management of gastroporesis diabeticorum. *Diabetes Care.* 1986;9:217–219.

25. Position statement: Nutrition recommendations and principles for people with diabetes mellitus. *Diabetes Care.* 1997;20:S14–S17.

26. Ray TK, Mansell KM, Knight LC, Malmud LS, et al. Long term effects of dietary fiber on glucose tolerance and gastric emptying in non insulin-dependent diabetic patients. *Am J Clin Nutr.* 1983;37:376–381.

27. Thomas BL, Laine DC, Goetz FC. Glucose and insulin response in diabetic subjects: acute effect of carbohydrate level and the addition of soy polysaccharide in defined-formula diets. *Am J Clin Nutr.* 1988;48:1048–1052.

28. Schafer RG, Bohannon B, Franz M, Freeman J, et al. Translation of the diabetes nutrition recommendations for health care institutions: technical review. *J Am Diet Assoc.* 1997;97:43–52.

29. Jenkins DJ, Goff DV, Leeds A, Wolever TM, et al. Unabsorbable carbohydrates and diabetes: decreased post prandial hyperglycemia. *Lancet.* 1976;11:172–174.

30. Blackburn NA, Redfern JS, Jarjis H, Holgate M, et al. The mechanism of action of guar gum in improving glucose tolerance in man. *Clin Sci.* 1984;66:329–336.

31. Schinnick FL, Hess RI, Fischer MH, Marlett JA, et al. Apparent nutrient absorption and upper gastrointestinal transit with fiber-containing enteral feedings. *Am J Clin Nutr.* 1989;49:471–475.

32. Schweizer TF, Bekhechi AR, Koellreutter B, Reimann S, et al. Metabolic effects of dietary fiber from dehulled soybeans in humans. *Am J Clin Nutr.* 1983;38:1–11.

33. Tsai AC, Vinik AI, Lasichiak A, Lo GS, et al. Effects of soy polysaccharide on postprandial plasma glucose, insulin, glucagon, pancreatic polypeptide, somatostatin and triglyceride in obese diabetic patients. *Am J Clin Nutr.* 1987;45:596–601.

34. Scheppach W, Burghardt W, Bartram P, Kaspar H, et al. Addition of dietary fiber to liquid formula diets: the pros and cons. *J Parenter Enter Nutr.* 1990;14:204–209.

35. Singer MV, Gyr KE, Sarles H. Revised classification of pancreatitis: report of the Second International Symposium on the Classification of Pancreatitis. *Gastroenterology.* 1985;89:683–685.

36. Piper-Bigelow C, Strocchi A, Levitt MD. Where does serum amylase come from and where does it go? *Gastroenterol Clin North Am.* 1990;19:793–807.

37. Steinberg WM. Predictors of severity of acute pancreatitis. *Gastroenterol Clin North Am.* 1990;19:849–860.

38. Koruda MJ, Feurer ID. Pancreatic fistulas. In: Blackburn GL, Bell SJ, Mullen JL, eds. *Nutritional Medicine: A Case Management Approach.* Philadelphia: WB Saunders Co; 1989:39–43.

39. Ranson JH, Rifkind KM, Roses DF, et al. Prognostic signs and the role of operative management in acute pancreatitis. *Surg Gynecol Obstet.* 1974;139:69–81.

40. Bank S. Chronic pancreatitis: clinical features and medical management. *Am J Gastroenterol.* 1986;81:153–167.

41. Guy O, Robles-Diaz G, Adrich Z, Sahel J, et al. Protein content of precipitates present in pancreatic juice of alcoholic subjects and patients with chronic calcifying pancreatitis. *Gastroenterology.* 1983;84:102–107.

42. Brugge WR, Goff JS, Allen NC, Allen RH. Development of a dual label Schilling test for pancreatic exocrine function based on the differential absorption of cobalamin bound to intrinsic factor and R protein. *Gastroenterology.* 1980;78:937–949.

43. Di Carlo V, Nespoli A, Chiesa R, Staudacher C, et al. Hemodynamic and metabolic impairment in acute pancreatitis. *World J Surg.* 1981;5:329–339.

44. Dickerson RN, Vehe KL, Mullen JL, Feurer IS, et al. Resting energy expenditure in patients with pancreatitis. *Crit Care Med.* 1991;19:484–490.

45. Sitzmann JV, Steinborn PA, Zinner MJ, Cameron JL, et al. Total parenteral nutrition and alternative energy substrates in treatment of severe acute pancreatitis. *Surg Gynecol Obstet.* 1989;168:311–317.

46. Grant JP, James S, Grabowski V, Trexler KM. Total parenteral nutrition in pancreatic disease. *Ann Surg.* 1984;200:627–631.

47. Sax HC, Warner BW, Talamini MA, Hamilton FN, et al. Early total parenteral nutrition in acute pancreatitis: lack of beneficial effects. *Am J Surg.* 1987;153:117–124.

48. Stabile BE, Borzatta M, Stubbs RS. Pancreatic secretory responses to intravenous hyperalimentation and intraduodenal elemental and full liquid diets. *J Parenter Enter Nutr.* 1984;8:377–380.

49. Guan D, Ohta H, Green GM. Rat pancreatic secretory response to intraduodenal infusion of elemental vs. polymeric defined-formula diet. *J Parenter Enter Nutr.* 1994;18:335–339.

50. Meyer JH, Kelly JA. Canine responses to intestinally perfused proteins and protein digests. *Am J Physiol.* 1976;231:682–691.

51. Kudsk KA, Campbell SM, O'Brien T, Fuller R, et al. Postoperative jejunal feedings following complicated pancreatitis. *Nutr Clin Pract.* 1990;5:14–17.

52. Cassim MM, Allardyce DB. Pancreatic secretion in response to jejunal feeding of elemental diet. *Ann Surg.* 1974;180:228–231.

53. Ragins H, Levinson SM, Signer R, Stamford W, et al. Intrajejunal administration of an elemental diet at neutral pH avoids pancreatic stimulation. *Am J Surg.* 1973;126:606–614.

54. Ertan A, Brooks FP, Ostrow JD, Arvan DA, et al. Effect of jejunal amino acid perfusion and exogenous cholecystokinin on exocrine pancreatic and biliary secretions in man. *Gastroenterology.* 1971;61:686–692.

55. Toskes P. Hyperlipidemic pancreatitis. *Gastroenterol Clin North Am.* 1990;19:783–792.

56. Buch A, Buch J, Carlson A, Schmidt A, et al. Hyperlipidemia and pancreatitis. *World J Surg.* 1980;4:307–314.

57. Guzman S, Nervi F, Llanos O, Leon P, et al. Impaired lipid clearance in patients with previous acute pancreatitis. *Gut.* 1986;26:888–891.

58. Farmer RG, Winkelman EI, Brown HB, Lewis LA. Hyperlipoproteinemia and pancreatitis. *Am J Med.* 1973;54:161–165.

59. Lashner BA, Kirsner JB, Hanauer SB. Acute pancreatitis associated with high concentration lipid emulsion during total parenteral nutrition therapy for Crohn's disease. *Gastroenterology.* 1986;90:1039–1041.

60. Buckspan R, Woltering E, Waterhouse G. Pancreatitis induced by intravenous infusion of a fat emulsion in an alcoholic patient. *South Med J.* 1984;77:251–252.

61. Noseworthy J, Colodny AH, Eraklis AJ. Pancreatitis and intravenous fat: an association in patients with inflammatory bowel disease. *J Ped Surg.* 1983;18:269–272.

62. Nelp WB. Acute pancreatitis associated with steroid therapy. *Arch Intern Med.* 1961;108:702–710.

63. A.S.P.E.N. Board of Directors. Guidelines for the use of parenteral and enteral nutrition in adult and pediatric patients. *J Parenter Enter Nutr.* 1993;17(suppl):16, 31–32.

64. Burns GP, Stein TA. Pancreatic enzyme secretion during intravenous fat infusion. *J Parenter Enter Nutr.* 1987;11:60–62.

65. Konturek SJ, Cieszkowski M, Tasler J, Jaworek J, et al. Intravenous amino acids and fat stimulate pancreatic secretion. *Am J Physiol.* 1979;236:678–684.

66. Edelman K, Valenzuela JE. Effect of intravenous lipid on human pancreatic secretion. *Gastroenterology.* 1983;85:1063–1068.

67. Stabile BE, Borzatta M, Stubbs RS, Debas HT, et al. Intravenous mixed amino acids and fats do not stimulate exocrine pancreatic secretion. *J Physiol.* 1984;246:G274–280.

68. Narins RG, ed. *Clinical Disorders of Fluid and Electrolyte Metabolism.* New York: McGraw-Hill; 1994;1021:1484–1485.

69. Warshaw AL, Lee KH, Napier TW, Fournier PO, et al. Depression of serum calcium by increased plasma free fatty acids in the rat: a mechanism for hypocalcemia in acute pancreatitis. *Gastroenterology.* 1985;89:814–820.

70. Izsak EM, Shike M, Roulet M, Jeejeebhoy KN, et al. Pancreatitis in association with hypercalcemia in patients receiving total parenteral nutrition. *Gastroenterology.* 1980;79:555–558.

71. Fernendez-del Castillo C, Rattner DW, Warshaw AL. Standards for pancreatic resection in the 1990's. *Arch Surg.* 1995;30:295–300.

72. Howard TJ, Maiden CL, Smith HG, Wiebke EA, et al. Surgical treatment of obstructive pancreatitis. *Surgery*. 1995;118:727–734.

73. Izbicki JR, Bloechle C, Knoefel WT, Kuechler T, et al. Duodenum-preserving resection of the head of the pancreas in chronic pancreatitis: a prospective, randomized trial. *Ann Surg.* 1995;221:350–358.

74. Yeo CJ. Management of complications following pancreaticoduodenectomy. *Surg Clin North Am.* 1995;75:913–924.

75. McLeod RS, Taylor BR, O'Connor BI, Greenberg GR, et al. Quality of life, nutritional status, and gastrointestinal hormone profile following the Whipple procedure. *Am J Surg.* 1995;169:179–185.

76. Dobrilla G. Management of chronic pancreatitis: focus on enzyme replacement. *Int J Pancreat.* 1989;5:17–29.

77. Andren-Sandberg A. Theory and practice in the individualization of oral pancreatic enzyme administration for chronic pancreatitis. *Int J Pancreat.* 1989;5:51–62.

78. Russell RM, Dutta SK, Oaks EV, Rosenberg IH, et al. Impairment of folic acid absorption by oral pancreatic extracts. *Dig Dis Sci.* 1980;25:369–373.

CHAPTER 10

Nutrition Management of the Adult with Liver Disease

Ka Wong, Barbara J. Visocan Klein, and Judith A. Fish

INTRODUCTION

The liver, a complex organ with hundreds of different known functions, plays a pivotal role in the maintenance of nutrition equilibrium within the body. It is uniquely involved in the digestion, storage, and metabolism of nutrients. Liver injury—whether by infection or mechanical or chemical insult—may result in functional impairment, with prominent effects on nutritional status.

Nutrition support of patients with liver disease is often critical in allowing the repair and regeneration of hepatocytes to proceed to eventual recovery of liver function. Provision of adequate nutrition care is based upon a thorough understanding of normal liver function and of the changes that result from various disease states. This chapter outlines the normal functions of the liver, the nutrition aberrations that result from hepatic insufficiency, the nutritional assessment of patients with liver disease, the appropriate nutrition therapy for various types of liver diseases, and guidelines for the delivery of enteral and parenteral nutrition in patients with hepatic insufficiency.

NORMAL FUNCTIONS OF THE LIVER

Numerous anabolic and catabolic processes that impact directly on nutritional status are dependent upon normal liver function. These include the metabolism of carbohydrate, fat, and protein, and the synthesis, transport, and storage of various vitamins and minerals.

Carbohydrate Metabolism

Through the processes of glycogen storage, glycogenolysis, and gluconeogenesis, the liver aids in maintaining normal blood glucose concentrations. Glycogenesis, the formation of glycogen from glucose, occurs postprandially when serum glucose rises. Glucose, which enters the liver via the portal circulation, must be phosphorylated prior to formation of glycogen. Fructose and galactose are also converted to glucose by the hepatocytes. When glycogen storage is maximized in the liver and muscle, glucose is then converted to fat. Glycogenolysis, the hydrolysis of glycogen back to glucose, takes place postabsorptively when blood glucose levels begin to fall or in the presence of glucagon. The process of gluconeogenesis, the formation of glucose from nonglucose substances, occurs mainly in the liver. This process is enhanced in the presence of glucocorticoids and lowered ratio of insulin to glucagon. Gluconeogenesis produces glucose principally from amino acids, lactate, and glycerol, which are mobilized from tissue proteins and fats. Metabolic pathways such as the alanine-glucose cycle and Cori cycle are examples of gluconeogenesis.

Fat Metabolism

The liver stores, synthesizes, and distributes lipids to plasma. It also produces bile, which is necessary for fat digestion. Bile salts, a component of bile, have an emulsifying function that breaks triglyceride into small globules enhancing digestion. The detergent-like properties of these salts increase the water solubility of fats, aiding their passage through the intestinal wall. Fatty acids are transported to the liver via the portal vein, with the exception of medium-chain triglyceride, which is delivered via the lymphatic system. Upon arrival in the liver, fatty acids are oxidized as an energy source by the hepatocytes, or reesterified to triglycerides for storage. Within the hepatocytes, fatty acids can also be converted to phospholipid and cholesterol. These two substances then can be combined with apoproteins and triglycerides to form lipoproteins, which are responsible for distributing lipids in the plasma. Hepatocytes also convert carbohydrates, fat, and protein in excess of body needs to lipid, which is released into the bloodstream in the form of very low-density lipoprotein for transport to adipose tissue and storage. Ketogenesis, which occurs primarily in hepatocytes, is the production of ketone bodies that serve as an energy source for protein preservation during prolonged starvation. This process is triggered by a lowered insulin to glucagon ratio. During ketogenesis, fatty acid oxidation accelerates and gives rise to acetyl coenzyme A. The majority of the acetyl coenzyme A is then converted to acetoacetic acid, which can be further transformed to beta-hydroxybutyric acid and acetone. These ketone bodies are exported to plasma circulation as energy substrates used primarily by the brain.

Protein Metabolism

The liver plays a unique and life-sustaining role in protein metabolism. Anabolic functions include transamination and the production of plasma proteins. All nonessential amino acids can be synthesized via hepatic transamination. This process involves the interconversion of available amino acids through the transfer of an amine group to a keto acid. Several clotting factors and all plasma proteins except gamma globulins, which are formed in lymph tissue, are produced in the liver. The three major types of plasma proteins are albumin, globulins, and fibrinogen. These proteins, particularly albumin, contribute to blood oncotic pressure and thus are critical to the maintenance of fluid balance, blood pressure, and normal circulation.

The catabolic process of deamination is also carried out in the liver and is regulated by the presence of catabolic hormones or when protein intake exceeds the body requirement. The removal of the amine group from amino acids (deamination) yields ammonia and a keto acid. This process must occur prior to protein interconversion to glucose or fat and before utilization as an energy source. Ammonia, a toxic byproduct of deamination, enters the urea cycle where it is converted to the intermediate product urea. Urea, in turn, is excreted as urine through the kidney.

Storage, Synthesis, and Transport of Vitamins and Minerals

The liver plays a central role in the storage, synthesis, and transport of various vitamins and minerals. It functions as a storage depot principally for vitamins A, D, and B_{12}, where up to 10-, 3-, and 12-month supplies, respectively, of these nutrients can accumulate and therefore prevent deficiency states. Hepatocytes store 15% to 30% of the body's total iron supply. Dietary iron, absorbed from the small intestine, is combined in the blood with the beta globulin transferrin and transported to all cells, but chiefly to the liver, for storage. When iron enters the hepatic circulation, the bond with transferrin is uncoupled. Apoferritin, a protein substance, forms a complex with iron to produce ferritin, the storage form of this mineral. Other micronutrients stored in the liver include copper, folate, riboflavin, niacin, pantothenic acid, vitamin B_6, vitamin E, vitamin K, and cobalt.

Additional hepatic functions include the conversion of carotene into an active form of vitamin A. This conversion also takes place in the intestine mucosa. The liver produces retinol-binding protein and prealbumin, which are required for the normal transport of vitamin A. Vitamin D is converted into its more active form of 25-hydroxyvitamin D in hepatocytes. Zinc and magnesium are also found in the hepatocytes and are necessary for enzymatic reactions of intermediary metabolism.

EFFECTS OF ETHANOL

Alcoholism is a major cause of hepatic insufficiency. Any discussion of liver disease would be incomplete without considering the nutrition consequences of ethanol. The effects of alcohol and the quantity necessary to produce hepatic damage have great individual variation. Not all alcoholics exhibit nutritional deficiencies. The development of malnutrition appears to have an economic and social component; affluent, employed drinkers who do not require or seek medical treatment generally are the least nutritionally impaired.[1,2]

Every alcoholic should be considered at nutritional risk, irrespective of histologic evidence of liver disease.[3] The etiology of alcohol-related nutritional deficits is multifactorial but includes suboptimal oral intake, malabsorption, decreased hepatocyte storage space, abnormalities in metabolism, and hyperexcretion.

Caloric imbalance is one consequence of alcohol abuse. Ethanol, when metabolized via the alcohol dehydrogenase system, yields 7.1 kcal/g. Theoretically, this calorically dense but nutrient-poor beverage can lead to obesity when consumed in excess of energy needs. However, no difference in weight has been found between drinkers and nondrinkers.[4-6] This observation may be attributable to an inefficient ethanol metabolism that occurs with chronic alcohol ingestion. This pathway, the microsomal ethanol-oxidizing system, instead of generating a high energy compound (NADH) during normal ethanol oxidation via alcohol dehydrogenase, consumes energy during the process.[7] Thus, it may even contribute to weight loss among alcohol abusers.

Ethanol may induce hypoglycemia in the absence of liver disease. Normal oxidation of ethanol yields an accumulation of NADH in the cells, which inhibits the entry of gluconeogenic precursors (such as the amino acids, glycerol, and lactate) into the gluconeogenic pathway.[8] Ethanol-induced hypoglycemia may be commonly seen in individuals who fast and deplete glycogen stores and then binge on alcohol.

Ethanol, which is metabolized in the liver, alters the normal metabolism of protein, fat, and carbohydrate. The major effect on protein metabolism is the inhibition of plasma protein and complement synthesis.[9] Increased susceptibility of alcoholic patients to infection seems to be related to the deficiency of complement. Ethanol ingestion causes a rapid rise in serum triglyceride level—which, in turn, increases the generation of very low-density lipoprotein, resulting in hyperlipidemia.[10] This serum triglyceride elevation usually decreases after ethanol is eliminated from the diet. Ethanol also inhibits galactose oxidation and suppresses gluconeogenesis.

Decreased food intake, a common finding in chronic alcoholics, is considered a major contributor to deficits of energy, macronutrients, vitamins, and minerals. Alcohol is believed to have a negative effect on appetite, secondary to decreased gastric emptying.[11] In general, depletions are corrected by cessation of ethanol and adequate food intake.

Studies suggest that serum depletion of biotin, vitamin B_{12}, and pantothenic acid are less commonly seen in patients with alcoholic liver disease; on the other hand, folate deficiency and deficiency of other vitamins such as thiamine, riboflavin, niacin, and pyridoxine are frequently identified.[12] Vitamin C deficiency is found in 47% of patients with alcoholic liver disease.[13] Alcohol ingestion can impair ascorbic acid absorption by affecting the sodium-dependent transport system in the intestine.[14] Folate deficiency may be attributable to malabsorption and decreased enterohepatic circulation due to ethanol inhibition.[15] In addition, ethanol interferes with the metabolism of vitamin A, thiamine, riboflavin, and pyridoxine by impeding the conversion of these vitamins from their inactive forms.[16] Ethanol induces catabolic loss of zinc, calcium, and urinary loss of magnesium.

Both acute and chronic ingestion of ethanol can lead to various acid-base and electrolyte disturbances that in extreme cases necessitate fluid- and electrolyte-replacement therapy. These include metabolic and respiratory acidoses and/or alkaloses, hyponatremia, hypokalemia, hypophosphatemia, and hypomagnesemia. Alcoholic ketoacidosis may develop; this requires intravenous glucose administration.[17]

NUTRITION ABERRATIONS IN HEPATIC INSUFFICIENCY

As discussed previously, the liver is involved in a myriad of functions of nutrient metabolism. Hepatic disease or injury can profoundly affect nutritional status via an alteration in the metabolism of carbohydrate, fat, protein, vitamins, and minerals. These derangements may be commonly seen in the clinical setting in patients with hepatic insufficiency.

Macronutrients

Adverse effects in carbohydrate metabolism include hypo- and hyperglycemia. Hypoglycemia is most frequently seen in acute hepatitis or fulminant liver failure, probably due to impaired glycogenesis, glycogenolysis, and/or gluconeogenesis. Injured hepatocytes have a reduced capacity to synthesize and store glycogen. The liver's capacity to induce gluconeogenesis seems to decrease the occurrence of hypoglycemia despite chronic liver disease. Blood sugar levels may also be sustained by gluconeogenesis in the kidney.[7] Despite reports of hyperinsulinemia in chronic liver disease,[18] hyperglycemia is a common clinical observation likely secondary to counteracting catabolic hormones and insulin resistance when superimposed by acute stress and injury. The digestion and absorption of carbohydrate generally are not affected.

Fat absorption may be impaired because of inadequate production of bile salts. This may lead to the development of steatorrhea, which, if excessive, leads to deficiencies of the fat-soluble vitamins and calcium.[19] Metabolic studies suggest that cirrhotic patients tend to burn fat as energy substrate more so than carbohydrate or protein, with demonstrated increase in lipid oxidation.[18,20,21] In addition, researchers have found elevated circulation of free fatty acids in the plasma, reflecting lipolysis.[18] The rise of plasma concentration of fatty acids may stimulate the hepatic uptake, which leads to the accumulation of triglycerides in the hepatocytes, precipitating fatty liver formation.

The effects of hepatic injury on protein metabolism are even more dramatic than the effects on carbohydrate and fat metabolism. When toxic ammonia, formed by bacteria in the gut and the process of deamination, cannot be converted adequately to urea by the injured liver, hepatic coma and death may ensue. This process is explained in greater detail later in this chapter. Transamination and the synthesis of plasma proteins may also be impaired. A decrease in the production of albumin, the major component of plasma protein, frequently leads to disturbances in blood oncotic pressure and fluid balance.

There is also a derangement in the metabolism of specific amino acids, namely the aromatic (phenylalanine, tryptophan, tyrosine) and the branched-chain amino acids (BCAAs) (valine, isoleucine, leucine). The only enzymes that metabolize aromatic amino acids (AAAs) are located in the hepatocytes. In hepatic insufficiency, there is a decrease in hepatic oxidation of AAA, leading to an increase in circulation of AAA in the plasma. In contrast, BCAAs are being metabolized primarily by the skeletal muscle. There is an increase in BCAA oxidation in the peripheral tissue during stress, causing a drop in plasma circulation.[21] Hepatitis, infection, and liver injury promote such a stress response.

Micronutrients

In addition to the direct insult of ethanol ingestion, malabsorption, decreased transport, storage, and altered metabolism of vitamins and minerals may occur in liver disease. Malabsorption may result from decreased bile salt level, dysfunction of the small intestine attributable to portal hypertension or lymph stasis, or because of drug-nutrient interaction. Steatorrhea and/or severe cholestasis may be associated with malabsorption of a specific form of vitamin D, cholecalciferol.[22,23] Neomycin sulfate and cholestyramine, drugs used in the treatment of chronic liver disease, may also lead to the malabsorption of fat-soluble vitamins.

Reduced hepatic concentrations of vitamins and minerals are likely in patients with liver disease because of decreased storage space due to deposition of fibrous tissue, fatty infiltration, and hepatocellular degeneration. Cirrhotic livers have been reported to store decreased levels of folate, riboflavin, niacin, pantothenic acid, vitamin B6, vitamin B12, vitamin A, zinc, and cobalt.[24] Also, hepatic injury limits the synthesis of the plasma proteins necessary for the normal transport of vitamins, thus limiting availability of vitamins to the peripheral tissue. For example, in liver disease, the normal transport of vitamin A is adversely affected by the decreased synthesis of retinol-binding protein and prealbumin so that a deficiency state results even in the face of adequate vitamin A status.

With decreased serum levels of albumin and transferrin, zinc is free from its visceral protein binding and is more prone to be excreted by the kidney at a higher rate than usual. Finally, the metabolism of certain micronutrients may be impeded, as exemplified by vitamin D metabolism. Vitamin D, whether derived from dietary sources or endogenously synthesized, must be hydroxylated in the liver to its more active form, a 25-hydroxy derivative. In chronic cholestatic liver disease, this reaction is impaired and may lead to a deficiency state and concomitant osteomalacia.[25] Despite the possibility of various vitamin and mineral deficiencies in alcoholics, supplements should not be administered indiscriminately; supplements should be prescribed only when a specific nutritional deficiency has been identified, because hepatic insufficiency may reduce the body's ability to clear certain nutrients from the body.

Vitamin K plays a key role in coagulation. It serves as a cofactor necessary for the production of biologically active clotting proteins: factors II (prothrombin), VII, VIIII, and X. In vitamin K deficiency, the lack of these clotting factors prolongs the time required or the rate at which prothrombin is converted to thrombin, thus hampering the coagulation process. Situations that induce a state of hypovitaminosis K include malabsorption with steatorrhea, dietary deficiency, impaired hepatic storage, and decreased gut flora production due to intake of antibiotics. Patients who fail to respond to vitamin K supplementation may have severe liver disease, causing inadequate production of clotting factors.

NUTRITIONAL ASSESSMENT OF PATIENTS WITH LIVER DISEASE

Several decades ago, protein malnutrition was once regarded as the primary culprit of liver injury in alcoholics.[26] Identification of malnutrition is important in the management of liver disease because it correlates with the mortality in cirrhotic patients.[27] Compromised nutritional status remains a common feature among patients with alcoholic liver disease. However, the reported prevalence varies between studies, probably due to the different nutrition parameters used. Determination of nutritional status in the presence of liver disease is often complex; many of the parameters commonly used are directly affected by liver injury, making laboratory and clinical findings difficult to interpret. Assessment parameters that are applicable and those of limited value to patients with hepatic insufficiency are outlined below.

Oral Intake Evaluation

Inadequate dietary intake is frequently documented in liver failure and can be attributed to a variety of factors, including disease-related anorexia, nausea, and vomiting; unpalatable therapeutic diets; ingestion of empty-calorie alcoholic beverages; and socioeconomic factors such as inadequate funds. Suboptimal oral intake is considered a major contributor to the high incidence of vitamin deficiencies and altered lean body mass and fat stores frequently reported in patients with alcoholic liver disease.[14] The focus of the nutrient evaluation interview should be on the details of typical daily food intake, use of over-the-counter drugs, and use of self- or medically prescribed nutrition supplements. If there is a history of alcohol abuse, the type, amount, proof, and average daily intake of these beverages must also be obtained. The number of calories derived from ethanol (7.1 kcal/g) in these beverages can be calculated easily by using the following formula[28]:

$$0.8 \times proof \times oz = kcal$$

Table 10–1 exemplifies the use of this formula for determining ethanol calories in liquor, wine, and beer. For alcoholic patients, reliability of the diet history depends on level of motivation, extent of confabulation and inebriation, and whether alcohol-induced psychosis (Korsakoff's psychosis) is present. For this reason, the patient's family and significant others are an invaluable source for clarifying and accumulating additional knowledge of dietary habits.[29]

Several studies published in the mid-1980s,[4,5,30] reported that healthy drinkers consumed more calories than nondrinkers due to the extra calories derived from alcohol. Investigators found that carbohydrate intake was lowest in heavy alcohol drinkers, suggesting that alcoholic calories replaced nutritive calories (carbohydrate) with increasing alcohol consumption. The majority of studies reported that healthy drinkers consumed extra calories without compromising other nutrient intake, but the findings were different for nutritional intake in patients with alcoholic liver disease. Mills et al[14] suggested a decreased intake of protein, folate, vitamin C, thiamine, and iron in alcoholic cirrhotic patients; other studies reported a deficit in caloric intake.[27]

Physical Evaluation

Techniques of nutrition diagnosis—including an evaluation of the hair, skin, eyes, mouth, and nails for signs and symptoms of nutritional deficiencies—should

---

Table 10–1 Calculation of Kilocalories Derived from Ethanol in Common Alcoholic Beverages

Quantity of Beverage Consumed	Calculation	Kilocalories from Ethanol
1 pt of 40% rum	0.8 × 80 proof* × 16 oz	1024
5 4-oz glasses of 12% wine	0.8 × 24 proof* × 20 oz	384
6 12-oz cans of 4% beer	0.8 × 8 proof* × 72 oz	461

*Double the percentage of alcohol to determine proof.

be included in the initial nutritional assessment. This is particularly true when liver disease is attributable to alcohol abuse, as nutritional examination may reveal signs of vitamin, mineral, protein, and calorie malnutrition. For instance, scurvy, which is rarely identified in the general population, is occasionally observed in patients with a history of alcoholism.[31] In patients with ascorbic acid deficiency, physical evaluation reveals the classic findings of perifollicular hemorrhages and "corkscrew" hairs, both diagnostic of scurvy. An in-depth discussion of nutritional diagnostic techniques is not presented here but is readily available in other references.[32,33]

Anthropometric Measurements

Patients with liver disease may develop peripheral edema, which can adversely affect anthropometric measurements. Fluid status varies and can be altered by presence of ascites or overzealous use of diuretics. However, Merli et al[34] found anthropometry to be a useful measure of nutritional status in liver disease if implemented after patients had been appropriately treated for fluid retention. Anthropometric measurements were not significantly correlated to the severity of liver disease and therefore were considered a more preferable nutrition index than visceral protein stores. An assessment of current weight, usual weight, recent weight change, triceps skinfold (fat stores), midarm circumference, and midarm muscle circumference (muscle mass) should be made. More recent studies done by Thuluvath and Triger[35] and Caregaro et al[36] reported a similar percentage of cirrhotic patients (35%) having depleted triceps skinfold and midarm muscle circumference of below the fifth percentile of standards. The observed reduction in body fat and body muscle store is further validated by measurement of total body potassium and total body water in another study.[37] Some researchers believe that preferred fat oxidation may contribute to body fat depletion commonly seen in patients with alcoholic liver disease.

Somatic and Visceral Protein Measurements

Because albumin, prealbumin, retinol-binding protein, and transferrin are synthesized in the liver, they may not serve as reliable parameters for nutritional assessment in hepatic insufficiency. Albumin may be found in large quantities in ascitic fluid, making serum levels even more unreliable. Transferrin levels are negatively affected by chronic alcohol abuse and are related to iron metabolism.[34,38] Mills et al[14] found that the withdrawal of alcohol leads to a rise in serum transferrin levels. As normal erythropoiesis resumes, there is a resultant increase in serum transferrin values. Indeed, numerous studies have reported a correlation between visceral protein status and severity of liver injury; serum levels decreased with progression of liver disease.[26,34] Clinicians should bear in mind, however, that only 25% of functional hepatocytes are needed to maintain normal albumin synthesis. It has also been reported that albumin synthesis may remain intact, despite serious liver injury.[39]

Studies on patients with advanced alcoholic cirrhosis reported albumin levels ranging from 2.8 to 3.7 g/dL.[13,34,40,41] A lower level of 2.5 g/dL is documented in patients with severe hepatitis and superimposed acute illness.[42] In clinical practice, the observed albumin level may even be lower than the referenced values, which should prompt further evaluation as to whether a true protein malnutrition is present.

Trends in albumin levels may reflect a patient's nutrition progress. Cabre et al[42] reported a significant increase in albumin level (17%) in cirrhotic patients who consumed adequate nutrition repletion for 23 days but found no significant improvement in those without nutrition supplements. This result was achieved despite the concomitant complications of infection in 44% of the patients, suggesting that albumin may reflect nutrition progress independent of medical progress. In a long-term study by Hirsch et al,[40] the albumin level of patients with alcoholic cirrhosis who consumed adequate oral supplements for a year increased by 23%, despite no changes observed in liver function parameters. An improvement in albumin level can be seen in cirrhotic patients, even though liver function or medical status remains unchanged; this improvement may reflect replenishing nutritional status. Other visceral proteins (transferrin, prealbumin, retinol-binding protein) also improve significantly in response to nutrition repletion.[43]

Certainly, all visceral protein indexes are influenced by acute stress or catabolic insult in all kind of patients, with or without underlying hepatic insufficiency. Furthermore, the depressed serum albumin level seen in hepatic insufficiency may be due to the increased volume (as in the case of ascites or edema) rather than impaired hepatic synthesis. Therefore, clinicians should use visceral protein stores judiciously in assessing nutritional status of patients with hepatic insufficiency.

Somatic protein stores can be assessed by using the creatinine-height index if fluctuations in dietary intake are not great.[44] Actual urinary creatinine excretion per 24-hour period is measured and compared with standards to calculate the creatinine-height index and thus obtain an estimation of muscle mass. Despite the fact that creatine, the precursor of creatinine, is synthesized in the liver and kidneys, hepatic insufficiency does not appear to affect adversely the results of this nutritional assessment parameter.[45] Using the creatinine-height index in conjunction with anthropometry can provide an accurate approximation of lean body mass.

Immunologic Response

The liver plays an important role in phagocytic function and can regulate the magnitude of immune response.[46] Hepatic insufficiency has been associated with altered cellular immunity, resulting in anergy and decreased total lymphocyte counts. These changes may be due to the liver disease itself or they may be indicative of a suboptimal nutritional state. Additionally, in patients with alcoholic liver disease, the alcohol itself has a deleterious effect on the immune defense system.[47] Mills et al[14] reported that 42% of the cirrhotic patients were anergic on delayed cutaneous hypersensitivity test and that there was no association between anergy and improved dietary intake or nutritional status during 2 weeks of monitoring. Other studies report a significant improvement in skin test after 3 months of nutrition repletion.[43] A more recent study reported 43% and 23% of the patients to be lymphopenic and anergic, respectively.[36] This study of 120 cirrhotic patients demonstrated that skin test score did not correlate with severity of liver disease.

It is difficult, in most cases, to attribute the alterations in immune function to specific disease process, protein-calorie malnutrition, or alcohol abuse. Thus, immune dysfunction may be regarded as a nonspecific indicator of nutritional status in liver disease and should be considered in conjunction with other parameters during nutritional assessment. Table 10–2 summarizes assessment parameters useful for determining the nutritional status of patients with liver disease. No single parameter should be used as the sole determinant of nutritional state, because of the influence that hepatic insufficiency or possible concomitant damage of other organs may have on these indexes. Thus, nutrition therapy decisions should be based upon a constellation of assessment parameters.

NUTRITION THERAPY IN LIVER DISEASE

Nutrition therapy for patients with liver disease may involve modulation of energy, macronutrient, vitamin, mineral, fluid, and electrolyte requirements. Although malnutrition does not correlate with the type of liver disease,[27] therapeutic modifications vary according to the type and severity of hepatic insufficiency. Generally, fatty liver requires little or no nutrition intervention, while cirrhosis necessitates major changes in the patient's nutrition regimen. Because one of the main goals of nutrition therapy in liver disease is the prevention and treatment of hepatic encephalopathy, a separate section is dedicated to the discussion of this disease process.

Steatosis/Fatty Liver Infiltration

Fatty liver (steatosis) develops when fatty acid mobilization from adipose tissue increases and hepatic fat oxidation or triglyceride synthesis decreases.[48] This disorder has been associated with obesity; diabetes mellitus; starvation; protein-calorie malnutrition; and drugs or toxins such as tetracycline, methotrexate, corticosteroids, and carbon tetrachloride. In the United States, however, it is most

Table 10–2 Nutritional Assessment Parameters in Liver Disease

Assessment Parameter	Utility in Liver Disease
Energy and nutrient intake	+ + +
Usual oral intake	Involve family if necessary
Vitamin/mineral supplements	
Physician/self-prescribed medications	
Ethanol	
Physical examination	+ + +
Hair, skin, eyes, mouth, nails	
Anthropometry	+ + +
Height	In absence of or with minimal
Current weight	fluid retention or dehydration
Usual body weight	
Recent weight change	
Triceps skinfold	
Midarm circumference	
Midarm muscle circumference	
Somatic protein stores	+ +
Urinary creatinine excretion	
(use to calculate creatinine-height index)	
Visceral protein stores	+ +
Albumin	Also use as monitor of nutrition
Prealbumin	progress
Retinol-binding protein	
Transferrin	
Immune response	+
Delayed cutaneous hypersensitivity	Could be altered by disease
Total lymphocyte count	process, protein-calorie
	malnutrition, or alcohol intake

+ Somewhat helpful
+ + More helpful
+ + + Most helpful

commonly caused by alcohol ingestion. As little as 20 to 40 mg of ethanol daily has been reported to lead to this condition,[49] which is characterized by a single large vacuole of fat displacing the hepatocyte nucleus. The presence of hepatic fat accumulation itself does not reflect liver disease or changes in liver function.[50] Nonalcoholic fatty liver does not necessarily progress into cirrhosis.

Patients with steatosis are generally asymptomatic, with nontender hepatomegaly noted upon routine physical examination. Imaging techniques, such as computed tomography or needle biopsy of the liver, are required for definitive diagnosis. Abnormal laboratory tests are few and are not specific to fatty liver, nor do they indicate the severity of the condition. Hyperbilirubinemia (up to 137 μmol/L) is present in 25% of steatosis patients, prothrombin time is prolonged by 2 seconds in 50% of cases, and alkaline phosphatase levels are elevated moderately (up to 200 U/L) in approximately 15% of cases.[48]

Fatty liver induced by ethanol usually resolves uneventfully after a few months of total abstinence from alcohol and provision of adequate nutrition. No specific dietary therapy is required. However, if this condition persists over time, inflammation, necrosis, and fibrosis can occur, and 90% of untreated patients develop alcoholic hepatitis.[49] When steatosis is due to other disorders, treatment of the underlying disease or withdrawal of the causative drug/toxin is required. In fatty liver attributable to obesity, weight reduction should be suggested. Nomura et al[51] reported that mean liver volume is reduced significantly after 3 months on a low-calorie diet. For patients with long-standing, diffuse fatty infiltration, the possibility of vitamin deficiencies should be investigated because of decreased storage space.[48]

Hepatic steatosis can be attributable to total parenteral nutrition (TPN). Although the exact pathogenic mechanism is unknown, certain proposed causes include the decreased export of fatty acids from liver secondary to carnitine and essential fatty acid deficiency, and increased hepatic lipid synthesis secondary to glucose and/or calorie overload with hyperinsulinemia.[7] Clinical findings include an elevation of serum alkaline phosphatase and aspartate transaminase in adults after as early as 2 weeks of TPN.[52] Adjusting the dextrose and total caloric delivery to an appropriate oxidative load, cycling down the hours of infusion of parenteral nutrition, and providing enteral trophic nutrition are suggested in the management of TPN-induced steatosis. Specific recommendations regarding TPN are discussed at the end of the chapter.

Hepatitis

Chronic hepatitis refers to a group of conditions that are characterized by an unresolved, necroinflammatory process that lasts more than 6 months.[53] Hepatitis can be caused by infectious agents including viruses, toxic substances, or an autoimmune process. Several viruses other than the hepatitis viruses can produce this condition, including cytomegalovirus and Epstein-Barr virus. Chronic hepatitis can be divided into two categories based on morphological features: (1) chronic, persistent hepatitis (CPH) is usually a benign, nonprogressive disease that does not require medical or nutrition therapy; (2) chronic, active hepatitis (CAH) results in patient symptoms and abnormal liver function tests. Frequently CAH progresses to cirrhosis, and patients may become candidates for liver transplantation.[54] These two morphological classifications, CPH and CAH, may be further refined by specifying their presumed etiology: chronic viral hepatitis, chronic autoimmune hepatitis, chronic cryptogenic hepatitis, etc. Patients with chronic hepatitis have preserved synthetic and clearance functions more than patients with cirrhosis. Alcohol hepatitis is a noninfectious, precirrhotic form of liver injury that is generally associated with protein-calorie malnutrition. This disease can range from a mild and asymptomatic form to a life-threatening condition with mortality rates exceeding 50%.[27] Acute hepatitis presents with variable degree of hepatocellular damage and usually resolves within 3 months of onset. However, it can progress to a more intense form of disease, fulminant hepatic failure, which is characterized by hepatic encephalopathy, coma, severe abnormality of coagulation and electrolyte balances, multisystem organ failure, and death.

Few studies have focused on the nutrition therapy of patients with hepatitis. Adequate calorie and protein intake, 30 to 35 kcal and at least 1 g of protein per kg of body weight, must be ensured to support hepatocyte repair and regeneration.[55] The presence of anorexia and fatigue may suppress appetite. Nausea and vomiting are reported in the afternoon hours; rearrangement of meals, such as providing a bigger breakfast and lunch than dinner, may enhance diet tolerance.[53] Small meals, high-calorie protein supplements, and snacks may be helpful, along with hard candy, carbonated beverages, and fruit juices.

Intravenous glucose infusions may be required to maintain euglycemia as hypoglycemia is frequently reported in patients with acute hepatitis and fulminant liver failure. Electrolyte replacement, especially potassium, may also be necessary. Vitamin and mineral supplements are not indicated for patients who were previously well nourished. The need for fat-soluble vitamin supplementation for patients with acute hepatitis has been suggested by a small study reporting depleted serum levels in eight subjects.[56]

Cirrhosis

Cirrhosis, the final and irreversible stage of liver injury, is characterized by fibrosis, nodular regeneration, increased hepatocyte size, and the deposition of collagen around the sinusoids. In the United States, 75% of all cases of cirrhosis are caused by alcohol abuse.[57] Cirrhosis may result from other conditions, including fatty liver, hepatitis, long-term obstruction of the bile ducts, chronic cholestasis, Wilson's disease, adverse drug reactions, metabolic injuries, and exposure to environmental toxins.

Protein-restricted diets are frequently used to prevent hepatic encephalopathy in hospitalized cirrhotic patients. However, such diets are unnecessary and may be deleterious in patients without impending or present encephalopathy. Patients with end-stage liver disease generally evidence accelerated protein catabolism, and hence a protein restriction may contribute to increased morbidity and possibly mortality. In cases where gastrointestinal hemorrhage or other factors lead to the development of encephalopathy, treatment of the underlying cause rather than protein restriction is the treatment of choice.[58] Excessive protein loads of more than 2g/kg/day should be avoided however.

Cirrhotic patients are often perceived as being hypermetabolic. Shanbhogue et al[59] studied 10 cirrhotic patients and demonstrated an increase in energy expenditure per unit of lean tissue mass, suggesting a state of hypermetabolism. While agreeing that there is a strong correlation between energy production rate and lean tissue mass, other researchers,[18,20] using a larger sample size ($N = 123$) of cirrhotic patients, have suggested a normal metabolic rate compared to healthy subjects. Numerous studies on indirect calorimetry[18,20,59,60] report that the measured resting energy requirement ranges from 21 to 27 kcal/kg of actual body weight. The majority of these studies, however, included patients with insignificant ascites and those with up to 3 liters of ascitic fluid, which may increase the body weight. The researchers also found no significant difference between the measured resting energy expenditure and basal energy expenditure (BEE) in projecting the energy need in stable cirrhotic patients. Estimation of caloric need based on calculated BEE may thus be applicable. Most studies found the measured energy need to be about 10% above BEE (BEE × 1.1). It should be emphasized that these reports were based on patients' resting state, which did not account for activity. Overall, energy expenditure is not associated with cause or clinical staging of liver disease.[60]

Portal hypertension, a common complication of end-stage liver disease, is directly related to increased pressures that develop because of disturbances in blood flow through the scarred, nodular cirrhotic liver. In an attempt to dissipate the increased pressure, portal-systemic collaterals develop. Esophageal and gastric varices are the most clinically significant of these collaterals, which divert flow away from the portal vein and aid in reducing pressure in the hepatic sinusoids. Varices, which are thin-walled veins, dilate and eventually lead to hemorrhage, a major cause of death in patients with cirrhosis.[61] For this reason, a diet modified in texture is often ordered for hospitalized patients to avoid traumatizing esophageal varices and precipitating bleeding. Although this measure is logical, no study exists that either confirms or refutes its efficacy. Clinicians must weigh the benefit of a modified diet in the prevention of esophageal bleed against the risk of further compromising the oral intake with an unpleasant diet. Medical management is required and may include a variety of techniques, such as administration of beta-blockers that decrease portal venous pressure; sclerotherapy; variceal band ligation; somatostatin; transjugular intrahepatic portal-systemic shunt; and surgical treatment.[62–64]

The formation of abdominal collaterals due to portal hypertension leads to the development of ascites when mounting pressures cause the hepatic lymphatic system to overflow into the peritoneal cavity.[65] Sodium and fluid retention is a contributing factor to reaccumulation of ascites due to the altered angiotensin-aldosterone system, and arginine vasopressin. The goal of medical therapy in ascites management is to maintain a negative sodium and fluid balance.[66] Of cirrhotic patients with ascites, 5% to 15% can be managed with sodium restriction and bed rest if life-threatening respiratory and cardiac complications are not present. Some researchers have suggested a very restricted sodium allowance (250 to 500 mg, or 10 to 22 mmol/day) for positive results to be achieved.[67] Because the unpalatability of very-low-sodium diet can compromise nutrition intake, typical sodium restriction can generally be liberalized to 2000 mg/day once diuretic therapy is instituted.[66] Gauthier et al[68] reported that sodium-restricted diets improved overall survival in cirrhotic patients with ascites. Fluid restriction may also be indicated, especially if edema is present. Daily fluid intake should be restricted to about 1500 mL if possible.[69]

Patients with cholestatic cirrhosis may have significant fat malabsorption as suggested by a study showing the average fecal fat to be 21.3 g/day upon consumption of a 100 g/day fat diet.[56] The reported serum levels of fat-soluble vitamins (vitamin A, D, E), however, was within the normal range, which could be explained by the well-preserved hepatic storage.[13,56] Overall, supplementation of fat-soluble vitamins up to 100% of the Recommended Dietary Allowance may be prescribed.

Liver Transplantation

Liver transplantation has become a practical therapeutic procedure for the management of adults and children with terminal liver failure. Since malnutrition has detrimental effects on surgical outcome, timely nutritional assessment and aggressive nutrition support should be considered early in the medical evaluation process of liver transplant candidates.[56]

Malnutrition remains prevalent in pretransplant patients. Some researchers reported a decrease in body fat and muscle store along with depletion of visceral protein status preoperatively.[56] Other authors, using subjective global assessment as a nutrition parameter, documented that about 71% of the patients were moderately to severely malnourished.[70] A review of the nutrition management of patients following liver transplant may be found in Chapter 15.[71,72]

NUTRITION CONSIDERATIONS IN HEPATIC ENCEPHALOPATHY

Definition

Hepatic encephalopathy is a neuropsychiatric disorder with clinical manifestation ranging from subtle changes in mental status to frank coma. It is characterized by a reversible altered state of consciousness, intellectual deterioration, and neurologic abnormalities.[73] This condition can be classified into four types, depending on rapidity of onset, severity of symptoms, and frequency of recurrence. (1) Acute or subacute encephalopathy, generally seen in patients with acute viral or toxic hepatitis or Reye's syndrome, is of rapid onset and short, intense duration, usually not lasting for more than a few days. (2) Recurrent acute or subacute encephalopathy is similar, but includes patients having more than one but not greater than a few episodes of encephalopathy. (3) Chronic recurrent encephalopathy generally occurs in cirrhotic patients with extensive portal collateral circulation; repeated occurrences and mental, emotional, and neurologic abnormalities that are controllable with proper treatment characterize this condition. (4) Chronic, permanent, hepatic encephalopathy is most common in cirrhotic patients with extensive portal collateral circulation or a surgically created portal-systemic shunt. Patients with this disorder generally develop permanent neurologic abnormalities.[74]

Pathogenesis

The precise pathogenesis of hepatic encephalopathy remains unclear. Five proposed theories have been identified, many of which were based on animal observation. The pathogenesis is undoubtedly multifactorial and more complex than this discussion indicates.

1. *Ammonia.* Ammonia, the principal byproduct of nitrogen metabolism, is considered a neurotoxin that is strongly linked to encephalopathy. The decreased ability of the damaged liver to synthesize urea from protein derived from dietary sources, luminal production, or gastrointestinal bleeding leads to hyperammonemia. Reduced blood flow to the liver due to portal-systemic shunt further impairs hepatic clearance of ammonia. Plasma ammonia levels are not elevated in all encephalopathic patients, however, and do not correlate well with the stage of encephalopathy. Hence, other metabolic abnormalities probably contribute to this condition.
2. *False neurotransmitters.* The brain, which detoxifies the elevated ammonia level by combining it with glutamic acid, yields a rise in the glutamine concentration as the byproduct. To maintain an equilibrium state, the brain effluxes the glutamine and, in exchange, an AAA is influxed into the brain.[75] When the AAA levels rise in the brain, the production of cerebral catecholamine is stimulated, which in turn increases the synthesis of the "false" neurotransmitters, octopamine and phenylethanolamine.[73] These replace dopamine, the "true" neurotransmitter in the brain, resulting in ineffective neurotransmission.
3. *Gamma-aminobutyric acid (GABA).* GABA is a major inhibitory neurotransmitter that is responsible for sedation. The theory that hepatic encephalopathy is related to the GABA neurotransmitter system was based on

an observation that GABA receptors increase by two-fold in animals sustaining hepatic coma.[73] Also, patients with fulminant hepatic coma have been reported to respond to a GABA-antagonistic drug, showing improvement in encephalopathy.[73]

4. *Synergism.* The synergism theory suggests that encephalopathy is caused by a summation of metabolic derangements. The levels of ammonia, short-chain fatty acids, and methanethiol are increased in plasma of patients with hepatic failure. They have been shown to induce a reversible coma in animals and interfere with the disposition of ammonia by depressing enzymes involved in urea synthesis.[74,76,77]

5. *Abnormal amino acids.* Despite a great deal of research in this area, the role of abnormal plasma amino acid patterns in encephalopathic patients remains unclear. An elevated concentration of the AAAs is frequently reported, while the BCAAs are found in lower than normal levels. The usual ratio of BCAA to AAA (3.5:1) is altered toward 1:1 in hepatic encephalopathy. Researchers have proposed that this leads to an increased delivery of phenylalanine to the brain (perhaps enhanced by increased permeability of the blood-brain barrier) which, in turn, decreases the conversion of tyrosine to the true neurotransmitter. Tyrosine may then be decarboxylated to the false neurotransmitter. Increased levels of plasma tryptophan may cross the blood-brain barrier and lead to the formation of the inhibitory neurotransmitter serotonin.[78,79] It is postulated that these false neurotransmitters induce encephalopathy. Although this explanation seems plausible, whether the altered amino acid profile is pathognomonic or merely a result of altered metabolic states remains undetermined.

Diagnosis

The diagnosis of hepatic encephalopathy is based almost entirely upon clinical findings and the severity of the condition. Five stages of encephalopathy have been defined based on these findings (see Exhibit 10–1). Laboratory findings are not as useful as the clinical examination in making a conclusive diagnosis. Standard liver function tests do not allow for differentiation between liver disease and liver disease accompanied by encephalopathy. Blood ammonia levels may be determined (the normal range is 20 to 40 µmol/L), but they are not elevated in all patients and do not correlate well with degree of illness. Cerebrospinal fluid glutamine, the end product of ammonia metabolism, is considered to be a more specific indicator of encephalopathy. This test requires a spinal tap, however, and is almost never used in actual practice. Abnormal electroencephalographic readings are characteristic of, but not specific to, hepatic encephalopathy. Patients generally show a slowing of cerebral electrical activity with high voltage and slow wave forms.[74,76]

Exhibit 10–1 Clinical Aberrations in Hepatic.Encephalopathy

Stage	Mental/Neuromuscular Abnormalities
0	None, no degree of encephalopathy present
1	Apathy, depression, inappropriate behavior, altered sleep patterns
2	Confusion, disorientation, drowsiness, asterixis
3	Sleeping most of the time but arousable, markedly confused, disoriented for place, asterixis
4	Semicomatose or comatose, flaccid limbs, depressed reflexes

Medical Therapy

Medical therapy revolves around the prevention or treatment of factors known to precipitate hepatic encephalopathy. Nitrogenous overload is the most important factor, whether it is of exogenous or endogenous origin. Gastrointestinal hemorrhage (from esophageal varices, gastritis, or peptic ulcer) precipitates encephalopathy twice as often as excessive dietary protein intake. Azotemia is the most frequent cause of this condition, leading to 29% of all cases. This can occur spontaneously or may be induced by excessive diuretic use. Sedatives, tranquilizers, narcotic analgesics, infection, and constipation can also precipitate this disorder.[74,76]

Lactulose (4-*O*-β-D-galactopyranosyl-D-fructose), a synthetic disaccharide that is neither absorbed nor hydrolyzed in the upper gastrointestinal tract, is the mainstay of therapy for encephalopathy. It passes unchanged into the colon, where it is metabolized to lactate by the bacteria. The lactate has an osmotic effect, simulating a laxative therapy. The beneficial effect may be in part due to acidification of the lumen, which leads to the conversion of ammonia to ammonium ion, which is not absorbed and is then excreted in the stool. In practice, the therapeutic effect is achieved when lactulose syrup is titrated to induce three bowel movements per day. Dose requirements vary, depending on individual response to therapy. Untoward effects of this drug include distention, flatulence, and abdominal discomfort. Excessive dosage can lead to diarrhea and loss of free water, resulting in hypernatremia. The unabsorbable antibiotic neomycin has also been used for treating encephalopathy for many years. It decreases the number of urease-producing bacteria in the gut, thereby reducing the production of ammonia from protein and amino acids. These drugs are generally used separately, although a few studies have shown a beneficial effect using them in combination.[78]

Nutrition Therapy

The provision of nutrition support to encephalopathic patients poses a unique challenge. An adequate energy and protein intake is required to satisfy energy needs to allow for hepatic regeneration and to prevent formation of endogenous sources of ammonia through the catabolism of lean body mass. Several decades ago, severe protein restriction of 20 g/day was suggested to ameliorate the symptoms of hepatic encephalopathy.[80,81] Recent data indicate that stable cirrhotic patients need and can tolerate a protein load equivalent to repletion needs of noncirrhotic patients with other medical diseases. Although the minimum protein requirement of cirrhotic patients is suggested to be 50 g/day,[82] protein intake of up to 70 g/day has been shown to be well tolerated without exacerbating encephalopathy.[42] Nitrogen balance is typically achieved when protein intake is at a level of no less than 1.2 g/kg/day in cirrhotic patients.[83] Furthermore, Bunout et al[84] and Kearns et al[85] demonstrated that hospitalized cirrhotic patients can tolerate protein intake of 1.5 g/kg/day without exacerbating hepatic encephalopathy while receiving adequate lactulose therapy. The majority of the studies mentioned above included cirrhotic patients without major acute stress; therefore, the protein requirement of acutely ill patients (in the intensive care setting) may be higher than 1.2 g/kg/day. Protein tolerance should be monitored closely when protein load is above 1.5 g/kg/day.

Based upon the altered plasma amino acid profile/false neurotransmitter theory, some have touted enteral and parenteral formulas decreased in AAAs and increased in BCAAs as the answer to the protein intolerance dilemma in encephalopathy. The theory was that administration of such formulas would correct the plasma amino acid abnormalities, improve nutritional status, and reverse observed mental changes. Early studies compared the provision of BCAA-enriched parenteral nutrition to neomycin or lactulose therapy alone or in combination with dextrose solutions. Some researchers found positive results in the BCAA-supported patients,[86,87] but it is impossible to determine whether this beneficial effect was attributable to the BCAAs or whether it was merely because these patients were provided with some rather than no protein. While the majority of the studies reported that plasma BCAA levels rise in response to BCAA supplement, conflicting data exist as to whether this corrected plasma profile correlates to improved encephalopathy. Wahren et al[88] reported that intravenous infusions of BCAAs corrected the abnormal amino acid profile but did not improve cerebral function or decrease mortality.

Conflicting results have also been obtained when standard dietary regimens are compared with diets identical in calorie and protein content but supplemented with BCAA. McGhee et al[89] and Christie et al[90] found no therapeutic advantage to a BCAA-supplemented diet. Horst and coworkers[91] also found no difference in achievement of positive nitrogen balance between groups receiving equivalent amounts of an intact protein diet and those receiving a BCAA-enriched enteral diet. Calvey et al[92] found no difference in nutrition parameters, mortality, or mental condition in patients with acute alcoholic hepatitis who received protein from conventional sources or from BCAA-enriched formulas.

There is a lack of well-controlled research that shows a distinct advantage to using BCAA-enriched enteral and parenteral formulas over standard ones in decreasing morbidity, achieving positive nitrogen balance, improving nutritional status, or enhancing mental status. The use of specialized hepatic products should be limited to patients who are catabolic but continue to have disabling encephalopathy despite maximized therapy with lactulose and neomycin.[82,93]

The theory that vegetable protein is less encephalogenic than animal protein was first mentioned in the 1970s. However, there are few proposed mechanisms to substantiate the theory.[11] A vegetable diet tends to have a higher carbohydrate to protein ratio, which may stimulate the production of insulin that, in turn, inhibits protein catabolism and endogenous generation of ammonia. Vegetable protein also has less methionine, the substance that increases the cerebral production of neurotransmission-blocking agents, mercaptans. In addition, it is postulated that fiber can simulate the lactulose effect by decreasing the gastrointestinal transit time and reducing nitrogen absorption in the colon.

Early work by Greenberger et al[94] and Uribe et al[95] supported the use of vegetable protein diets. DeBruijn and coworkers[96] studied eight patients with subclinical portal-systemic encephalopathy, providing them with equal amounts of mixed, animal, and vegetable protein diets in a crossover design. They reported no statistically significant difference between the three diets with regard to apparent nitrogen balance, improvement in mental status, or ammonia level. However, this study provided patients with only 50 g of protein/day, which may have led to endogenous protein breakdown, contributing to ammonia accumulation. A different result is reported in another study of similar design.[97] Bianchi et al[97] reported a significant improvement in the mental status in patients on vegetable diet, while ensuring a provision of 70 g protein/day (1g/kg/day) and a diet compliance rate exceeding 90%. Compliance problems were reported in a metabolic study conducted by Shaw et al.[98] Patients were given 40 g of animal protein and 40 g of vegetable protein in a crossover design. Again, investigators observed no significant difference between the diets in regard to enhanced mental status or nitrogen balance. Keshavarzian et al[99] found that patients with chronic stable portal-systemic encephalopathy could tolerate 80 g of protein from vegetable sources. However, because these researchers compared this regimen with a 40-g animal protein diet, it is not possible to conclude that a vegetable protein diet is more efficacious.

The superiority of vegetable protein diets in the treatment of hepatic encephalopathy remains inconclusive, in part due to the small sample size involved in the study. Considering that vegetable protein diets do not induce major harmful side effects, they may be attempted in patients with refractory forms of encephalopathy rather than an overall protein restriction. The mentioned studies adopted a 70% to 90% replacement of protein from vegetable origin. Early satiety, abdominal distention, and flatulence were common complaints when patients received the vegetable diet, and extensive encouragement was required for the meals to be consumed in their entirety. Individual tolerance in terms of gastrointestinal distress should be monitored, and intake of vegetable protein should be titrated accordingly.

GUIDELINES FOR NUTRITION SUPPORT

Therapeutic modifications are summarized in Table 10–3 and serve as a guide for developing nutrition regimens. Aspects of nutrition care of patients with liver failure that pertain directly to tube feeding and parenteral nutrition are discussed below. Provision of aggressive nutrition support has not been shown to reduce mortality in patients with liver disease.[40,85] The aim of nutrition support is to reduce nutrition-related complications such as infection.[40] Patients with moderate or severe protein-calorie malnutrition and those with moderately severe liver disease benefit most from vigorous nutrition support.[43,93]

Tube Feeding

Numerous enteral formulas are commercially available for oral and tube feeding supplementation that are appropriate for patients with liver disease. In general, clinicians should adopt formulas that are low in sodium and fluid content for patients who are prone to develop ascites and/or edema. Occasionally, tube-fed patients may develop diarrhea due to the administration of lactulose. In such a case, electrolyte abnormalities or deteriorating nutritional status may necessitate nutrition via the parenteral route. Furthermore, clinicians need to identify fat malabsorption as a potential cause of diarrhea. Substituting the standard formula with a low-fat, medium-chain triglyceride–based product may be helpful in aiding absorption.

Some studies have reported that isotronic formulas (1 kcal/1 mL) with sodium content ranging from 450 mg to 600 mg per 1000 kcal are well tolerated and do not exacerbate preexisting ascites.[40,84] Calorically dense enteral formulas are also well tolerated by cirrhotic patients without diarrhea.[42,85] Smith et al[100] used a ready-prepared product providing 2.0 kcal/mL and 500 mg of sodium per 1000 kcal to aliment 10 subjects with ascites due to alcoholic liver disease or postnecrotic cirrhosis. Nine patients were able to tolerate the formula without adverse effects and evidenced improvement in serum albumin, creatinine-height index, and anthropometric measurements.

Large-bore feeding tubes are considered to be inappropriate for patients with esophageal varices, although no controlled studies have been conducted in this area. Fine-bore feeding tubes are reported to be safe, even in the presence of variceal bleeding,[42,85] and are recommended for such patients in an attempt to prevent hemorrhage.[101] Serum glucose levels should be determined frequently to detect hyperglycemia, as carbohydrate intolerance may be present in patients with chronic liver failure. Specialized hepatic products (BCAA-enriched) should be

Table 10–3 Nutrition Therapy in Liver Disease

Type of Hepatic Disease	Therapeutic Measure
Fatty liver/steatosis	• Abstinence from ethanol • Weight reduction if attributable to obesity • Reduce calorie and dextrose intake especially in TPN
Hepatitis (acute/chronic/alcoholic)	• At least 30 kcal/kg and 1g protein/kg • Small meals plus snacks and oral supplements if anorexia and nausea are present • High-fat foods generally not restricted • Tube-feeding or parenteral nutritional support if oral intake is inadequate • IV dextrose infusion and electrolyte replacement
Cirrhosis	• 27 to 30 kcal/kg; may use BEE × 1.1 to 1.3 in stable patients • Protein: 1.2 to 1.5g/kg
Esophageal varices Ascites	• Liberal diet consistency is often tolerated • Sodium restriction: 2 g/day with diuretics • Fluid restriction: 1.5 L/day • Fat-soluble vitamin supplement up to 100% RDA may be necessary in cholestatic cirrhosis
Liver transplantation	• 33 to 40 kcal/kg of IBW • Protein: 1.5 g/kg • Replace K, Mg, Phos, Ca, and other electrolytes and minerals as needed
Hepatic encephalopathy	• 27 to 30 kcal/kg • Protein intake: 1.2 to 1.5 g/kg • Vegetable protein: 70% to 90% replacement • Enteral and parenteral products with high BCAA content may be attempted in refractory patients who are catabolic

BCAA—branched-chain amino acid
BEE—basal energy expenditure
IBW—ideal body weight
RDA—Recommended Dietary Allowance

used only in refractory encephalopathy patients who have been given a trial of an appropriate standard formula.

Parenteral Nutrition

Indications for parenteral feeding in patients with liver failure include gastrointestinal hemorrhage or an inability to gain enteral access during active variceal bleeding.

The choice between peripheral and central parenteral nutrition depends on the patient's nutritional needs, metabolic status, and fluid tolerance. In the face of ascites or edema that requires severe fluid restriction of 1 to 1.5 L/day, peripheral parenteral nutrition is unlikely to provide adequate nutrients for the protein sparing.

Standard parenteral solutions can be easily modified to meet the specific nutritional needs of cirrhotic patients. A more concentrated solution of dextrose, amino acids, and lipid may be used when fluid restriction is required. In patients with fatty liver infiltration/steatosis, dextrose and total kilocalorie delivery should be adjusted to avoid overfeeding. Dextrose should be provided at the rate of no more than 3 to 5 mg/kg/minute (or 5–7 g/kg/day), and blood glucose level should be monitored for tolerance. Indirect calorimetry can be used in determining energy expenditure in patients, especially those who are critically ill. As with tube feeding, BCAA solutions for liver failure should be reserved for patients who have refractory hepatic encephalopathy despite maximized medical therapy while receiving standard amino acids.

Even though studies have shown preferred lipid oxidation in stable cirrhotic patients, parenteral lipid should be used with caution. Muscaritoli et al,[102] using a 10% intravenous lipid emulsion, found that maximal clearing capacity for exogenous triglycerides was impaired in 10 cirrhotic patients. The study, however, provided lipid over a period of 3 hours, which is unusual in clinical practice. Lipid was cleared by the bloodstream at a normal rate when moderate amounts of fat were delivered. Other researchers reported fewer episodes of hepatic encephalopathy when alcoholic-cirrhotic patients were randomized to a high-lipid administration compared to the group who received glucose alone.[103] Overall, lipids are safe in liver disease if patients are given appropriate amounts and infusion rates.

The delivery of electrolytes is tailored to each patient, and sodium is generally administered in reduced amounts or eliminated in cirrhotic patients with ascites or edema. Because copper and manganese are principally excreted via the bile, accumulation of such trace minerals may be possible, causing damage to the liver in patients with cholestatic liver disease. A study of 20 patients with primary biliary cirrhosis showed serum copper levels were significantly elevated. Current clinical practice is to provide copper and manganese no more than three times per week in patients with cholestatic cirrhosis or biliary obstruction while monitoring blood levels. Vitamin K (5–10 mg/day) is usually administered intravenously up to three doses when prothrombin time is prolonged.[55] Thiamine is generally provided as a 100-mg intravenous dose. Carbohydrate load can precipitate Wernicke's encephalopathy within minutes in patients with marginal thiamine stores.[104]

CONCLUSIONS

Nutrition management of the adult with liver disease remains a challenge due to the pivotal role of the liver in the metabolism of both macro- and micronutrients.

Although not all alcoholics are malnourished, the impact of ethanol ingestion is significant in each aspect of nutrition delivery—from suppressing appetite to impairing nutrient metabolism. Nutrition intervention is vital, because malnutrition is closely related to mortality in patients with cirrhosis. A successful nutrition regimen begins with an accurate nutritional assessment. A reliable diet history and physical examination are especially informative, given that many biochemical data are influenced by the degree of liver damage. The goal of nutrition intervention in cirrhosis is to prevent undesirable side effects of therapy (hepatic encephalopathy, ascites/edema, steatosis) while maintaining or repleting the patient's nutritional status. Dietary modifications include an appropriate restriction of sodium and fluid intake that is palatable to patients. Although caloric requirements may not be elevated in cirrhotic patients, the protein intake should be increased to aid in nutrition repletion while monitoring tolerance to the nitrogen load. The clinical effectiveness of BCAA supplements and vegetable-protein diets remains inconclusive. Tube-feeding can be safely instituted, and a standard, concentrated formula is well tolerated by the majority of patients. When parenteral nutrition is indicated, central delivery is preferred over peripheral due to the need for volume restriction commonly encountered in cirrhotic patients with ascites.

REFERENCES

1. Rissanen A, Sarlio-Lahteen Korva S, Alfthan G, Gref CG, et al. Employed problem drinkers: a nutritional risk group? *Am J Clin Nutr.* 1987;45:456–461.
2. Dickson BJ, Delaney CG, Walker RD, Hutchinson M, et al. Visceral protein status of patients hospitalized for alcoholism. *Am J Clin Nutr.* 1983;37:216–220.
3. Roe DA. Nutritional concerns in the alcoholic. *J Am Diet Assoc.* 1981;78:17–27.
4. Jones BR, Barrett-Connor E, Criqui MH, Holbrook MJ, et al. A community study of calorie and nutrient intake in drinkers and nondrinkers of alcohol. *Am J Clin Nutr.* 1982;35:135–139.
5. Gruchow HW, Sobocinski KA, Barboriak JJ, Scheller JG, et al. Alcohol consumption, nutrient intake and relative body weight among U.S. adults. *Am J Clin Nutr.* 1985;42:289–295.
6. Fisher M, Gordon T. The relation of drinking and smoking habits to diet: the lipid research clinics prevalence study. *Am J Clin Nutr.* 1985;41:623–630.
7. Lieber CS. Biochemical and molecular basis of alcohol-induced injury to liver and other tissues. *N Engl J Med.* 1988;319:1639–1650.
8. Nanji AA, Zakim D. Alcoholic liver disease. In: Zakim D, Boyer TD, eds. *Hepatology.* Philadelphia: WB Saunders Co; 1996:891–961.
9. Isselbacher KJ. Metabolic and hepatic effects of alcohol. *N Engl J Med.* 1977;296:612–616.
10. DeLuca JR, ed. *Fourth Special Report to the U.S. Congress on Alcohol and Health.* Rockville, MD: US Dept of Health and Human Services; 1981.
11. Feinman L, Lieber CS. Nutrition and diet in alcoholism. In: Shils ME, Olson JA, Shike M, eds. *Modern Nutrition in Health and Disease.* Philadelphia: Lea & Febiger; 1994:1081–1101.
12. Schenker S, Halff GA. Nutritional therapy in alcoholic liver disease. *Semin Liver Dis.* 1993;13:196–209.

13. Halsted CH, Robles EA, Mezey E. Decreased jejunal uptake of labeled folic acid in alcoholic patients: roles of alcohol and nutrition. *N Engl J Med*. 1971;285:701–706.

14. Mills PR, Shenkin A, Anthony RS, McLelland AS, et al. Assessment of nutritional status and in vivo immune responses in alcoholic liver disease. *Am J Clin Nutr*. 1983;38:849–859.

15. Fazio V, Flint DM, Wahlqvist ML. Acute effects of alcohol on plasma ascorbic acid in healthy subjects. *Am J Clin Nutr*. 1981;34:2394–2396.

16. Patek AJ. Alcohol, malnutrition, and alcoholic cirrhosis. *Am J Clin Nutr*. 1979;32:1304–1312.

17. Bluntzer ME, Blachley JD. Acid-base and electrolyte disturbances induced by alcohol. *J Crit Illness*. 1986;1:19–32.

18. Merli M, Riggio O, Romiti A, Ariosto F, et al. Basal energy production rate and substrate use in stable cirrhotic patients. *Hepatology*. 1990;12:106–112.

19. Gabuzda GJ. Nutrition and liver disease: practical considerations. *Med Clin North Am*. 1970;54:1455–1472.

20. Muller MJ, Lautz HU, Plogmann B, Burger M, et al. Energy expenditure and substrate oxidation in patients with cirrhosis: the impact of cause, clinical staging and nutritional state. *Hepatology*. 1992;15:782–794.

21. Mullen KD, Denne SC, McCullough AJ, Savin SM, et al. Leucine metabolism in stable cirrhosis. *Hepatology*. 1986;6:622–630.

22. Davies M, Mawer EB, Krawitt EL. Comparative absorption of vitamin D_3 and 25-hydroxyvitamin D_3 in intestinal disease. *Gut*. 1980;21:287–292.

23. Sitrin MD, Bengoa JM. Intestinal absorption of cholecalciferol and 25-hydroxycholecalciferol in chronic cholestatic liver disease. *Am J Clin Nutr*. 1987;46:1011–1015.

24. Russell RM. Vitamin and mineral supplements in the management of liver diease. *Med Clin North Am*. 1979;63:537–544.

25. Herlong HF, Recker RR, Maddrey WC. Bone disease in primary biliary cirrhosis: histologic features and response to 25-hydroxyvitamin D. *Gastroenterology*. 1982;83:103–108.

26. Achord JL. Malnutrition and the role of nutritional support in alcoholic liver disease. *Am J Gastroenterol*. 1987;82:1–7.

27. Mendenhall CL, Tosch T, Weesner RE, Garcia-Pont P, et al. VA cooperative study on alcoholic hepatitis, II: prognostic significance of protein-calorie malnutrition. *Am J Clin Nutr*. 1986; 43:213–218.

28. Gastineau CF. Nutrition note: alcoholic and calories. *Mayo Clin Proc*. 1976;51:88.

29. Visocan BJ. Nutritional management of alcoholism. *J Am Diet Assoc*. 1983;83:693–696.

30. Herbeth B, Didelot-Barthelemy L, Lemoine A, Le Devehat C, et al. Dietary behavior of French men according to alcohol drinking pattern. *J Stud Alcohol*. 1987;49:268–272.

31. Scully RE, Mark EJ, McNeely BU. Case records of the Massachusetts General Hospital: case. *N Engl J Med*. 1986;315:503–508.

32. Dreizen S. Systemic significance of glossitis. *Postgrad Med*. 1984;75:207–215.

33. Jelliffe DB. *The Assessment of the Nutritional Status of the Community*. Geneva: World Health Organization; 1966. Monograph 53.

34. Merli M, Romiti A, Riggio O, Capocaecia L, et al. Optimal nutritional indexes in chronic liver disease. *J Parenter Enter Nutr*. 1987;11:130S–134S.

35. Thuluvath P, Triger DR. Evaluation of nutritional status by using anthropometry in adults with alcoholic and nonalcoholic liver disease. *Am J Clin Nutr*. 1994;60:269–273.

36. Caregaro L, Alberino F, Amodio P, Merkel C, et al. Malnutrition in alcoholic and virus-related cirrhosis. *Am J Clin Nutr*. 1996;63:602–609.

37. Crawford DH, Shepherd RW, Halliday JW, Cooksley GW, et al. Body composition in nonalcoholic cirrhosis: the effect of disease etiology and severity on nutritional compartments. *Gastroenterology*. 1994;106:1611–1617.

38. Gofferje H. Prealbumin and retinol-binding protein-highly sensitive parameters for the nutritional state in respect of protein. *Med Lab*. 1978;5:38–44.

39. Donohue TM, Tuma DJ, Sorrell MF. Plasma protein metabolism. In: Zakim D, Boyer TD, eds. *Hepatology*. Philadelphia: WB Saunders Co; 1996:130–161.

40. Hirsch S, Bunout D, De La Maza P, Iturriaga H, et al. Controlled trial on nutrition supplementation in outpatients with symptomatic alcoholic cirrhosis. *J Parenter Enter Nutr*. 1993;17:119–124.

41. Ballmer PE, Walshe D, McNurlan MA, et al. Albumin synthesis rates in cirrhosis: correlation with child-turcotte classification. *Hepatology*. 1993;18:292–297.

42. Cabre E, Gonzalez-Huix F, Abad-Lacruz A, Esteve M, et al. Effect of total enteral nutrition on the short-term outcome of severely malnourished cirrhotics. *Gastroenterology*. 1990;98:715–720.

43. Mendenhall CL, Moritz TE, Roselle GA, Morgan TR, et al. Protein energy malnutrition in severe alcoholic hepatitis: diagnosis and response to treatment. *J Parenter Enter Nutr*. 1995;19:258–265.

44. Lukaski HC. Methods for the assessment of human body composition: traditional and new. *Am J Clin Nutr*. 1987;46:537–556.

45. Heymsfield SB, Artega C, McManus C. Measurement of muscle mass in humans: validity of the 24-hour urinary creatinine method. *Am J Clin Nutr*. 1983;37:478–494.

46. Buschenfelde KH. Immune mechanisms in the production of liver disease. In: Zakim D, Boyer TD, eds. *Hepatology*. Philadelphia: WB Saunders Co; 1996:1243–1258.

47. MacGregor RR. Alcohol and immune defense. *JAMA*. 1986;256:1474–1479.

48. White HM, Alpers DH, Sabesin SM. Fatty liver: biochemical and clinical aspects. In: Schiff L, Schiff ER, eds. *Diseases of the Liver*. Philadelphia: JB Lippincott Co; 1993:825–855.

49. Pimstone NR. The spectrum of alcoholic liver disease. *Hosp Med*. October 1986;22:23–46.

50. Zakim D. Metabolism of glucose and fatty acids by the liver. In: Zakim D, Boyer TD, eds. *Hepatology*. Philadelphia: WB Saunders Co; 1996:58–91.

51. Nomura F, Ohniski K, Ochiai T, Okuda K. Obesity-related nonalcoholic fatty liver: CT features and follow-up studies after low calorie diet. *Radiology*. 1987;162:845–847.

52. Clarke PJ, Ball MJ, Kettlewell MG, Chir M, et al. Liver function tests in patients receiving parenteral nutrition. *J Parenter Enter Nutr*. 1991;15:54–59.

53. Seeff LB. Diagnosis, therapy, and prognosis of viral hepatitis. In: Zakim D, Boyer TD, eds. *Hepatology*. Philadelphia: WB Saunders Co; 1996:1067–1145.

54. Boyer JL, Reuben A. Chronic hepatitis. In: Schiff L, Schiff ER, eds. *Diseases of the Liver*. Philadelphia: JB Lippincott Co; 1993:586–637.

55. Koff RS, Galambos JT. Viral hepatitis. In: Schiff L, Schiff ER, eds. *Diseases of the Liver*. Philadelphia: JB Lippincott Co; 1993:492–577.

56. DiCecco SR, Wieners EJ, Wiesner RH, et al. Assessment of nutritional status of patients with end stage liver disease undergoing liver transplantation. *Mayo Clinic Proc*. 1989;64:95–102.

57. Mitchell MC, Herlong HF. Alcohol and nutrition: caloric value, bioenergetics, and relationship to liver damage. *Ann Rev Nutr.* 1986;6:457–474.

58. Antonow DR, McClain CJ. Nutritional support in alcoholic liver disease. *J Parenter Enter Nutr.* 1985;9:566–567.

59. Shanbhogue RLK, Bistrian BK, Jenkins RL, Jones C, et al. Resting energy expenditure in patients with end stage liver disease and in normal population. *J Parenter Enter Nutr.* 1987;11:305–308.

60. Muller MJ, Fenk A, Lautz HU, Selberg O, et al. Energy expenditure and substrate metabolism in ethanol-induced liver cirrhosis. *Am J Physiol.* 1991;23:E338–E344.

61. Groszmann RJ, Atterbury CE. Measurement and manifestations of portal hypertension. *Med Times.* 1984;112:42–49.

62. Pascal JP, Cales P. Propranolol in the prevention of first upper gastrointestinal tract hemorrhage in patients with cirrhosis of the liver and esophageal varices. *N Engl J Med.* 1987;317:856–861.

63. Resnick RH. Treatment of bleeding varices: controversy and opportunity. *Hosp Pract.* April 1984;19:54A, 54D–54E, 54H.

64. Cello JP, Grass RA, Grendell JH, Trunkey DD, et al. Management of the patient with hemorrhaging esophageal varices. *JAMA.* 1986;256:1480–1484.

65. Strauss RM, Boyer TD. Diagnosis and management of cirrhotic ascites. In: Zakim D, Boyer TD, eds. *Hepatology.* Philadelphia: WB Saunders Co; 1996:764–791.

66. Roberts LR, Kamath PS. Ascites and hepatorenal syndrome: pathophysiology and management. *Mayo Clin Proc.* 1996;71:874–881.

67. Rocco VK, Ware AJ. Cirrhotic ascites: pathophysiology, diagnosis, and management. *Ann Intern Med.* 1986;105:573–585.

68. Gauthier A, Levy VG, Quinton A, Michel H, et al. Salt or no salt in the treatment of cirrhotic ascites: a randomized study. *Gut.* 1986;27:705–709.

69. Gitlin N. Nutritional support in liver disease. *Nutr Supp Serv.* 1984;4:14–18.

70. Hasse JM. Nutritional implications of liver transplantation. *Henry Ford Hosp Med J.* 1990;38:235–240.

71. Delafosse B, Faure JL, Bouffard Y, et al. Liver transplantation-energy expenditure, nitrogen loss, and substrate oxidation rate in the first two postoperative days. *Transplant Proc.* 1989;21:2453–2454.

72. Reilly J, Mehta R, Teperman L, et al. Nutritional support after liver transplantation: a randomized prospective study. *J Parenter Enter Nutr.* 1990;14:386–391.

73. Gitlin N. Hepatic encephalopathy. In: Zakim D, Boyer TD, eds. *Hepatology.* Philadelphia: WB Saunders Co; 1996:605–617.

74. Conn HO. Hepatic encephalopathy. In: Schiff L, Schiff ER, eds. *Diseases of the Liver.* Philadelphia: JB Lippincott Co; 1993:1036–1060.

75. James JH, Ziparo V, Jeppsson B, Fischer JE, et al. Hyperammonemia, plasma amino acid imbalance, and blood-brain amino acid transport: a unified theory of portal-systemic encephalopathy. *Lancet.* 1979:772–776.

76. Schenker S, Hoyumpa AM. Pathophysiology of hepatic encephalopathy. *Hosp Pract.* September 1984;19:99–121.

77. Souba WW. Interorgan ammonia metabolism in health and disease: a surgeon's view. *J Parenter Enter Nutr.* 1987;11:569–579.

78. Fraser CL, Arieff AI. Hepatic encephalopathy. *N Engl J Med.* 1985;313:865–873.

79. Millikan WJ, Henderson JM, Warren WD, Riepe SP, et al. Total parenteral nutrition with F080 in cirrhotics with subclinical encephalopathy. *Ann Surg*. 1983;197:294–304.

80. Sherlock S, Summerskill WHJ, White LP, Phear EA. Portal systemic encephalopathy. Neurological complication of liver disease. *Lancet*. 1954;267:453–457.

81. McDermott WV, Adams RD. Episodic stupor associated with an Eck fistula in the human with particular reference to the metabolism of ammonia. *J Clin Invest*. 1954;33:1–9.

82. Crossley IR, Williams R. Progress in the treatment of chronic portasystemic encephalopathy. *Gut*. 1984;25:85–98.

83. Kondrup J, Nielsen K, Hamberg O. Nutritional therapy in patients with liver cirrhosis. *Europ J Clin Nutr*. 1992;46:239–246.

84. Bunout D, Aicardi V, Hirsch S, Peterman M, et al. Nutritional support in hospitalized patients with alcoholic liver disease. *Europ J Clin Nutr*. 1989;43:615–621.

85. Kearns PJ, Young H, Garcia G, Blaschke T, et al. Accelerated improvement of alcoholic liver disease with enteral nutrition. *Gastroenterology*. 1992;102:200–205.

86. Cerra FB, Cheung NK, Fischer JE, Kaplowitz N, et al. Disease-specific amino acid infusion (F080) in hepatic encephalopathy: a prospective, randomized, double-blind, controlled trial. *J Parenter Enter Nutr*. 1985;9:288–295.

87. Rossi-Fanelli F, Angelico M, Cangiano C, Cascino A, et al. Effect of glucose and/or branched chain amino acid imbalance in chronic liver failure. *J Parenter Enter Nutr*. 1981;5:414–419.

88. Wahren J, Denis J, Desurmont P, Eriksson LS, et al. Is intravenous administration of branched chain amino acids effective in the treatment of hepatic encephalopathy? A multicenter study. *Hepatology*. 1983;3:475–480.

89. McGhee A, Henderson JM, Millikan WJ, Bleier JC, et al. Comparison of the effects of hepatic-aid and casein modular diet on encephalopathy, plasma amino acids, and nitrogen balance in cirrhotic patients. *Ann Surg*. 1983;197:288–293.

90. Christie ML, Sack DM, Pomposelli J, Horst D, et al. Enriched branched chain amino acid formula versus a casein-based supplement in the treatment of cirrhosis. *J Parenter Enter Nutr*. 1985;9:671–678.

91. Horst D, Grace ND, Conn HO, Schiff E, et al. Comparison of dietary protein with an oral, branched chain-enriched amino acid supplement in chronic portal-systemic encephalopathy: a randomized controlled trial. *Hepatology*. 1984;4:279–287.

92. Calvey H, Davis M, Williams R. Controlled trial of nutritional supplementation, with and without branched chain amino acid enrichment, in treatment of acute alcoholic hepatitis. *J Hepatol*. 1985;1:141–151.

93. Nompleggi DJ, Bonkovsky HL. Nutritional supplementation in chronic liver disease: an analytical review. *Hepatology*. 1994;19:518–533.

94. Greenberger NJ, Carley J, Schenker S, Bettinger I, et al. Effect of vegetable and animal protein diets in chronic hepatic encephalopathy. *Dig Dis Sci*. 1977;22:845–855.

95. Uribe M, Marquez MA, Ramos G, Ramos-Uribe MH, et al. Treatment of chronic portal-systemic encephalopathy with vegetable and animal protein diets: a controlled crossover study. *Dig Dis Sci*. 1982;27:1109–1116.

96. DeBruijn KM, Blendis LM, Zilm DH, Carlen PL, et al. Effect of dietary protein manipulations in subclinical portal-systemic encephalopathy. *Gut*. 1983;24:53–60.

97. Bianchi GP, Marchesini G, Fabbri A, Rondelli A, et al. Vegetable protein diet and hepatic encephalopathy. *J Intern Med*. 1993;233:385–392.

98. Shaw S, Worner TM, Lieber CS. Comparison of animal and vegetable protein sources in the dietary management of hepatic encephalopathy. *Am J Clin Nutr.* 1983;38:59–63.

99. Keshavarzian A, Meek J, Sutton C, Emery VM, et al. Dietary protein supplementation from vegetable sources in the management of chronic portal systemic encephalopathy. *Am J Gastroenterol.* 1984;79:945–949.

100. Smith J, Horowitz J, Henderson JM, Heymsfield S. Enteral hyperalimentation in undernourished patients with cirrhosis and ascites. *Am J Clin Nutr.* 1982;35:56–72.

101. Jones BJM. Enteral feeding: techniques of administration. *Gut.* 1986;27(suppl 1):47–50.

102. Muscaritoli M, Cangiano C, Cascino A, Ceci F, et al. Exogenous lipid clearance in compensated liver cirrhosis. *J Parenter Enter Nutr.* 1986;10:599–603.

103. Glynn MJ, Powell-Tuck J, Reaveley DA, Murray-Lyon IM, et al. High lipid parenteral nutrition improves portasystemic encephalopathy. *J Parenter Enter Nutr.* 1988;12:457–461.

104. Schenker S, Henderson GI, Hoyumpa AM, McCandless DW. Hepatic and Wernicke's encephalopathies: current concepts of pathogenesis. *Am J Clin Nutr.* 1980;33:2719–2726.

CHAPTER 11

Renal Function

Carol Liftman

INTRODUCTION

The nephron is the functional unit of the kidney. Each kidney contains approximately 1 million nephrons. Each nephron is composed of a vascular component—the glomerulus, which produces an ultrafiltrate of the plasma—and a tubular component. The tubule is composed of a single layer of epithelial cells that differ in structure and function along the length of the tubule.

The tubule starts as a blind sac called Bowman's capsule, one side of which is associated with the glomerulus. The other, highly coiled, side is the proximal convoluting tubule. The next portion of the tubule contains a sharp, hairpin loop—the loop of Henle. The tubule becomes coiled again—the distal convoluting tubule—and finally straightens into the collecting duct. Collecting ducts combine, forming larger ducts that empty into the renal pelvis. The renal pelvis becomes the ureter, which empties into the bladder.

Blood enters the kidney via the renal artery, which divides into smaller and smaller branches, leading to the capillaries that form the glomerulus. Blood in the glomerulus is separated from Bowman's capsule by a thin layer of tissue that allows the blood to filter from the capillaries to Bowman's capsule.

The glomerular capillaries recombine to form another set of arterioles that are associated with the remaining portion of the tubule. Eventually, they rejoin to form the venous system leaving the kidney.

URINE FORMATION

The glomerular filtrate in Bowman's capsule is basically protein-free plasma that contains small-molecular-weight crystalloids (ie, glucose, sodium, potassium, hydrogen ions, urea, creatinine, phosphorus, and uric acid) in the same concentration as in blood. As the filtrate flows through the tubule, it is altered by two

239

processes. In the first process—tubular reabsorption—water and solutes move from the tubular lumen to the peritubular capillaries. In the second process—tubular secretion—movement occurs in the opposite direction. The rates at which these processes occur regulate the internal environment. Tubular reabsorption and tubular secretion can be active or passive. Active transport systems require energy, and they may become saturated and able to carry only limited amounts of material at one time.

The entire plasma volume passes through the kidneys about 60 times daily, concentrating about 180 L of ultrafiltrate into 1 to 2 L of urine. Approximately 99% of water and solute filtered by the kidney is reabsorbed.

SODIUM AND FLUID REGULATION

Sodium ions are found primarily in the extracellular fluid, as they are excluded from the cells by active transport. Sodium and its major ions, chloride and bicarbonate, comprise 90% of the solute in extracellular fluid, determining extracellular fluid volume. The kidney is the primary regulator of sodium, water, and extracellular fluid volume. Sodium and water balance can be maintained with sodium intakes ranging from 50 mg to 25 g and water intakes ranging from 400 mL to 25 L.

There is no tubular secretion of sodium, chloride, or water. Of the sodium and chloride, 99% is reabsorbed as the ions pass through the tubule. Sodium is actively transported by a carrier against a concentration gradient. The reabsorption of water and chloride by passive diffusion depends on sodium reabsorption.

The water permeability of the distal portion of the tubule is controlled by antidiuretic hormone (ADH). In the absence of ADH, water permeability is very low, so that sodium is reabsorbed but water cannot follow. ADH increases water permeability but has no effect on sodium reabsorption. The tubular response to ADH allows for fine adjustment.

Of the filtered sodium, 75% is reabsorbed in the proximal tubule. Aldosterone, a hormone produced by the adrenal cortex, is the major control for the absorption of sodium in the distal tubule. The remaining sodium is absorbed in the loop of Henle.

POTASSIUM REGULATION

Most of the potassium in the body is intracellular (only 2% is extracellular). Intracellular potassium establishes the resting membrane potential of the cells. As with sodium, the kidney is the major regulator of potassium. Potassium is completely filtered by the glomerulus, and almost all of the potassium in the filtrate is reabsorbed by active transport. The amount of potassium excreted in the urine is regulated by changes in potassium secretion. An elevated potassium intake increases the potassium content of all cells, including the renal tubular cells. Concentrated cellular potassium levels increase potassium secretion into the lumen of the tubule, and it is subsequently lost in urine. Aldosterone enhances tubular secretion of potassium.

CALCIUM REGULATION

Extracellular calcium is regulated in kidney, bone, and the gastrointestinal tract. The calcium concentration of the extracellular fluid controls parathyroid hormone (PTH) production, which mediates the renal response. PTH stimulates the kidneys to decrease phosphate reabsorption and increase calcium reabsorption in the tubule. In the kidney, PTH also stimulates conversion of vitamin D to its most active metabolite, 1,25-dihydroxycholecalciferol.

ACID-BASE BALANCE

Acid-base balance, or pH, is under respiratory or metabolic control. Respiratory control of pH is discussed in detail in Chapter 6. In metabolic acidosis or alkalosis, an alteration in the concentration of plasma bicarbonate (HCO_3) leads to a change in plasma pH. The kidney controls HCO_3 concentration by reclaiming filtered HCO_3 or by secreting acid. This process is regulated in the tubules without hormonal mediators.

RENAL DISEASE

Assessment of Patients with Renal Disease

One of the most useful tools for nutritional assessment of a patient with renal disease is a detailed dietary history for evaluation of calorie, protein, potassium, sodium, phosphorus, and fluid intake. The impact of medications and vitamin or mineral supplements is also considered. This information then serves as a guide for individualized nutrition therapy.

Edema invalidates weight and other anthropometric data, making interpretation of these measurements difficult. Plasma albumin levels are lowered by fluid overload and are temporarily unreliable when salt-poor albumin is given. Prealbumin and retinol-binding protein levels are elevated as a result of impaired renal function.[1,2] The serum transferrin concentration, therefore, is the best biochemical index of nutritional status in renal failure. In predialysis patients, a low serum transferrin level has been shown to correlate with poor nutritional status.[3] However, iron deficiency or iron overload alters transferrin levels independently of nutritional status. With iron deficiency, transferrin levels rise; with iron overload, they fall.[3,4]

Excess iron is stored as ferritin, making measurement of this substance the most useful tool for assessing iron status.[5,6] Iron deficiency may occur secondary to blood losses during dialysis, and iron overload may result from multiple blood transfusions. These factors must be considered when using serum transferrin levels to evaluate nutritional status.

Laboratory Assessment of Renal Function

Because dietary therapy differs according to the severity of renal disease, the dietitian should be familiar with the laboratory indices of renal function. The most precise measurement of renal function is the glomerular filtration rate (GFR); however, its routine measurement is not practical. A reliable and practical index to renal failure is the serum creatinine level. For every 50% reduction in GFR, the serum creatinine level doubles. For example, with a GFR of 100 mL/min, the serum creatinine concentration is 1.0 mg/dL. As GFR decreases to 50 mL/min, the serum creatinine level increases to 2.0 mg/dL. Another fairly simple and reliable indicator of renal function is creatinine clearance, which estimates GFR. The level of blood urea nitrogen (BUN) is an often-used but less-accurate measure of renal function, because it rises with increased protein intake, dehydration, fever, or infection.[7]

Clinical Symptoms in Renal Failure

Azotemia may be defined as the accumulation of nitrogen waste products. Uremia is the symptom complex and clinical effect of severe azotemia. Uremic symptoms usually occur when the GFR falls below 25 mL/min. Urea itself is not the cause of the adverse manifestations of chronic renal failure, but it may be partially responsible for nausea, vomiting, headache, and bleeding disorders. In more advanced renal failure, uremic stomatitis, dry mucous membranes, and ulcerative lesions may be seen.

NUTRITION MANAGEMENT OF PATIENTS WITH CHRONIC RENAL FAILURE

Protein Requirements

Catabolism of dietary protein and the breakdown of body stores liberate nitrogen, which is converted almost entirely to urea. Based on the concept that protein catabolism produces uremic toxin, patients with renal failure historically have been placed on low-protein diets. However, restricting protein in early renal failure to prevent or slow further deterioration may have a slightly different mechanism. When renal function is compromised, a high-protein diet seems to increase

GFR in remaining nephrons.[8] This "hyperfiltration" response in single nephrons becomes maladaptive and causes further damage. A high-protein diet also increases renal blood flow, which may cause further damage.[9] Another theory suggests that the accumulation of phosphorus—found abundantly in high-protein foods—whether alone or by causing secondary hyperparathyroidism, may also damage the kidney.[10,11]

The goal of nutrition therapy in early renal failure (serum creatinine 2 to 6 mg/dL) is to preserve remaining kidney function. A protein restriction of 0.6 g/kg of body weight with 75% of the protein of high biological value has been shown to slow or even stop the progression of the disease.[11-15] If adequate calories are given (35 to 40 kcal/kg of body weight), nutritional status is not compromised.[11-16]

For patients with moderate renal insufficiency in the multicenter Modification of Diet in Renal Disease Study, a slower decline in renal function was seen 4 months after starting on a low-protein (0.58 g/kg) diet compared to a usual-protein diet (1.3 g/kg). For patients with more severe renal insufficiency, a very-low-protein (0.28 g/kg) diet with keto acid amino acid supplements did not further slow the progression of renal disease when compared to the low-protein diet (0.58 g/kg).[17] Other studies have successfully used keto acid analogs of essential amino acids combined with a 20–30 g protein diet to delay dialysis while maintaining or improving nutritional status.[18,19] However, these products are not yet commercially available in the United States.

The major cause of chronic renal failure is chronic glomerulonephritis. It may be primary or secondary to a systemic illness such as diabetes mellitus or amyloidosis. Proteinuria is common in glomerular diseases.[7] Researchers have reported that patients with glomerulonephritis have a better prognosis on protein-restricted diets.[15,20-22] However, in another study investigators found that patients with nonglomerular diseases benefit most from the diet.[23]

In advanced renal failure, diet can no longer be used to preserve renal function. The goal of nutrition therapy is to maintain metabolic status as near normal as possible, while relieving uremic symptoms, until dialysis is started or transplantation is performed. A very-low-protein diet of 0.3 g/kg of body weight has been advocated.[24] However, patients who follow a very-low-protein diet for more than a short period of time become malnourished. Compliance is also a problem.

Once dialysis is begun, protein needs increase because of amino acid losses during dialysis. In hemodialysis, 6 to 8 g of free amino acids and 3 to 4 g of bound amino acids are lost per treatment.[25] Loss of amino acids increased 50% during the sixth reuse of a dialyzer membrane compared to the first.[26] With peritoneal dialysis, as much as 9 g of protein[24] and 3 to 4 g of amino acids[27,28] may be lost in 24 hours.

The recommended protein requirement for patients on hemodialysis is 1.1 to 1.4 g/kg of body weight.[26,27] With peritoneal dialysis, the protein recommendation is 1.2 to 1.5 g/kg of body weight.[27-32]

Nephrotic Syndrome

In nephrotic syndrome, the glomerular membrane allows passage of excess protein, especially albumin, into the lumen of the tubule. This protein is then lost in the urine. The resulting hypoalbuminemia can lead to edema from salt and water retention. Sodium restriction may minimize edema. Hypotension from hypoalbuminemia is corrected by using salt-poor albumin; otherwise this agent is of no benefit.

When proteinuria is present, one tends to think of giving a high-protein diet. However, protein-restricted diets have been shown to reduce proteinuria without compromising nutritional status.[33] The recommended protein intake (0.5 to 1.0 g/kg of body weight)[9,15,21,23,33] may be calculated by adding the number of grams of protein lost in the urine to the calculated protein requirement. For each gram of protein lost in the urine, 0.5 to 1.43 g of protein is added to the above figures.[24,34] The author has successfully used 0.6 g of protein per kg of body weight plus an amount equal to urinary protein losses.

Diabetes Mellitus

Because of altered carbohydrate metabolism, 70% of uremic patients are glucose-intolerant.[7] Fasting blood glucose levels may be elevated, but a glucose tolerance test usually reveals that only postprandial levels are elevated. Peripheral insulin resistance with impaired glucose uptake has been noted.[35–38]

For patients with diabetes mellitus without renal disease, the American Association recommends a diet in which 10% to 20% of total calories are from high-quality protein. This protein allowance is significantly greater than the Recommended Dietary Allowance (RDA) (0.8 g/kg of body weight) and obviously in excess of appropriate amounts for patients with compromised renal function. For example, on a standard diabetic diet, a 70-kg man requiring 2000 kcal/day would be given 60 to 100 g of protein. In chronic renal failure, 0.6 g of protein per kg of body weight would be given, resulting in a protein intake of 42 g. Insulin-dependent diabetic patients with chronic renal failure have been shown to benefit from protein-restricted diets.[39–42] They are able to tolerate higher carbohydrate loads while maintaining acceptable serum glucose levels.[42,43] In patients with non–insulin-dependent diabetes mellitus (NIDDM), Summerson et al[44] did not find a correlation between the appearance or changes in proteinuria or microalbuminuria with the dietary protein intake. However, in a random cross-over trial with NIDDM patients, a moderate protein restriction (0.8 g/kg) compared to an isocaloric high-protein diet (2.0 g/kg) resulted in a decrease in urinary albumin excretion without affecting glycemic control.[45] The unanswered question is whether diabetic patients with the potential for developing renal disease should limit their protein intake prophylactically. Of patients who have had insulin-dependent diabetes mellitus for more than 20 years, 50% develop renal failure.[7] Therefore, it might be prudent to design diabetic diets in which 10% to 12% of calories are from protein, approximating the RDA.

Calorie Needs

Adequate calories are essential to prevent catabolism both before and after dialysis is initiated. A diet containing 30–35 kcal/kg of ideal body weight is usually recommended.[16,29,31,32] With individual variations, patients may absorb up to 800 kcal/day from the peritoneal dialysate.[31]

Lipid Metabolism

Hypercholesterolemia is common in nephrotic syndrome, but it rarely responds to dietary treatment. In chronic renal failure without nephrotic syndrome, an increase in triglycerides may be noted, but elevated cholesterol levels are seen infrequently. Hyperinsulinemia may play a role in increased hepatic production of triglycerides. Patients with fasting levels of cholesterol and triglycerides significantly greater than normal need appropriate dietary treatment.

Potassium

Hyperkalemia is frequently noted because of a reduction in the renal excretion of potassium. In less advanced renal failure, hyperkalemia may be a result of reduced levels of renin and aldosterone. This condition, hyporeninemic hypoaldosteronism, is most common in patients with diabetes mellitus and interstitial nephritis. Without hyporeninemic hypoaldosteronism, hyperkalemia does not occur until late in the course of chronic renal failure because of the increased ability of remaining nephrons to excrete potassium. Potassium levels can be maintained within normal limits until the creatinine clearance declines to 5 mL/min.

Hyperkalemia may be the result of exogenous dietary potassium or potassium supplements given with potassium-sparing diuretics. Endogenous potassium sources include the products of muscle and red blood cell breakdown, which release potassium into plasma. The result is an increase in serum potassium levels as potassium is forced to leave the cells to maintain electrical neutrality.

The major toxic effect of hyperkalemia is on the cell membrane of excitable tissue such as muscle and nerves. Electrocardiographic changes are best used to monitor these effects. Chronic hyperkalemia is better tolerated than an acute rise in serum potassium. However, a serum potassium level greater than 6.5 to 6.7 mmol/L requires treatment. If the electrocardiogram is unchanged or limited to peak T waves, potassium restriction of about 2000 mg should be initiated. Advanced electrocardiographic changes mandate more aggressive therapy. Intravenous calcium may be administered to counteract the neuromuscular effects of the high serum potassium concentration. This treatment works quickly, but the results are short-lived. Sodium bicarbonate or glucose and insulin may be administered to redistribute potassium from the extracellular fluid to the intracellular fluid.

Patients on chronic hemodialysis may need a potassium restriction of 2500 to 3000 mg/day or 40 mg/kg/ideal body weight. With peritoneal dialysis, potassium may be unrestricted. If a restriction is necessary, 3000 to 4000 mg/day should be adequate. Potassium restrictions vary with the degree of residual renal function and should be evaluated with serum potassium levels.

In end-stage renal disease, nondiabetic patients often have reduced total body potassium. The body adapts very well as kidney function declines. The patient may have a normal serum potassium but a depletion of intracellular potassium. (Acidosis forces potassium out of cells.) Diuretics contribute to urinary losses of potassium. Potassium intake may be reduced in end-stage disease because of poor appetite and poor intake. Potassium is also lost during vomiting and diarrhea.

Sodium

As renal disease progresses, remaining nephrons excrete increasing amounts of sodium to maintain sodium balance unless sodium intake is excessive. If sodium intake is suddenly decreased, the nephrons cannot adapt, and sodium depletion occurs. Therefore, increased sensitivity to sodium intake should be noted. Reducing sodium intake by 2 to 4 grams daily may help control thirst, edema, and hypertension.

Calcium and Phosphorus

The causes of bone disease are altered vitamin D, calcium, and phosphorus metabolism with high levels of PTH. As the GFR declines and nephron destruction occurs, phosphorus is retained in the body. The serum phosphorus concentration rises with a reciprocal fall in the serum calcium level. The fall in the serum calcium level stimulates PTH secretion, which results in an increase in renal phosphorus secretion and mobilization of calcium from the bone. By this process, serum calcium and phosphorus are normalized but at the expense of chronically high levels of PTH, leading to hyperparathyroid bone disease. When GFR falls below 30 mL/min, phosphorus secretion can no longer maintain a normal level of phosphorus in the blood. The results are high levels of serum phosphorus, extremely high serum PTH, and low serum calcium.

Metabolic acidosis in chronic renal failure also contributes to bone disease as calcium is mobilized to buffer retained acid. Eventually a negative calcium balance and osteoporosis result.

Bone disease is a common and difficult problem to treat in patients with chronic renal failure. Patients may be asymptomatic or severely disabled as a result of pathologic fractures and bone pain. Bone disease can be reversed in early renal disease and controlled in end-stage disease.[47] Serum calcium and phosphorus concentrations need to be maintained within normal limits to prevent secondary hyperparathyroidism. To accomplish this, dietary phosphorus can be restricted, along with aluminum-containing antacids, calcium supplements and the active form of vitamin D_3. The administration of intravenous calcitriol (active form of vitamin D_3) during hemodialysis treatment may suppress PTH with less hypercalcemia. Sample protocols for calcitrol administration are available.[47,48]

For patients on chronic dialysis, a low-phosphorus diet does not allow sufficient protein. Each gram of protein contains at least 10 mg of phosphorus. With a 70 g protein diet, consumption of 700 mg of phosphorus is inevitable. The phosphorus content of the diet can be reduced by limiting foods that are very high in phosphorus, such as bran cereal, liver, and milk products.

Aluminum-containing antacids have been successfully used to bind dietary phosphorus and reduce intestinal absorption. However, aluminum is absorbed and can play a role in bone disease and dementia.

Calcium carbonate supplements can be used to control serum levels of calcium and phosphorus.[51] The mean dosage of calcium carbonate is 9.2 g/day.[50] This dosage is usually divided into three doses, one given after each meal. If hypercalcemia occurs, the calcium concentration in the dialysate can be reduced to less than 3 mEq/L.[50] Recently, calcium acetate has been found to be a more potent phosphate binder than calcium carbonate when given with meals.[51–53] A combination of aluminum-containing antacids and calcium carbonate may also be used.[52–54]

Vitamins and Minerals

The primary cause of anemia in chronic renal failure is the inadequate production of endogenous erythropoietin. Iron deficiency was rarely seen prior to the use of recombinant human erythropoietin (r-HuEPO). Because of the previous need for multiple transfusions, iron overload was common. Oral iron supplementation is often not sufficient to maintain iron balance with r-HuEPO therapy. An assessment of iron stores would include serum ferritin, iron concentrations and transferrin saturation. Intravenous iron dextran infusion during hemodialysis treatment has become a common practice. Also essential to the production of red blood cells is adequate folic acid and vitamin B_{12}.[54]

Vitamin deficiencies can develop in dialysis patients for many reasons: inadequate food intake because of poor appetite or altered taste sensation, avoidance of vitamin-rich fruits and vegetables because of their high potassium content, loss of water-soluble vitamins from soaking or boiling vegetables to reduce their potassium content, alterations in the metabolism or utilization of vitamins, and loss of water-soluble vitamins during the dialysis treatment. The most common vitamin deficiencies seen are deficiencies of pyridoxine (vitamin B_6), ascorbic acid (vitamin C), and folic acid.[55]

Vitamin C should be supplemented at 60 mg daily, with the total daily intake from food about 140 to 150 mg per day. Recommendations for folic acid are 800–1000 mg and pyridoxine are 10 mg. The remaining B vitamins can be supplemented at the RDA level. Jahnke et al[56] found that elevated plasma vitamin A (retinol) levels were independent of dietary intake of vitamin A or carotenoids and that plasma vitamin E levels were comparable to the general population. Therefore, fat-soluble vitamins usually do not need to be supplemented.

In chronic hemodialysis patients, serum zinc was found to be in the low-normal range; this was not corrected by supplementation. A low serum zinc level may be related to the disease process and not necessarily reflect zinc status. Still, a trial of 25 mg elemental zinc may be useful for poor taste acuity.[57–58] Deficiencies of selenium,[60] iron, chromium, and manganese have been reported.[61]

Fluid

Fluid restrictions usually are not indicated until dialysis is necessary. For patients on hemodialysis, a fluid intake equal to urine output, if any, plus 500 mL has been recommended. Most patients can tolerate up to 1000 mL, resulting in a weight gain of 2 lb/day. For patients on peritoneal dialysis, a fluid intake equal to the urine output plus 2000 mL/day is recommended.

Fiber

A high-fiber diet may be beneficial to patients with chronic renal failure. One study has reported an increase in fecal nitrogen excretion of 39% with a high-fiber diet. Fiber also appears to reduce colonic bacterial ammonia production, which in turn reduces hepatic synthesis of urea.[62] Supplementation with 50 g gum arabic fiber resulted in a 41% increase in fecal nitrogen excretion and a 12% decrease in BUN in patients on a low-protein diet compared to 1 g pectin.[63]

Malnutrition in Chronic Renal Failure

Chronic malnutrition is common in patients on dialysis. Thunberg et al[30] found that 60% of patients on maintenance hemodialysis had a serum transferrin level less than 150 mg/dL and a serum albumin in the low-normal range. Hobbs et al[64] reported that dialysis patients with albumin levels less than 4.0 g/dL had a fivefold increase in the incidence of sepsis as compared with patients with serum albumin levels greater than 4.0 g/dL. A threefold increase in the incidence of sepsis was seen with a serum transferrin level less than 220 mg/dL.

Poor intake may be a result of dietary restrictions that eliminate favorite or familiar foods. A poor appetite may persist because of the emotional impact of dialysis. A skilled dietitian can help patients overcome these problems by teaching them to incorporate favorite foods into their meal patterns. Diet instructions should emphasize foods that are allowed, rather than those that are restricted.

Adequacy of Dialysis

Adequacy of hemodialysis can be estimated by urea kinetic equations that calculate the clearance of waste products. A KT/V (amount of plasma cleared of urea during the dialysis time divided by the urea distribution volume) of at least 1.20 is considered adequate.[65] Several large studies have suggested that mortality decreases as KT/V increases to 1.30 or higher. A higher KT/V also appears to improve albumin and mortality rates.[66] In peritoneal dialysis, clearance is calculated based on the amount of solute removed from drained dialysate.

Tube Feeding

For patients receiving dialysis, standard concentrated enteral formulas are usually well tolerated. Specialty formulas are available if necessary but are usually more costly.

Parenteral Nutrition

Amino acid solutions containing essential and nonessential amino acids are appropriate for patients with chronic renal failure requiring total parenteral nutrition. The amount of calcium, phosphorus, sodium, and potassium in the solution needs to be individualized. Concentrated dextrose and lipids may be used for energy.

Intradialytic parenteral nutrition (IDPN) allows the infusion of amino acids, glucose, and lipids during the hemodialysis treatment.[67,68] The correction of hypoalbuminemia with IDPN has been shown to reduce mortality rates in hemodialysis patients.[69–71] However, no clear indications have been established for the use of IDPN.[72] Intraperitoneal parenteral nutrition (IPN) is the replacement of a glucose exchange with a 1% amino acid–based solution.[73–76] Reimbursement from third-party payers is not uniformly provided for IDPN and IPN.

NUTRITION MANAGEMENT OF PATIENTS WITH ACUTE RENAL FAILURE

Acute renal failure is not a homogeneous clinical entity. At one end of the spectrum are medical patients with acute renal failure secondary to nephrotoxic agents or postpartum renal failure. In this group of patients, morbidity and mortality are minimal. The gastrointestinal tract is usually functioning, and aggressive nutrition therapy is rarely needed.[77] When the patient is expected to recover from acute renal failure, a protein-restricted diet is not indicated. A low-protein diet may actually slow the rate of recovery, as protein is needed to heal the injured kidney. Fluid and electrolyte management is the mainstay of treatment.

In contrast, surgical patients with acute, postoperative renal failure have a 40% to 60% chance of survival.[77] The routine use of dialysis has not improved survival rates,[1,71–81] as patients usually die of the underlying disease or its complications rather than renal failure.[77] In this group of patients, nutritional intervention plays a major role in the prognosis. Because most of these patients have multisystem failure, they are not able to ingest and absorb nutrients. Parenteral nutrition is usually indicated.

The consequences of malnutrition are the same in patients with acute renal failure as in other stressed patients: loss of body weight, increased susceptibility to infection, poor wound healing, hypoproteinemic edema, and prolonged recovery from illness.[82] Conceivably, correcting malnutrition and maintaining a normal nutritional status in patients with acute renal failure will prevent these complications and improve survival rates. Nutrition therapy in acute renal failure should also reduce uremic toxicity and metabolic derangement while facilitating healing of the injured kidney.[83]

Protein

In the past, patients with acute renal failure were given parenteral solutions containing essential amino acids and glucose. The use of only essential amino acids was based on the theory that nitrogen obtained from urea could be used for the synthesis of nonessential amino acids. However, an insignificant amount of urea nitrogen is used for protein synthesis.[84–88] Therefore, formulas containing essential as well as nonessential amino acids are recommended.[89]

Many patients with acute renal failure are catabolic, with enhanced protein breakdown. The rate of protein breakdown may be as great as 70 g/day. Dialysate losses increase the protein requirement.[90] For stressed patients, the daily protein requirement may be 2.0 to 2.5 g/kg of body weight.[91]

Energy Requirements

Researchers have found that the resting energy requirement in patients with acute renal failure is 20% to 50% greater than normal.[92] These patients probably need 40 to 50 kcal/kg of body weight per day.[92,93] Hypertonic dextrose (70%) can be used to help meet the energy requirements.[89]

About half of all patients with acute renal failure who receive parenteral nutrition require exogenous insulin. The glucose intolerance may be exacerbated by diabetes mellitus, sepsis, pancreatic insufficiency, or exogenous steroid administration. With peritoneal dialysis, glucose is also absorbed transperitoneally. It is recommended that insulin be added directly to the intravenous solution so that a constant glucose-insulin ratio can be maintained.[77]

An emulsion of 20% lipids offers a high-calorie substrate in a reduced amount of fluid. Patients need to be monitored carefully because of impaired triglyceride metabolism.[94]

Sodium

In the absence of extraordinary surgical losses of sodium (such as occurs in nasogastric suction and fistula drainage), patients with acute renal failure usually have an increase in total body sodium because of inadequate excretion. The presence of hyponatremia rarely represents an absolute sodium deficit. Severe hyponatremia (less than 125 mmol/L) is managed by restriction of free water intake or removal of fluid during dialysis.

Potassium

An increase in serum potassium levels may be seen in acute renal failure as a result of decreased renal excretion, metabolic acidosis, and catabolism. As with chronic renal failure, a patient with a serum potassium level greater than 6.5 mmol/L with electrocardiographic changes needs to be treated.

Hypokalemia may occur as the patient is nutritionally replenished. In general, potassium does not need to be added to the parenteral solution until the serum potassium is less than 3 mmol/L. No more than 5 mmol of potassium (as chloride, acetate, or phosphate) per hour[77] or a concentration of 10 to 15 mmol/L should be given.[81]

Phosphate

Progressive hyperphosphatemia is commonly seen in acute renal failure. With nutritional repletion, the serum phosphorus level falls. By the fifth to eighth posttreatment day, supplementation may be needed. In general, 5 to 15 mEq of potassium phosphate should be given.[77]

Calcium

As with chronic renal failure, abnormalities of calcium and vitamin D metabolism occur in acute renal failure. Calcium can be added to the parenteral solution as calcium gluconate.[77]

Vitamins and Trace Elements

Water-soluble vitamins need to be supplemented to compensate for dialysate losses. Folic acid and pyridoxine requirements are especially high. The requirements for fat-soluble vitamins are still undetermined.[81,89] Iron, zinc, manganese, copper, and chromium may be deficient.[59,61] Although data are still limited, trace elements should probably be added to parenteral solutions.

CONCLUSIONS

Malnutrition is just as serious a problem for patients with renal failure as it is for any other group of patients. In chronic renal failure, diets need to be kept as liberal as medically possible. It is important to consider the patient's ability to comply with the diet. The sodium, potassium, fluid, calcium, phosphorus, protein, and calorie requirements need to be individualized.

With acute renal failure, adequate calories and protein are needed to help heal the injured kidneys. Normally, as many calories and as much protein are given as the fluid allowance permits. Electrolyte and mineral requirements vary with each patient. It may be necessary to start dialysis to allow for adequate nutrition support.

REFERENCES

1. Blumenkrantz M, Kopple J, Koffler A, Komdar A, et al. Total parenteral nutrition in the management of acute renal failure. *Am J Clin Nutr.* 1978;31:1831–1839.

2. Carpentier Y, Barthel J, Bruyns J. Plasma protein concentrations in nutritional assessment. *Proc Nutr Soc.* 1982;41:405–417.

3. Young G, Oli H, Davidson AM, et al. The effects of calorie and essential amino acid supplementation on plasma proteins in patients with chronic renal failure. *Am J Clin Nutr.* 1978;31:1802–1807.

4. Ingerbleek Y, VonDen Schrieck H, DeNayer P, DeVisscher M. Albumin, transferrin, and the thyroxine-binding prealbumin/retinol-binding protein (TBPA-RBP) complex in assessment of malnutrition. *Clin Chim Acta.* 1975;63:61–67.

5. Wilms J, Batey R. Effect of iron stores on hepatic metabolism of transferrin-bound iron. *Am J Physiol.* 1983;244:G138–G144.

6. Moreb J, Poportzer M, Friedlaender M, Konigm A, et al. Evaluation of iron status in patients on chronic hemodialysis: relative usefulness of bone marrows, hemosiderin, serum ferritin, transferrin saturation, mean corpuscular volume, and red cell protoporphyrin. *Nephron.* 1983;35:196–200.

7. Alfrey A. Chronic renal failure: manifestations and pathogenesis. In: Schrier R, ed. *Renal and Electrolyte Disorders.* 3rd ed. Boston: Little Brown & Co; 1986:461.

8. Brenner BM, Meyer T, Hostetter TH. Dietary protein intake and the progressive nature of kidney disease: the role of hemodynamically mediated glomerular injury in the pathogenesis of progressive glomerular sclerosis in aging, renal ablation, and intrinsic renal disease. *N Engl J Med.* 1982;307:652–659.

9. Zakar G. Effects of dietary protein restriction on the course of early renal failure. *Proc Eur Dial Transplant Assoc Eur Ren Assoc.* 1984;21:600–603.

10. Mitch W. The influence of the diet on the progression of renal insufficiency. *Annu Rev Med.* 1984;35:249–264.

11. Barsotti G. The decline of renal function slowed by very low phosphorus intake in chronic renal patients following a low nitrogen diet. *Clin Nephrol.* 1984;21:54–59.

12. Maschio G, Oldrizzi L, Tessitore N, D'Angelo A, et al. Effects of dietary protein and phosphorus restriction on the progression of early renal failure. *Kidney Int.* 1982;22:371–376.

13. Maschio G, Oldrizzi L, Tessitore N, D'Angelo A, et al. Early dietary protein and phosphorus restriction is effective in delaying progression of chronic renal failure. *Kidney Int.* 1983;24(suppl):273–277.

14. Frohling P, Schmicker R, Kokat F, Vetter K, et al. Influence of phosphate restriction, keto-acid, and vitamin D on the progression of chronic renal failure. *Proc Eur Dial Transplant Assoc Eur Ren Assoc.* 1984;21:561–566.

15. Rosman J, ter Wee PM, Meijers S, Piers-Becht TP, et al. Prospective randomized trial of early dietary protein restriction in chronic renal failure. *Lancet.* 1984;2:1291–1296.

16. Kopple J, Monteon F, Shaib J. Effect of energy intake on nitrogen metabolism in nondialyzed patients with chronic renal failure. *Kidney Int.* 1986;29:734–742.

17. Klahr S, Levey AS, Beck GH, Caggiula AW, et al. The effects of dietary protein restriction and blood-pressure control on the progression of chronic renal disease. *N Engl J Med.* 1994;220:877–884.

18. Mitch W, Abras E, Walser M. Long-term effects of a new keto-acid: amino acid supplement in patients with chronic renal failure. *Kidney Int.* 1982;22:48–53.

19. Mitch W, Walser M, Steinman T, Hill S, et al. The effect of a keto-acid: amino acid supplement to a restricted diet on the progression of chronic renal failure. *N Engl J Med.* 1984;311:623–629.

20. Westberg G. Protein restriction in chronic renal failure. *Lancet.* 1985;3:102.

21. Oldrizzi L, Rugin C, Valvo E, Lupo A, et al. Progression of renal failure in patients with renal disease of diverse etiology on protein restricted diet. *Kidney Int.* 1985;27:553–557.

22. Schaap GH, Bilo HJG, Van der Meulen J, Oe PL, at al. Effect of changes in daily protein intake on renal function in chronic renal insufficiency: differences in reaction according to disease entity. *Nephrol.* 1993;64:207–215.

23. El Nahas AM, Masters-Thomas A, Brady S, Farrington K, et al. Selective effect of low protein diets in chronic renal diseases. *Br Med J.* 1984;289:1337–1341.

24. Holiday M. Nutritional therapy in renal disease. *Kidney Int.* 1986;30(suppl):3–6.

25. Kopple JD. Dietary requirements. In: Mossry SG, Sellers AL, eds. *Clinical Aspects of Uremia and Dialysis.* Chicago: Charles C Thomas; 1976:453.

26. Ikizler JA, Flakoll PJ, Parker RA, Hakin RM. Amino acid and albumin losses during hemodialysis. *Kidney Int.* 1994;46:830–837.

27. Blumenkrantz M, Kopple J, Moran J, Coburn JW. Metabolic balance studies and dietary protein requirements in patients undergoing continuous ambulatory peritoneal dialysis. *Kidney Int.* 1982;21:849–861.

28. Kopple J, Blumenkrantz M, Jones M, Moran J, et al. Plasma amino acid levels and amino acid losses during continuous ambulatory peritoneal dialysis. *Am J Clin Nutr.* 1982;36:395–402.

29. Kluthe R, Luttgen F, Capetianu T, Heinz V, et al. Protein requirements in maintenance hemodialysis. *Am J Clin Nutr.* 1978;31:1812–1820.

30. Thunberg B, Swamy A, Cestero R. Cross-sectional and longitudinal nutritional measurements in maintenance hemodialysis patients. *Am J Clin Nutr.* 1981;34:2005–2012.

31. Bodnar D. Rationale for nutritional requirements for patients on continuous ambulatory peritoneal dialysis. *J Am Diet Assoc.* 1982;80:247–249.

32. Stover J, ed. *A Clinical Guide to Nutrition Care in End Stage Renal Disease.* Chicago: The American Dietetic Association; 1994.

33. Kaysen G, Gambertoglio J, Jiminez I, Jones H, et al. Effect of dietary protein intake on albumin hemostasis in nephrotic patients. *Kidney Int.* 1986;29:572–577.

34. Giordano C, Madias N. Protein restriction in chronic renal failure. *Kidney Int.* 1982;22:401–408.

35. Frohlich J, Schollmeyer P, Gerok W. Carbohydrate metabolism in renal failure. *Am J Clin Nutr.* 1978;31:1541–1546.

36. Maillet C, Garber A. Skeletal muscle amino acid metabolism in chronic uremia. *Am J Clin Nutr.* 1980;33:1343–1353.

37. DeFronzo R, Alvestrand A. Glucose intolerance in uremia: site and mechanism. *Am J Clin Nutr.* 1980;33:1483–1445.

38. Oshida Y. Studies on glucose intolerance in chronic renal failure: estimation of insulin sensitivity before and after initiation of hemodialysis. *Clin Nephrol.* 1978;28:35–38.

39. Zeller K, Whittaker E, Sullivan L, Raskin P, et al. Effect of restricting dietary protein on the progression of renal failure in patients with insulin-dependent diabetes mellitus. *N Engl J Med.* 1991;324:78–84.

40. Walker JD, Bending JJ, Dodds RA, Mattock MB, et al. Restriction of dietary protein and progression of renal disease in diabetic nephropathy. *Lancet.* 1989;2:1411–1415.

41. Brouhard BH, LaGrone L. Effect of dietary protein restriction on functional renal reserve in diabetic nephropathy. *Am J Med.* 1990;89:427–431.

42. Ciavarella A, DiMizio G, Stefoni S, Borguinol L, et al. Reduced albuminuria after dietary protein restriction in insulin-dependent diabetic patients with clinical nephropathy. *Diabetes Care.* 1987;10:407–413.

43. Attman P, Bucht H, Larsson O, Uddebom G. Protein-reduced diet in diabetic renal failure. *Clin Nephrol.* 1983;19:217–220.

44. Summerson JH, Bell RA, Konen JC. Dietary protein intake, clinical proteinuria, and microalbuminuria in non-insulin-dependent diabetes mellitus. *J Renal Nutr.* 1996;6:89–93.

45. Pomerleau J, Verdy M, Garrel DR, Houde Nadeau M. Effect of protein intake on glycemic control and renal function in type 2 (non-insulin-dependent) diabetes mellitus. *Diabetologia.* 1993;36:829–834.

46. Cushner H, Adams N. Review: renal osteodistrophy: pathogenesis and treatment. *Am J Med Sci.* 1985;290:234–245.

47. DeTar SJ, Patel C, Valdin J. A practical approach to administration of intravenous calcitriol in an outpatient dialysis setting. *J Renal Nutr.* 1991;1:182–186.

48. McCann L. Protocol for the administration of intravenous calcitriol. *J Renal Nutr.* 1994;4:143–148.

49. Gokal R, Ramos J, Ellis H, Parkinson I, et al. Histological renal osteodistrophy, and 25-hydroxycholecalciferol and aluminum levels in patients on continuous ambulatory peritoneal dialysis. *Kidney Int.* 1983;23:15–21.

50. Mactier R, VanStone J, Cox A, Van Stone M, et al. Calcium carbonate is an effective phosphate binder when dialysate calcium concentration is adjusted to control hypercalcemia. *Clin Nephrol.* 1987;28:222–226.

51. Mai ML, Emmett M, Sheikh MS, Santa Ana CA, et al. Calcium acetate, an effective phosphorus binder in patients with renal failure. *Kidney Int.* 1989;36:690–695.

52. Schiller LR, Santa Ana CA, Sheikh MS, Emmett M, et al. Effect of the time of administration of calcium acetate on phosphorus binding. *N Engl J Med.* 1989;210:1110–1113.

53. Emmett M, Sirmon MD, Kirkpatrick WG, Nolan CR, et al. Calcium acetate control of serum phosphorus in hemodialysis patients. *Am J Kidney Dis.* 1991;5:544–550.

54. VanBeber AD, Peraglie C, Smith RD, Liepa GU. The effect of recombinant human erythropoietin therapy in anemia kidney patients: a nutritional emphasis. *J Renal Nutr.* 1991;2:96–104.

55. Makoff R. Water-soluble vitamin status in patients with renal disease treated with hemodialysis on peritoneal dialysis. *J Renal Nutr.* 1991;1:56–73.

56. Jahnke MG, Rock CL, Carter CM, Kelly MP, et al. Antioxidant vitamins and carotenoids in hemodialysis and peritoneal dialysis patients. *J Renal Nutr.* 1996;6:79–88.

57. Reid DJ, Barc SI, Leichter J. Effects of folate and zinc supplementation on patients undergoing chronic hemodialysis. *J Am Diet Assoc.* 1992;92:574–579.

58. Mahajan S, Praod A, Lambujon J, Abbasi AA, et al. Improvement of uremic hypogeusia by zinc: a double blind study. *Am J Clin Nutr.* 1980;33:1517–1521.

59. Burge J, Schemmel R, Park H, Greene JA. Taste acuity and zinc status in chronic renal disease. *J Am Diet Assoc.* 1984;84:1203–1209.

60. Dworkin B, Weseley S, Rosenthal W, Schwartz EM, et al. Diminished blood selenium levels in renal failure patients on dialysis: correlation with nutritional status. *Am J Med Sci.* 1987;293:6–12.

61. Sanstead H. Trace elements in uremia and hemodialysis. *Am J Clin Nutr.* 1980;33:1501–1508.

62. Rampton D, Cohen S, Crammond V, Gibbons J, et al. Treatment of chronic renal failure with dietary fiber. *Clin Nephrol.* 1984;21:159–163.

63. Bliss DZ, Stein TP, Schleifer CR, Settle RG. Supplementation with gum arabic fiber increases fecal nitrogen excretion and lowers serum urea nitrogen concentration in chronic renal failure patients consuming a low protein diet. *Am J Clin Nutr.* 1996;63:392–398.

64. Hobbs C, Murray T, Mullen J. Implications of malnutrition in chronic renal hemodialysis patients. *J Parenter Enter Nutr.* 1979;3:27. Abstract.

65. Kopple JD, Hakin RM, Held JP, Keane WE, et al. Recommendations for reducing the high morbidity and mortality of U.S. maintenance dialysis patients. *Am J Kidney Dis.* 1994;24:968–973.

66. Yang CS, Chan SW, Chaing CH, Wang M, et al. Effects of increasing dialysis dose on serum albumin and mortality in hemodialysis patients. *Am J Kidney Dis.* 1996;27:380–386.

67. Wolfson M, Jones M, Kopple J. Amino acid losses during hemodialysis with infusion of amino acids and glucose. *Kidney Int.* 1982;21:500–506.

68. Piraino A, Firpo J, Powers D. Prolonged hyperalimentation in catabolic chronic dialysis therapy patients. *J Parenter Enter Nutr.* 1981;5:463–475.

69. Capelli JP, Kushner H, Camiscioli TC, Chen SM, et al. Effect of intradialytic parenteral nutrition on mortality rates in ESRD care. *Am J Kidney Dis.* 1994;23:808–816.

70. Chertow GW, Ling J, Lew N, Lazarus JM, et al. The association of intradialytic parenteral nutrition administration with survival in hemodialysis patients. *Am J Kidney Dis.* 1994;24:912–920.

71. Burrowes JD, Lyonds TA, Kaufman AM, Levin NW. Improvement in serum albumin with adequate hemodialysis. *J Renal Nutr.* 1993;3:171–176.

72. Wolfson M, Foulks C. Intradialytic parenteral nutrition: a useful therapy? *Nutr Clin Pract.* 1996;11:5–11.

73. Bruno M, Bagnis C, Marangella M, Rovera L, et al. CAPD with an amino acid dialysis solution: a long-term cross-over study. *Kidney Int.* 1989;3:1189–1194.

74. Arfeen S, Goodship THJ, Kirkwood A, Wood MK. The nutritional/metabolic and hormonal effects of 8 weeks of continuous ambulatory peritoneal dialysis with a 1% amino acid solution. *Clin Nephrol.* 1990;4:192–199.

75. Young GA, Dibble JB, Hobson SM, Tompkins L, et al. The use of an amino-acid-based CAPD fluid over 12 weeks. *Nephrol Dial Transplant.* 1989;4:285–292.

76. Oren A, Wu G, Anderson GH, Marliss E, et al. Effective use of amino acids dialysate over four weeks in CAPD patients. *Perit Dial Bull.* 1983;2:66–73.

77. Abel R. Nutritional support in the patient with acute renal failure. *J Am Coll Nutr.* 1983;2:33–44.

78. Knochel J. Complications of total parenteral nutrition. *Kidney Int.* 1985;27:489–496.

79. Stott R, Cameron J, Ogg C, Bewick M, et al. Why the persistently high mortality in acute renal failure? *Lancet.* 1972;2:75–79.

80. Berne T, Barbour B. Acute renal failure in general surgical patients. *Arch Surg.* 1971;102:594–597.

81. Mirtallo J, Kidsk K, Ebbert M. Nutritional support of patients with renal disease. *Clin Pharm.* 1984;3:253–263.

82. Lee H. The management of acute renal failure following trauma. *Br J Anesth.* 1977;49:697–705.

83. Kopple J, Cianiciaruso B. Nutritional management of acute renal failure. In: Fischer JE, ed. *Surgical Nutrition.* Boston: Little Brown & Co; 1983:567.

84. Walser M. Nutritional support in renal failure: future directions. *Lancet.* 1983;1:340–341.

85. Mitch W, Lietman P, Walser M. Effects of oral neomycin and kananycin in chronic uremic patients, I: urea metabolism. *Kidney Int.* 1977;11:116–122.

86. Mitch W, Walser M. Effects of oral neomycin and kananycin in chronic uremic patients, II: nitrogen balance. *Kidney Int.* 1977;11:123–127.

87. Varcoe AR, Halliday D, Carson E, Richards P, et al. Anabolic role of urea in renal failure. *Am J Clin Nutr.* 1978;31:1601–1607.

88. Mitch W. Effects of intestinal flora on nitrogen metabolism in patients with chronic renal failure. *Am J Clin Nutr.* 1978;31:1594–1600.

89. Feinstein E. Total parenteral nutritional support of patients with acute renal failure. *Nutr Clin Pract.* 1988;3:3–9.

90. Giordano C, DeSanto N, Senatore R. Effects of catabolic stress in acute and chronic renal failure. *Am J Clin Nutr.* 1978;31:1561–1571.

91. Steffe W. Nutrition support in renal failure. *Surg Clin North Am.* 1981;61:661–670.

92. Spreiter S, Myers B, Swenson R. Protein-energy requirements in subjects with acute renal failure receiving intermittent hemodialysis. *Am J Clin Nutr.* 1980;33:1433–1437.

93. Teschan P. Acute renal failure versus nutrition: no free lunch in the ICU. *Transplantation.* 1983;29:764–769.

94. Druml W, Laggner A, Widdhalm K, Kleinberger G, et al. Lipid metabolism in acute renal failure. *Kidney Int.* 1983;24:S139–S142.

CHAPTER 12

Respiratory Disease and Mechanical Ventilation

Denise B. Schwartz

RESPIRATORY SYSTEM FUNCTION

It is important to understand the normal structure and function of the respiratory system prior to determining the impact of malnutrition on disease processes and the effects of various nutrient substrates on this system. The respiratory system exists for the purpose of gas exchange. The respiratory system has three subdivisions: a drive mechanism controlled by the central nervous system, a pump serviced by the respiratory muscles, and a gas-exchanging organ facilitated by the lungs.[1,2]

The drive mechanism attempts to maintain homeostasis by various feedback controls. Respiration is adjusted by the nervous system to satisfy physiologic demands. The respiratory center in the brain, which consists of the medulla oblongata and the pons, directs the contraction and relaxation of the respiratory muscles. Depth and rhythm of respiration are controlled by the Hering-Breuer reflex, which also prevents overinflation of the lungs. Response to the reflex occurs when nerve impulses are transmitted from stretch receptors in the bronchi and bronchioles to the respiratory center in the brain. Carbon dioxide, oxygen, and hydrogen ion concentrations determine the rate of respiration by acting directly on the respiratory center in the brain or on the chemoreceptors located in the carotid arteries and the aorta. These control mechanisms stabilize blood oxygen and carbon dioxide.[3]

Respiratory muscles function as a pump system. The diaphragm is the principal muscle of respiration, but abdominal muscles can act in conjunction with the diaphragm. Many factors other than neural stimuli affect respiratory muscle movement and volume displacement. These include the mechanical factors against which the respiratory muscle is working—such as resistance and compliance of the lungs and chest wall, the resting length of the muscle, speed of the contraction, the mechanical advantage of the muscle attachments on the chest wall, the cooperation of other muscles, and muscle fatigue and training.[4]

Diaphragm and intercostal muscles interact dynamically to reduce intrathoracic pressure and expand the lung. Intercostal muscles assist in pulling the rib cage outward and upward. During inspiration, the chest cavity increases in size as the ribs rise and the diaphragm lowers. During exhalation, the ribs swing down and the diaphragm returns to a relaxed position; this is predominantly a passive process.[5] Loss of both intercostal and abdominal wall muscles in quadriplegia severely decreases inspiratory efficiency, even when diaphragmatic function is intact. In the absence of diaphragmatic function, intercostal and strap muscles in the upper rib cage can be used for inspiration, but not without extensive training.[6]

The respiratory system controls the gas exchange between the atmosphere and the body. The lungs provide the surface that allows oxygen to move from the external environment into the body and the carbon dioxide produced in the tissues to exit the body. As air moves into the lungs through the nose and mouth, it is filtered, humidified, and adjusted to the body temperature. Organs involved in the gas exchange are the nose, pharynx, larynx, trachea, bronchi, secondary bronchi, bronchioles, terminal bronchioles, and alveolar sacs. The walls of the alveolar sacs, the alveoli, are covered by a capillary network of arterioles and venules. The alveoli are the functional units of the lungs responsible for the exchange of gases between air and blood.[3,6]

Three concurrent processes permit gas exchange during respiration: ventilation, diffusion, and perfusion. *Ventilation* is the movement of air between the atmosphere and the alveoli. This process is the result of the contraction and relaxation of the respiratory muscles, primarily the diaphragm, that compress and distend the lung and cause the rise or fall of pressure in the alveoli. Inspiration occurs when the pressure in the alveoli is less than atmospheric pressure. *Diffusion* is the process by which oxygen and carbon dioxide cross the alveolar capillary membrane. Oxygen, at a higher concentration in alveolar air than in blood, and carbon dioxide, at a higher concentration in blood than in alveolar air, move from their respective regions of higher concentration to regions of lower concentration. *Perfusion* is the injection of blood into an artery that supplies blood to an organ or tissue.[3]

ROLE OF MALNUTRITION IN THE RESPIRATORY DISEASE PROCESS

Adequate respiratory muscle strength and endurance are prerequisites for normal ventilation.[7] Energy utilization and visceral protein synthesis are maintained by degradation of skeletal muscle during prolonged malnutrition. Human studies indicate that diseases associated with somatic wasting cause atrophy of respiratory muscles. Prolonged diet-induced malnutrition is associated with atrophy of diaphragm muscle fibers and a decrease in muscle force output. Specifically, the dry and wet weight and muscle thickness of the diaphragm decrease in proportion to decreases in body weight. Thus, the respiratory muscles are not spared from atrophy during severe nutritional deprivation.[8]

In cachectic subjects, diaphragmatic muscle mass and thickness are reduced as measured at autopsy. In addition, maximal static inspiratory and expiratory pressures and substantial maximal voluntary ventilation are reduced in cachectic subjects, indicating a decrease in respiratory strength and endurance.[9] The adverse impact of malnutrition on muscle function may contribute to the abnormalities of lung function that are associated with emphysema. Malnutrition impairs muscle function by reducing the availability of energy substrates and by altering the structure of the muscle fiber.[7] Malnutrition is a cofactor in many diseases; however, its effects on the respiratory muscles are most pronounced in three groups of patients: those with severe burns, trauma, or infection; those on mechanical ventilation because of respiratory failure; and those with chronic obstructive pulmonary disease (COPD).[10]

Malnutrition and Respiratory Immunity

Malnourished patients are particularly vulnerable to pulmonary infection. Nutrition plays a significant role in the lung defense system in three areas: the antioxidant defense system, surfactant production, and immunologic competence. Nutritional deficiencies that may impair antioxidant protective mechanisms are lack of sulfur-containing amino acids, copper, selenium, iron, and vitamins. The damaging effect of oxygen, at least as it relates to free radical mechanisms, occurs directly through reactions with cellular lipids, proteins, and nucleic acids and indirectly through inflammatory cells that are attracted to the area of injury and have the capacity to form additional free radicals or to release proteolytic enzymes into surrounding tissue.[8]

Pulmonary surfactant function is important in maintaining alveolar stability, in reducing the work of breathing, and perhaps in protecting against fluid transudations. In malnutrition, decreased production of surfactant, a mucoprotein, leads to decreased compliance, pulmonary collapse, and pneumonia.[11] In experimental malnutrition, there is a marked initial reduction in surfactant phospholipid production within type II cells of the lung, which eventually returns to normal.[8]

Nutrition is an important factor in immunologic defenses of the lungs, and possibly other pulmonary defenses. Lung mucosa is constantly exposed to contaminants, pathogens, and sensitizing substances, which, by a variety of defense mechanisms, are prevented from entering the lung tissue or systemic sites. Malnutrition may impair local defenses and increase the incidence, severity, and duration of respiratory diseases.[8]

Low serum albumin levels lead to a decrease in colloid osmotic pressure and possible pulmonary edema. Malnutrition may reduce replication of pulmonary epithelium, resulting in laryngeal ulceration and pulmonary infection with prolonged intubation. These factors—in addition to impaired cell-mediated immunity and decreased surfactant production—contribute to decreased inspiratory force, decreased vital capacity, decreased functional residual capacity, and impaired oxygenation, necessitating increased minute ventilation (the measurement of total air inspired and expired in a minute). These conditions are detrimental to weaning from mechanical ventilation.

Incidence of Malnutrition in Patients with Respiratory Disease

There remain several unresolved issues concerning both the cause and effect of malnutrition in patients with COPD. Hypermetabolism alone does not appear to be the sole reason for weight loss in patients with COPD. Other causes of moderate hypermetabolism, such as hyperthyroidism, are not ordinarily associated with wasting, as patients are easily able to increase their intake appropriately. Inadequate food intake or inability to utilize nutrients must also be present.[8]

Hunter and associates[12] designed the first study to evaluate the nutritional status of patients with COPD. The degree of malnutrition was based on dietary intake, anthropometric measurements, biochemical analyses, and immunologic testing.[12] These investigators found that the nutrient intake of patients with COPD was comparable to or greater than the Recommended Dietary Allowance (RDA) for all of the nutrients analyzed. From these results, the researchers concluded that the nutrient requirements of patients with COPD exceed the RDA.[12] Weight loss, even to the point of cachexia, in patients with COPD was confirmed in subsequent studies.[12-16] The incidence of weight loss among patients with COPD varied between 25% and 65% of the populations studied.[15]

There are several possible reasons for weight loss and poor nutritional status in patients with COPD. A decrease in caloric intake might be the result of dyspnea while eating. Exercise intolerance could limit food procurement and preparation for individuals who must perform these tasks themselves. Gastrointestinal symptoms could be related to the high incidence of peptic ulcer disease in patients with COPD, to abdominal discomfort caused by bronchodilator drugs or corticosteroids, or to early satiety caused by flattened diaphragms or air swallowing.[15]

Another possible reason for poor nutrition is malabsorption of ingested food. The increased work of breathing might increase basal energy demands and result in lower body weights. Hormonal differences between undernourished and well-nourished patients might be partially responsible for weight differences; yet, the work of breathing is probably a major contributor to the weight loss and poor nutritional status of this patient group.[15]

Depleted triceps skinfold, midarm circumference, midarm muscle circumference, and creatinine-height index have been reported in patients with COPD,[12-14,16] and these patients appear to have deficits in subcutaneous fat stores and lean body mass. However, intact visceral proteins have been noted.[12] Driver and colleagues[13] studied the likelihood of preexisting nutritional deficits in patients with acute respiratory failure and found significant reductions in serum levels of transferrin and retinol-binding protein.

Openbrier and associates[14] compared the nutritional status of patients with emphysema and chronic bronchitis and examined the relationship between lung dysfunction and nutritional depletion in emphysematous patients. They found no evidence of nutritional depletion in patients with chronic bronchitis. In contrast, patients with emphysema had lower values for percentage of ideal body weight, arm muscle circumference, and triceps skinfold. The creatinine-height index was also lower in the emphysematous group, but the difference was not significant. There was a good correlation between somatic depletion and the degree of airflow obstruction. These results suggest that nutritional depletion contributes to lung dysfunction in emphysema.

Hunter and associates[12] found more than the standard total lymphocyte count in their patients with COPD, indicating intact cellular immunity. However, 9 of 38 subjects were anergic. Although inconclusive, these results suggest the potential for immunocompetence.

EFFECTS OF NUTRITION ON PULMONARY FUNCTION

Nutritional repletion increases respiratory muscle workload by increasing the neural ventilatory drive and the metabolic rate.[9] The interaction of nutrition and ventilatory drive seems to be a direct function of the influence of nutrition on metabolic rate. In general, conditions that reduce the metabolic rate reduce the ventilatory drive, and conditions that increase the metabolic rate increase the ventilatory drive.[2]

Starvation is associated with a decreased metabolic rate, which returns to normal with refeeding. Semistarvation in normal men over a 10-day period has been shown to decrease the metabolic rate and to diminish the ventilatory response to hypoxia and hypercapnia. With increased protein intake, patients receiving parenteral nutrition have an enhanced ventilatory response to carbon dioxide.[2] However, increasing the ventilatory drive by increasing protein intake may have therapeutic limits. Some patients receiving high-protein formulas are dyspneic with increased levels of ventilation, and carbon dioxide values may drop below normal. Patients with dyspnea have been shown to have increased neuromuscular drive. Increasing the ventilatory drive in patients with pulmonary dysfunction may lead to an unnecessary increase in respiratory effort as the patient attempts to decrease the resting level of carbon dioxide. Those with severe lung dysfunction may be particularly susceptible to an increase in workload resulting from an increase in chemosensitivity.[2]

The effect of nutrition on ventilation control is not well understood. Changes in hypoxic drive may occur very rapidly after nutrient intake. The response to malnutrition in patients with emphysema who depend on a hypoxic drive for adequate ventilation may be maladaptive in that it might predispose them to respiratory failure. It seems justifiable to conclude that the quality of food intake affects the ventilation drive, but the mechanism is unclear.[7]

IMPACT OF ENERGY SUBSTRATES ON PULMONARY FUNCTION

The major function of the respiratory system is to provide adequate oxygen to meet metabolic demands and to allow for the efficient elimination of carbon dioxide. Therefore, it is important to understand the effects of various nutrients on oxygen consumption and carbon dioxide production. To provide energy, each of the three nutrients uses a different quantity of oxygen and carbon dioxide. The volume ratio of carbon dioxide and oxygen is termed the *respiratory quotient.* The respiratory quotients of the fuels are lipid, 0.7; protein, 0.8; and carbohydrate, 1.0. Conversion of carbohydrate to fat occurs with a respiratory quotient of approximately 8.0. Obviously, the formation of fat from carbohydrate—lipogenesis—results in a large amount of carbon dioxide production in relation to the oxygen consumption. The respiratory system must be able to eliminate carbon dioxide, or respiratory failure will result.[17]

The influence of caloric intake on oxygen consumption and carbon dioxide production must be considered in determining the best nonprotein calorie source for patients with respiratory failure. Studies have demonstrated increased carbon dioxide production in patients receiving parenteral nutrition when glucose is the primary source of nonprotein calories.[18] In patients with sepsis, there is increased oxygen consumption as well. Additionally, patients who are hypermetabolic secondary to injury and infection seem to have a response to glucose that differs from the response of normal or nutritionally depleted patients. In these patients, glucose does not completely suppress lipolysis or fat oxidation, and urinary norepinephrine excretion is markedly increased. These patients have an increased clearance and oxidation of exogenous lipids. The increase in catecholamine excretion may contribute to a decrease in lung recoil pressure.[2]

The workload imposed by carbon dioxide production may precipitate respiratory distress in patients with compromised pulmonary function. Changes in carbon dioxide production and oxygen consumption induced by parenteral nutrition using either glucose as the entire source of nonprotein calories or fat emulsion as 50% of the nonprotein calories have been analyzed in patients with chronic nutritional depletion and in patients who are acutely ill secondary to injury and infection. In patients with chronic nutritional depletion, shifting from the lipid to the glucose system caused a 20% increase in carbon dioxide production that resulted in a 26% increase in minute ventilation. In acutely ill patients who received the glucose system, carbon dioxide production was significantly higher than in those who received the lipid system.[18]

Carbohydrate

The effect of carbohydrate on ventilation depends on the amount administered and the clinical condition of the patient. Carbohydrate increases respiratory work when administered in amounts that equal or exceed the daily energy expenditure. Large amounts of carbohydrate may change ventilatory chemosensitivity.[18]

The responses of patients with sepsis or injury to high glucose intake differ from the responses of nutritionally depleted patients. Depleted patients respond to glucose intake above energy requirements by synthesizing fat from carbohydrate. Gas exchange under these circumstances results in a respiratory quotient above 1.0 with a minimal rise in resting energy expenditure, which presumably reflects the low energy cost of lipogenesis. In contrast, when hypermetabolic patients are given large infusions of glucose, there is a minimal reduction in net lipolysis, an increase in norephinephrine excretion and resting energy expenditure, and continuing fat oxidation. The result is a large increase in carbon dioxide production and oxygen consumption while the total and nonprotein respiratory quotient remains below 1.0. The increased carbon dioxide production can be predicted accurately in nutritionally depleted patients by an increase in respiratory quotient; in hypermetabolic patients, the rise in respiratory quotient may not accurately reflect changes in carbon dioxide production.[18]

Fat

Fat emulsions produce less carbon dioxide than do isocaloric amounts of glucose.[18] Lipids are usually well tolerated by patients with impaired pulmonary function.[17] Abbott and associates[19] evaluated the respiratory and metabolic consequences of fat calories, provided both continuously and discontinuously, in excess of resting energy expenditure. No significant changes in respiratory mechanics, oxygen consumption, carbon dioxide production, resting energy expenditure, serum substrates, liver function, or nitrogen balance were noted when 500 kcal of lipid emulsion was added to dextrose calories sufficient to meet energy requirements. The respiratory quotient declined significantly with the 12- and 24-hour lipid infusions, but the decline persisted for the entire 24 hours only with the 24-hour infusion. The sustained, increased oxidation of lipid with a 24-hour infusion suggests that a continuous infusion of lipid is preferable to a discontinuous infusion.[19]

Glucose/Fat Systems

In a randomized, double-blind study, patients with COPD and hypercapnia were fed low-, moderate-, and high-carbohydrate diets to determine the effect on metabolic and ventilatory values. The low-carbohydrate, high-fat diet resulted in lower carbon dioxide production and respiratory quotient than did diets with higher carbohydrate and lower fat levels. This study confirms previous results in critically ill patients.[20]

Protein

Weissman and associates[21] studied eight normal subjects to determine the effect of parenteral solutions containing glucose and amino acids on respiration. Prolonged use of 5% dextrose as the sole nutrient resulted in decreases in metabolic rate and ventilatory drive. These reductions may be detrimental in patients with a primary decrease in neurogenic respiratory drive. Amino acids administered parenterally to semistarved patients in amounts commonly used in clinical practice increased metabolic rate, resting minute ventilation, and the threshold to carbon dioxide. Thus, caution should be used not only when administering large glucose loads but also when infusing amino acids to acutely ill patients. Because the administration of glucose and amino acids to patients with respiratory disease may be limited, institution of nutrition support early and in modest quantities is suggested.[21]

Protein and amino acids have been shown to alter respiratory patterns by inducing alterations in ventilatory drive. An increase in the large neutral amino acid plasma concentration may decrease the cerebral tryptophan concentration and lead to increased sensitivity to carbon dioxide. Also, the effect of protein intake on ventilatory drive appears to be dose-related.[17]

Overfeeding

Covelli and colleagues[22] noted acute respiratory failure in three patients on ventilatory support within hours after parenteral nutrition was begun. They postulated that the high carbohydrate load in the parenteral solution resulted in increases in carbon dioxide production and the respiratory quotient. Because these patients had a relatively fixed ventilatory response, hypercapnia ensued. Excessive carbohydrate loading may precipitate respiratory acidosis in patients unable to improve their alveolar ventilation adequately when compensating for increased carbon dioxide production.

In patients receiving parenteral nutrition with glucose as the primary source of calories, small increases in carbon dioxide production occur, causing the respiratory quotient to rise to 1.0 or above. There has been much speculation that respiratory distress can be precipitated by the high carbohydrate load of parenteral nutrition, presumably because of the patient's inability to increase ventilation in response to the increased carbon dioxide production. It is not yet clear whether the increased carbon dioxide production from high carbohydrate loads is clinically important in patients without preexisting respiratory failure.[23]

Heymsfield and associates[24] found that the rates at which carbon dioxide production, minute ventilation, and heat production increased with advancing energy infusion were greater for high-carbohydrate than for high-fat enteral formulas. The physiologic changes caused by continuous intragastric feeding are therefore a function of formula infusion rate and composition. Knowledge of these changes can be applied to patients treated for semistarvation who suffer respiratory or cardiac insufficiency.

Enteral Feeding

A study in three hospitals of similar size in different regions of the country reported that patients with diseases of the respiratory system were more often fed enterally instead of parenterally.[25] Therefore, evaluating the specific effects of enteral feeding on pulmonary function is highly desirable. The respiratory effects of enteral feeding relate to an increase in formula-induced tissue oxygen demands and carbon dioxide production. Two groups of patients deserve special emphasis: patients with chronic lung disease and weight loss and patients maintained on mechanical ventilation.

Patients with chronic lung disease and weight loss suffer pulmonary cachexia. As in cardiac cachexia, the diminishing oxygen reserve is paralleled by a fall in lean tissue mass. This semistarvation state, combined with a reduction in metabolically active tissue, tends to lower the workload of the failing organ and other involved systems. Counterbalancing these effects of underfeeding are such factors as the increased work of breathing and elevated cardiac demands secondary to pulmonary hypertension. Hence, a symmetry exists between weight loss and organ failure. Nutritional repletion can disrupt this balance, worsening organ failure.[26]

The key consideration is limitation of the increase in carbon dioxide production related to fuel infusion. This is accomplished by supplying a conservative energy infusion rate and avoiding formulas that can produce more carbon dioxide when metabolized. Sodium and fluids are minimized, since patients with lung disease often suffer cardiac or renal insufficiency.[26]

For patients maintained on mechanical ventilation, substrate tolerance is extremely important. The most critical phase in managing these patients is the weaning period. Overfeeding an elemental formula, which can result in more carbon dioxide production because of its low fat content, is a recognized cause of worsening hypercapnia and metabolic acidosis. Cautious infusion of energy and associated carbohydrate is recommended during this period. During the period of active respiratory support, adjustment in mechanical ventilation can compensate for formula-induced effects on gas exchange.[26]

A large carbohydrate-induced increase in carbon dioxide production, whether delivered enterally or parenterally, is most likely to affect patients with weak inspiratory muscles and an increased breathing workload, but it can also affect patients already on mechanical ventilators if the ventilator rate and tidal volume are not adjusted to compensate for the increased ventilatory requirement. An important criterion for the clinical value of nutritional repletion is whether it can strengthen the respiratory muscles to the point where ventilator-dependent patients can resume spontaneous breathing. Studies suggest that successful weaning from mechanical ventilation can be facilitated by appropriate nutrition support.[9]

Hunker and colleagues[27] studied patients over a 24-hour period for oxygen uptake, carbon dioxide production, respiratory quotient, and urinary urea nitrogen. Indirect calorimetry measurements were compared with the calories administered. The parenterally alimented group had a mean respiratory quotient of 1.23, which was significantly greater than the nonalimented group, whose respiratory quotient was 0.88. The increased carbon dioxide noted in the parenterally alimented group may have been secondary to a high carbohydrate intake with fat synthesis. Patients in this study received an average of 2.6 times the measured energy expenditure, which would explain the higher respiratory quotients obtained.

The provision of adequate nutrition support to ventilator-dependent patients, although important, is still overlooked in many hospitals. In a retrospective review, Bassili and Deitel[11] found that 54% of 33 nonfed patients were weaned from the ventilator, compared with 93% of nutritionally supported patients. Larca and Greenbaum[28] conducted a retrospective evaluation of 14 viable ventilator-dependent patients; these investigators found that ventilator-dependent patients who responded to nutrition support with an increase in protein synthesis were more likely to be weaned from mechanical ventilation than those who did not.

Herve and associates[29] studied gas-exchange and blood gas values in six patients with chronic respiratory failure who were ventilated at low and high minute ventilation during three randomized nutrition regimens. The risk of parenteral alimentation-induced carbon dioxide retention was lower if minute ventilation was increased before parenteral nutrition was begun. However, this precaution may be difficult to institute because the resultant increase in carbon dioxide depends not only on the amount and source of nutrients but also on the type of stress, pulmonary function, and cardiovascular status.

The respiratory muscles of critically ill patients are subject to a host of adverse factors, including hypoxemia, hypercapnia, electrolyte imbalance, fever, and other nonnutritional catabolic consequences of infection, trauma, and disuse. Current intensive care regimens are directed at correcting the underlying disturbances. Nonetheless, it is difficult to separate the effects of nutritional repletion from those of respiratory muscle rest, pharmacologic intervention such as administration of aminophylline (which enhances respiratory muscle contractility), and inspiratory muscle training.[7]

RECOMMENDATIONS FOR NUTRITION SUPPORT

The overall aim of nutritional intervention in patients with chronic lung disease is to maintain or improve pulmonary function. The objectives will vary, however, according to the underlying metabolic and nutritional status of each patient. Ideally, nutritional status should be maintained in adequately nourished patients and improved in nutritionally depleted patients.[23]

Guidelines for standards of care for patients with acute respiratory failure on mechanical ventilatory support were developed by the Task Force on Guidelines of the Society of Critical Care Medicine. These guidelines state that "nutritional support (enteral and parenteral) shall be utilized at intervals to be determined by individual circumstances."[30] The American Association for Respiratory Care developed clinical practice guidelines for metabolic measurement using indirect calorimetry during mechanical ventilation. These guidelines indicate specific objectives of metabolic measurements by indirect calorimetry, limitations of the procedure, assessment of test quality and outcome, and additional data.[31]

An aggressive nutrition support regimen should improve respiratory muscle function. However, it may also increase metabolic demand, thereby increasing the respiratory workload and ultimately causing clinical deterioration. The goal in designing a nutrition regimen for patients with lung disease is to provide a diet that will minimize metabolic demands while maximizing functional improvements.[32] While ventilatory support may not necessarily determine the need for nutrition, it may, on occasion, alter the amounts and types of nutrients needed.[33]

Nutritional supplementation has been recommended for patients with uncomplicated acute respiratory failure and previously normal pulmonary status when mechanical ventilation has been used for 72 hours. Nutritional supplementation should be started earlier if acute respiratory failure is accompanied by severe trauma, multisystem organ failure, sepsis, or previous malnutrition. Early nutritional supplementation is recommended in most patients with COPD, because many are malnourished and reversal of respiratory muscle fatigue may play a significant role in successfully weaning them from mechanical ventilation.[33]

Refeeding patients with COPD must be done as a preventive measure at the start of weight loss. Patients with long-term weight loss and end-stage COPD appear unable to tolerate any increase in metabolic demand; consequently, respiratory and skeletal muscle function cannot be improved by refeeding.[32]

Patients should be fed according to their metabolic needs. Acutely ill patients who are not depleted benefit from an intake that approaches caloric and nitrogen equilibrium. Efforts to achieve a positive caloric and nitrogen balance should be reserved until the objective is to rebuild tissue. The metabolic rate should be measured whenever possible. Sedation, controlled ventilation, and muscle relaxants may depress the metabolic rate, whereas sepsis and stressful procedures may increase it.[17]

When the intent is maintenance of lean body mass, nutrition support should be designed to attain caloric and nitrogen equilibrium. This requires an energy intake of 1 to 1.2 times the energy expenditure and a minimum protein intake of 1.0 g/kg of body weight. For restoration of lean body tissue, the nutrition regimen should be designed to achieve a positive caloric and nitrogen balance. Minimum energy intake should be 1.4 times the energy expenditure, and the protein intake should be 1.5 g/kg of body weight. Additional increases in protein should be determined by measuring nitrogen balance. Ideally, caloric requirements should be determined by measuring resting energy expenditure. If these measurements are not available routinely, caloric requirements can be estimated at 25 kcal/kg of body weight for maintenance therapy and 35 kcal/kg of body weight for repletion therapy.[34,35] However, when patients are critically ill and especially during attempts at weaning from the ventilator, the goal would be to aliment, meeting nutrient requirements, but avoid excessive substrates.

Significantly higher energy expenditures are found in mechanically ventilated patients than in spontaneously breathing patients. The Ireton-Jones formula for ventilator-dependent patients correlated better predicted calorie than most formulas in a study of mechanically ventilated, obese patients. The Ireton-Jones formula for ventilator dependent patients is: VEE = 1784 − 11(A) + 5(ABW) + 241(S) + 239(T) + 804(B) where A is age (years), ABW is actual body weight (kg), S is sex (male = 1, female = 0), T is trauma (present = 1, absent = 0), B is burn (present = 1, absent = 0).[36] For patients with Swan-Ganz catheters, the reverse Fick equation can be used to determine oxygen consumption and therefore caloric expenditure. The original equation has been modified for patients with pulmonary disease as follows[37]:

$$\textbf{REE} = CO \times Hgb \times (SaO_2 - SmvO_2) \times 105$$

Where:
CO = cardiac output from Swan-Ganz in liters per minute
Hgb = hemoglobin in grams per 100 mL
SaO_2 = arterial oxygen saturation expressed as percent
SmvO_2 = mixed venous oxygen saturation expressed as percent

Amino acids increase oxygen consumption, minute ventilation, and the response to both hypoxia and hypercapnia. Therefore, high amino acid intakes in patients with marginal respiratory function may result in breathlessness.[17]

The nature of the energy source in respiratory disease remains the subject of continued debate. Formulations high in fat and low in carbohydrate have been developed for enteral tube feeding or oral supplementation. In one study, patients with emphysema and severe airflow obstruction had no adverse effects from diets containing 50% carbohydrate.[23]

Carbohydrate given in hypocaloric amounts decreases metabolic rate, minute ventilation, and response to hypoxia. Hypercaloric amounts result in increased carbon dioxide production, minute ventilation, and response to hypoxia. Substituting lipid for some carbohydrate reduces carbon dioxide production. Patients receiving lipid emulsion, specifically neonates and patients with adult respiratory distress syndrome, should be observed regularly for decreased arterial oxygenation of hyperlipidemia.[17]

The nitrogen-sparing effects of glucose, lipid, or glucose plus lipid parenteral nutrition mixtures appear similar. However, it seems appropriate to avoid the extremes of either 100% glucose or 100% fat as the calorie source. A wide range of fuel mixtures can maintain protein balance.[23]

Fluid intake must be controlled carefully to avoid unsuspected fluid loading, as patients on mechanical ventilation have an increased tendency to retain fluid.[17] Nutritional status and its effect on body fluid compartments and serum protein levels also appear to affect lung water homeostasis and the development of respiratory failure.[38]

Hypophosphatemia impairs the contractile properties of the diaphragm during acute respiratory failure.[39] Supplements are given as necessary to maintain normal serum inorganic phosphate levels in such patients.

There is a great deal of interest in the role of nutrition support in weaning patients from mechanical ventilation. The optimal conditions for the patient who is to be weaned from mechanical ventilation include absence of fluid loading, adequate respiratory drive, a normal acid-base balance, and carbohydrate intake appropriate to minimizing carbon dioxide production.[17]

Many investigators have attempted to identify weaning predictors and weaning models for use in long-term (exceeding 3 days) mechanically ventilated patients, but there is limited consensus on the exact parameters. Preliminary survey results of the members of the American Thoracic Society revealed that some practices of mechanical ventilation are changing and the underlying beliefs are being reexamined. The process of weaning needs to be viewed as a dynamic continuum. It is difficult to define a specific time frame because patients tolerate weaning differently. Care delivery systems that focus on systemic, comprehensive, and coordinated care are promising because outcome studies demonstrate that these systems decrease ventilator time, length of stay, and costs. Recently, approaches to weaning have been reported that include computer-assisted weaning plans; the use of collaborative, interdisciplinary weaning teams to increase timely communication and promote a comprehensive approach; and special care units that use protocols and critical pathways focused on standardized, consistent, and progressive planning.[40-44]

Specific guidelines for nutrition during weaning and extubation have not been identified. The initial goal is to provide optimal nutrition therapy to the mechanically ventilated patient to prevent malnutrition from contributing to weaning failure. However, clinicians may tend to overfeed malnourished patients during the weaning and extubation phases. This practice could be more detrimental than underfeeding for a short period of 1 to 2 days for some patients, such as those who retain carbon dioxide. For nasogastrically alimented patients, holding feeding for 4 to 6 hours prior to extubation is appropriate to avoid aspiration.[45]

In the immediate postweaning phase, the objective is to maintain nutritional needs. Aggressive feeding is suspended during this period to avoid increasing the respiratory workload through high caloric intake. At the same time, semi-starvation should be avoided because acute deprivation may also precipitate respiratory distress. During this phase, patients are usually able to eat, but appetite may be poor and sufficient intake may be difficult because of dysphagia from prior intubation. Oral intake should be monitored for several days to ensure adequacy. Supplemental feedings may be necessary. The postweaning phase is also the time to begin patient and family education. The educational program should focus on the relation between nutrition and pulmonary function; the importance of a balanced diet; ways to increase caloric intake; and management of dyspnea, fatigue, and early satiety.[46]

REFERENCES

1. Alspach JG, Williams SM. *Core Curriculum for Critical Care Nursing.* 3rd ed. Philadelphia: WB Saunders Co; 1985:2–97.

2. Askanazi J, Weissman C, Rosenbaum AH, et al. Nutrition and the respiratory system. *Crit Care Med.* 1982;10:163–172.

3. Nurse's Reference Library. *Diagnostics.* 2nd ed. Springhouse, PA: Springhouse Corp; 1986:627–667.

4. Whitelow WA. The respiratory pump. In: Guenter C, ed. *Pulmonary Medicine.* 2nd ed. Philadelphia: JB Lippincott Co; 1982:42–189.

5. Katch FI, McArdle WD. *Nutrition, Weight Control, and Exercise.* Philadelphia: Lea & Febiger; 1988:74–81.

6. Cerra FB. *Manual of Critical Care.* St. Louis, MO: CV Mosby Co; 1987:34–73, 341–358.

7. Rogers RM, Dauber JH, Sanders MH, et al. Nutrition and COPD: state-of-the-art minireview. *Chest.* 1984;85(suppl):63–66.

8. Edelman NH, Rucker RB, Peavy HH. NIH workshop summary, nutrition and the respiratory system: chronic obstructive pulmonary disease. *Am Rev Respir Dis.* 1986;134:347–352.

9. Rochester DF. Malnutrition and the respiratory muscles. *Clin Chest Med.* 1986;7:91–99.

10. Lewis MI, Sieck GC, Fournier M, Belman MJ, et al. Effect of nutritional deprivation on diaphragm contractility and muscle fiber size. *J Appl Physiol.* 1986;60:596–603.

11. Bassili HR, Deitel M. Effect of nutritional support on weaning patients off mechanical ventilators. *J Parenter Enter Nutr.* 1981;5:161–163.

12. Hunter AMB, Carey MA, Larsh HW. The nutritional status of patients with chronic obstructive pulmonary disease. *Am Rev Respir Dis.* 1981;124:376–381.

13. Driver AG, McAlvery MT, Smith JL. Nutritional assessment of patients with chronic obstructive pulmonary disease and acute respiratory failure. *Chest.* 1982;82:568–571.

14. Openbrier DR, Irwin MM, Rogers RM, Gottlieb GP, et al. Nutritional status and lung function in patients with emphysema and chronic bronchitis. *Chest.* 1983;83:17–22.

15. Brown SE, Light RW. When COPD patients are malnourished. *J Respir Dis.* 1983;4:36–50.

16. Braun SR, Keim NL, Dixon RM, et al. The prevalence and determinants of nutritional changes in chronic obstructive pulmonary disease. *Chest.* 1984;86:558–563.

17. Kinney JM, Weissman C, Askanazi J. Influences of nutrients on ventilation. *Rev Clin Nutr.* 1984;54:917–929.

18. Askanazi J, Nordenstrom J, Rosenbaum SH, Elwyn DH, et al. Nutrition for the patients with respiratory failure: glucose vs. fat. *Anesthesiology.* 1981;54:373–377.

19. Abbott WC, Grakauskas AM, Bistrian BR, Rose R, et al. Metabolic and respiratory effects of continuous and discontinuous lipid infusions. *Arch Surg.* 1984;119:1367–1371.

20. Angelillo VA, Bedi S, Durfee D, Dahl J, et al. Effects of low and high carbohydrate feedings in ambulatory patients with chronic obstructive pulmonary disease and chronic hypercapnia. *Ann Intern Med.* 1985;103:883–885.

21. Weissman C, Askanazi J, Rosenbaum S, et al. Amino acids and respiration. *Ann Intern Med.* 1983;98:41–44.

22. Covelli HD, Black JW, Olsen MS, Beekman JF, et al. Respiratory failure precipitated by high carbohydrate loads. *Ann Intern Med.* 1981;95:579–581.

23. Wilson DO, Rogers RM, Hoffman RM. State of the art nutrition and chronic lung disease. *Am Rev Respir Dis.* 1985;132:1347–1365.

24. Heymsfield SB, Head CA, McManus CB, Seitz S, et al. Respiratory, cardiovascular, and metabolic effects of enteral hyperalimentation: influence of formula dose and composition. *Am J Clin Nutr.* 1984;40:116–130.

25. *St. Joseph Medical Center Nutritional Support: Cost and Quality Analysis.* Colley R, Stamus C, eds. Deerfield, IL: Clintec Nutrition Co; 1987.

26. Heymsfield SB, Erbland M, Casper K, Grossman G, et al. Enteral nutritional support, metabolic, cardiovascular, and pulmonary interrelations. *Clin Chest Med.* 1986;7:41–67.

27. Hunker FD, Bruton CW, Hunker EM, Durham RM, et al. Metabolic and nutritional evaluation of patients supported with mechanical ventilation. *Crit Care Med.* 1980;8:628–632.

28. Larca L, Greenbaum D. Effectiveness of intensive nutritional regimens in patients who fail to wean from mechanical ventilation. *Crit Care Med.* 1982;10:297–300.

29. Herve P, Simonneau G, Girard P, Cerrina J, et al. Hypercapnic acidosis induced in mechanically ventilated patients: glucose vs fat. *Crit Care Med.* 1985;13:537–540.

30. Task Force on Guidelines, Society of Critical Care Medicine. Guidelines for standards of care for patients with acute respiratory failure on mechanical ventilatory support. *Crit Care Med.* 1991;19:275–278.

31. American Association for Respiratory Care clinical practice guidelines: metabolic measurement using indirect calorimetry during mechanical ventilation. *Respir Care.* 1994;39:1169–1175.

32. Goldstein SA, Thomashow B, Askanazi J. Functional changes during nutritional repletion in patients with lung disease. *Clin Chest Med.* 1986;7:141–151.

33. Norwood SH, Andrassy RJ. Nutritional support in patients requiring mechanical ventilation. *Contemp Surg.* 1986;29:45–52.

34. Bell LP, Shronts EP. Nutritional support in respiratory failure. In: Lang CE, ed. *Nutritional Support in Clinical Care*. Rockville, MD: Aspen Publishers Inc; 1987:329–343.

35. Schwartz DB. Pulmonary failure. In: Matarese L, Gottschlich M, Shronts E, eds. *Nutrition Support Dietetics Core Curriculum*. Springfield, MD: A.S.P.E.N.; 1993:251–260.

36. Amato P, Keating KP, Quercia RA, Karbonic J. Formulaic methods of estimating calorie requirements in mechanically ventilated obese patients: a reappraisal. *Nutr Clin Pract*. 1995;10:229–232.

37. Grant JP. Nutrition care of patients with acute and chronic respiratory failure. *Nutr Clin Pract*. 1994;9:11–17.

38. Starker PM, Gump FE. Nutrition and lung water. *Clin Chest Med*. 1986;7:127–130.

39. Aubier M, Murciano D, Lecocguic Y, Vires N, et al. Effects of hypophosphatemia on diaphragmatic contractility in patients with acute respiratory failure. *N Engl J Med*. 1985;313:420–424.

40. Burns SM, Clochesy JM, Goodnough Hanneman SK, Ingersoll GE, et al. Weaning from long-term mechanical ventilation. *Am J Crit Care*. 1995;4:4–22.

41. Carmichael LC, Wheeler AP. Current practices in mechanical ventilation for ARDS. *Contemp Intern Med*. 1996;8:53–65.

42. Trego B. Care of long-term ventilator patients. *TCM*. October-November-December 1995;6(5): 77–82.

43. Ideno KT, Sabau D, Randall C. Managing respiratory patients' nutritional outcomes. *J Respir Care Pract*. April-May 1995;111–118.

44. Pierson DJ. Nonrespiratory aspects of weaning from mechanical ventilation. *Respir Care*. 1995;40:263–270.

45. Sharar SR. Weaning and extubation are not the same thing. *Respir Care*. 1995;40:230–243.

46. Irwin MM, Openbrier DR. A delicate balance: strategies for feeding ventilated COPD patients. *Am J Nurs*. 1985;85:274–280.

CHAPTER 13

Bone Marrow Transplantation

Paula M. Charuhas

INTRODUCTION

Bone marrow transplantation (BMT) is a recognized therapeutic modality for the treatment of malignant and nonmalignant disorders of the bone marrow.[1,2] Malignant diseases such as acute leukemia, chronic myelogenous leukemia, and lymphoma have been treated successfully with marrow transplantation.[3] Aplastic anemia, thalassemia major, and immunologic deficiency diseases are other conditions amenable to transplantation.[3] The objective is to replace the malignant or defective marrow to restore hematopoietic and immunologic function.

Preparation for BMT consists of a myeloablative conditioning regimen, which includes cytotoxic chemotherapy with or without total body irradiation (TBI), directed at eradicating the malignancy or defective stem cells, and providing immunosuppression. An infusion of autologous (patient receives own marrow), syngeneic (patient receives marrow from an identical twin), or allogeneic (marrow is from a human leukocyte antigen compatible related or unrelated donor) marrow follows.[3]

Because the transplant recipient is devoid of functioning marrow for 2 to 3 weeks following the marrow infusion, neutropenia and thrombocytopenia ensue. Transfusions of platelets, erythrocytes, and growth factors are often required to prevent hemorrhage and infection. Most patients receive some form of infection prophylaxis, which routinely includes antibiotic therapy and may also include ultraisolation in laminar air flow rooms and low-microbial diets. Indication of marrow engraftment is reflected by rising granulocyte and platelet counts.

The number of transplants performed over the last two decades has increased significantly.[1] This is due, in part, to the increased availability of unrelated donors through the National Donor Marrow Program.[4] Moreover, hematopoietic peripheral blood stem cell transplants are being used with increased frequency.[5] Finally, successful transplants using human umbilical cord blood have also been reported and have the potential to make transplantation available to an even larger number of individuals.[6]

Although BMT represents a potentially curative therapy for patients with hematologic disorders, life-threatening complications, high morbidity, and long-term health problems often ensue. The histologic effects of high-dose cytotoxic and immunosuppressive medications in addition to supralethal TBI may result in gastrointestinal damage with multiple nutritional complications.[7] Infections, major organ toxicities, and graft-versus-host disease (GVHD) are also common and further impact the patient's nutritional status.

This chapter addresses the nutritional implications associated with marrow transplantation. Guidelines for nutrition management of transplant-related complications and nutrition support practices are also discussed.

NUTRITION ASSESSMENT

The nutritional assessment should begin before the transplant and continue throughout the transplant course to ensure optimum nutrition support.[8] The nutritional assessment for marrow transplant patients is essentially the same as for other patients as described in Chapter 1. However, some components of the assessment for transplant patients should be highlighted.

The nutrition history should include a thorough evaluation of current oral and gastrointestinal symptoms and recent weight changes. This information will help to identify those patients in need of aggressive nutritional intervention. Routine anthropometric measurements (including height, weight, and in some patient populations skinfold measurements) should be obtained before the transplant and provide landmark data for serial measurements.[9] From this information, the ideal body weight, adjusted ideal body weight for obese patients, and body surface area—which are used in calculating medication dosages—can be determined.[9]

Baseline laboratory values are recommended and provide objective information regarding fluid and electrolyte balance, renal and hepatic function, and visceral protein status. Hematologic indices, such as hemoglobin, hematocrit, and total lymphocyte count, are readily affected by hematologic disorders and prior therapy; therefore, they are not valid parameters for assessment of this population.

NUTRIENT REQUIREMENTS

Energy

Energy requirements are increased in the first 30 to 50 days posttransplant to account for the physiologic stress induced by the conditioning regimen, fever, sepsis, acute GVHD, and other metabolic complications.[10] An early study by Szeluga et al[11] estimated calorie needs by predictive equations based on nitrogen balance at 37 to 42 kcal/kg/day and as high as 45 to 50 kcal/kg/day in adults with acute GVHD. A more recent study by Geibig and associates,[12] using indirect calorimetry in a small group of allogeneic and syngeneic transplant patients, suggested a much lower requirement of 30 to 35 kcal/kg/day, which is more consistent with current practice.

The Harris-Benedict equation[13] for basal energy expenditure (BEE) and the basal metabolic rate (BMR) table,[14] which is appropriate for children ≤45 kg, are other tools used to estimate energy requirements. Energy needs during the early postgrafting period are estimated at BEE × 1.5 for adults and BEE or BMR × 1.6 for children, to provide additional nutrition support for growth.[10] Energy needs may be further increased if metabolic complications persist; however, requirements should generally be no more than a maximum of BEE × 1.7 for adults and BEE or BMR × 1.8 for children.[10] Energy needs are adjusted downward for patients with evidence of hematologic engraftment without metabolic complications to BEE × 1.3 for adults and BEE or BMR × 1.4 for children.[10] However, basal needs may need to be adjusted higher in patients with increased activity, when weight loss has occurred, in patients with increased metabolic complications, or in patients who require nutritional repletion.[10]

Protein

Protein needs are increased during marrow transplantation to provide substrate for tissue repair after cytoreductive therapy, for maintenance of nitrogen balance, and for synthesis of lean body mass.[8] Protein needs are estimated at 1.5 g/kg ideal body weight for adults and twice the Recommended Dietary Allowance (range 1.8 to 3.0 g/kg ideal body weight) for children.[10,15] During catabolic corticosteroid therapy, protein needs may be further increased to spare muscle breakdown. Protein intake may be modified if hepatic, renal, or neurological function is altered.[9]

Fat

Intravenous lipids are provided to supply a concentrated source of calories and essential fatty acids. Although lipids can influence host immunity, they have not been shown to increase the incidence of infections in marrow transplant recipients who are at high risk for bacterial and fungal infections.[16] Clemans et al[17] reported essential fatty acid deficiency within 21 days of transplantation in marrow graft recipients maintained on fat-free parenteral nutrition. Another study by the same investigators suggested that an amount of 250 mL/day of 10% lipid emulsion was insufficient to prevent this deficiency.[18] The optimal amount of lipid calories for marrow transplant patients is unknown. A minimum of 4% to 8% of total energy should be provided as lipids to prevent essential fatty acid deficiency.[19] The maximum amount of lipid provided should be no greater than 60% of total energy intake.[8] For pediatric patients, the maximum lipid dosage is 4 gm/kg/day.[20]

Prior to instituting intravenous lipids, a baseline fasting triglyceride level should be obtained. Elevated baseline levels have been observed in patients treated with high-dose corticosteroids and may necessitate a lower lipid dose.

Fluid

Fluid requirements are highly individualized and depend upon the patient's clinical status. Suggested guidelines are provided in Exhibit 13–1.[10] Fever, gastrointestinal losses, high-output renal failure, and nephrotoxic medications increase fluid needs.[21] During cytoreductive therapy, hydration needs are increased by 1.5 to 2 times the maintenance requirements when nephrotoxic agents such as cyclophosphamide are used. Conditions such as oliguria, hepatorenal failure, or volume overload often require fluid restriction.[21]

Vitamins

Parenteral vitamin recommendations for marrow graft recipients are based on guidelines provided by the Nutrition Advisory Group of the American Medical Association.[22] Additional vitamin C (500 mg/day for patients ≥31 kg and 250 mg/day for patients <31 kg) is provided to promote tissue recovery via collagen bio-

---

Exhibit 13–1 Fluid Guidelines

<10 kg:
100 mL/kg/24 hr

11–20 kg:
1000 mL (plus 50 mL/kg for each kg > 10 kg)/24 hr

21–40 kg:
1500 mL (plus 20 mL for each kg > 20 kg)/24 hr

>40 kg:
1500 mL/m^2/24 hr

Source: Data from J.A. Kerner, *Manual of Pediatric Nutrition,* © 1983, John Wiley & Sons, Inc.

synthesis following cytoreductive therapy.[23] Vitamin K is not included in current adult multiple vitamin preparations and is provided at weekly doses of 10 mg (5 mg for patients <11 kg) and infused separately from other vitamins to avoid incompatible interactions. Vitamin K deficiency has been reported in a marrow transplant patient receiving parenteral nutrition.[24] Because thiamin deficiency in association with lactic acidosis has been observed in a child following BMT for acute leukemia, thiamine should be routinely supplemented.[25] Decreased plasma vitamin E and beta-carotene levels have also been reported in marrow transplant patients.[26] Further research is needed to determine specific vitamin requirements for marrow transplant patients. Oral multivitamin supplementation is recommended for all patients following discontinuation of parenteral nutrition for 1 year following transplant.

Trace Minerals

Trace mineral requirements during marrow transplantation have been sparsely studied. Suggested recommendations are presented in Table 13–1.[27] Zinc losses may be increased in patients with diarrhea and may contribute to negative nitrogen balance and immune dysfunction. Additional zinc should be provided at a suggested replacement dose of 17 mg/L stool output.[27] Copper and manganese, trace minerals excreted in bile, should be removed from parenteral nutrition solutions if obstructive biliary disease develops. Manganese toxicity has been reported in a marrow transplant recipient with hyperbilirubinemia and cholestasis.[28] Fredstrom and colleagues[28] suggest the need to reevaluate routine manganese supplementation in marrow transplant patients as manganese toxicity may be unrecognized. Because hemosiderosis may develop due to frequent blood product administration, iron supplementation for marrow transplant patients is not recommended.

Table 13–1 Parenteral Trace Mineral Recommendations

Mineral	Adult Dose	Pediatric Dose
Zinc	2.5–4.0 mg/day	100 µg/kg
Copper	0.5–1.5 mg/day	20 µg/kg
Chromium	10–15 µg/day	0.14–0.2 µg/kg
Manganese	0.15–0.8 mg/day	2–10 µg/kg

Source: Adapted with permission from B.A. Cunningham, Parenteral Management, in *Nutritional Assessment and Management During Marrow Transplantation: A Resource Manual,* P. Lenssen and S.N. Aker, eds., pp. 45–61, © 1985, Fred Hutchinson Cancer Research Center.

Electrolytes

Electrolyte requirements vary widely among individuals. Exhibit 13–2 outlines suggested initial parenteral nutrition electrolyte recommendations.[23] Magnesium wasting is frequently observed in marrow transplant patients treated with cyclosporine and FK-506, necessitating increased magnesium supplementation.[29,30] Hypokalemia occurs with potassium-wasting diuretics, corticosteroids, and amphotericin and is also associated with gastrointestinal losses.[31] Potassium-sparing diuretics and renal insufficiency often induce hyperkalemia.[31] Close monitoring of serum electrolyte levels is recommended to enable adjustments in parenteral dosing. Daily alterations in parenteral nutrition electrolyte additives are frequently necessary.

NUTRITION SUPPORT

Following the nutritional assessment and estimation of nutrient requirements, nutrition support can be instituted. The goals of nutrition support in hypermetabolic marrow transplant patients are to maintain or improve nutritional status and to provide the nutrients necessary for the recovery of the hematopoietic and immune systems.[32]

Parenteral Nutrition

Because of the adverse oral and gastrointestinal manifestations associated with intense cytoreductive therapy, parenteral nutrition is often included as standard supportive care. At many transplant centers, parenteral nutrition is instituted in the conditioning phase or when the patient is unable to consume adequate calories to

---

Exhibit 13–2 Suggested Initial Parenteral Nutrition Electrolyte Recommendations*

Calcium gluconate	8 mEq
Magnesium sulfate	16 mEq
Potassium chloride	25 mEq
Potassium phosphate	15 mEq
Sodium chloride	30 mEq

*Standard electrolyte additives per liter of parenteral nutrition solution.

Source: Adapted with permission from B.A. Cunningham, Parenteral Management, in *Nutritional Assessment and Management During Marrow Transplantation: A Resource Manual,* P. Lenssen and S.N. Aker, eds., pp. 45–61, © 1985, Fred Hutchinson Cancer Research Center.

maintain weight. Monitoring the patient's tolerance to parenteral nutrition, as described in Chapter 21, is essential throughout the transplant course to prevent metabolic complications. Carbohydrate, in the form of dextrose, typically comprises 50% to 60% of total calories; however, administration must be individualized. Patients treated with corticosteroids should be closely monitored for hyperglycemia and may require insulin additive or a lower concentration of dextrose to maintain euglycemia.

Protein, in the form of crystalline amino acids, comprises about 15% to 20% of total calories. Specialized pediatric solutions have been developed and provide an amino acid profile similar to breast milk.[33] These formulas typically contain increased concentrations of histidine, taurine, and tyrosine, and may be used in marrow transplant patients up to 2 years of age.

The use of modified amino acid parenteral nutrition formulas during BMT has been reported. Recent studies suggest glutamine is a conditionally essential amino acid in the tumor-bearing state.[34] Ziegler and coworkers[35] reported improved nitrogen balance, reduced infectious complications, and decreased hospitalization in marrow transplant patients supplemented with glutamine-enriched parenteral nutrition formulas. Although glutamine-supplemented nutrition support may be beneficial to marrow transplant recipients, larger, controlled clinical trials are needed before specific recommendations can be made.

Formulas enriched with branched-chain amino acid have also been explored in marrow graft recipients. Branched-chain amino acid therapy has been shown to improve nitrogen balance during surgery and trauma,[36] but this has not been demonstrated in the marrow transplant population.[37]

Clinical benefits of parenteral nutrition during marrow transplantation are well documented. Weisdorf and associates[38] found that marrow transplant recipients supported with parenteral nutrition prophylactically engrafted more rapidly than those not given parenteral nutrition. Improved visceral protein status[39] and maintenance of body weight[40] have been observed in pediatric transplant patients maintained on parenteral nutrition. Another study by Weisdorf et al[41] demonstrated improved outcome in a prospective clinical trial of well-nourished marrow transplant patients randomized to receive parenteral nutrition or 5% dextrose during cytoreductive therapy. Allogeneic patients who received prophylactic parenteral nutrition had a longer estimated 2-year survival as well as a longer time to disease relapse.[41] Improved disease-free survival was not demonstrated in the autologous patients in this study.[41]

Enteral Nutrition

Enteral alimentation provided during the acute phases of many critical illnesses has been shown to decrease infection rates in critically ill patients who are fed early.[42] The theory is that intraluminal fuels, such as enteral feedings, help to maintain integrity of intestinal mucosa and prevent translocation of gut bacteria.[43] Because the pathogenesis of GVHD may be due, in part, to bacteria gaining entry to the blood through a compromised intestinal barrier,[44] maintenance of gastrointestinal mucosa with enteral nutrition may have significant importance. Other advantages of enteral feedings include convenience, safety, and lower cost than parenteral feedings.[33]

Despite these benefits, enteral feedings have been used infrequently in the marrow transplant population. Gastrointestinal dysfunction associated with regimen-related toxicities, thrombocytopenia, and neutropenia have precluded this method of nutrition support early in the transplant course. Two studies, however, have reported the combined use of enteral feedings with parenteral nutrition to take advantage of the mucosal-preserving aspects of enteral alimentation and the more physiological nutrition support of parenteral alimentation.[45,46] Szeluga et al[45] conducted a randomized clinical trial comparing a parenteral to an enteral feeding program in the first month posttransplant in 57 allogeneic patients. These investigators observed improved maintenance of body composition in the parenteral nutrition group; however, they reported no difference in rate of hematopoietic recovery, length of hospitalization, or short-term survival between the groups.[45] They concluded that parenteral nutrition was not superior to an enteral feeding program.[45] Mulder and coworkers[46] reported the use of total or partial parenteral nutrition with enteral feedings in 22 autologous patients and suggested that this combined method of feeding was an acceptable alternative.

In recent years, issues surrounding cost containment and reduced length of hospitalization have renewed interest in the use of enteral feedings during BMT. Several anecdotal case studies have been reported.[47–50] Enteral tube feedings in marrow transplant patients have been used as early as 6 days after transplant,[47] and a gastrostomy tube placed as early as 63 days posttransplant.[48] Formulas used have included high-nitrogen, isotonic polymeric solutions; partially hydrolyzed formulas; and concentrated infant formulas.[47–50] Issues such as optimal time for initiation of feedings, types of tubes, methods of delivery, and appropriate formulas are currently being explored and provide new research opportunities.

Oral Feedings

Infection can be a major source of morbidity and mortality in immunosuppressed patients, and food is a potential infection source. For this reason, sterile or low-microbial diets are provided to marrow transplant patients.[51] Currently, most transplant centers restrict foods with high bacterial content. The degree of modification may range from a regular hospital diet without raw fruits and vegetables to a more strict diet of low microbial content. An example of diet guidelines for immunosuppressed marrow transplant patients is presented in Exhibit 13–3. The

Exhibit 13–3 Diet Guidelines for Immunosuppressed Patients

These guidelines are intended to minimize the introduction of pathogenic organisms into the gastrointestinal tract by food while maximizing healthy food options for immunosuppressed patients. The diet consists of foods that have been shown by culture to be safe when properly prepared in the home and hospital kitchen. High-risk foods identified as potential sources of organisms known to cause infection in immunosuppressed patients are restricted.

In general, autologous transplant patients follow the diet during the first three months after marrow transplant. Allogeneic transplant patients should follow the diet until off all immunosuppressive therapy.

Food Restrictions

- No raw and undercooked meat (including game), fish, shellfish, poultry, eggs, hot dogs, tofu, sausage, and bacon
- No cold smoked fish (salmon) and lox, pickled fish
- No unpasteurized and raw milk and milk products including cheese and yogurt
- No aged cheese (eg, brie, camembert, blue, roquefort, sharp cheddar, Stilton, etc)
- No refrigerated cheese-based salad dressings (eg, blue cheese) that are not shelf-stable
- No Mexican hot (eg, hot chili pepper) cheese, farmer's cheese, feta cheese
- No *unwashed* raw vegetables and fruits and those with visible mold
- No raw or unpasteurized honey
- No miso products (eg, miso soup); tempeh; mate'tea
- No moldy and outdated food products
- No well water, unless tested yearly and found safe

Courtesy of the Clinical Nutrition Department, Fred Hutchinson Cancer Research Center, Seattle, Washington.

protective benefits of a low-microbial diet for this population are unknown, however, and warrant further study.

NUTRITIONAL CONSIDERATIONS DURING BONE MARROW TRANSPLANTATION

Oral and Gastrointestinal Complications

Taste alterations, including dysgeusia (impaired taste) and hypogeusia (diminished taste), are common following transplant. Changes in taste acuity are primarily an effect of the TBI. Chemoradiotherapy conditioning regimens and antiemetic medications often induce xerostomia.[30] After TBI, saliva production diminishes and becomes thick and viscous. Patients recover their sense of taste 30 to 50 days following transplant.[52]

Ulcerative oral and esophageal mucositis are major complications associated with myeloablative chemoradiotherapy. The mucosal ulcerations may develop as early as 4 days after the preparative chemotherapy and several days after the first doses of TBI.[9] Healing generally begins with marrow engraftment and the return of neutrophils.[9] Efforts to minimize the severity of mucositis, in an attempt to decrease the need for parenteral nutrition, have included the use of oral glutamine supplementation. A recent report by Jebb and associates,[53] however, showed no significant differences in incidence or severity of mucositis in 24 autologous transplant patients treated with 16 g/day of oral glutamine.

Nausea and vomiting may occur soon after initiation of the preparative conditioning regimen. Medications such as trimethoprim-sulfamethoxazole, cyclosporine, immunomodulators (such as interleukin-2), and antibiotics often induce gastrointestinal symptoms. Viral intestinal infections, GVHD, and fluid and electrolyte imbalances are also associated with nausea and vomiting.[9,54]

Anorexia is another major nutritional complication of marrow transplantation. Nausea, vomiting, taste alterations, xerostomia, and psychological issues may affect a patient's desire to eat. Parenteral nutrition has also been associated with anorexia and delayed resumption of oral intake.[55] In a clinical trial of 258 marrow transplant recipients randomized to receive parenteral nutrition or intravenous hydration at hospital discharge, patients who received intravenous hydration resumed oral intake sooner and parenteral nutrition delayed refeeding posttransplant.[55]

High-dose cytoreductive therapy may cause intestinal mucosal damage resulting in diarrhea. Oral antibiotics, intestinal infection, and acute GVHD may also cause diarrheal illness.[56]

Because of these multiple oral and gastrointestinal manifestations, oral intake posttransplant is often impaired and prolongs dependence on parenteral nutrition. Oral feedings must be highly individualized to the patient's tolerance, and regular nutrition counseling is essential. Guidelines for management of oral and gastrointestinal transplant-related problems are provided in Exhibit 13–4.[30]

Infection

Following cytoreduction, the patient is profoundly neutropenic for 2 to 3 weeks until marrow engraftment. The patient is at increased risk for bacterial and fungal infections. The damaged intestine may serve as a portal of entry for infection or can itself be affected with bacterial or fungal overgrowth. Patients are placed on antibiotics and antiviral therapy as prophylaxis against infection. These agents may impact the patient's nutritional status by inducing anorexia, nausea, vomiting, diarrhea, or fluid and electrolyte imbalances.

Lipids have been implicated as immunosuppressive by altering the reticuloendothelial system and impairing neutrophil function.[57] To determine whether lipids

Exhibit 13–4 Dietary Management of Common Nutrition Problems Posttransplant

Nausea and vomiting
- High-carbohydrate foods and fluids (crackers, toast, gelatin); nonacidic juices
- Small, frequent feedings
- Cold, clear liquids and solids
- No overly sweet or high-fat foods

Dysgeusia (taste alterations)
- Flavored poultry, fish, eggs, dairy products
- Herbs, spices, flavor extracts, and marinades to enhance food taste
- Cold, nonodorous foods
- Fruit-flavored beverages
- Highly aromatic foods
- Good oral hygiene

Xerostomia (oral dryness)
- Moist foods (stews, casseroles, canned fruit) and liquids
- Extra sauces, gravies, margarine, butter, and broth added to foods
- Liquids with meals
- Vinegar and pickles added to foods to help lessen xerostomia
- Sucking lemon-flavored, sugarless candy to stimulate saliva
- Good oral hygiene
- Commercial saliva substitutes

Thick, viscous saliva and mucous
- Adequate fluid intake
- Clear liquids (tea, Popsicles, slushes)
- Good oral hygiene

Anorexia
- Small, frequent meals of foods high in calories and protein
- Carbohydrate supplements and protein powders
- A pleasant mealtime atmosphere created with enhancing food aromas, colorful place settings, varied color and textures of foods, and soft music
- Patient participation in grocery shopping and meal planning
- Relaxation techniques and light exercise before meals

Oral and esophageal mucositis (inflammation of the mucous membranes of the oral mucosa and esophagus)
- Soft- or puree-textured diet
- Smooth, bland, moist foods (custard, cream soups, mashed potatoes)
- Soft, nonirritating, cold foods (Popsicles, ice cream, frozen yogurt, slushes)

continues

Exhibit 13–4 continued

> - Liquid diets
> - Good oral hygiene
>
> **Diarrhea**
> - Low-fat, low-fiber diet
> - No caffeine and alcohol
> - Cold or room-temperature foods and beverages
> - Low-lactose intake
> - Adequate fluids to prevent dehydration
>
> *Source:* Reprinted with permission from P.M. Charuhas, Introduction to Marrow Transplantation, *Oncology Nutrition, A Newsletter of Oncology Nutrition Dietetic Practice Group,* Vol. 2, No. 3, pp. 2–9, © 1994.

could affect incidence of infection during BMT, Lenssen et al[16] conducted a large clinical trial of marrow transplant patients with hematologic malignancies who were randomized to receive 6% to 8% or 25% to 30% of total calories from lipids. The results showed no increased incidence of bacterial or fungal infections in the group who received the higher lipid dose.[16]

Hepatic Veno-Occlusive Disease

Hepatic veno-occlusive disease (VOD) is the leading cause of morbidity and mortality in the first 2 months posttransplant.[58] VOD is characterized by a fibrous obstruction of the hepatic venules and is associated with radiation preparation.[59] The incidence is 1% to 2% in patients with thalassemia but may be as high as 50% in high-risk patients.[58] Patients with a history of hepatitis or those undergoing a second marrow transplant are at increased risk of developing VOD.[58,59] Clinical characteristics of VOD include elevated bilirubin, weight gain with ascites, jaundice, and hepatomegaly; in severe cases, encephalopathy may develop.[58,59]

Nutrition management of VOD entails fluid and sodium restriction, the administration of exogenous albumin, and diuretics to mobilize fluids.[9] Concentration of parenteral nutrition fluids is often necessary, and sodium may be eliminated from parenteral solutions to minimize fluid retention. Nattakom et al[60] suggest that administration of vitamin E and glutamine may also be effective in the management of VOD, because administration of these nutrients reverses biochemical and clinical signs of severe hepatic dysfunction.

Administration of intravenous fat emulsion and lipid utilization should be closely monitored in patients who develop VOD or other hepatic dysfunction (eg, bilirubin >10 mg/dL).[10] Measuring the clearance of lipid emulsion particles during infusion by nephelometric techniques should be evaluated.[61] If evidence of poor lipid clearance is present, the rate of infusion and/or lipid dose should be decreased. If encephalopathy develops, a plasma amino acid profile should be drawn.[10] When elevated serum aromatic amino acids are present, a solution that is high in branched-chain amino acids and low in aromatic amino acids should be considered.[9]

Renal Complications

The majority of BMT patients experience some degree of renal compromise. While renal function may be normal before transplant, renal insult is frequently experienced during BMT and is multifactorial in etiology. Renal compromise may be associated with the preparative regimen, VOD, sepsis, or nephrotoxic medications such as cyclosporine and amphotericin.

Nutrition management of renal-compromised BMT patients includes provision of adequate fluid support during renal insufficiency. If acute renal failure develops, nutrition support should be maximized within fluid allowance with correction of electrolyte imbalances. Should dialysis be required, modification of vitamin supplementation is necessary to prevent fat-soluble vitamin toxicity.[9,10] Protein requirements also may be modified, and lipid utilization should be monitored.

Graft-versus-Host Disease

GVHD is a T-cell–mediated immunologic reaction of engrafted lymphoid cells against the host tissues. Acute GVHD occurs within the first 100 days posttransplant. The incidence varies and depends upon the degree of histocompatibility; there is an 80% to 90% probability among mismatched and unrelated donor transplants.[62,63] GVHD generally manifests itself in three major organs: the skin, the liver, and the gastrointestinal tract.

Skin GVHD usually occurs first and is the most common. It is characterized by a pruritic, maculopapular, erythematous rash, typically originating on the palms and soles. In its most advanced form, generalized blistering and desquamation may occur.

Liver GVHD generally appears later. It is characterized by abnormal liver function tests, jaundice, and hepatomegaly; in severe cases, encephalopathy may develop.

Intestinal GVHD is characterized by nausea; vomiting; severe abdominal pain and cramping; and large-volume, secretory diarrhea. In its advanced stage, the diarrhea may exceed several liters per day and is associated with severe malabsorption and fluid and electrolyte imbalances. Mucosal degeneration associated with GVHD induces gastrointestinal protein losses.[7]

Adequate nutrition support is a vital adjunctive to the immunosuppressive therapy used to treat gastrointestinal symptoms. Nutrition management includes a specialized five-phase dietary regimen as shown in Table 13–2.[64]

Table 13–2 Gastrointestinal GVHD Diet Progression

Phase	Clinical Symptoms	Diet	Clinical Symptoms of Diet Intolerance
1. Bowel rest	GI cramping Large volume of watery diarrhea Depressed serum albumin Severely reduced transit time Small-bowel obstruction or diminished bowel sounds Nausea and vomiting	*Oral:* NPO *IV:* emphasize energy and protein requirements	
2. Introduction of oral feeding	Minimal GI cramping Diarrhea less than 500 mL/day Guaiac-negative stools Improved transit time (minimum 1.5 hours) Infrequent nausea and vomiting	*Oral:* isosmotic, low-residue, low-lactose beverages, initially 60 mL every 2–3 hours, for several days *IV:* as for Phase 1	Increased stool volume or diarrhea Increased emesis Increased abdominal cramping
3. Introduction of solids	Minimal or no GI cramping Formed stool	*Oral:* allow introduction of solid food, once every 3–4 hours; minimal lactose,[a] low fiber, low fat (20–40 g/day),[b] low total acidity, no gastric irritants *IV:* as for Phase 1	As in Phase 2
4. Expansion of diet	Minimal or no GI cramping Formed stool	*Oral:* minimal lactose,[a] low fiber, low total acidity, no gastric irritants; if stools indicate fat malabsorption: low fat[b] *IV:* as needed to meet nutritional requirements	As in Phase 2

| 5. Resumption of regular diet | No GI cramping
Normal stool
Normal transit time
Normal albumin | *Oral:* progress to regular diet by introducing one restricted food per day: acid foods with meals, fiber-containing foods, lactose-containing foods; order of addition will vary, depending on individual tolerances and preferences; patients no longer exhibiting steatorrhea should have the fat restriction liberalized slowly.
IV: discontinue when oral nutritional intake meets estimated needs | As in Phase 2 |

[a]Lactose is one of the last disaccharidases to return following villous atrophy. A commercially prepared lactose solution (Lactaid®) is used to reduce the lactose content of milk by >90%. Lactaid® milk (100% lactose-free) is also commercially available.

[b]Additional calories may be provided by commercially available medium-chain triglycerides, which do not exacerbate symptoms.

Source: Reprinted with permission from J. Darbinian and M.M. Schubert, Special Management Problems, in *Nutritional Assessment and Management During Marrow Transplantation. A Resource Manual*, P. Lenssen and S.N. Aker, eds., pp. 63–80, © 1985, Fred Hutchinson Cancer Research Center.

Therapeutic measures used to prevent or treat GVHD usually include multidrug immunosuppressive therapy. Methotrexate, cyclosporine, corticosteroids, and FK-506 are commonly used medications. Many of these agents, however, have nutritional implications, as described in Exhibit 13–5.[30]

LONG-TERM COMPLICATIONS

As the number of patients surviving BMT increases, late effects related to transplantation have become evident.

Chronic Graft-versus-Host Disease

Chronic GVHD generally develops after 70 days following transplant. The incidence is 30% in matched sibling transplants, with increased frequency in nonidentical, related transplants and unrelated donor patients, who often require multidrug therapy.[65] There is a high prevalence of nutrition-related problems among recipients of allogeneic marrow transplant who develop chronic GVHD. In a retrospective review, Lenssen and colleagues[66] observed that at 1 year posttransplant, several patients still reported problems with weight gain, weight loss, oral sensitivity, xerostomia, stomatitis, and anorexia.[66] Diarrhea, steatorrhea, taste alterations, esophageal stricture, shortness of breath, and contractures were also reported.[66] Bone density loss has also been observed in patients with chronic GVHD.[67] These findings suggest the need for ongoing nutrition monitoring following discharge from transplant centers.[66]

Pediatric Growth and Development Issues

Growth and development problems frequently occur in pediatric patients who have undergone BMT. Myeloablative conditioning therapy can affect endocrine gland function. With cyclophosphamide alone, thyroid function, growth rates, and pubertal maturation are normal.[68] Decreased growth velocity, growth hormone deficiency, and delayed onset of puberty have been observed in children treated with busulfan or TBI.[68] All children who receive marrow transplants should have regular evaluations to detect endocrine gland dysfunction. Initiation of appropriate hormonal therapy, when abnormal endocrine function is detected, may improve growth and development.

CONCLUSIONS

Marrow transplantation is now being used to treat a variety of hematologic malignant and nonmalignant disorders of the bone marrow with a wide range of re-

Exhibit 13–5 Medications for GVHD Prophylaxis and Treatment

Medication	Classification	Mechanism of Action	Nutritional Implications
Anti-thymocyte globulin (ATG)	Immunosuppressant	May eliminate antigen-reactive T cells (T lymphocytes) in peripheral blood and/or alteration of T cell function	Must infuse with normal saline over 8–10 hours, thus interfering with parenteral nutrition support; may cause nausea, vomiting, diarrhea, and stomatitis
Azathioprine (Imuran®)	Immunosuppressant	Suppresses hypersensitivities of the cell-mediated type and causes variable alterations in antibody production	Nausea and vomiting; anorexia and diarrhea when drug is given in large doses; mucosal ulceration; esophagitis; steatorrhea
Beclomethasone dipropionate	Synthetic glucocorticoid	Produces anti-inflammatory and vasoconstrictor effects	Xerostomia; dysgeusia; adrenal insufficiency; nausea
Corticosteroids (Methylprednisone®) (Solu-Medrol®) (Prednisone®) (Dexamethasone®)	Synthetic glucocorticoid	Produces anti-inflammatory effects	Sodium and fluid retention resulting in weight gain or hypertension; hyperphagia; weight gain; hypokalemia; skeletal muscule catabolism and atrophy; gastric irritation and peptic ulceration; osteoporosis; growth retardation in children; decreased insulin sensitivity and impaired glucose tolerance, resulting in hyperglycemia or steroid-induced diabetes; hypertriglyceridemia
Cyclosporine	Immunosuppressant	Prevents or ameliorates GVHD by suppressing T cell function	Nausea and vomiting; renal insufficiency, magnesium wasting, potassium wasting
FK-506 (Prograf®)	Macrolide immunosuppressant	Suppresses cell-mediated and humoral immune responses	Nephrotoxicity; hyperglycemia; hyperkalemia; hypomagnesemia
Methotrexate	Antimetabolite	Interferes with DNA synthesis by antagonizing folic acid; given intravenously for GVHD prophylaxis and intrathecally for the prevention of central nervous system relapse	Nausea and vomiting (mild to moderate); anorexia, mucositis, and esophagitis (severe); diarrhea, renal and hepatic implications; decreased absorption of vitamin B_{12}, fat, and D-xylose; hepatic fibrosis; change in taste acuity

continues

Exhibit 13–5 continued

Medication	Classification	Mechanism of Action	Nutritional Implications
Mycophenolate mofetil	Immunosuppressant	Enhances availability of mycophenolic acid, which inhibits recruitment of leukocytes	Vomiting and diarrhea
PUVA/Psoralen	Photosensitizer	Used in treatment of skin GVHD; modulates immune system (ie, number and function of circulating lymphocytes, monocytes, and macrophages)	Nausea, hepatotoxicity
Sirolumus (Rapamycin®)	Immunosuppressant	Inhibits T cell proliferation	Weight loss; hyperglycemia; anorexia; hypertriglyceridemia
Thalidomide (investigational)	Glutamic acid derivative	Alters T cell function	Constipation, nausea, xerostomia; teratogen
Trimetrexate (TMTX) (investigational)	Folate analogue	Dihydrofolate reductase inhibitor; used for prophylaxis of GVHD in patients receiving 2 or 3 antigen mismatches	Mucositis; nausea and vomiting; diarrhea
Ursodeoxycholic acid (UDCA) (Actigall®)	Bile acid	Used in treatment of liver GVHD; displaces retained toxic bile acids in cholestatic or inflammatory hepatic diseases	Nausea and vomiting; diarrhea, dyspepsia

Source: Reprinted with permission from P.M. Charuhas, Introduction to Marrow Transplantation, *Oncology Nutrition, A Newsletter of Oncology Nutrition Dietetic Practice Group,* Vol. 2, No. 3, pp. 2–9, © 1994.

sults depending on the disease, stage of the disease, and type of transplant. As new information and new treatment modalities become available, marrow transplantation may become more widely employed in the treatment of other diseases. Advances in nutrition support will parallel these improvements, making better care of marrow transplant patients possible.

REFERENCES

1. Bortin MM, Horowitz MM, Rimm AA. Increasing utilization of allogeneic bone marrow transplantation: results of the 1988–1990 survey. *Ann Intern Med.* 1992;116:505–512.

2. Franco T, Gould DA. Allogeneic bone marrow transplantation. *Semin Oncol Nurs.* 1994;10:3–11.

3. Thomas ED. Bone marrow transplantation. *CA Cancer J Clin.* 1987;37:291–301.

4. Welte K. Matched unrelated transplants. *Semin Oncol Nurs.* 1994;10:20–27.

5. Lowry PA, Tabbara IA. Peripheral hematopoietic stem cell transplantation: current concepts. *Exp Hematol.* 1992;20:937–942.

6. Wagner JE, Broxmeyer HE, Byrd RL, Zehnbauer B, et al. Transplantation of umbilical cord blood after myeloablative therapy: analysis of engraftment. *Blood.* 1992;79:1874–1881.

7. McDonald GV, Shulman HM, Sullivan KM, Spencer GD. Intestinal and hepatic complications of human bone marrow transplantation: part I. *Gastroenterology.* 1986;90:460–477.

8. Cunningham BA, Lenssen P, Aker SN, Gittere KM, et al. Nutritional considerations during marrow transplantation. *Nurs Clin North Am.* 1983;18:585–595.

9. Aker SN. Bone marrow transplantation: nutrition support and monitoring. In: Bloch AS, ed. *Nutrition Management of the Cancer Patient.* Rockville, MD: Aspen Publishers, Inc; 1990:199–225.

10. Fred Hutchinson Cancer Research Center, Swedish Medical Center, Veterans Administration Medical Center. *BMT/PBSCT Nutrition Care Criteria.* Seattle, WA: Fred Hutchinson Cancer Research Center; 1995.

11. Szeluga DJ, Stuart RK, Brookmeyer R, Utermohlen V, et al. Energy requirements of parenterally fed bone marrow transplant recipients. *J Parenter Enter Nutr.* 1985;9:139–143.

12. Geibig CB, Owens JP, Mirtallo JM, Bowers D, et al. Parenteral nutrition for marrow transplant recipients: evaluation of an increased nitrogen dose. *J Parenter Enter Nutr.* 1991;15:184–188.

13. Harris JA, Benedict FG. *Biometric Studies of Basal Metabolism in Man.* Washington, DC: Carnegie Institution of Washington; 1919. Publication 279.

14. Altman PL, Dittmer DS, eds. *Metabolism.* Bethesda, MD: Federation of American Societies for Experimental Biology; 1968.

15. National Research Council. Committee on Dietary Allowances. Food and Nutrition Board. *Recommended Dietary Allowances.* 10th ed. Washington, DC: National Academy of Sciences; 1989.

16. Lenssen P, Bruemmer B, Aker S, Bowden R, et al. Relationship between IV lipid dose and incidence of bacteremias and fungemias in 492 marrow transplant (MT) patients. *J Parenter Enter Nutr.* 1994;18:22S.

17. Clemans GW, Yamanaka W, Flournoy N, Aker SN, et al. Plasma fatty acid patterns of bone marrow transplant patients primarily supported by fat-free parenteral nutrition. *J Parenter Enter Nutr.* 1981;5:221–225.

18. Yamanaka WK, Tilmont G, Aker SN. Plasma fatty acids of marrow transplant recipients on fat-supplemented parenteral nutrition. *Am J Clin Nutr.* 1984;39:607–611.

19. McCrae JD, O'Shea R, Udine LM. Parenteral nutrition: hospital to home. *J Am Diet Assoc.* 1993;93:664–673.

20. American Academy of Pediatrics. Committee on Nutrition. Commentary on parenteral nutrition. *Pediatrics.* 1983;71:547–552.

21. Sherry MEG, Aker SN, Cheney CL. Nutrition assessment and management of the pediatric cancer patient. *Top Clin Nutr.* 1987;2:38–48.

22. American Medical Association. Department of Foods and Nutrition. Multivitamin preparations for parenteral use: a statement by the Nutrition Advisory Group. *J Parenter Enter Nutr.* 1979;3:258–262.

23. Cunningham BA. Parenteral management. In: Lenssen P, Aker SN, eds. *Nutritional Assessment and Management during Marrow Transplantation: A Resource Manual.* Seattle, WA: Fred Hutchinson Cancer Research Center; 1985:45–61.

24. Carlin A, Walker WA. Rapid development of vitamin K deficiency in an adolescent boy receiving total parenteral nutrition following bone marrow transplantation. *Nutr Rev.* 1991;49:179–183.

25. Rovelli A, Bonomi M, Murano A, Locasciulli A, et al. Severe lactic acidosis due to thiamine deficiency after bone marrow transplantation in a child with acute monocytic leukemia. *Haematologica.* 1990;75:579–581.

26. Clemens MR, Ladner C, Ehninger G, Einsele H, et al. Plasma vitamin E and beta-carotene concentrations during radiochemotherapy preceding bone marrow transplantation. *Am J Clin Nutr.* 1990;51:216–219.

27. American Medical Association. Department of Foods and Nutrition. Guidelines for essential trace element preparations for parenteral use: a statement by an expert panel. *JAMA.* 1979;241:2051–2054.

28. Fredstrom S, Rogosheske J, Gupta P, Burns LJ. Case report. Extrapyramidal symptoms in a BMT recipient with hyperintense basal ganglia and elevated manganese. *Bone Marrow Transplant.* 1995;15:989–992.

29. June CH, Thompson CB, Kennedy MS, Nims J, et al. Profound hypomagnesemia and renal magnesium wasting associated with the use of cyclosporine for marrow transplantation. *Transplantation.* 1985;39:620–624.

30. Charuhas PM. Introduction to marrow transplantation. *Oncol Nutr Diet Pract Group Newslet.* 1994;2:2–9.

31. McDonald RA. Disorders of potassium balance. *Pediatr Ann.* 1995;24:31–37.

32. Dezenhall A, Curry-Bartley K, Blackburn SA, Delamerens S, et al. Food and nutrition services in bone marrow transplant centers. *J Am Diet Assoc.* 1987;87:1351–1353.

33. Marian M. Pediatric nutrition. *Nutr Clin Pract.* 1993;8:199–209.

34. Souba WW. Glutamine and cancer. *Ann Surg.* 1993;218:715–728.

35. Ziegler TR, Young LS, Benfell K, Scheltinga M, et al. Clinical and metabolic efficacy of glutamine-supplemented parenteral nutrition after bone marrow transplantation: a randomized, double-blind controlled study. *Ann Intern Med.* 1992;116:821–828.

36. Echenique MM, Bistrian BR, Moldawer LL, Palombo JD, et al. Improvement in amino acid use in the critically ill patient with parenteral formulas enriched with branched chain amino acids. *Surg Gynecol Obstet.* 1984;159:233–241.

37. Lenssen P, Cheney CL, Aker SN, Cunningham BA, et al. Intravenous branched chain amino acid trial in marrow transplant recipients. *J Parenter Enter Nutr.* 1987;11:112–118.

38. Weisdorf S, Hofland C, Sharp HL, Teasley K, et al. Total parenteral nutrition in bone marrow transplantation: a clinical evaluation. *J Pediatr Gastroenterol Nutr.* 1984;3:95–100.

39. Uderzo C, Rovelli A, Bonomi M, Fomia L, et al. Total parenteral nutrition and nutritional assessment in leukaemic children undergoing bone marrow transplantation. *Eur J Cancer.* 1991;27:758–762.

40. Yokoyama S, Fujimoto T, Mitomi T, Yabe M, et al. Use of total parenteral nutrition in pediatric bone marrow transplantation. *Nutrition.* 1989;5:27–30.

41. Weisdorf SA, Lysne J, Wind D, Haake RJ, et al. Positive effect of prophylactic total parenteral nutrition on long-term outcome of bone marrow transplantation. *Transplantation.* 1987;43:833–838.

42. Moore FA, Moore EE, Jones TN, McCroskey BL, et al. TEN versus TPN following major abdominal trauma: reduced septic morbidity. *J Trauma.* 1989;29:916–923.

43. American Gastroenterology Association. American Gastroenterology Association medical position statement: guidelines for the use of enteral nutrition. *Gastroenterology.* 1995;108:1280–1281.

44. Fegan C, Poynton CH, Whittaker JA. The gut mucosal barrier in bone marrow transplantation. *Bone Marrow Transplant.* 1990;5:373–377.

45. Szeluga DJ, Stuart RK, Brookmeyer R, Utermohlen V, et al. Nutritional support of bone marrow transplant recipients: a prospective, randomized clinical trial comparing total parenteral nutrition to an enteral feeding program. *Cancer Res.* 1987;47:3309–3316.

46. Mulder POM, Bouman JG, Gietema A, van Rijsbergen H, et al. Hyperalimentation in autologous bone marrow transplantation for solid tumors. Comparison of total parenteral versus partial parenteral plus enteral nutrition. *Cancer.* 1989;64:2045–2052.

47. Davies S, McCorkle N. Transition to oral feeds using enteral nutrition in pediatric bone marrow transplant patients. *Marrow Transplant Nutr Network Newslet.* 1994;2:1–2.

48. Ringwald-Smith K, Krance R, Stricklin L. Enteral nutrition support in a child after bone marrow transplantation. *Nutr Clin Pract.* 1995;10:140–143.

49. Miller J. Enteral nutrition in marrow transplant patients. *Marrow Transplant Nutr Network Newslet.* 1994;2:1.

50. Barron MA. Successful use of percutaneous endoscopic gastrostomy (PEG) tube feeding pre- and post-bone marrow transplant (BMT). American Society for Parenteral and Enteral Nutrition 19th Clinical Congress, Miami Beach, FL. January 15–18, 1995. Poster 156.

51. Aker SN, Cheney CL. The use of sterile and low microbial diets in ultraisolation environments. *J Parenter Enter Nutr.* 1983;7:390–397.

52. Barale K, Aker SN, Martinsen CS. Primary taste thresholds in children with leukemia undergoing marrow transplantation. *J Parenter Enter Nutr.* 1982;6:287–290.

53. Jebb SA, Marcus R, Elia M. A pilot study of oral glutamine supplementation in patients receiving bone marrow transplants. *Clin Nutr.* 1995;14:162–165.

54. Charuhas PM. Dietary management during antitumor therapy of cancer patients. *Top Clin Nutr.* 1993;9:42–53.

55. Charuhas PM, Fosberg KL, Bruemmer B, Aker SN, et al. A double-blind randomized trial comparing outpatient parenteral nutrition with intravenous hydration: effect on resumption of oral intake after marrow transplantation. *J Parenter Enter Nutr.* 1997;21:157–161.

56. Cox GJ, Matsui SM, Lo RS, Hinds M, et al. Etiology and outcome of diarrhea after marrow transplantation: a prospective study. *Gastroenterology.* 1994;107:1398–1407.

57. Wan JMF, Teo TC, Babayan VK, Blackburn GL. Lipids and the development of immune dysfunction and infection. *J Parenter Enter Nutr.* 1988;12:43S–52S.

58. Shulman HM, Hinterberger W. Hepatic veno-occlusive disease: liver toxicity syndrome after bone marrow transplantation. *Bone Marrow Transplant.* 1992;10:197–214.

59. Baglin TP. Veno-occlusive disease of the liver complicating bone marrow transplantation. *Bone Marrow Transplant.* 1994;13:1–4.

60. Nattakom TV, Charlton A, Wilmore DW. Use of vitamin E and glutamine in the successful treatment of severe veno-occlusive disease following bone marrow transplantation. *Nutr Clin Pract.* 1995;10:16–18.

61. Carlson LA, Rossner S. A methodological study of an intravenous fat tolerance test with intralipid® emulsion. *Scan J Clin Lab Invest.* 1972;29:271–280.

62. Beatty PG, Clift RA, Mickelson EM, Nisperos BB, et al. Marrow transplantation from related donors other than HLA-identical siblings. *N Engl J Med.* 1985;313:765–771.

63. Beatty PG, Hansen JA, Longton GM, Thomas ED, et al. Marrow transplantation from HLA-matched unrelated donors for treatment of hematological malignancies. *Transplantation.* 1991;51:443–447.

64. Darbinian J, Schubert MM. Special management problems. In: Lenssen P, Aker SN, eds. *Nutritional Assessment and Management during Marrow Transplantation: A Resource Manual.* Seattle, WA: Fred Hutchinson Cancer Research Center; 1985:63–80.

65. Sullivan KM. Graft-versus-host disease. In: Forman SJ, Blume KG, Thomas ED, eds. *Bone Marrow Transplantation.* Boston: Blackwell Scientific Publications; 1994:339–360.

66. Lenssen P, Sherry ME, Cheney CL, Nims JW, et al. Prevalence of nutrition-related problems among long-term survivors of allogeneic marrow transplantation. *J Am Diet Assoc.* 1990;90:835–842.

67. Stern JM, Chesnut CH III, Bruemmer B, Sullivan KM, et al. Bone density loss during treatment of chronic GVHD. *Bone Marrow Transplant.* 1996;17:395–400.

68. Sanders JE. Growth and development after bone marrow transplantation. In: Forman SJ, Blume KG, Thomas ED, eds. *Bone Marrow Transplantation.* Boston: Blackwell Scientific Publications; 1994:527–537.

CHAPTER 14

Solid Organ Transplantation

Jeanette M. Hasse and Sara Reek DiCecco

INTRODUCTION

Transplantation is indicated when individuals suffer from end-stage organ failure that no longer responds to medical or surgical treatment. Thousands of individuals undergo transplantation of the kidney, heart, lung, liver, pancreas, and/or small bowel every year. In 1997, approximately 53,000 people in the United States awaited a transplant.[1] In 1996, 3926 patients died while waiting for a transplant.[1] Many factors affect a patient's outcome both before and after transplantation; poor nutritional status is one factor that can be reversible. Therefore, nutrition therapy must be an integral part of any transplant patient's care.

PRETRANSPLANT PHASE

Nutritional Assessment

The first part of nutrition therapy is nutritional assessment. Nutritional assessment can be difficult to perform in patients undergoing organ transplantation because symptoms of end-stage organ disease often affect interpretation of common assessment parameters.[2–5] Fluid retention occurs in many patients awaiting heart, kidney, and liver transplantation. Excess fluid dilutes serum concentrations of nutrition-related laboratory parameters and inflates body weight. Serum protein production is depressed in liver failure, and excretion is increased in wasting conditions such as nephrotic syndrome, blood loss, or gastrointestinal loss. Immunosuppressive medications such as corticosteroids render interpretation of serum albumin and transferrin values invalid. When objective measures are invalid, subjective global assessment (SGA) is the preferred technique for nutritional assessment.[2,6–10] Chapter 1 describes nutritional assessment techniques that can be adapted for use with transplant candidates.

Malnutrition among Transplant Recipients

A majority of transplant patients suffer from some degree of malnutrition. The pattern and severity of malnutrition partially depend upon the type of organ failure. Grady and Herold[11] evaluated 65 cardiac transplant patients using anthropometric measurements and skin antigen tests. Over one third of the patients had depressed somatic protein stores and were anergic. The average pretransplant weight was 90% of usual body weight. In another study, SGA and several other objective parameters were used to assess 35 patients undergoing lung transplantation.[12] Although mean serum albumin and transferrin levels were normal, 60% of the patients were moderately to severely malnourished according to the SGA technique. In addition, body mass index (BMI) was subnormal in patients with emphysema and cystic fibrosis.

Several studies have evaluated the frequency of malnutrition in kidney failure and kidney transplant recipients. Miller et al[13] studied 24 diabetic and 21 nondiabetic kidney transplant patients. Of these patients, 36% were below 85% of their desirable body weight; 38% had midarm muscle circumference values below the 5th percentile, and the remainder had circumferences greater than the 50th percentile. In another study, 95 renal patients were assessed using several objective tests.[14] The researchers found that patients with the lowest glomerular filtration rates had the lowest energy intakes, serum transferrin concentrations, and creatinine-height ratios. Researchers who conducted a small study evaluating six patients undergoing maintenance hemodialysis reported that serum total protein and albumin levels were normal, but body weight was only 88.6% of usual weight.[15] In a multicenter trial of 224 patients who received continuous ambulatory peritoneal dialysis, nutritional assessment revealed that 8% of patients were severely malnourished, 32.6% were mildly to moderately depleted, and 59.4% were well nourished.[16]

Malnutrition is prevalent among liver transplant recipients as well. DiCecco and colleagues obtained diet histories and performed biochemical, anthropometric, and immunocompetence evaluations on 74 liver transplant candidates.[17] The researchers concluded that malnutrition was present in all patients but with varying degrees and with characteristics distinct to specific types of liver disease. Depleted fat and muscle stores with retained visceral protein stores characterized patients with primary biliary cirrhosis. Patients with sclerosing cholangitis had the lowest muscle stores of all patients but retained their body fat stores. Moderate depletion of all nutritional assessment parameters existed among patients with chronic active hepatitis. However, the severest degree of malnutrition occurred in patients with acute hepatitis. In another report, 13 liver transplant candidates were evaluated using anthropometric, serum albumin, and skin antigen measurements.[18] The mean triceps skinfold measurement was 40% ± 25% of standard; arm muscle circumference was 78% ± 9% of standard; mean serum albumin concentration was below standard; and 60% of the patients were anergic.

Two studies used the SGA technique to assess liver transplant candidates. Pikul et al[10] assessed 68 patients and determined a 79% rate of mild to severe malnutrition. Hasse and colleagues[19] reported a 70% rate of moderate to severe malnutrition in a group of 500 liver transplant patients assessed according to SGA. The causes of malnutrition among transplant recipients are listed in Table 14–1.[4,5,11,12,20–28]

Table 14–1 Factors Contributing to Malnutrition in Organ Transplant Recipients

Contributing Factor	Possible Treatment
Decreased food intake	
Anorexia	• Encourage patient to try favorite foods and consider eating as part of treatment.
	• Encourage patient to eat nutrient-dense foods.
	• Consider use of appetite stimulants.
Dysgeusia	• Encourage patient to try variety of foods with different flavors.
Nausea and vomiting	• Try antinausea medications; consider tube-feeding if vomiting is persistent.
Diarrhea	• Evaluate cause; patient may need alteration in medications (eg, patient may be taking too much lactulose) or treat with antidiarrheals.
Early satiety	• Encourage small, frequent meals.
Mental depression	• Consider treatment for depression.
Restricted diets	• Liberalize diet as much as possible.
Increased nutrient losses	
Drug-nutrient interactions altering absorption and utilization of food	• Plan administration of interfering drugs and food at separate times to avoid interaction.
Increased stool and urine losses; depressed gastrointestinal absorptive capacity; increased muscle protein degradation; reduced circulatory function impairing nutrient delivery to tissues	• Encourage increased intake to account for some losses; support with oral supplements, tube feeding, or total parenteral nutrition as necessary.
Pancreatic insufficiency	• Have patient take pancreatic enzymes.
Increased nutrient needs	
Hypermetabolism due to pretransplant disease state	• Encourage increased intake; support with oral supplements, tube feeding, or total parenteral nutrition as necessary.

Source: Data from refs 4, 5, 11, 12, 20–28.

Malnutrition in transplant recipients has been shown to increase posttransplant morbidity and mortality rates. Among 52 heart transplant recipients, death occurred in 50% of severely malnourished patients, 23% of marginally nourished patients, and 21% of adequately nourished patients.[21] Likewise, loss of body cell mass was associated with increased mortality in 123 liver transplant recipients.[29] In addition, two other studies have found that malnutrition among liver transplant recipients led to prolonged ventilatory support and increased incidence of tracheostomy,[10] prolonged intensive care and hospital stays,[10,19] and significantly higher hospitalization costs.[19] Studies have not shown malnutrition to affect infection or rejection rates, so one could speculate that extended intensive care unit stays may be due to prolonged ventilatory support, and the overall increased length of stay may be due to malnourished patients' inability to recuperate quickly from this major surgery.

Pretransplant Obesity

Although many patients are undernourished before transplantation, some transplant candidates are obese. Obesity is considered a relative contraindication to organ transplantation due to theoretical complications such as the difficulty of performing a transplant in an obese abdomen, increased wound infections, and decreased graft survival. Table 14–2 summarizes several studies that have evaluated the risks of transplanting obese patients.[30-35] Because some risk is associated with transplanting obese patients, these patients should be counseled to lose weight before transplantation, if possible. Weight loss should include caloric restriction with adequate protein for muscle sparing. Activity and exercise should be a part of the weight-loss program; however, many patients with end-stage organ failure are unable to exercise due to weakness and fatigue. Patients awaiting a kidney, pancreas, or small-intestine transplant may have time to lose weight before transplantation because life-sustaining treatments such as dialysis, insulin therapy, and total parenteral nutrition (TPN) are available while patients lose weight. Patients who need a heart, lung, or liver transplant may be so critically ill that they may not be able to lose enough weight to have a transplant, and there is not a viable alternative for survival for these patients.

Pretransplant Nutrition Therapy

Pretransplant nutrition therapy should focus on (1) maintaining or improving nutritional status, and (2) treating symptoms of organ failure through dietary changes. Other chapters in this book describe in detail the appropriate nutritional care of patients with organ failure. The paramount point is that aggressive pretransplant nutrition support should prevent further deterioration and enhance

Table 14–2 Effect of Obesity on Transplant Outcomes

Researchers	Study Design	Results
Merion et al[30]	263 renal transplant patients were evaluated retrospectively.	• 15% of patients were >120% of ideal body weight. • Obese patients had a significantly increased rate of wound infections. • Obese patients gained significantly more weight by 1-year posttransplant than nonobese subjects.
Holley et al[31]	46 obese renal transplant patients were compared with a control group of 50 nonobese patients.	• Obese patients had significantly higher rates of wound complications, intensive care unit admissions, reintubations, and new onset of diabetes mellitus compared with nonobese controls. • Obese patients had significantly lower patient and graft survival rates compared with nonobese controls. • Obese patients had significantly worse immediate graft function compared with controls.
Pirsch et al[32]	584 renal transplant recipients were classified according to body mass index (BMI).	• 20% of patients were obese (BMI >27.5 kg/m^2). • Obese patients had significantly higher rates of urologic and wound complications compared with nonobese patients. • Patients with BMI >30 had delayed graft function and greater immunologic graft loss significantly more often than patients with BMI <30.
Winters et al[33]	Failed human heart allografts from 15 subjects were studied; luminal narrowing was related to 40 individual risk factors.	• BMI was the single most predictive risk factor of luminal narrowing.
Keefe et al[34]	18 severely or morbidly obese liver transplant patients were studied.	• Obesity significantly increased incidences of wound infection, diabetes mellitus, and hypertension.

continues

Table 14–2 continued

Researchers	Study Design	Results
Blue et al[35]	390 liver transplant patients were classified according to BMI and evaluated retrospectively.	• 23.5% were obese (≥27.5 kg/m²). • Severely obese patients required significantly longer intensive care unit stays than nonobese patients. • No difference in rates of infection or rejection, duration of ventilatory support, or hospital length of stay was detected between the two groups.

posttransplant outcomes. Sodium or fluid restrictions may be necessary to ameliorate organ failure symptoms, but these restrictions should be as liberal as possible to allow for the greatest nutrient intake. Pretransplant diets often must consist of small, frequent, nutrient-dense meals. Oral liquid nutrition supplements may be used to fortify a patient's diet. More patients than in the past require tube feeding as waiting times to transplant increase. Patients who are awaiting small-bowel transplants should be maintained on TPN until they have functioning transplanted intestines.

IMMEDIATE POSTTRANSPLANT PHASE

Acute Posttransplant Nutrition Therapy

The immediate posttransplant phase is characterized by a highly catabolic state. In the acute posttransplant phase, corticosteroids are administered in high doses, resulting in protein catabolism. It is during this acute phase that patients most often experience infections, graft rejection, and vascular or other surgical problems. Other posttransplant problems that can prevent patients from eating include delayed organ function, missed meals because of medical tests, altered mental status, bleeding, and inability to wean from ventilatory support. When patients are able to eat, they frequently are unable to eat adequate amounts due to poor appetite, taste changes from medications, gastrointestinal disturbances, early satiety, or mental confusion. Aggressive nutrition therapy, therefore, must be considered for transplant recipients. Exhibit 14–1 lists some general guidelines for oral diet, tube feeding, and TPN in transplant recipients.[2,36–38]

Acute Posttransplant Nutrient Requirements

In general, caloric requirements for organ transplant patients in the postoperative phase have been estimated to be 35 calories/kg or 130% to 150% of the basal energy

Exhibit 14–1 General Nutrition Support Guidelines for Organ Transplant Recipients in the Acute Posttransplant Phase

Oral diet
- Initiate oral diet when patient passing flatus and/or having bowel movements.
- Advance diet as quickly as possible to a solid food diet.
- Avoid dietary restrictions as much as possible to allow adequate intake of necessary calories and protein.
- Diabetic diets are recommended for patients with hyperglycemia.
- Sodium or fluid restrictions may be needed for uncontrolled fluid retention or hyponatremia.
- Small, frequent meals and/or liquid nutrition supplements often help patients achieve nutrient goals.

Tube feeding
- Consider placing feeding tube in patient during surgery if patient is malnourished or if complications are anticipated posttransplant.
- Small-bore, nasointestinal feeding tubes and continuous pump feeding are best tolerated.
- High-nitrogen, polymeric formulas usually are well tolerated. Semielemental formulas may be required if digestion or absorption is impaired. Calorically dense formulas are indicated when volume needs to be restricted. Specialty products for hyperglycemia or renal failure can be used as indicated.
- When patients are eating approximately 50% of their protein and calorie needs, tube feeding can be reduced to nocturnal infusion only.

Total parenteral nutrition (TPN)
- TPN is indicated only when the gut is not functional, such as in ileus, pancreatitis, small-bowel obstruction, or immediately following small-bowel transplantation.
- The TPN solution may need to be concentrated.
- A typical TPN solution for a transplant patient would consist of 70% of nonprotein calories as carbohydrate and 30% as lipid. Dextrose and lipid content is adjusted depending upon serum glucose and triglyceride levels.
- If a patient has significant hyperglycemia, initiate the TPN at a reduced dextrose concentration and increase dextrose only after glucose control is achieved.
- Shift patient to tube feeding and oral diet as soon as possible. Central catheters are a potential source of infection in an already immunosuppressed patient.

Source: Data from refs 2, 36–38.

expenditure (BEE) calculated by the Harris-Benedict equation.[2,9,20,21,24,25,27,36,39–41] Dry or ideal body weight should be used in these calculations when patients are retaining fluid or are overweight.[25] Fever or infection may elevate caloric requirements.[21,25] In the short-term phase, nonprotein calories usually are provided as 70% from carbohydrate sources and 30% from lipid sources. Hyperglycemia is a common complication resulting from surgical stress as well as effects from three immunosuppressive agents: cyclosporine, tacrolimus, and corticosteroids. Serum glucose levels should be monitored frequently (every 6 hours) in the first few days after transplantation. Many patients initially require insulin therapy. However, if a patient is still hyperglycemic when he or she approaches discharge from the hospital, clinicians should assume that the patient has developed, at least temporarily, posttransplant diabetes and should treat and educate the patient accordingly. It is imperative to achieve blood sugar control, because hyperglycemia leads to delayed wound healing and increased susceptibility to opportunistic infections.

In cases where hyperglycemia is difficult to control, carbohydrate intake can be decreased and lipid intake increased until glucose control is achieved. In some instances, elevated fasting serum triglyceride levels may indicate lipid intolerance. The lipid content of the diet may be reduced temporarily and, if tolerated, the carbohydrate content of the diet increased.

Protein goals are 1.2 to 2.0 g/kg body weight to account for a posttransplant catabolic state.[2,7,9,14,21,24,36,38,40–42] Protein malnutrition in a posttransplant patient increases the likelihood of complications such as delayed wound healing, infection, skin breakdown, ulceration, osteopenia, and myopathy.[26] Protein needs are increased due to the catabolic effects of corticosteroids used as immunosuppressive agents and surgical stress.[26] The protein catabolic rate seems to be related to the corticosteroid dose, as the former increases with increased steroid use and causes negative nitrogen balance and protein deficits.[43,44] Whittier et al[45] compared the effects of a standard protein diet (1 g/kg body weight) with an isocaloric, high-protein (3 g/kg body weight), low-carbohydrate, high-fat diet. The latter diet appeared to promote nitrogen balance and reduce cushingoid symptoms. However, the practical use of this diet is limited; most patients are unable to eat 3 g protein/kg, and the diet contradicts long-term recommendations of a low-fat diet. Newer immunosuppressive regimens using powerful drugs such as cyclosporine, tacrolimus, and mycophenolate mofetil require lower corticosteroid doses than were used in many early studies.

A nucleotide-free diet administered to rats suppressed cell-mediated immunity and prolonged heart transplant survival when the rats also were given cyclosporine.[46,47] This regimen has not been studied in humans and is not used widely.

Other nutrient requirements often depend upon the type of transplant performed, the current condition of the patient, and posttransplant complications. Fluid requirements are individualized, depending on the patient's fluid intake and output. Hyperkalemia is a common side effect of immunosuppressive medications and impaired renal function after transplantation. Dietary potassium restriction may be necessary until renal function improves. On the other hand, potassium, phosphorus, and magnesium can deplete rapidly during diuresis and refeeding; cyclosporine also causes magnesium wasting.[38] Other vitamin and mineral requirements are linked to previous nutriture and current losses. Although not studied, other nutrients such as arginine may have beneficial effects in wound healing (see Chapter 18 on surgery and wound healing). Nutritional recommendations are, to a degree, specific to the type of organ that was transplanted. Guidelines for each type of organ transplant population are discussed below.

Posttransplant Nutrition Monitoring

In the acute posttransplant phase, the most important monitoring tools are nutrient-intake analyses and observation of clinical improvement in functional status and wound healing. Whether patients are receiving nutrition support or are eating, it is critical to monitor intake to ensure that patients are receiving adequate nutrients. Nutrition monitoring suggestions are listed in Table 14–3.

NUTRITIONAL CONCERNS AND SPECIFIC TRANSPLANT PROCEDURES

Heart and Lung Transplantation

Patients who have undergone heart transplantation with or without lung transplantation should be able to eat 3 to 4 days after transplantation once their nasogastric tubes are removed. Postoperative nutrition support is not indicated if it

---

Table 14–3 Nutrition Monitoring Tools for Organ Transplant Recipients during the Immediate Posttransplant Phase

Monitoring Tool	Suggested Frequency
Indirect calorimetry	When it is difficult to estimate caloric needs and when a patient is receiving adequate nutrition according to estimates but is not thriving
Body weight	Daily
Fluid intake and output	Every 8 to 12 hours and daily
Nutrient intake	Daily until adequate
Serum glucose concentration	Every 6 hours initially, less when level normalizes
Serum potassium concentration	Daily
Serum phosphorus level	At least twice per week
Serum bicarbonate level	Daily for small-intestine and pancreas transplant recipients
Serum magnesium level	Once or twice per week

Source: Data from ref 37.

is anticipated that a patient will be able to eat by this time and the patient previously has shown that he/she can eat well. When a patient is eating well, a low-fat, heart-healthy diet can be initiated.

Tube feeding is indicated when a patient requires prolonged ventilatory support or for some other reason is unable to eat adequate amounts to meet his or her needs. If a patient has not eaten well before the transplant procedure and is malnourished, tube feeding should be initiated as soon after transplantation as possible. Nasointestinal tubes are the tubes of choice because they pose little risk for infection compared to surgically placed tubes; they are easily removed; and, if the tip is placed into the third portion of the duodenum, early postoperative feeding can be initiated. Reduced-carbohydrate, high-fat formulas should be considered if hypercarbia prevents ventilator weaning.[37] Patients who received a lung transplant for cystic fibrosis may experience fat malabsorption and require a low-fat formula or treatment with pancreatic enzymes.

TPN is restricted to patients who have failed tube feeding or who do not have adequate gastrointestinal function. Typically, a concentrated solution is required to provide adequate calories and protein in minimal volume. Exhibit 14–2 provides a sample of a TPN solution.

Kidney Transplantation

Kidney transplant recipients almost always eat the day after their transplant; rarely is tube feeding or TPN required.[9,38] Many renal-failure patients are accustomed to restricting their fluid, potassium, and phosphorus intake. Because fluids and electrolytes are lost when a transplanted kidney begins to produce significant

---

Exhibit 14–2 Typical TPN Solution for an Organ Transplant Patient

Patient: 45-year-old male, 5'10" tall, 70 kg
Estimated requirements: 2100 kilocalories (1.3 × BEE), 105 g protein (1.5 g/kg body weight)

Substrate and Initial Concentration	Volume
15% amino acids	700 mL
$D_{70}W$	500 mL
20% lipid solution	240 mL

Sample TPN solution infused at 60 mL/hour for 24 hours provides 2090 kilocalories, 105 g protein, 71% of nonprotein calories as dextrose.

amounts of urine, many patients must be encouraged to increase fluid intake when their kidney begins to function. Depending upon the degree of renal function and the effect of immunosuppressive drugs, dietary potassium and phosphorus intakes may need to be altered.

Liver Transplantation

Nutritional requirements of liver transplant recipients have been studied more thoroughly than those of other organ transplant populations. Resting energy expenditure (REE) measured by indirect calorimetry and nitrogen excretion measured by urinary urea nitrogen (UUN) have been studied by several researchers. Delafosse et al[48] evaluated 8 patients and found REE to be 36% to 38% above the predicted BEE, with UUN values of 20.1 and 24.6 g, respectively, on the first two posttransplant days. Another group's evaluation of 11 patients determined REE to be 7% above BEE, with UUN excretion of 12.9 ± 4.4 g on the third postoperative day.[49] Plevak and colleagues[50] determined REE and nitrogen balance in 28 patients pretransplant and on posttransplant days 1, 3, 5, 14, and 28. The REE did not change significantly over time, and the BEE + 20% met measured REE needs. Nitrogen excretion peaked at day 3 and returned to preoperative levels by posttransplant day 28; mean nitrogen balance was negative during the study period, despite administration of nutrition support. In a study by Hasse et al,[51] 31 patients underwent measurement of REE and UUN on posttransplant days 2, 4, 7, and 12. The mean REE rose gradually during the study period, and the greatest REE was 27% above the calculated BEE. Daily UUN losses ranged from 9.6 ± 5.1 g to 11.7 ± 6.3 g for unfed patients and 2.9 ± 4.3 g to 15.0 ± 7.7 g for tube-fed patients.

Achievement of adequate oral intake usually takes several days in liver transplant recipients. As with other transplant types, snacks and supplements frequently are required to help patients achieve adequate intake. With shortened hospitalizations, many outpatients should continue to be monitored for adequate intake.

Benefits of early posttransplant tube feeding have been studied by three groups of researchers. First, Wicks and colleagues[52] compared enteral to parenteral nutrition support in 24 liver transplant recipients. The patients were randomized to receive either tube feeding via a nasojejunal feeding tube 18 hours after surgery (N = 14) or TPN. Up to 60 hours were required to initiate TPN. No significant differences between the groups were found in relation to time of initiation of oral diet, intestinal absorption capacity, anthropometric measurements, or infection rates. In a second study, surgically placed jejunostomies were used for tube feeding in 108 liver transplant patients, and a retrospective evaluation was reported.[53,54] A full-strength, semielemental formula was initiated within 12 to 48 hours after transplantation, with a goal achieved 24 to 48 hours later. The researchers concluded that jejunal feeding was well tolerated and reduced the need for TPN. However, 18 complications from the jejunostomy tube occurred in 16 patients (6 kinked tubes, 6 infections or perforations, 2 tube displacements, 2 intestinal obstructions, 2 miscellaneous complications). In seven instances, surgery was required to correct the complications. In a third study of early posttransplant patients, tube feeding ($N = 14$) using nasointestinal tubes placed during surgery was compared with diet and intravenous fluid ($N = 17$).[51] Tube feeding was initiated 12 hours posttransplant using a semielemental formula at 20 mL/hr. Goal rates were reached 36 to 48 hours later. All patients began to eat by about the third posttransplant day. The tube-fed group had greater initial calorie and protein intakes and a more rapid improvement in nitrogen balance compared with controls. In addition, infection rates (viral, bacterial, overall) tended to decrease in the tube-fed population.

For liver transplant recipients, as with other transplant patients, TPN is limited to patients with nonfunctioning gastrointestinal tracts. Initiation of immediate posttransplant tube feeding seems to decrease the use of TPN.

Pancreas Transplantation

Frequently, pancreas transplants are performed at the same time as kidney transplants in diabetic patients. Patients usually are not allowed to eat until about 5 days posttransplant,[55] and slow dietary progression may be required. Many pancreas transplant patients have a history of diabetic gastroparesis, and delayed gastric emptying commonly occurs after transplantation; anesthesia and analgesia exacerbate this complication.[56] Diabetic diets are not required unless the patient experiences hyperglycemia.

Some centers propose administering TPN to pancreas transplant recipients until oral intake is adequate.[55] Parenteral nutrition may be required if a patient develops pancreatitis requiring gut rest. The initiation of TPN may be delayed a few days after transplantation to prevent hyperglycemia. Because hyperglycemia is one symptom of a poorly functioning pancreas transplant, it is important to avoid confusing symptoms of poor graft function with symptoms of high-dextrose infusion.

Some centers place nasointestinal tubes during surgery to allow for early postoperative tube feeding during the period when oral intake is inadequate. Tube feeding also is indicated when oral intake remains inadequate but gut function is acceptable.

Some nutritional considerations are unique to pancreas transplant recipients. Exocrine secretions of the transplanted pancreas are commonly diverted through the bladder and urinary system; the head of the pancreas is connected to the recipient's bladder, using a segment of the donor duodenum.[55,56] The resulting loss of bicarbonate requires replacement. Patients can lose 2 to 3 liters of fluid per day through pancreatic-urinary drainage. Without adequate fluid replacement, dehydration will occur. Patients may require up to 5 liters of fluid per day. Some patients may require intravenous fluid administration, if they are unable to drink enough fluid. Exocrine juice production usually slows by the third posttransplant month.[55] Pancreas transplant recipients may develop posttransplant diabetes from drugs such as cyclosporine, tacrolimus, or corticosteroids.

Small-Bowel Transplantation

Small-bowel transplantation is an alternative for individuals who are TPN dependent. During the immediate posttransplant phase, TPN is required until gut function begins (about 1 to 2 weeks after transplantation). Function of the gut is noted by the establishment of output from the terminal ileostomy.[57,58] During rejection and infection episodes, intestinal function declines, and TPN may be required.

The goal of intestinal transplantation is to allow normal digestion and absorption of food. Once gut function is established, a clear liquid diet usually is initiated. Full liquid diets should be avoided; fat malabsorption can occur because the lacteals and lymphatics, used for long-chain fatty acid absorption, are severed during the transplant.[59] In addition, lactase can be deficient in the early posttransplant phase, affecting lactose digestion. A low-fat diet is the next step in the progression to a general diet. Patients often have long histories of food aversions, so achieving adequate oral intake after small-bowel transplantation can be difficult. Tube feeding may be required as a transition between TPN and oral diet.

Many types of feeding tubes have undergone trials with small-bowel transplant recipients—nasogastric, nasoduodenal, gastric with postpylorus extensions, and jejunostomy tubes.[57,60] A semielemental formula supplemented with glutamine theoretically may be the best-tolerated formula,[59] but intact protein and elemental formulas also have been used.[57,60]

Other nutrition concerns are particular to small-bowel transplant recipients. Nutrient absorption can be inconsistent, with intestinal transit time varying from 30 minutes to 5 hours.[60] Likewise, ostomy output can range from minimal to greater than 4 liters per day. Fluid, zinc, electrolytes, and bicarbonate must be replaced.[60]

IMMUNOSUPPRESSION

While the body's immune system is very complex and effective in warding off infection and disease, rejection can mean loss of graft and life for some recipients. Therefore, controlling the rejection response is a primary goal following organ transplantation. Immunosuppressive drugs (see Table 14–4) act in a variety of ways to affect or change the body's normal immune response to the foreign material (transplanted graft).

Table 14–4 Immunosuppressive Medications, Mechanisms of Action, and Side Effects

Drug	Mechanism of Action	Side Effects
Cyclosporin A (Sandimmune, Neoral)	Inhibits the response of cytotoxic T cells to interleukin-2 (IL-2) and prevents helper T lymphocytes from producing IL-2	Nephrotoxicity Neurotoxicity (eg, headache, tremor, seizure) Hypertension Hyperglycemia Hyperlipidemia Hyperkalemia Hypomagnesemia Gingival hyperplasia
Tacrolimus (Prograf, FK506)	Inhibits the proliferation of cytotoxic T cells and the synthesis of IL-2	Nephrotoxicity Neurotoxicity Hypertension Hyperglycemia (diabetogenic effects) Hyperkalemia Nausea and vomiting Gastrointestinal symptoms (eg, diarrhea)
Corticosteroids (prednisone, prednisolone, Solu-Medrol, Solu-Cortef)	Anti-inflammatory response at the arterial site Inhibits IL-1 and decreases IL-2, which suppresses lymphocyte proliferation and decreases circulating lymphocytes	Altered fluid/electrolyte balance Hypertension Adrenal-axis suppression Mood swings (depression, euphoria) Peptic ulcer disease Hyperphagia Hyperglycemia Osteoporosis Hyperlipidemia Poor wound healing Cataracts

continues

Table 14–4 continued

Drug	Mechanism of Action	Side Effects
Azathioprine (Imuran)	Inhibits RNA and DNA synthesis to prevent cytotoxic T cell and B cell proliferation and antibody production	Bone marrow suppression (leukopenia, thrombocytopenia, pancytopenia) Nausea and vomiting Diarrhea Macrocytic anemia Hepatotoxicity
Mycophenolate mofetil (Cellcept, RS-61443)	Decreases lymphocyte activation and replication by suppressing enzymes in the purine salvage pathway, creating a purine deficiency thus inhibiting T and B cell proliferation Suppressed antibody formation	Gastrointestinal symptoms (eg, nausea, vomiting, diarrhea) Leukopenia
Antithymocyte globulin (ATGam)	Decreases circulating lymphocytes	Anaphylactic reaction Fever and chills Nausea and vomiting Leukopenia
Muromonab-CD3 (Orthoclone OKT3)	Binds to mature T cells to decrease their effector function	Anaphylactic reaction Pulmonary edema (usually first dose only) Severe flu-like symptoms Headache Increased incidence of lymphoproliferative disorders
Sirolimus (Rapamycin)	Inhibits T and B cell proliferation while not affecting IL-2 production	Possible hyperglycemia Possible gastrointestinal symptoms Hyperlipidemia
15-Deoxysperagualin	Inhibits T and B lymphocytes	Leukopenia Thrombocytopenia Gastrointestinal symptoms

Source: Data from refs 61, 62–67.

The immune system includes a nonspecific, innate response by providing barriers such as skin, mucous membranes, ciliated cells, gastric acid, and natural immunoglobulins. The specific or acquired immune response is provided by T and B lymphocytes. T lymphocytes mediate the acute cellular rejection that occurs in the vast majority of patients. Helper T lymphocytes and recipient macrophages recognize the graft's foreign antigens, initiating increased production of T lymphocytes, interleukins, and antibodies, and eventually causing anti-inflammatory cells to attach to the donor endothelium. Fortunately, several immunosuppressive drugs can stop this process at different metabolic sites.[61] B lymphocytes, as part of the humoral immune response, react by producing antibodies to destroy foreign antigens. These antibodies are the primary cause of chronic rejection, as they activate the complement system and attract platelets. These platelets and fibrin attach to the graft's vascular system, causing ischemia, chronic rejection, and eventually graft loss.[61]

In patients with preformed antibodies, a hyperacute rejection response can occur within a very short time after recirculation of the graft; this is most commonly seen in renal transplantation. While prevention of hyperacute rejection includes avoidance of positive lymphocyte crossmatches and elimination of transplanting among different ABO blood groups, the only treatment is removal of the graft.[61]

A wide variety of immunosuppressive drug combination therapies is used, depending upon the organs transplanted, patient and graft health status, drug action and side effects, and program philosophy. The most commonly used drugs, mechanism of action, and side effects are listed in Table 14–4.[61,62–67]

Given the necessity of immunosuppressive drugs for patient and graft survival, one of the dietitian's roles on the transplant team is to treat or help patients adapt to nutritional changes caused by drug side effects. The side effects with nutritional implications can generally be divided into three categories: gastrointestinal, metabolic, and hematological. These side effects, along with general suggestions for nutritional intervention, are listed in Table 14–5.

Posttransplant infections are somewhat predictable based on the length of time since transplant. Infections in the initial posttransplant period (1 month) tend to be bacterial (wound, pneumonia, and intravenous-line related). Subsequent infections can be categorized as persistent (cytomegalovirus, Epstein-Barr virus, or hepatitis B or C viruses), community-acquired (influenza and bacteria), and opportunistic (cryptococcus, pneumocystis, aspergillosis, etc).[68–70] The lung is a frequent site of infection in thoracic transplant recipients due to the poor cough response with denervated organs.[70] Chronic viral hepatitis (B or C) in liver transplant recipients, whether newly acquired or recurrent, is a long-term management issue, often requiring decreases in immunosuppressive therapy.

Table 14–5 Immunosuppressive Medication Side Effects and Dietary Management

Side Effects	Potential Nutrition Therapy
Gastrointestinal	
Nausea and vomiting	Diet as tolerated
	Antiemetics
Anorexia	Diet as tolerated
	Six small feedings per day
	Nutrient-dense food choices
	Nutritional supplements
Increased appetite	Structured eating habits
(hyperphagia)	Behavior-modification techniques
	Avoidance of high-calorie foods
Altered taste perception	Varied food flavors and textures
Diarrhea	Diet as tolerated
	Adequate fluid intake
	Antidiarrheals if stool culture negative
Sore mouth/throat	Diet as tolerated
	Adequate fluid intake
Gingival hypertrophy	Diet as tolerated
	Appropriate dental hygiene
Abdominal pain/cramps	Six small feedings per day
	Limited air swallowing (straw use)
Peptic ulcer disease	Diet as tolerated
Metabolic	
Hypertension	Low-sodium diet (2 to 3 g/day)
	Regular exercise program
	Maintain appropriate weight
Hyperkalemia	Potassium-restricted diet (30 to 40 mEq/1000 calories)
Hyperlipidemia	American Heart Association Step 1 diet
	Maintain or reach appropriate weight
	Regular exercise program
Hyperglycemia	Calorie-appropriate, balanced diet
	Maintain or reach appropriate weight
	Regular exercise program
	Insulin or oral hypoglycemic agent
Hypercalciuria	Increase calcium intake
Hypophosphatemia	Increase phosphorus intake or take supplement
Hypomagnesemia	Increase magnesium intake or take supplement

continues

Table 14–5 continued

Side Effects	Potential Nutrition Therapy
Osteoporosis/osteopenia	1500 mg calcium per day
	Regular exercise program
	Maintain appropriate weight
Increased protein	
catabolism	Increase protein intake
Hematologic	
Leukopenia	
Thrombocytopenia	
Macrocytic anemia	Folate supplement

Source: Data from refs 61, 62–67.

LONG-TERM POSTTRANSPLANT NUTRITIONAL CONCERNS

Long-Term Posttransplant Nutritional Requirements

The objective of the dietitian in the long-term posttransplant phase is to help patients achieve and maintain good nutritional status and healthy lifestyles. Too often, recipients' long-term health and lifestyles are compromised by one or several of the following common nutrition-related complications: obesity or excessive weight gain, hyperlipidemia, diabetes, hypertension, osteoporosis, and renal insufficiency. These complications can decrease a recipient's quality of life significantly or result in death. Table 14–6 lists the usual nutrient requirements in the long-term posttransplant period.[20,39,71–74]

Obesity or Excessive Weight Gain

Causes

Because many transplant recipients are malnourished pretransplant, they often need to regain some weight posttransplant to help return them to good health. However, many patients exceed their goal weight or fail to maintain an appropriate weight. Reasons for this include increased appetite and dietary intake, resolved anorexia or other eating difficulties, liberalized diet restrictions, poor eating habits, the "I can eat anything I want" or "It won't happen to me" attitude, steroid-induced hyperphagia, increased participation in food-centered social events, resolved maldigestion and malabsorption, inadequate activity and exercise, and genetic predisposition. A primary predictive factor for posttransplant obesity is preexisting pretransplant obesity.[75] A review of the natural history of weight gain

Table 14–6 General Long-Term Posttransplant Nutritional Requirements

Nutrient	Recommendation
Calories	Estimated basal energy expenditure + 20%
	Adjust for activity, weight gain or loss
Protein	1.0–1.2 g/kg body weight
	Adjust for decreased renal function
Fat	<30% of total calories as fat
	<10% of total calories as saturated fat
	Low cholesterol (<300 mg/day)
Carbohydrates	50–60% calories
	Limit simple sugars
Sodium	2–4 g/day
Calcium	1200–1500 mg/day
Vitamin/minerals	Adjust or supplement according to individual needs

Source: Adapted with permission from J. Hasse, Nutritional aspects of liver transplantation. In: R.W. Bussttil, G.B. Klintman, eds. *Transplantation of the Liver,* pp. 359–367, © 1996, Philadelphia: W.B. Saunders Company.

in 28 patients pre- and post-liver transplant found that 11 out of 28 (39.3%) patients were overweight (based on dry weight) pretransplant, while 18 out of 28 (64.3%) were overweight posttransplant (at 7 to 96 months' follow-up).[76] All 11 patients who were obese before transplant were obese after transplant.

Treatment

Obesity is common among all organ transplant populations,[12,30,77–82] and it is a concern because of its interrelationship with hyperlipidemia, cardiac disease, posttransplant diabetes, increased pressure on often fragile bones, and general mobility issues. For normal or underweight patients, prevention of obesity following transplant, while difficult, is easier than subsequent weight loss. Success seems to entail careful, moderately disciplined eating habits (including decreased snacking) and steady progress in an aerobic exercise program. Obese patients who are successful in maintaining or decreasing weight posttransplant do so by embarking on a very disciplined approach to eating, employing a variety of behavior-modification techniques, and participating in a regular exercise program for at least 30 minutes per day.

The evolution of immunosuppressive drug therapy may help in the control of weight gain in transplant patients. The US Multicenter FK506 Liver Transplant Study Group reported a decreased tendency for weight gain in liver transplant patients in the first posttransplant year if they were taking tacrolimus (FK506) instead of cyclosporine, presumably due to the decreased prednisone dose associated with tacrolimus.[75]

Hyperlipidemia

Causes

Posttransplant hyperlipidemia has become a major focus in solid organ transplantation. Pretransplant lipid levels, basal hyperinsulinism, diet, renal function, proteinuria, beta-blockers, and diuretics are theorized to contribute to posttransplant hyperlipidemia. Immunosuppressive agents also predispose transplant recipients to elevated serum lipid levels. Hepatic lipoprotein production and adipocyte hormone-sensitive lipase are stimulated by corticosteroids, and hepatic lipoprotein synthesis is fueled by free fatty acids released from stored triglycerides.[83] In addition, corticosteroids increase lipoprotein lipase activity and interfere with low-density lipoprotein cholesterol receptor function. In the presence of cyclosporine, free cholesterol excretion can be blocked through an inhibition of bile acid production; an abnormal interaction between low-density lipoprotein receptors and their ligands also can occur.[83] There seems to be a greater incidence of hyperlipidemia among cyclosporine-treated versus tacrolimus-treated patients; still unknown is whether this finding is caused by a single drug effect on lipid metabolism or is the result of tacrolimus patients receiving less corticosteroids.[84]

Prevalence

Development of hyperlipidemia following cardiac transplant has been well described as an important risk factor affecting the development of coronary vasculopathy (intimal thickening) and eventual graft loss. Hyperlipidemia is also common following renal transplant (70%), with cardiovascular disease being the second major cause of morbidity and mortality after infection. This condition often is aggravated or accentuated by concurrent diabetes and preexisting atherosclerosis. Patients receiving a pancreas-renal transplant generally experience a decrease in serum cholesterol and triglyceride levels; however, the lipoprotein profile still may not match that of the normal population (increased very-low-density lipoprotein particles and low-density and high-density lipoprotein triglycerides). Continued insulin resistance and altered peripheral and hepatic insulin levels are the proposed mechanisms causing lipid abnormalities.[85]

As long-term (10 years and beyond) success is being achieved in the liver transplant population, more attention is being devoted to the issues of hyperlipidemia and cardiovascular disease, including the occurrence rates, successful therapies, and whether implications are the same on patient survival as in the heart and renal transplant populations. The literature suggests increased cholesterol levels and increased triglycerides occur in post-liver transplant patients.[78,80,86]

Treatment

Some success in reducing serum lipid levels in renal transplant patients has been reported,[87,88] but traditional diet therapy often is inadequate in producing meaningful changes in lipid levels. Researchers have hypothesized that withdrawal of corticosteroids reduces serum cholesterol levels; however, randomized studies have shown that even though cholesterol levels decline with steroid withdrawal, high-density lipoprotein levels also decrease, resulting in no change to cardiac risk.[89] Traditional drug therapies are used with care because of side effects. For example, cholestyramine binds cyclosporine unless taken at least 4 hours after or 1 hour before cyclosporine; niacin can be hepatotoxic; and HMG-CoA reductase inhibitors (pravastatin, simvastatin, lovastatin) can cause rhabdomyolysis.[83,86] Kobashigawa et al[90] reported that aggressive therapy with low-dose (20–40 mg/day) pravastatin from the time of heart transplant resulted in lower cholesterol levels, fewer episodes of rejection with hemodynamic compromise, better 1-year survival, and a lower incidence of vasculopathy, as compared with a nontreatment group. Bastani et al[91] found that a low-calorie, low-fat, low-cholesterol diet can help stabilize cholesterol levels and weight while not actually significantly decreasing these levels. They found that diet therapy and gemfibrozil (fibric acid derivative) minimally decreased cholesterol and modestly decreased hypertriglycerides. In another study, Pollock and colleagues[92] found that simvastatin was beneficial in decreasing cholesterol levels (mean reduction, 16.5%) and triglyceride levels (mean reduction, 21%) in 43 patients over a range of 7 to 30 months following renal transplant.[92] Research on the benefits and risks of drug therapies continues to be reported in the literature. As with any posttransplant complication, all of the risk factors that promote hyperlipidemia should be reviewed and treated appropriately.

Diabetes

Causes

The development of posttransplant diabetes mellitus probably is due to the mechanisms of steroid-induced insulin resistance and/or cyclosporine and tacrolimus inhibition of pancreatic islet cell function and insulin release.[93] The diabetogenicity of tacrolimus is probably slightly higher than cyclosporine; the percentage of patients who develop diabetes from these two drugs is equal, but the effects of steroids are not as pronounced in tacrolimus patients because of the lower dosage.[94] Risk factors for the development of posttransplant diabetes mellitus include increased body weight, a positive family history, recipient of a cadaveric renal transplant, older age, and black or Hispanic ethnicity.[95]

Prevalence

Posttransplant diabetes mellitus occurs in 3% to 46% of transplant patients, depending upon the transplanted organ, length of follow-up, and criteria used. Over one half of the incidences of posttransplant diabetes are diagnosed within the first few weeks after transplantation. Pancreas transplant recipients can develop posttransplant diabetes that is seen in other organ transplant groups. This outcome is often a sign of pancreas graft rejection or ischemia.[93] Patients may also reacquire diabetes as a side effect of immunosuppressive drugs.[72,93]

Treatment

Treatment includes the traditional diabetes management tools of diet therapy, weight maintenance or reduction, a regular exercise program, and hypoglycemic agents and/or insulin. Minimizing immunosuppressive drug dosages also can be beneficial in bringing blood glucose levels under control, as shown by the quantity of patients who only require drug therapy for a short time until they reach stable maintenance levels of their immunosuppressants. Achieving control of diabetes also can decrease serum triglyceride levels.

Hypertension

Posttransplant hypertension (sustained blood pressure levels >140/90 mm Hg) has been well documented as a significant complication in all types of solid organ transplantation, occurring in 50% to 80% of patients on cyclosporine-based immunosuppression. Less hypertension is seen in pancreas-renal transplant recipients, presumably due to the large volume of exocrine secretions lost via the bladder, with subsequent large sodium bicarbonate requirements.[70] The development of hypertension is related to an underlying renal insufficiency and the nephrotoxic side effects of immunosuppressive drugs; most noteworthy are cyclosporine and tacrolimus. Cyclosporine and tacrolimus are thought to cause hypertension via widespread vasoconstriction, which produces systemic hypertension and decreases the renal blood flow.[70,96–98] Hypertension is usually diagnosed in the first few weeks posttransplant. Dietary treatment includes modest sodium restriction (2–4 g/day) and maintenance of appropriate weight through diet and exercise.[96]

Although many patients require drug therapy for hypertension following transplant, side effects of the drugs often impede quality of life, due to severe edema, headache, and/or postural intolerance. Drug therapy must be adapted to individual needs.

Osteoporosis/Osteopenia

Osteopenic bone disease is a common morbidity factor in solid organ transplantation. Many patients already have some degree of pretransplant osteopenic bone disease due to the disease process itself and to decreased physical activity, extensive diuretic use, smoking, decreased estrogen levels in women, hyperparathyroidism, and poor nutritional status. Patients' conditions are often aggravated posttransplantation by the chronic administration of corticosteroids and cyclosporine, which cause a high-turnover osteopenia.

The occurrence of osteopenia in cardiac transplantation has not been well defined. Van Cleemput et al[99] prospectively reviewed bone mineral density (BMD) in 33 males undergoing cardiac transplantation and found that values for lumbar spine BMD were 90% of expected at the time of hospital dismissal following transplant. BMD decreased further when remeasured 1-year posttransplantation, with an 8.5% further decrease in lumbar spine and 10.4% decrease in femoral neck BMD. Also, 5 of the 33 patients suffered vertebral compression fractures during the first year posttransplantation. Many patients with chronic renal failure also have decreased BMD due to the renal osteodystrophy process. Again, their conditions are exacerbated by corticosteroid administration posttransplantation. Patients undergoing combined pancreas and renal transplantation probably have the same concerns about bone disease, based on their renal failure. The natural history of osteodystrophy after combined transplant has not been well documented. Researchers have described osteopenic bone disease occurring in the setting of chronic liver disease, especially primary biliary cirrhosis, primary sclerosing cholangitis, and some autoimmune chronic active hepatitis (due to steroids).[100,101] For patients on cyclosporine-prednisone-azathioprine antirejection therapy, BMD decreases further posttransplantation in primary biliary cirrhosis and primary sclerosing cholangitis patients with the low point occurring from 3 to 6 months posttransplantation.[102] Then BMD appears to stabilize and improve over subsequent years of follow-up. However, patients transplanted for other diseases who start with a relatively good BMD may experience a decrease in BMD over time. Avascular necrosis of hips and knees also plagues liver transplant recipients. Suggested therapies for prevention and management of osteopenia are listed in Exhibit 14–3.

Renal Insufficiency

Evaluation of posttransplant renal insufficiency is important for its role in predicting the development or exacerbation of hypertension, diabetes, and hyperlipidemia. Such an evaluation is characterized by a normal urine volume and the absence of proteinuria. However, tests indicate a decreased glomerular filtration glomerulofiltration rate, increased serum creatinine concentration, decreased urea secretion with increased azotemia, increased serum potassium and urate levels due to decreased renal excretion, renal tubular acidosis with decreased bicarbonate resorption, and decreased urinary sodium excretion leading to a sodium avid state.[70]

Management of renal insufficiency in transplant recipients involves the traditional therapy. Evaluation and treatment of renal artery stenosis or other mechanical or structural defects, especially in renal recipients, should be completed. Re-

Exhibit 14–3 Appropriate Therapy for Prevention and Maintenance of Osteopenic Bone Disease

- adequate calcium intake of 1200 to 1500 mg/day via diet and supplements
- well-balanced diet
- adequate vitamin D intake
- minimal use of corticosteroids posttransplantation
- hormonal-replacement therapy when appropriate
- regular exercise program
- education regarding appropriate body mechanics
- timely management of fractures and avascular necrosis
- moderate sodium intake
- no smoking

Source: Data from refs 99, 100.

ductions in immunosuppressants without precipitating rejection can be helpful. Several groups studied the effects of reduced-protein diets on renal insufficiency (primarily renal transplants) and found that such diets may result in a decrease in the glomerular growth rate, thereby enabling the patients to avoid glomerulo-hypertrophy. Restricting dietary protein intake while maintaining nitrogen balance and adequate caloric intake and weight can be a struggle.[101,102]

Nutritional Concerns and Small-Bowel Transplantation

Long-term posttransplant issues for small-bowel transplant recipients are much different than those for recipients of other solid organs. Nutrition therapy is based on graft function and the patient's ability to tolerate enteral feedings, overcome food aversions, and eat adequately. Graft-versus-host disease, infection, and rejection are the primary causes of graft loss. Long-term nutritional implications are yet to be determined.[60,103,104]

CONCLUSIONS

The nutritional care and feeding of solid organ transplant recipients through each of the three phases of the transplant process can be particularly challenging. The dietitian's role in the assessment and subsequent maintenance, prevention, and therapy for the potential nutritional problems is vast and varied. Optimal pretransplant nutritional status and initial posttransplant nutrition therapy can positively affect patient outcome. Long-term nutritional complications and the side effects of immunosuppressive drugs require aggressive prevention and maintenance to ensure long-term survival.

REFERENCES

1. U.S. organ transplants in 1996 show little increase. *UNOS Bull.* 1997;2:2.

2. Hasse JM. Nutritional implications of liver transplantation. *Henry Ford Hosp Med J.* 1990;38:235–240.

3. Shronts EP, Teasley KM, Thoele SL, Cerra FB. Nutrition support of the adult liver transplant candidate. *J Am Diet Assoc.* 1987;87:441–451.

4. Shronts EP. Nutritional assessment of adults with end-stage hepatic failure. *Nutr Clin Pract.* 1988;3:113–119.

5. Munoz SJ. Nutritional therapies in liver disease. *Semin Liver Dis.* 1991;11:278–291.

6. Hasse J, Strong S, Gorman MA, Liepa GU. Subjective global assessment: alternative nutritional assessment technique for liver transplant candidates. *Nutrition.* 1993;9:339–343.

7. Detsky AS, McLaughlin JR, Baker JP, Johnston N, et al. What is subjective global assessment of nutritional status? *J Parenter Enter Nutr.* 1987;11:8–13.

8. Baker JP, Detsky AS, Wesson DE, Woman SL, et al. Nutritional assessment: a comparison of clinical judgment and objective measurements. *N Engl J Med.* 1982;306:969–972.

9. Blue LS. Nutrition considerations in kidney transplantation. *Top Clin Nutr.* 1992;7(3):17–23.

10. Pikul J, Sharpe MD, Lowndes R, Chent CN. Degree of preoperative malnutrition is predictive of postoperative morbidity and mortality in liver transplant recipients. *Transplantation.* 1994;57:469–472.

11. Grady KL, Herold LS. Comparison of nutritional status in patients before and after heart transplantation. *J Heart Transplant.* 1988;7:123–127.

12. Madill J, Maurer JR, deHoyas A. A comparison of preoperative and postoperative nutritional status of lung transplant recipients. *Transplantation.* 1993;56:347–350.

13. Miller DG, Levine SE, D'Elia JA, Bistrian BR. Nutritional status of diabetic and nondiabetic patients after renal transplantation. *Am J Clin Nutr.* 1986;44:66–69.

14. Kopple JD, Berg R, Houser H, Steinman TI, et al. Nutritional status of patients with different levels of chronic renal insufficiency. *Kidney Int.* 1989;36(suppl 27):S184–S194.

15. Slomowitz LA, Monteon FJ, Grosvenor M, Laidlaw SA, et al. Effect of energy intake on nutritional status in maintenance hemodialysis patients. *Kidney Int.* 1989;35:704–711.

16. Young GA, Kopple JD, Lindholm B, Vonesh EF, et al. Nutritional assessment of continuous ambulatory peritoneal dialysis patients: an international study. *Am J Kidney Dis.* 1991;17:462–471.

17. DiCecco SR, Wieners EJ, Wiesner RH, Southorn PA, et al. Assessment of nutritional status of patients with end-stage liver disease undergoing liver transplantation. *Mayo Clin Proc.* 1989;64:95–102.

18. Hehir DJ, Jenkins RL, Bistrian BR, Blackburn GL. Nutrition in patients undergoing orthotopic liver transplant. *J Parenter Enter Nutr.* 1985;9:695–700.

19. Hasse JM, Blue LS, Crippin JS, Goldstein RM, et al. The effect of nutritional status on length of stay and clinical outcomes following liver transplantation. *J Am Diet Assoc.* 1994;94(suppl):A-38.

20. Poindexter SM. Nutrition support in cardiac transplantation. *Top Clin Nutr.* 1992;7(3):12–16.

21. Frazier OH, Van Buren CT, Poindexter SM, Waldenberger F. Nutritional management of the heart transplant recipient. *J Heart Transplant.* 1985;4:450–452.

22. Hasse JM. Nutrition considerations in liver transplantation. *Top Clin Nutr.* 1992;7(3):24–33.

23. Williams JW. Early postoperative care. In: Williams JW, ed. *Hepatic Transplantation.* Philadelphia: WB Saunders Co; 1990:137–162.

24. Ragsdale D. Nutritional program for heart transplantation. *J Heart Transplant.* 1987;6:228–233.

25. Poindexter SM. Nutrition in heart transplantation. *Support Line.* 1992;14:8–9.

26. Rosenberg ME, Hostetter TH. Nutrition. In: Toledo-Pereya LH, ed. *Kidney Transplantation.* Philadelphia: FA Davis Co; 1988:169–186.

27. Evans MA, Shronts EP, Fish JA. A case report: nutrition support of a heart-lung transplant recipient. *Support Line.* 1992;14:1–8.

28. Porayko MK, DiCecco S, O'Keefe SJD. Impact of malnutrition and its therapy on liver transplantation. *Semin Liver Dis.* 1991;11:305–314.

29. Muller MJ, Lautz HU, Plogmann B, Burger M, et al. Energy expenditure and substrate oxidation in patients with cirrhosis: the impact of cause, clinical staging and nutritional state. *Hepatology.* 1992;15:782–794.

30. Merion RM, Twork AM, Rosenberg L, Ham JM, et al. Obesity and renal transplantation. *Surg Gynecol Obstet.* 1991;172:367–376.

31. Holley JL, Shapiro R, Lopatin WB, Tzakis AG, et al. Obesity as a risk factor following cadaveric renal transplantation. *Transplantation.* 1990;49:387–389.

32. Pirsch JD, Armbrust MJ, Knechtle SJ, D'Allesandro AM, et al. Obesity as a risk factor following renal transplantation. *Transplantation.* 1995;59:631–633.

33. Winters GL, Kendall TJ, Radio SJ, Wilson JE, et al. Posttransplant obesity and hyperlipidemia: major predictors of severity of coronary arteriopathy in failed human heart allografts. *Transplantation.* 1990;9:364–371.

34. Keefe EB, Gettys C, Esquivel CO. Liver transplantation in patients with severe obesity. *Transplantation.* 1994;57:309–311.

35. Blue LS, Hasse JM, Levy ML, Jennings LW. Effect of obesity on clinical outcomes in liver transplantation. *J Am Diet Assoc.* 1993;93(suppl):A-49.

36. Hasse J. Role of the dietitian in the nutrition management of adults after liver transplantation. *J Am Diet Assoc.* 1991;91:473–476.

37. Hasse JM, Blue LS, Watkins LA. Solid organ transplantation. In: Gottschlich MM, Matarese LE, Shronts EP, eds. *Nutrition Support Dietetics Core Curriculum.* 2nd ed. Silver Spring, MD: American Society for Parenteral and Enteral Nutrition; 1993:409–421.

38. Hasse J. Nutritional management of renal transplant patients. *Dietetic Curr.* 1993;20:21–24.

39. Edwards MS, Doster S. Renal transplant diet recommendations: results of a survey of renal dietitians in the United States. *J Am Diet Assoc.* 1990;90:843–846.

40. Zabielski P. What are the calorie and protein requirements during the acute postrenal transplant period? *Support Line.* 1992;14:11–13.

41. Kowalchuk D. Nutritional management of the pancreas transplant patient. *Support Line.* 1992;14:10–11.

42. Kumar MR, Coulston AM. Nutritional management of the cardiac transplant patient. *J Am Diet Assoc.* 1983;83:263–265.

43. Hoy WE, Sargent JA, Hall D, McKenna BA, et al. Protein catabolism during the postoperative course after renal transplantation. *Am J Kidney Dis.* 1985;5:186–190.

44. Hoy WE, Sargent JA, Freeman RB, Pabico RC, et al. The influence of glucocorticoid dose on protein catabolism after renal transplantation. *Am J Med Sci.* 1986;291:241–247.

45. Whittier FC, Evans DH, Dutton S, Ross G, et al. Nutrition in renal transplantation. *Am J Kidney Dis.* 1985;6:405–411.

46. Van Buren CT, Kulkarni A, Rudolph F. Synergistic effect of a nucleotide-free diet and cyclosporine on allograft survival. *Transplant Proc.* 1983;15(suppl 1):2967–2968.

47. Van Buren CT, Kulkarni AD, Schandle VB, Rudolph FB. The influence of dietary nucleotides on cell-mediated immunity. *Transplantation.* 1983;36:350–352.

48. Delafosse B, Faure JL, Bouffard Y, Viale JP, et al. Liver transplantation: energy expenditure, nitrogen loss, and substrate oxidation rate in the first two postoperative days. *Transplant Proc.* 1989;21:2453–2454.

49. Shanbhogue RLK, Bistrian BR, Jenkins RL, Randall S, et al. Increased protein catabolism without hypermetabolism after human orthotopic liver transplantation. *Surgery.* 1987;101:146–149.

50. Plevak DJ, DiCecco SR, Wiesner RH, Porayko MK, et al. Nutritional support for liver transplantation: identifying caloric and protein requirements. *Mayo Clin Proc.* 1994;69:225–230.

51. Hasse JM, Blue LS, Liepa GU, Goldstein RM, et al. Early enteral nutrition support in patients undergoing liver transplantation. *J Parenter Enter Nutr.* 1995;19(6):437–443.

52. Wicks C, Somasundaram S, Buarnason I, Menzies IS, et al. Comparison of enteral feeding and total parenteral nutrition after liver transplantation. *Lancet.* 1994;344:837–840.

53. Pescovitz MD, Mehta PL, Leapman SB, Milgrom ML, et al. Tube jejunostomy in liver transplant recipients. *Surgery.* 1995;117:642–647.

54. Mehta PL, Alaka KJ, Filo RS, Leapman SB, et al. Nutrition support following liver transplantation: a comparison of jejunal versus parenteral routes. *Clin Transplant.* 1995;344:837–840.

55. Bartucci MR, Loughman KA, Moir EJ. Kidney-pancreas transplantation: a treatment option for ESRD and type I diabetes. *Am Nephrol Nurs Assoc J.* 1992;19:467–474.

56. Bass M. Pancreas transplantation: detecting rejection and patient care. *Am Nephrol Nurs Assoc J.* 1992;19:476–482.

57. Reyes JD, Tzakis AG, Todo S, Abu-Elmagd K, et al. Post-operative care of small bowel transplant recipients. *Care Critically Ill.* 1993;9:193–194, 196–198.

58. Todo S, Tzakis A, Abu-Elmagd K, Reyes J, et al. Clinical intestinal transplantation. *Transplant Proc.* 1993;25:2195–2197.

59. Nour B, Reyes J, Tzakis A, Todo S, et al. Intestinal transplantation with or without other abdominal organs: nutritional and dietary management of 50 patients. *Transplant Proc.* 1994;26:1432–1433.

60. Reyes J, Tzakis AG, Todo S, Nour B, et al. Nutritional management of intestinal transplant recipients. *Transplant Proc.* 1993;25:1200–1201.

61. Wahrenberger A. Pharmacologic immunosuppression: cure or curse? *Crit Care Nurs Q.* 1995;17:27–36.

62. Ohara MM. Immunosuppression in solid organ transplantation: a nutrition perspective. *Top Clin Nutr.* 1992;7(3):6–11.

63. Manez R, Jain A, Marino IR, Thomson AW. Comparative evaluation of tacrolimus (FK506) and cyclosporine A as immunosuppressive agents. *Transplant Rev.* 1995;9:63–76.

64. Klintmalm GB. FK506: an update. *Clin Transplant.* 1994;8:207–210.

65. Gonwa TA. Mycophenolate mofetil for maintenance therapy in kidney transplantation. *Clin Transplant.* 1996;10:128–130.

66. Mueller AR, Platz KP, Blumhardt G, Bechstein WO, et al. The superior immunosuppressant according to diagnosis: FK506 or cyclosporine A. *Transplant Proc.* 1995;27:1117–1120.

67. Browne BJ, Kahan BD. Transplantation 1994: the year in review. In: Teraski PI, Cecka JM, eds. *Clinical Transplants 1994.* Los Angeles: UCLA Tissue Typing Laboratory; 1994:317–340.

68. Rubin RH. Infectious disease problems. In: Maddrey WS, ed. *Current Topics in Gastroenterology: Transplantation of the Liver.* New York: Elsevier. In press.

69. Dominguez EA. Long-term infectious complications of liver transplantation. *Semin Liver Dis.* 1995;15:133–138.

70. Miller LW. Long-term complications of cardiac transplantation. *Prog Cardiovasc Dis.* 1991;33: 229–282.

71. Fish JA, Mandt J, Brunzell C. Nutritional implications in pancreas transplant recipients. *Top Clin Nutr.* 1993;8:64–73.

72. Vizioli TL, Ishkanian I. Nutrition in pancreas-renal transplantation. *J Renal Nutr.* 1992;2:161–164.

73. Maurer JR. Therapeutic challenges following lung transplantation. *Clin Chest Med.* 1990; 11:279–290.

74. Zetterman RK, McCashland TM. Long-term follow-up of the orthotopic liver transplantation patient. *Semin Liver Dis.* 1995;15:173–180.

75. Mor E, Facklam D, Hasse J, Sheiner P, et al for the US Multicenter FK506 Study Group. Weight gain and lipid profile changes in liver transplant recipients: long-term results of the American FK506 Multicenter Study. *Transplant Proc.* 1995;27:1126.

76. Palmer M, Schaffner F, Thung SN. Excessive weight gain after liver transplantation. *Transplantation.* 1991;51:797–800.

77. Lake KD, Reutzel TJ, Pritzker MR, Jorgenson CR, et al. The impact of steroid withdrawal on the development of lipid abnormalities and obesity in heart transplant recipients. *J Heart Lung Transplant.* 1993;12:580–590.

78. Mathe D, Adam R, Malmendier C, Gigou M, et al. Prevalence of dyslipidemia in liver transplant recipients. *Transplantation.* 1992;54:167–170.

79. Munoz SJ, Deems RO, Moritz MJ, Martin P, et al. Hyperlipidemia and obesity after orthotopic liver transplantation. *Transplant Proc.* 1991;23:1480–1483.

80. Stegall MD, Everson G, Schroter G, Bilir B, et al. Metabolic complications after liver transplantation. *Transplantation.* 1995;60:1057–1060.

81. Larsen JL, Stratta RJ, Ozaki CF, Taylor RJ, et al. Lipid status after pancreas-kidney transplantation. *Diabetes Care.* 1992;15:35–42.

82. Perkins JD, Frohnert PP, Service FJ, Wilhelm MP, et al. Pancreas transplantation at Mayo: III. multidisciplinary management. *Mayo Clin Proc.* 1990;65:496–508.

83. Perez R. Managing nutrition problems in transplant patients. *Nutr Clin Pract.* 1993;8:28–32.

84. Aboujoud MS, Levy MF, Klintmalm GB, and the US Multicenter Study Group. Hyperlipidemia after liver transplantation: long-term results of the FK506/cyclosporine. A US Multicenter trial. *Transplant Proc.* 1995;27:1121–1122.

85. LaRoca E, Secchi A, Parlavecchia M, Bonfatti D, et al. Lipoprotein profile after combined kidney pancreas transplantation in insulin-dependent diabetes mellitus. *Transplant Int.* 1995;8:190–195.

86. Munoz SJ. Hyperlipidemia and other coronary risk factors after orthotopic liver transplantation: pathogenesis, diagnosis and management. *Liver Transplant Surg.* 1995;1(suppl 1):29–38.

87. Moore RA, Callahan MF, Cody M, Adams PL, et al. The effect of the American Heart Association Step One Diet on hyperlipidemia following renal transplantation. *Transplantation.* 1990;49:60–62.

88. LaRocca E, Ruotolo G, Parlavecchia M, Librenti MC, et al. Dietary advice and lipid metabolism in insulin-dependent diabetes mellitus kidney- and pancreas-transplanted patients. *Transplant Proc.* 1992;24:848–849.

89. Hricik DE, Bartucci MR, Mayes JT, Schulak JA. The effects of steroid withdrawal on the lipoprotein profiles of cyclosporine-treated kidney and kidney-pancreas transplant recipients. *Transplantation.* 1992;54:868–871.

90. Kobashigawa JA, Katznelson S, Laks H, Johnson JA, et al. Effect of pravastatin on outcomes after cardiac transplantation. *N Engl J Med.* 1995;333:621–627.

91. Bastani B, Robinson S, Heisler T, Puntney G, et al. Post-transplant hyperlipidemia: risk factors and response to dietary modification and gemfibrozil therapy. *Clin Transplant.* 1995;9:340–348.

92. Pollock CA, Mahoney JF, Ong CS, Caterson RJ, et al. Hyperlipidemia in renal transplant recipients: does it matter and can we treat it? *Transplant Proc.* 1995;27:2152–2153.

93. Jindal RM. Posttransplant diabetes mellitus—a review. *Transplantation.* 1994;58:1289–1298.

94. Senniger N, Golling M, Datsis K, Sido B, et al. Glucose metabolism following liver transplantation and immunosuppression with cyclosporine A or FK 506. *Transplant Proc.* 1995;27:1127–1128.

95. Friedman EA, Shyh T, Beyer MM, Manis T, et al. Posttransplant diabetes in kidney transplant recipients. *Am J Nephrol.* 1985;5:196–202.

96. Textor SC, Canzenello VJ, Taler SJ, Schwartz L, et al. Hypertension after liver transplantation. *Liver Transplant Surg.* 1995;1(suppl 1):20–28.

97. Luke RG. Pathophysiology and treatment of posttransplant hypertension. *J Am Soc Nephrol.* 1991;2(suppl 1):S37–S44.

98. Monsour HP, Wood RP, Dyer CH, Galati JS, et al. Renal insufficiency and hypertension as long-term complications in liver transplantation. *Sem Liver Dis.* 1995;15:123–132.

99. Van Cleemput J, Daenen W, Nijs J, Geusens P, et al. Timing and quantification of bone loss in cardiac transplant recipients. *Transplant Int.* 1995;8:196–200.

100. Hay JE. Bone disease after liver transplantation. *Liver Transplant Surg.* 1995;1(suppl 1):55–63.

101. Koote AMM, Paul LC. Cyclosporine therapy or dietary protein manipulation in chronic renal allograft rejection. *Transplant Proc.* 1988;20(suppl 3):821–826.

102. Salahudeen AK, Hostetter TH, Raatz SK, Rosenberg ME. Effects of dietary protein in patients with chronic renal transplant rejection. *Kidney Int.* 1992;41:183–190.

103. Tsakis AG, Todo S, Reyes J, Abu-Elmagd K, et al. Clinical intestinal transplantation: focus on complications. *Transplant Proc.* 1992;24:1238–1240.

104. Meijssen MAC, Heineman E. Functional aspects of small bowel transplantation: past, present and future. *Gut.* 1994;35:1338–1341.

CHAPTER 15

HIV and AIDS

Stacey J. Bell, Leah M. Gramlich, Christine Wanke,
Judith C. Hestnes, and Bruce R. Bistrian

INTRODUCTION

Human immunodeficiency virus (HIV) infection is often accompanied by malnutrition, irrespective of the patient's progression toward acquired immune deficiency syndrome (AIDS). The wasting syndrome—weight loss of greater than 10% of usual body weight (UBW) in less than one month—occurs in approximately 80% of AIDS patients at some stage during their illness.[1,2] At present, 17% of HIV-positive patients in the United States are classified as having AIDS with diarrhea and/or wasting as the AIDS-defining illness. This weight loss has significant pathophysiologic and immunologic consequences. In AIDS patients, there is a close correlation between weight loss and mortality: Death occurs at approximately 66% of ideal body weight (54% of lean body mass),[3] and survival times are significantly shortened with weight loss of greater than 20% of UBW.[4] Researchers have suggested that immunodeficiency associated with malnutrition contributes to the immunodeficiency aspect of AIDS.[5,6] With appropriate nutrition support, it may be possible for clinicians to prevent weight loss associated with HIV infection or AIDS. Weight maintenance not only improves survival, but it also gives patients an improved sense of well-being.

MECHANISMS OF WEIGHT LOSS

Weight maintenance requires that energy intake and absorption equal energy expenditure. During AIDS, there is impairment of both energy intake and absorption, in conjunction with altered protein and energy metabolism. During chronic HIV infection, there are also recurrent secondary infections, which contribute to the development of malnutrition (see Exhibit 15–1). Cytokine activity is heightened as a result of the HIV infection and secondary infections and by the presence of tumors in an attempt to fight off these insults. However, the side effects of increased cytokine activity include increased muscle proteolysis and anorexia, which contribute further to malnutrition.[7]

Anorexia

Decreased caloric intake, especially during secondary infections, is the most significant cause of weight loss in patients with AIDS.[8,9] Many factors contribute to poor oral intake. Anorexia is present in 18% to 61% of patients.[4,10] Anorexia may be cytokine-mediated, which can have both central and local effects to reduce intake,[7] especially in the presence of secondary infections. More commonly, severe anorexia may be related to oroesophageal disease associated with secondary viral or fungal infections that alter taste sensation or cause dysphagia (see Table 15–1). Many medications used in the treatment of HIV infection and its related complications also contribute significantly to the development and perpetuation of anorexia and gastrointestinal dysfunction (see Table 15–2). Precipitation of gastrointestinal symptomatology (such as diarrhea and abdominal pain) from an oral diet can lead to a fear of eating (sitophobia) by negative conditioning, which further compromises caloric intake. Central nervous system involvement in AIDS can be associated with problems of chewing and swallowing. In addition, depression may cause a decrease in oral intake.

Exhibit 15–1 Causes of Malnutrition in AIDS

Impairment of Energy Intake and/or Absorption
- impaired oral intake
  - anorexia
  - oroesophageal disease
  - dyschezia, sitophobia
  - depression
- malabsorption
  - small-bowel disease/diarrhea
  - pancreatic insufficiency
  - biliary obstruction/cholestastic
  - HIV enteropathy/HIV infection of the small bowel

Alteration of Energy Metabolism
- hypermetabolism
- protein wasting
- cytokine-mediated effects

Table 15–1 Oral and Esophageal Manifestations of AIDS that Interfere with Food Intake

Condition	Signs and Symptoms
Candidiasis	Pain, dysphagia, odynophagia, nausea, decreased salivation
Cytomegalovirus	Dysphagia, odynophagia, esophagitis, esophageal ulcer
Herpes simplex virus	Dysphagia, odynophagia, esophagitis
Kaposi's sarcoma	Dysphagia, obstruction
Non-Hodgkins lymphoma	Dysphagia
Aphthous ulcers	Pain, dysphagia, odynophagia

Diarrhea

Diarrhea is common in patients with HIV and may be seen at some point in the course of the disease in 30% of 80% of North American and European patients infected with HIV.[11] Diarrhea is a nonspecific term that describes a change in stool frequency or consistency, which may be caused by a wide variety of etiologic factors[12] (see Table 15–3). Diarrhea may present as either large- or small-bowel dysfunction, or it may be caused by a known or unknown pathogen (pathogen negative). Dramatic weight loss accompanies loss of fluids and electrolytes when small-bowel damage is severe and prolonged enough that the small-bowel function begins to deteriorate and malabsorption occurs.[13–16] Macronutrients—particularly fat and lactose, but also carbohydrates and protein—as well as vitamins and micronutrients are malabsorbed. Pathogens (such as mycobacteria or fungi) or tumors that infiltrate the small bowel can also lead to malabsorption, as can pancreatic insufficiency and abnormal enterohepatic circulation of bile acids related to obstructive cholangiopathy. Some patients present with small-bowel dysfunction of unknown etiology; they are pathogen negative.

Diarrhea from large-bowel dysfunction is commonly caused by more invasive and inflammatory diarrheal pathogens than are present in the small bowel. Because the colon serves as more of a storage organ and loss of a nutrient absorptive organ, the weight loss that accompanies colitic diarrhea is often related to the systemic effects of the pathogenic process, such as fever or cytokine release, and the behavioral response to avoid painful or unpleasant symptoms.

Metabolism

Metabolic disturbances that contribute to the development of wasting in AIDS include hypermetabolism and dysregulation of substrate utilization due primarily

Table 15–2 Effects of Drugs Frequently Used in the Treatment of AIDS and AIDS-Related Infections

Drug	Use	Possible Side Effects or Nutrition Interaction
Azidothymidine (AZT)	HIV infection	Nausea, dysgeusia, edema of tongue and lips, mouth ulcers, constipation, reduced serum vitamin B_{12}, diarrhea
Didanosine	HIV infection	Pancreatitis, nausea, diarrhea
Zalcitabine (ddC)	HIV infection	Nausea, diarrhea
Stavudine (d4T)	HIV infection	Nausea, diarrhea
Acyclovir	Herpes simplex	Diarrhea, nausea, vomiting, fatigue, sore throat, dysgeusia, nephrotoxity
Ganciclovir	Cytomegalovirus, resistant herpes viruses	Anorexia
Foscarnet	Cytomegalovirus, hepatitis B, herpes viruses	Nausea, headache, fatigue, neurologic impairment, calcium imbalance, hypophosphatemia, hypomagnesemia, hypokalemia
Rifabutin	*Mycobacterium avium* complex	Possible liver dysfunction, dysgeusia, headache, anorexia, fatigue, malabsorption
Clarithromycin	*Mycobacterium avium* complex	Nausea, diarrhea
Rifampin	*Mycobacterium avium* complex	Hepatitis
Sulfadiazine	*Toxoplasma gondii, pneumocystis carinii*	Nausea, vomiting, anorexia, diarrhea, abdominal pain, altered taste, dyspepsia
Clindamycin	*Toxoplasma gondii*	Nausea, *Clostridium difficile*
Pentamidine	*Pneumocystis carinii*	Nephrotoxicity, nausea, vomiting, hypoglycemia, pancreatitis, folate deficiency, dysgeusia, possible diabetes
Atovaquone	*Pneumocystis carinii*	Drug failure, poorly absorbed in patients with diarrhea; nausea, vomiting, abdominal pain

continues

Table 15–2 continued

Drug	Use	Possible Side Effects or Nutrition Interaction
Amphotericin	Cryptococcal meningitis, fungal infections	Possible decreased potassium and magnesium levels, weight loss, anorexia, nausea, vomiting, diarrhea, severe nephrotoxicity
Fluconazole	Fungal infections	Nausea, abdominal pain, diarrhea
Ketoconazole	Esophageal and oral candidiasis	Nausea, vomiting, abdominal pain, decreased serum sodium
Itraconozole	Antifungal	Hepatitis, nausea, vomiting, diarrhea, hypoalbuminemia
Nystatin	Candidiasis	Diarrhea, nausea, vomiting, fever, gastrointestinal distress
Dapsone	*Pneumocystis carinii*	Nausea, vomiting, oral lesions
Trimethoprim, Sulfamethoxazole	*Pneumocystis carinii*	Pancreatitis, anorexia, hyperkalemia, glucose intolerance, folate deficiency, glossitis, stomatitis, hepatitis

to the presence of cytokines.[7] Energy expenditure has been studied in different stages of HIV infection. Most investigators have found that there is an increase in resting energy expenditure (REE), even in the absence of acute infections.[10,17,18] This metabolic response (increased REE) is abnormal in the setting of semistarvation. Normally, there is a decrease in REE in order to preserve lean body mass (LBM).[3,8] This decrease in REE is an inappropriate response to semistarvation and suggestive of cytokine-mediated cachexia. Excessive production of cytokines (eg, tumor necrosis factor, interferon, and interleukin-1), particularly through their autocrine and paracrine effects, are thought to mediate many of these abnormal metabolic responses in HIV-infected patients.

It is likely that many factors underlie significant weight loss in advanced AIDS. Macallan et al[9] prospectively looked at patterns of weight change and found a close association between acute weight loss episodes and opportunistic infections, particularly those characterized by a marked systemic illness. These infections are likely accompanied by both hypermetabolism and reduction in food intake, ultimately leading to acute weight loss. Chronic progressive weight loss is more commonly associated with gastrointestinal symptoms. It is likely that a combination of impaired intake and malabsorption of nutrients is the prominent reason for this latter pattern of weight loss. Weight gain is also possible after successful treatment of the opportunistic infection and resumption of oral intake.

Table 15–3 Differential Diagnosis of Diarrhea in Patients with HIV

Cause	Small Bowel	Colon/Terminal Ileum
Bacteria	Salmonella*	Campylobacter*
	*Escherichia coli**	Shigella*
	Mycobacterium avium	*Clostridium difficile*
	intracellulare complex*	Yersinia
	*Mycobacterium tuberculosis**	Aeromonas
	Mycobacterium genevenese	
Fungi	Histoplasma*	
	Cryptococcus*	
	Candida	
Viruses	Rotavirus	Cytomegalovirus*
	HIV	Adenovirus
		Herpes simplex
Parasites	*Cryptosporidium parvum**	*Entamoeba histolytica*
	Isopora belli	
	Cyclospora cayatenensis	
	Giardia lamblia	
	Blastocystic hominis	
	Microsporidium	
	*Enterocytozoon bieneusi**	
	*Septata intestinalis**	
Noninfectious	Kaposi's sarcoma*	
	Lymphoma	

*Organism or process can involve both the small bowel and large bowel or the entire gastrointestinal tract, but most commonly occurs in location listed.

NUTRITIONAL ASSESSMENT

Patients with HIV infection or AIDS can be assessed using standard techniques similar to those used with other malnourished patients.[2,18–21] Typical assessment measures are weight, height, body mass index (kg/m^2) percent weight loss, upper arm anthropometry, serum protein (albumin and, less often, prealbumin or retinol-binding protein), and 24-hour urinary creatinine used to calculate a creatinine-height index. However, each measurement needs to be interpreted with caution. Weight is usually reliable if edema is not present. Serum proteins can fluctuate, depending upon total body water or the presence of inflammation, and they can drop abruptly when patients have a secondary infection.[20]

Prevalence of Malnutrition

Hospitalized Patients

About half of all medical and surgical patients routinely seen in urban teaching hospitals are malnourished as measured by standard assessment techniques and criteria.[22,23] For patients with HIV, the percentage is higher. For example, the nutritional status of 49 HIV admissions to a Boston tertiary-referral hospital were evaluated for weight change and serum albumin concentrations. The average weight loss was 15%, with a mean albumin level of 3.2 g/dL; 84% of patients were malnourished, about 34% more than typically seen in non-HIV populations.[2]

Outpatients

If hospitalized patients with AIDS represent a more critically ill group of patients, then outpatients with AIDS might be expected to be less severely malnourished. Chlebowski and collaborators[4] evaluated the nutritional status of 71 AIDS patients from the University of California at a Los Angeles clinic. Of those surveyed, 98% had lost weight, with 68% experiencing weight loss in excess of 10%. Almost half (42%) of these patients were classified as having moderate to severe malnutrition. The hypoalbuminemia seen in hospitalized patients was present in 83% of this group as well. Most (60%) of the patients had serum albumin concentrations in a suboptimal range of 2.5 to 3.5 g/dL. Fewer (23%) were severely hypoalbuminemic; mean albumin levels were 2.9 g/dL. Hypoalbuminemia at these very low concentrations in the hospital and outpatient setting could be associated with an acute infectious episode or chronic exposure to HIV, or both. Serum albumin levels fall as a result of the acute phase response to infection as a consequence of reduced rates of albumin synthesis and increased catabolic rates, but the falling levels are principally due to extracellular extravasation to achieve a new and lower intravascular to extravascular equilibrium.[24] Additionally, the presence of HIV infection for a period of several years may produce hypoalbuminemia. Serum albumin concentrations have been shown to be lower in patients with AIDS than in those with HIV that has not progressed to AIDS.[10] Nonetheless, serum albumin levels should be obtained every 6 months, and abnormal values should be evaluated to explain their etiology (malnutrition versus infection).

Body Composition

A group of German investigators[25] established that the bioelectric impedance analysis (BIA) method (RJL model 109, RJL Systems, Detroit, Michigan) was extremely sensitive to subtle changes in body composition of HIV-seropositive patients who had not developed AIDS. The study included 193 HIV-seropositive patients of whom 82 fell within the Walter Reed (WR) classification for AIDS (WR-6). Those in WR-2 had significantly reduced body cell mass (BCM), despite unchanged weight and body mass index (BMI). Moreover, the group's extracellular mass (ECM) and the ratio of ECM to BCM was significantly increased, indicating that lean tissue was lost. It is likely that BCM was replaced with water, which explains why weight and BMI could remain constant. Body fat became significantly reduced only in the WR-6 group. The authors of this study attempted to explain the loss of BCM by the presence of diarrhea but found a correlation only when the number of stools exceeded 20 per day. They concluded that the use of simple, relatively inexpensive BIA methods accurately detected changes in body composition. It appears prudent to assess the body composition of HIV-seropositive patients before weight loss to establish whether there are increases in ECM or decreases in BCM and in body fat. If any of these changes have occurred, aggressive nutrition support should be considered.

NUTRITIONAL REQUIREMENTS

Macronutrients

Many patients with HIV infection or the AIDS syndrome experience alterations in metabolic processes and declines in caloric intake. It appears prudent to provide the patients with at least enough calories to meet the estimated or measured REE, plus an activity factor (typically a 20% to 30% increase), and to cover the influence of HIV infection and secondary infections (a 5% to 10% increase). It is possible for patients with HIV infection to regain weight after acute weight loss, but the weight increases are usually increases in body fat, because cytokine activity persists and leads to systemic response to the illness. When anorexia due to a response to gastrointestinal symptoms is the principal reason for the development of BCM, lean tissue repletion is possible when adequate nutrition is provided.

Protein requirements vary, depending upon the presence of a secondary infection or a systemic response to primary HIV infection. AIDS patients without secondary infections have a decreased rate of whole body protein turnover,[26] reflecting their malnutrition and the absence of an injury response. Such individuals should maintain lean tissue balance with modest intakes of protein at the Recommended Dietary Allowance (RDA), or slightly higher (1.0 g/kg). Patients experiencing a secondary infection or a systemic response to HIV are likely to have increased catabolic rates and less efficient dietary protein utilization. Although higher protein intakes up to 1.5 g/kg may overcome this inefficiency in some patients with an elevated catabolic response, it is unlikely, if not impossible, for accrual of LBM during active infection without anabolic therapies[8] such as growth hormone.[27] Thus, it is prudent to provide at least the RDA of protein (0.8 g/kg).[27]

For an extra measure of protection, it may be reasonable to recommend that patients receive twice the RDA (1.5 g protein/kg) when weight loss has begun or during active secondary infection. The rationale behind the high-protein diet is similar to the rationale for its use in septic patients: It may help maintain protein stores but not completely prevent protein losses.

The exact proportions of carbohydrate and fat requirements are unknown. The essential fatty acid requirement for linoleic acid is approximately 1% of total calories, and for linolenic acid, less than 1%. There is little evidence to suggest altering the usual ratio of calories: 20% protein, 40% to 60% carbohydrate, 20% to 40% fat. Although there is generally little difficulty in maintaining carbohydrate intake, fat intake may be limited by gastrointestinal intolerance when malabsorption is present. Fluid needs approximate normal values (30 mL/kg). However, patients with diarrhea or vomiting require significantly more fluids to prevent dehydration.

Micronutrients

It is important to provide patients with at least the RDA for all nutrients.[19,28,29] Ideally, this should be done with natural food sources, but it is practical to suggest supplemental multivitamin capsules with trace elements and perhaps beta-carotene.[30] Generally, single vitamins or minerals have not proved efficacious unless there are documented deficiencies. Electrolyte needs are normal, unless there are small- or large-bowel dysfunctions resulting in extraordinary losses. In these patients, sodium, potassium, and bicarbonate needs increase and parenteral supplementation may be warranted. The di- and trivalent cations (calcium, magnesium, and zinc) may become depleted when the patient presents with severe diarrhea.[11] Thus, their concentration should be monitored during periods of severe diarrhea. Unfortunately serum levels of calcium and magnesium are lowered only after severe depletion, and serum zinc levels (which normally reflect intake) also fall with any infection or inflammatory response. It is therefore reasonable to supplement calcium, magnesium, and zinc to a total of 1.5 to 2 times the RDA when severe diarrhea exceeds 1 L/day.

In an extensive study where associations were made between different levels of dietary intake of micronutrients and the progression of HIV infection to AIDS, high intakes of vitamin C, thiamin, and niacin were associated with a significant reduction in the progression to AIDS.[30] In contrast, high zinc intakes were significantly associated with increased progression of disease.

HIV patients have been noted to have low serum selenium levels[31,32]; with supplementation, serum values are normalized. Other studies have identified deficient levels of vitamin C, beta-carotene, zinc, calcium, and magnesium.[33] However, it is not known how often or even whether low serum levels for various nutrients reflect deficiency. More research is needed to determine the optimal regimen of micronutrients.

NUTRITION SUPPORT

Oral Diet

Many HIV patients resort to alternative diet therapies.[28,34,35] As many as one third of 122 HIV-seropositive patients assessed in South Florida used alternative therapies.[36] These included herbs, teas, megadoses of vitamins and minerals, bee propolis, amino acids, cod liver oil, lecithin, and glandular extracts (eg, thymus gland). Of the patients who used excessive doses (over twice the RDA) of vitamins and minerals, 38% also used other unproven nutrition therapies for HIV infection.

As with any therapy, conventional or otherwise, the first objective is to cause no harm. Many alternative therapies meet this criterion, but a dietitian should explore dietary habits using food frequency questionnaires and 24-hour recall to establish safety. Of course the cost-effectiveness of alternative therapies versus conventional diets should be examined. There are no acceptable scientific data to support the use of herbal medicines, garlic, coenzyme Q, immune power diets, yeast-free diets, maximal-immunity type diets, or macrobiotic diets. Moreover, macrobiotic diets can lead to deficiencies of calories, protein, calcium, iron, and vitamin B_{12}.

Anorexia is a common complaint among HIV-positive patients. Many patients have reported that marijuana acts as both an antiemetic and an appetite stimulant. Recently, Dronabinol has been released as an appetite stimulant for AIDS patients and as an antiemetic for oncology patients. Megestrol acetate (Megace®) induces weight gain, but it is significantly more costly than Dronabinol and the weight gain appears to be principally fat.[37] A large, multicenter, randomized clinical trial of growth hormone in AIDS patients with malnutrition recently reported improvement in weight, lean tissue, performance, and quality of life following a 3-month trial.[38]

Oral Supplements

Patients without diarrhea or other symptoms of gastrointestinal dysfunction may benefit from standard oral supplements.[39] These formulas typically contain delactosed milk solids, sugar, and vegetable oils. During the early stages of AIDS, patients who received an oral supplement containing hydrolyzed protein and omega-3 rich fish oil had better weight maintenance and fewer hospitalizations during a 6-month period compared with patients consuming a standard formula.[40] Although these results appear promising, a disproportionate number of patients had contracted HIV infection through intravenous drug use in the fish oil supplement group, which may have biased the results.[41] Circulating cytokine concentrations were shown to be higher in patients who used intravenous drugs (regardless of HIV infection) compared to HIV-infected patients who contracted the disease through homosexual behavior.[42] Supplemental fish oil has been shown to decrease cytokine production from peripheral blood mononuclear cells in normal volunteers,[43] and this same action could have occurred in these HIV-infected patients. As cytokines have been associated with the wasting syndrome, dietary fish oil may have been one factor that accounted for the improvement in nutritional status and decreased morbidity.

In a recent randomized, prospective study, HIV-infected patients without evidence of secondary infections received food bars containing 10 g of either fish oil or safflower oil.[44] After 6 weeks, the fish oil supplemented group showed significant incorporation of the omega-3 fatty acid, docosahexaenoic acid, in the plasma phospholipid fatty acid pools. The fish oil group experienced a significant reduction in the concentration of one of the dienoic eicosanoids and an increase in cytokines released from stimulated peripheral blood mononuclear cells. More work is needed before widespread use of fish oil can be recommended.

Oral supplements may also play a role as an intervention in symptomatic and HIV-infected patients with chronic diarrheal disease. A randomized, double-blinded prospective study[45] was conducted comparing the use of nutritional formulas with medium-chain triglycerides (MCT) to long-chain triglycerides (LCT). Twenty-four patients with chronic diarrhea (greater than 1 month duration) and fat malabsorption received their total daily caloric intake for 12 days from the nutritionally complete liquid diets. All patients demonstrated a favorable response, with an overall 45% decrease in the number of stools, and significantly decreased stool fat and weight at the end of the study compared to baseline determinations. Patients who received the nutritional supplement containing MCT as the source of fat demonstrated a decrease in fecal fat that was significantly greater than that seen in the patients who received the LCT product. In the group of patients who received the MCT product, mean stool fat normalized over the 12-day study period. Of the study participants, 10 patients had one of the two intestinal species of microsporidium as the cause of diarrheal disease; 9 patients had no identifiable cause of diarrheal disease after extensive evaluation. The patients with and without identifiable pathogens were randomized equally to both supplement groups. Patients with microsporidia were more severely malnourished than the patients with no identifiable pathogen. Both groups responded favorably to the dietary intervention. These findings suggest (1) the use of low-residue supplements may improve the diarrheal symptoms in HIV-infected patients with chronic diarrhea; (2) the more easily digested MCT may promote the maintenance of nutritional status for patients with fat malabsorption. Additional studies are needed to clarify the role that these kinds of dietary interventions play in the long-term maintenance of nutritional status in HIV-infected patient populations with and without diarrhea and with and without overt fat malabsorption. For patients with untreatable diarrheal pathogens, patients who have no identifiable pathogen, and patients for whom no other therapy is available, dietary or nutritional interventions with such specific supplements may be beneficial.

Tube-Feeding Diets

Before selecting a tube-feeding diet—instead of or in combination with an oral diet—it is necessary to evaluate gastrointestinal function, estimated length of time required for nutritional repletion, cost, patient acceptance, and feasibility of home use.[46] Formula selection may vary, depending upon the integrity of the small bowel, its absorptive capacity, documentation of carbohydrate or fat malabsorption, and antibiotic use. If malabsorption is present, it is prudent to begin with low-fat, elemental formula or a diet rich in short-chain peptides and MCTs. AIDS patients with documented fat malabsorption showed significant increases in total body potassium with these diets, and some patients showed improvement in serum albumin concentration and functional capacity.[47] Methods for formula administration are described in Chapter 20. Given the substantial malabsorption of fat, protein, and several micronutrients in many AIDS patients, enteral nutrition by tube is often considered to be an appropriate means of nutrition support. Tube feedings are appropriate for patients with anorexia who have failed appetite stimulants and have no documented malabsorption, but it is necessary to conduct individual trials to determine their efficacy in patients with substantial diarrhea.

Parenteral Nutrition

The use of oral or enteral routes for nutritional supplementation is preferred to the use of parenteral nutrition unless the enteral route is not possible. In the short term (less than 10 days), nasoenteric supplementation should be considered. If longer support (greater than 8 to 10 weeks) is anticipated, percutaneous tube enterostomies are preferable. Parenteral nutrition should be considered when enteral supplementation is not possible (eg, if the patient is at increased risk for aspiration, if the patient has significant small-bowel disease, or if there was a poor response to an enteral trial).

Peripheral parenteral nutrition (PPN) may be sufficient for short-term support but is more limited in terms of nutrient delivery by the tolerance of peripheral veins to highly osmotic solutions and the larger volumes required to deliver the nutrients peripherally. When longer support is needed, total parenteral nutrition (TPN) can be considered. TPN should only be considered if it is anticipated that such therapy may bring about a substantial improvement in quality of life (eg, a patient with severe diarrhea refractory to all treatment that is worsened by oral intake). As with other critically ill patients, rigorous nutrition support would be less appropriate in patients who have multiple complications of their HIV disease or are near death.

Parenteral nutrition support should be considered in the following AIDS patients: patients who have failed attempts at enteral nutrition supplementation, patients with bowel obstruction, patients with severe refractory diarrhea or intractable upper gastrointestinal symptoms such as nausea or vomiting, and patients who have been compromised acutely by an active, but treatable, opportunistic infection (see Table 15–3 and Exhibit 15–2). The potential to improve quality of life by decreasing the severity and/or frequency of gastrointestinal symptoms may also affect the decision to institute parenteral nutrition. In the short term, PPN may meet volume, protein, and energy requirements, but if the need for parenteral feeding is anticipated to exceed this period, central venous access should be attained to facilitate provision of nutrient requirements. Although the efficacy of long-term home parenteral nutrition (HPN) in AIDS patients remains to be proven, several studies support its use in terms of altering morbidity and mortality. Singer et al[48,49] reported that 17 out of 21 patients receiving HPN gained weight. Kotler et al[50] documented that HPN in AIDS patients with altered intake or absorption could produce weight gain and significantly replete LBM.

CONCLUSIONS

The AIDS epidemic has given most primary care providers exposure to a complex disease characterized by the prevalence of protein-calorie malnutrition. Nutritional knowledge is required in order to (1) distinguish who is malnourished, (2) determine the response depending on the presumed etiology of the lean tissue loss, and (3) determine the amount of nutrients required and the means to accom-

---

Exhibit 15–2 Indications for Parenteral Nutrition Support in AIDS

Severe Refractory Diarrhea
  Cryptosporidium
  Microsporidium
  Mycobacterium avium intracellulare complex
  Lymphoma
Bowel Obstruction
  Kaposi's sarcoma
  Lymphoma
  Refractory upper gastrointestinal symptoms
  Esophageal cytomegalovirus/candidiasis
  Pancreatitis
  Biliary tract disease/cholestasis, cryptosporidium, cytomegalovirus
Failure of Enteral Support
  Persistent or severe diarrhea with elemental diet feeding or diet rich in medium-
    chain triglycerides
  Aspiration
  Intractable vomiting

plish their intake. Because it is presumed that nutritional status influences the quality of life and probably improves survival of AIDS patients, a basic understanding of clinical nutrition is an integral component of optimal patient care.

REFERENCES

1. Beach RS, Mantero-Atinga E, Van Roel F, Eideufer C, et al. Implications of nutritional deficiencies in HIV infection. *Arch AIDS.* 1989;3:287–305.

2. Trujillo EB, Borlase BC, Bell SJ, Gruenther KJ, et al. Assessment of nutritional status, nutrient intake, and nutrition support in AIDS patients. *J Am Diet Assoc.* 1992;92:477–478.

3. Kotler DP, Tierney AR, Wang J, Pierson RN. Magnitude of body-cell-mass depletion and the timing of death from wasting in AIDS. *Am J Clin Nutr.* 1989;50:444–447.

4. Chlebowski RT, Grosvenor MB, Bernhard NH, Morales LS, et al. Nutritional status, gastrointestinal dysfunction, and survival in patients with AIDS. *Am J Gastroenterol.* 1989;84:1288–1293.

5. Blatt SP, Hendrix CW, Butzin CA, Freeman TM, et al. Delayed-type hypersensitivity skin testing predicts progression to AIDS in HIV-infected patients. *Ann Intern Med.* 1993;199:177–184.

6. Moseson M, Zeleniunch-Jaquotte A, Belsito DV, Shore RE, et al. The potential role of nutritional factors in the induction of immunologic abnormalities in HIV-positive homosexual men. *J AIDS.* 1989;2:235–247.

7. Grunfeld C, Feingold KR. Metabolic disturbances and wasting in the acquired immunodeficiency syndrome. *N Engl J Med.* 1992;327:329–337.

8. Grunfeld C, Pang M, Shimizu L, Shigenaga JK, et al. Resting energy expenditure, caloric intake, and short-term weight change in human immunodeficiency virus infection and the acquired immunodeficiency syndrome. *Am J Clin Nutr.* 1992;55:455–460.

9. Macallan DC, Noble C, Baldwin C, Foskett M, et al. Prospective analysis of patterns of weight change in stage IV human immunodeficiency virus infection. *Am J Clin Nutr.* 1993;58:417–424.

10. Dworkin BM, Wormser GP, Axelrod F, Pierre N, et al. Dietary intake in patients with acquired immunodeficiency syndrome (AIDS), patients with AIDS-related complex, and serologically positive human immunodeficiency virus patients: correlations with nutritional status. *J Parenter Enter Nutr.* 1990;14:605–609.

11. Smith PD, Quinn TC, Strober W, Janoff E, et al. Gastrointestinal infections in AIDS. *Ann Intern Med.* 1992;116:63–77.

12. Mayer HB, Wanke CA. Diagnosis strategies in HIV-infected patients with diarrhea. *AIDS.* 1994;8:1639–1648.

13. Gillin JS, Shike M, Alcock N, Urmacher C, et al. Malabsorption and mucosal abnormalities of the small intestine in the acquired immunodeficiency syndrome. *Ann Intern Med.* 1985;102:619–622.

14. Miller TL, Orav EJ, Martin SR, Cooper ER, et al. Malnutrition and carbohydrate malabsorption in children with vertically transmitted human immunodeficiency virus 1 infection. *Gastroenterology.* 1991;100:1296–1302.

15. Ulrich R, Zeitz M, Heise W, L'age M, et al. Small intestine structure and function in patients infected with human immunodeficiency virus (HIV): evidence for HIV-induced enteropathy. *Ann Intern Med.* 1989;111:15–21.

16. Lambl BB, Federman M, Pleskow D, Wanke CA. Malabsorption and wasting in AIDS patients with microsporidia and pathogen-negative diarrhea. *AIDS.* 1996;10:739–744.

17. Hommes MJ, Romijn JA, Endert E, Sauerwein HP. Resting energy expenditure and substrate oxidation in human immunodeficiency virus (HIV)-infected asymptomatic men: HIV affects host metabolism in the early asymptomatic stage. *Am J Clin Nutr.* 1991;54:311–315.

18. Rakower D, Galvin TA. Nourishing the HIV-infected adult. *Holistic Nurs Pract.* 1989;3:26–37.

19. Dwyer JT. Nutrition support of HIV positive patients. *Henry Ford Hosp Med J.* 1991;39:60–65.

20. Raiten DJ. Nutrition and HIV infection: a review and evaluation of the extant knowledge of the relationship between nutrition and HIV infection. *Nutr Clin Pract.* 1991;6:1S–94S.

21. O'Sullavin P, Linke RA, Dalton S. Evaluation of body weight and nutritional status among AIDS patients. *J Am Diet Assoc.* 1985;85:1483–1484.

22. Bistrian BR, Blackburn GL, Hallowell E, Heddle R. Protein status of general surgery patients. *JAMA.* 1974;230:858–860.

23. Blackburn GL, Bistrian BR, Maini BS, Schlamm HT, et al. Nutritional and metabolic assessment of the hospitalized patient. *J Parenter Enter Nutr.* 1977;1:11–22.

24. Doweiko JP, Nompleggi DJ. The role of albumin in human physiology and pathophysiology, part III: albumin and disease states. *J Parenter Enter Nutr.* 1991;15:476–483.

25. Ott M, Lembeke B, Fischer H, Jager R, et al. Early changes of body composition in human immunodeficiency virus-infected patients: tetrapolar body impedance analysis indicates significant malnutrition. *Am J Clin Nutr.* 1993;57:15–19.

26. Stein TP, Nutinsky C, Condoluci D, Schluter MD, et al. Protein and energy substrate metabolism in AIDS patients. *Metabolism.* 1990;39:876–881.

27. Galvin TA. Micronutrients: implications in human immunodeficiency virus disease. *Top Clin Nutr.* 1992;7:63–73.

28. Resler SS. Nutrition care of AIDS patient. *J Am Diet Assoc.* 1988;88:828–832.

29. Gorgach SL, Knox TA, Roubenoff R. Interactions between nutrition and infection with human immunodeficiency virus. *Nutr Rev.* 1993;51:226–234.

30. Tang AM, Grahan NM, Kirby AJ, McCall D, et al. Dietary micronutrient intake and risk of progression to acquired immunodeficiency syndrome (AIDS) in human immunodeficiency virus type 1 (HIV-1)-infected homosexual men. *Am J Epidemiol.* 1993;138:937–951.

31. Dworkin BM, Rosenthal WS, Wormser GP, Weiss L. Selenium deficiency in the acquired immunodeficiency syndrome. *J Parenter Enter Nutr.* 1986;10:405–407.

32. Olstead L, Schrauzer GN, Flores-Arce M, Dowd J. Selenium supplementation of symptomatic human immunodeficiency virus infected patients. *Bio Trace Elem Res.* 1989;20:59–65.

33. Bogden JD, Baker H, Frank O, Perez G, et al. Micronutrient status and human immunodeficiency virus (HIV) infection. *Ann N Y Acad Sci.* 1990;587:189–195.

34. Henry K. Alternative therapies for AIDS. *Minn Med.* 1988;71:297–299.

35. Dwyer JT, Bye RL, Holt PL, Lauze SR. Unproven nutrition therapies for AIDS: what is the evidence? *Nutr Today.* 1988;Mar/Apr:25–33.

36. Bandy CE, Guyer LK, Perkin JE, Probart CK, et al. Nutrition attitudes and practices of individuals who are infected with human immunodeficiency virus and who live in South Florida. *J Am Diet Assoc.* 1993;93:70–72.

37. Von Roenn JH, Armstrong D, Kotler DP, Cohn DL, et al. Megestrol acetate in patients with AIDS-related cachexia. *Ann Intern Med.* 1994;121:393–399.

38. Shambelan M, Grunfeld C, Mulligan K. Serona Symposia, USA Inc; 1995.

39. Stack J, Bell SJ, Burke PA, Forse RA. High energy, high protein, oral, liquid, nutrition supplementation in patients with HIV infection: effect of weight status in relation to incidence of secondary infection. *J Am Diet Assoc.* 1996;96:337–341.

40. Chlebowski RT, Beall C, Grosvenor MB, Lillington L, et al. Long-term effects of early nutritional support with new enterotropic peptide-based formula vs. standard enteral formula in HIV-infected patients: randomized prospective trial. *Nutrition.* 1993;9:507–511.

41. Blackburn GL, Bell SJ. Eutrophia in patients with HIV infection and early AIDS with novel nutrient "cocktail": is this the first food for special medical purpose? *Nutrition.* 1993;9:554–556.

42. Reddy MM, Sorrell SJ, Lange M, Grieco MH. Tumor necrosis factor and HIV P24 antigen levels in serum of HIV-infected populations. *J AIDS.* 1988;1:436–440.

43. Endres S, Ghorbani R, Kelley VE, Georgillis K, et al. The effect of dietary supplementation with n-3 polyunsaturated fatty acids on the synthesis of interleukin-1 and tumor necrosis factor by mononuclear cells. *N Engl J Med.* 1989;320:265–271.

44. Bell SJ. Dietary fish oil, cytokine and eicosanoid production during human immunodeficiency virus infection. *J Parenter Enter Nutr.* 1996;20:43–49.

45. Wanke CA, Pleskow D, DeGirolami PC, Lambl BB, et al. A medium chain triglyceride-based diet in patients with HIV and chronic diarrhea reduces diarrhea and malabsorption: a prospective, controlled trial. *Nutrition.* 1996;12:766–771.

46. Task Force on Nutrition Support in AIDS. Guidelines for nutrition support in AIDS. *Nutrition.* 1989;5:39–46.

47. Kotler DP, Tierney AR, Ferraro R, Cuff P, et al. Enteral alimentation and repletion of body cell mass in malnourished patients with AIDS. *Am J Clin Nutr.* 1991;53:149–154.

48. Singer P, Rothkopf MM, Kvetan V, Kirvela O, et al. Risks and benefits of home parenteral nutrition in the acquired immunodeficiency syndrome. *J Parenter Enter Nutr.* 1991;15:75–79.

49. Smith PD, Quinn TC, Strober W, Janoff E, et al. Gastrointestinal infections in AIDS. *Ann Intern Med.* 1992;116:63–77.

50. Kotler DP, Tierney AR, Culpepper-Morgan JA, Wang J, et al. Effect of home parenteral nutrition on body composition in patients with acquired immunodeficiency syndrome. *J Parenter Enter Nutr.* 1990;14:454–458.

CHAPTER 16

Burns

Theresa Mayes and Michele M. Gottschlich

INTRODUCTION

Thermal injury is characterized by unique disturbances in the hormonal, immunologic, and metabolic environment resulting in hypercatabolism, bacterial invasion, and erosion of energy and protein stores. Specific nutritional provisions must be implemented postburn to counteract the impact of the metabolic milieu on nutrient utilization and requirements. Decisions regarding optimal nutrient provision for burn patients dictate a thorough understanding of the etiology of hypermetabolism and ensuing catabolism, nutrient requirements, and nutritional assessment guidelines. This chapter reviews nutritional considerations distinctive to burns. It discusses current information to assist the clinician in the formulation of a treatment plan that promotes tissue repair, immunocompetence, and survival.

ETIOLOGY OF HYPERMETABOLISM

Thermal injury interrupts multiple regulatory systems that collectively cause unique alterations in metabolism leading to increased calorie requirements. Therefore, acute energy needs following burns exceed those associated with any other form of trauma.[1] Energy demands positively correlate with the percentage of the body with open wound, reaching a ceiling when approximately 50% of body surface area is affected. Postburn days 7 to 12 are associated with an energy climax, following which calorie needs decelerate to normal as the wound is covered by reepithelialization or skin grafting.[2] The observed rise in initial metabolism may be reincited with the occurrence of infection or multisystem organ failure. A number of processes contribute to postburn hypermetabolism and are discussed below.

Neuroendocrine changes, specifically the persistent rise in catecholamines following burn injury, appear to exercise the strongest influence on energy requirements. The steady escalation of adrenal catecholamines postburn immediately cause energy needs to accelerate. The release of the hormone cortisol following injury appears to maintain a similar property of invoking the hypermetabolic response.

Further influences on postburn energy demands include nonhormonal factors such as evaporative water loss, early enteral feeding, and sleep deprivation. The loss of the skin organ that characterizes thermal injury is associated with an interruption of the mechanism that normally maintains body temperature. Increased evaporative water loss leads to heat loss by means of the open wound. The increase in heat production in order to maintain body temperature appears to cause a rise in metabolism.[3,4] In addition, initiation of enteral feedings within hours postburn has been associated with reduced energy needs in animal[5,6] and clinical models.[7–10] Gottschlich et al confirm the existence of sleep deprivation in pediatric patients following thermal injury and suggest that it may drive hypermetabolism as well.[11]

Caregivers may exercise control over some of the factors that affect metabolic rate. For example, occlusive dressings[12] and elevated ambient temperature[13] help to lower energy needs. Also, early excision of burned eschar with subsequent grafting appears to decrease hypermetabolism.[14,15] Finally, adequate medications for pain, anxiety, and sleep deprivation impact calorie needs as does minimizing fear and anxiety by offering a thorough explanation for procedures prior to induction.

NUTRITIONAL REQUIREMENTS

Energy

The assessment of energy needs and the ability to meet those requirements is critical to a burn victim's survival. Multiple mathematical equations exist to aid in the determination of calorie needs postburn[16–30] (see Table 16–1). Formulas typically incorporate two or more of the following variables: age, weight, body surface area, body surface area burn, or basal metabolic rate. The reliability of energy equations in the burn population has been widely criticized.[28,31,32] Factors such as body weight (often skewed by edema), changes in wound size over time, and elevation of core temperature are among many variables that can confound results.

Nevertheless, a survey conducted by Williamson[33] indicates that burn clinicians most often rely on a single formula. The Curreri equation[16,18,19] or the Long's Modified Harris-Benedict equations[21] appear to be the most popular means for predicting calorie requirements.

The determination of calorie requirements from formulas is better handled by considering the calculated recommendations derived from several equations and then deducing a goal that is comfortable for the clinician. For example, the authors use the following formulas to establish a caloric goal in pediatrics: the Recommended Dietary Allowance[29] and Estimated Resting Energy Expenditure (REE),[30]

Table 16–1 Formulas for Calculating Energy Requirements for Burn Patients

Formula Name	Sex	Age (Years)	Calorie Prediction
Curreri[16,18,19]	M & F	< 1	Basal + (15 × % burn)
		1–3	Basal + (25 × % burn)
		4–15	Basal + (40 × % burn)
		16–59	(25 × kg) + (40 × % burn)
		> 60	Basal + (65 × % burn)
Galveston 1990[15]	M & F	< 12	($1800/m^2$ body surface area) + ($1300/m^2$ body surface area burn)
Long's Modified Harris-Benedict equation[21]	M	All ages	$66.47 + (13.75 \times kg) + (5 \times cm)$ (height) $- (6.76A^c) \times$ (activity factor^a) × (injury factor^b)
	F	All ages	$655.1 + (9.56 \times kg) + (1.85\ cm)$ (height) $- (4.68A^c) \times$ (activity factor^a) × (injury factor^b)
Mayes[28]	M & F	< 3	$108 + (68 \times kg) + (3.9 \times \%\ burn)$
		5–10	$818 + (37.4 \times kg) + (9.3 \times \%\ burn)$
Resting Energy Expenditure[30]	M	0–3	$(60.9 \times kg) - 54$
		3–10	$(22.7 \times kg) + 495$
		10–18	$(17.5 \times kg) + 651$
	F	0–3	$(61.0 \times kg) - 51$
		3–10	$(22.5 \times kg) + 499$
		10–18	$(12.2 \times kg) + 746$
Recommended Dietary Allowances[29]	M & F	0.0–0.5	108 cals/kg
		0.5–1.0	98 cals/kg
		1–3	102 cals/kg
		4–6	90 cals/kg
		7–10	70 cals/kg
	M	11–14	55 cals/kg
		15–18	45 cals/kg
	F	11–14	47 cals/kg
		15–18	40 cals/kg

[a]Activity factor: Confined to bed: 1.2; Out of bed: 1.3
[b]Injury factor: Severe burns: 2.1
[c]A = age in years
M = male, F = female

the Curreri and Mayes[28] formulas,[16–18] and the revised Galveston equation[15] (see Table 16–1). Overfeeding and underfeeding can have deleterious effects,[34] so assessment parameters should be diligently monitored. Furthermore, periodic recalculation of requirements is necessary to accommodate changes in wound size and, hence, metabolism.

Because of the ambiguity of burn energy equations, indirect calorimetry is invaluable during the acute phase of injury. Indirect calorimetry provides an individualized account of calorie needs by incorporating differences in weight, burn size, core temperature, infection, sex, and other variables into the calculation of REE. Factors known to increase energy needs above resting conditions (such as physical therapy, dressing changes, temperature spikes, pain) necessitate the addition of a multiplier to measured REE. For most patients, a calorie goal of 20% to 30% above REE appears adequate for maintenance of weight and other outcome parameters.[35,36] Metabolic testing is optimally repeated two to three times per week as transitory alterations in energy needs continue until wounds are healed. As indicated, adjustments in the nutrition support regimen routinely accompany indirect calorimetry results.

Carbohydrate

In order to promote nitrogen sparing, carbohydrate is the most important energy-yielding nutrient in the postburn state. Provision of 60% to 65% of calories as carbohydrate is a reasonable goal, assuming that this amount does not exceed the described 5 mg/kg/min maximum oxidation rate.[37] Hyperglycemia and glycosuria should be monitored in severely burned patients. However, it is not necessary to alter nutrition regimens automatically to accommodate this expected postinjury consequence. Rather, exogenous insulin is often administered to maximize systemic uptake of glucose.

Protein

Increased nitrogen requirements are necessary postburn in order to replete losses through integumentary exudate and to provide conditions favorable for wound healing. Studies support enteral protein fortification in burns because of the relationship between high protein intake and improved nitrogen balance, immune function, and survival.[38,39] Alexander and colleagues[38] recommend approximately 23% to 25% of calories as protein for patients with serious burns.[38] Additional formulas for determining protein requirements are available as well.[20,25,27,40–43] The administration of elevated levels of protein may contribute to a high renal solute load, especially in infants and elderly patients, dictating routine monitoring of fluid status, blood urea nitrogen, and serum creatinine levels.

Researchers have recently examined the supplementation of individual amino acids in burns, specifically, arginine and glutamine. Following trauma, dietary arginine is associated with benefits that could also be appreciated in the postburn state: improved nitrogen retention,[44,45] wound healing,[46,47] and immune function[48–50]; and an increase in the anabolic hormones insulin and growth hormone.[51,52] In an animal model, Saito and associates[50] found that a total of 2% of energy needs in the form of arginine correlated with improved immune function and survival. This amount was subsequently tested clinically with similar beneficial results.[49]

Glutamine supplementation following trauma is associated with maintenance of gut metabolism, structure, and function.[53–55] Furthermore, Parry-Billings and colleagues demonstrate that plasma glutamine levels decline postburn and may contribute to an already depressed immune system.[56] Although glutamine fortification in burns is at the preliminary stages of investigation, it appears to decrease the incidence of bacterial translocation.[57] Glutamine supplementation in the burn population appears promising; however, the optimum means of delivery has not been determined.

Fat

Fat is necessary in the diet of burn patients because it serves as a carrier of the fat-soluble vitamins and the essential fatty acids—linoleate and alpha linoleate. In the past, the caloric density of fat was viewed favorably, and fat was used regularly as a major energy source for burn patients. However, recent investigations have questioned the overuse of fat in the burn diet because of its immunosuppressive characteristics.[48,58,59] Furthermore, excessive delivery of lipid can be detrimental in burns because, unlike carbohydrate, fat does not spare nitrogen[60] nor does it induce the production of the anabolic hormone insulin. Provision of 5% to 15% of nonprotein calories as lipid is currently recommended postburn.[58]

Linoleic acid, an omega-6 fatty acid, is the precursor of several inflammation-inducing arachidonic acid metabolites. These metabolites are also associated with immunosuppression[61,62] and increased muscle wasting.[58,63] On the other hand, omega-3 fatty acids, primarily of marine origin, are rich in alpha linolenic acid and are known for their anti-inflammatory, immune-enhancing,[64,65] and vasodilator qualities.[66] Therefore, it is suggested that the standard postburn diet, historically high in the long-chain fatty acid, linoleate, should be replaced with increasing quantities of a marine source of alpha linoleate. Alexander and colleagues[61] confirmed the benefits of omega-3 fatty acids in an animal model, documenting less weight loss, improved muscle mass, and enhanced immune parameters in the supplemented group of burned animals. Based on evidence of enhanced immune response, decreased length of stay, improved muscle mass, decreased incidence of diarrhea, and improved glucose tolerance in the clinical setting, Gottschlich et al recommended the fortification of a low-fat regimen with omega-3 fatty acids in burn patients.[49]

Most commercially available enteral products do not meet the unique needs of burn patients. All contain greater than the recommended fat content and most have a high rate of linoleic acid to alpha linolenic acid. The careful examination of the total fat and omega-6 and omega-3 fatty acid content of enteral formulas is essential to optimize postinjury nutrition therapy.

Micronutrients

Micronutrient requirements following burn injury are not as well defined as macronutrient needs.[67,68] Vitamins and minerals not only function as coenzymes and cofactors that allow energy and protein to be more efficiently employed, but also are an integral component of wound healing and immunocompetence. Enhanced losses from wound exudate and alterations in metabolism predispose burn patients to an increased need for micronutrient replacement. Enrichment of a daily multivitamin with additional vitamin A, vitamin C, and zinc is recommended (see Table 16–2).

Table 16–2 Micronutrient Requirements Following Burn Injury

Adults and Children ≥ 3 yr		Children < 3 yr	
Major Burn	Minor Burn (<20%) or Reconstructive Patient	Major Burn	Minor Burn (<10%) or Reconstructive Patient
1 multivitamin (qd)	1 multivitamin (qd)	1 children's multivitamin (qd)	1 children's multivitamin (qd)
500 mg ascorbic acid (bid)*		250 mg ascorbic acid (bid)*	
10,000 IU vitamin A (qd)		5000 IU vitamin A (qd)	
220 mg zinc sulfate (qd)*		110 mg zinc sulfate (qd)*	

*Recommended delivery in suspension for tube feeding, as orally administered vitamin C and zinc in large doses may precipitate nausea or vomiting.

qd = daily
bid = 2 times daily

Source: Adapted with permission from M.M. Gottschlich and G.D. Warden. Vitamin Supplementation in the Patient with Burns. *J Burn Care Rehabil,* Vol. 11, pp. 275–279, © 1990, Mosby-Year Book, Inc.

Disorders of electrolyte balance are common following severe thermal injury.[69] Daily monitoring of serum levels of sodium, potassium, chloride, phosphorus, calcium, and magnesium is required. Electrolyte manipulation during the acute postburn phase is most often accomplished using the intravenous route.

NUTRITIONAL ASSESSMENT

Assessment of nutritional status at regular intervals is an essential component of the postburn nutrition therapy program. Perhaps the most important initial and ongoing determination is the success by which the patient's actual intake (from all sources) meets the calorie and protein recommendation. Other assessment tools help ascertain if the nutrition regimen is sufficient or needs adjustment. Because thermal injury affects multiple organ systems, the typical assessment parameters used in other types of trauma may not apply in burns.[70] Body weight, visceral protein status, and respiratory quotient (RQ) are frequently used following thermal injury and support the most reliable and convenient means of nutritional assessment.

Body Weight

Although weight is skewed by edema in severely burned individuals for the initial 2 to 3 weeks postburn, monitoring weight over time is useful in assessing the adequacy of the nutrition program. Considering that factors such as amputations, bulky dressings, and orthopaedic devices affect weight status, it is recommended that weights be obtained directly following the removal of burn dressings to ensure that nude weights are recorded. A goal of 90% to 110% of preburn weight as recollected from the patient/family, or dry weight as obtained on admission, represents optimal ongoing nutrition support.

Visceral Protein Status

Serum albumin levels are often distorted in the thermally injured patient due to wound losses, fluid shifts, intravenous albumin infusions, and infection. Because albumin has a relatively long half-life (approximately 20 days), trends in daily albumin levels should be observed over time.

Serum transferrin offers a more dependable appraisal of nutritional status than albumin. Transferrin typically decreases within 1 to 3 days of initial injury as plasma proteins seep through the open wound. However, the prompt initiation and ongoing provision of adequate nutrition support will potentially replete stores, reflected by increasing serum values over time. Given its relatively short half-life of 8 days, a weekly transferrin measurement is usually sufficient to monitor trends.

Prealbumin is characterized as an acute-phase reactant; as a result, serum levels plummet in the initial postburn period. However, because prealbumin has a half-life of 2 to 3 days and values are not affected by intravenous albumin infusions, trends in serum levels are considered a reliable, sensitive indicator of nutritional status into and throughout convalescence. A weekly serum prealbumin assessment is sufficient to observe the adequacy of the nutrition support program.

Additionally, nitrogen balance may be used to assess visceral protein status. Interpretation of nitrogen balance requires consideration of the nitrogen lost through the open wound. A formula that estimates wound nitrogen losses is available to help determine postburn nitrogen balance.[71] However, the use of this formula requires evaluation of the percentage of the body surface that is open wound, because wound size changes with reepithelialization, grafting, and wound sepsis. In the event that reassessment of wound size does not occur, the standard nitrogen-balance formula, which allots 4 grams of nitrogen for insensible losses, may be applied to burns. However, nitrogen balance greater than 5 grams is needed to support anabolism.

Respiratory Quotient

Indirect calorimetry elucidates energy requirements while simultaneously revealing the adequacy of the current nutrition regimen through the documentation of RQ. Proper interpretation of RQ aids in the assessment of substrate utilization in order to avert the negative consequences of over- or underfeeding. An RQ between 0.80 and 0.95 represents optimal macronutrient delivery. Any deviation from this range requires careful scrutiny to determine if an increase or decrease in calories is necessary.

NUTRITION SUPPORT GUIDELINES

Enteral Nutrition

Because of the multiple disadvantages of parenteral alimentation[72] and because the small intestine maintains its digestive and absorptive properties,[73,74] enteral support is the preferred method of nutrient delivery postburn. In addition, there is no evidence to support a delay in enteral feeding until the resuscitation period has ended. In fact, enteral support that is initiated within 24 hours of injury appears to have beneficial effects.[5–10]

An intact protein formula is indicated and is well tolerated postburn. Only in the case of associated gut trauma or severe malabsorption is a predigested formula considered. In this rare instance, a peptide-based formula is recommended over free amino acids because of evidence that supports the role of peptides in improving absorption of water and electrolytes.[75,76]

Patients with burns that are less than 20% of total body surface area are usually capable of orally consuming sufficient nutrients to avert the use of enteral tube feedings. Adequacy of oral intake for this category of patients should be reevaluated after 24 to 48 hours. Pediatric or geriatric patients with less than 20% involvement require a detailed nutrition evaluation before the recommendation for supplemental enteral feeding is forgone, because these populations are at particular risk for malnutrition and dehydration.

In most instances, patients with burns involving greater than 20% of the body's surface area or requiring prolonged ventilator support require supplemental enteral nutrition. Currently, full-strength initiation of a high-intact-protein, high-carbohydrate, low-fat, low-linoleic acid product is recommended. Because nutrition support is a priority postburn, the regimen should be advanced hourly as tolerated so that the tube feeding goal rate is achieved within 12 to 24 hours of initiation.

To augment early enteral alimentation, the continuation of enteral feedings throughout operative procedures has been safely demonstrated in burn patients.[77,78] Intraoperative enteral feeding in the thermally injured population has been correlated with a reduction in calorie deficit, albumin requirement, and wound infection.[77] This practice permits maximum nutrient provision at a time when the metabolic demands of the patient increase substantially.

Parenteral Nutrition

Due to procedural, metabolic, and immunosuppressive complications, intravenous feedings are reserved for patients with prolonged dysfunction of the digestive tract.[79,80] For the infrequent occasion when total parenteral nutrition is necessary, several guidelines are respected. First, the length of time that parenteral nutrition is used should be minimized. Second, as medically permitted, trophic enteral feedings should continue throughout intravenous alimentation in an attempt to preserve and improve gut function. And third, conservative intravenous lipid administration is recommended because of its immunosuppressive characteristics. If the enteral regimen provides the essential 1% to 2% of total calorie requirements as linoleate and another 1% to 2% of calories from a lipid source rich in omega-3 fatty acids, then additional fat as part of the parenteral regimen is not necessary.

CONCLUSIONS

Burn trauma elicits particular pathophysiological aberrations that potentially impact all organ systems. Consequently, burn patients experience unique nutrient deviations that require aggressive nutrition intervention. The introduction of early, continuous enteral feedings with high-calorie, high-protein, high-carbohydrate, and low-fat content represents the current nutrient recommendation for burn patients. Multivitamin supplementation along with pharmacologic doses of vitamins

A and C and zinc is also indicated. In addition, ongoing monitoring and adjustment of the nutrition care plan is essential to achieve outcome goals. Recent studies have concentrated on the effects of supplemental arginine and glutamine and determination of optimal lipid provision and growth factor involvement, in an effort to direct the future of nutrient pharmacology in burns. Preliminarily, the manipulation of various nutrients appears to be involved in beneficial immunologic and reparative sequelae postburn. As researchers continue to discern the ultimate nutrition regimen following thermal injury, refined nutrient recommendations are anticipated.

REFERENCES

1. Long CL, Schaffel N, Geiger JW, Schiller WR, et al. Metabolic response to injury and illness: estimation of energy and protein needs from indirect calorimetry and nitrogen balance. *J Parenter Enter Nutr.* 1979;3:452–457.
2. Kagan RJ, Gottschlich MM, Jenkins ME. Nutritional support in the burn patient. In: Nuhaus LM, ed. *Problems in General Surgery.* Philadelphia: JB Lippincott Co; 1991:57–75.
3. Birke G, Carlson LA, von Euler US, Liljedahl SO, et al. Lipid metabolism, catecholamine excretion, basal metabolic rate and water loss during treatment of burns with warm dry air. *Acta Chir Scand.* 1972;138:321–333.
4. Harrison HN, Moncrief JA, Duckett JW, Mason AD. The relationship between energy metabolism and water loss from vaporization in severely burned patients. *Surgery.* 1964;56:203–211.
5. Dominioni L, Trocki O, Mochizuki H, Fang CH. Prevention of severe postburn hypermetabolism and catabolism by immediate intragastric feeding. *J Burn Care Rehabil.* 1984;5:106–112.
6. Mochizuki H, Trocki O, Dominioni L. Mechanisms of prevention of postburn hypermetabolism and catabolism by early enteral feeding. *Ann Surg.* 1984;200:297–310.
7. Jenkins M, Gottschlich M, Alexander JW, Warden GD. An evaluation of the effect of immediate enteral feeding on the hypermetabolic response following severe burn injury. *J Parenter Enter Nutr.* 1989;13(suppl):12.
8. Chiarelli A, Enzi G, Casodei A, Baggio B. Very early supplementation in burned patients. *Am J Clin Nutr.* 1990;51:1035–1039.
9. McDonald WS, Clarborne WS, Dietch EA. Immediate enteral feeding in burn patients is safe and effective. *Ann Surg.* 1991;213:177–183.
10. Hansbrough WB, Hansbrough JF. Success of intragastric feeding of patients with burns. *J Burn Care Rehabil.* 1993;14:512–516.
11. Gottschlich MM, Jenkins ME, Mayes T, Khoury J, et al. A prospective clinical study of the polysomnographic stages of sleep following burn injury. *J Burn Care Rehabil.* 1994;15:486–492.
12. Caldwell FT, Bowser BH, Crabtree JH. The effect of occlusive dressings on the energy metabolism of severely burned children. *Ann Surg.* 1981;193:579–591.
13. Danielsson V, Arturson G, Wennberg L. The elimination of hypermetabolism in burned patients. *Burns.* 1976;2:110–114.
14. Cone JB, Wallace BH, Caldwell FT. The effect of staged burn wound closure on the rates of heat production and heat loss of burned children and young adults. *J Trauma.* 1988;28:968–972.

15. Hildreth MA, Herndon DN, Desai MH, Broemeling LD. Current treatment reduces calories required to maintain weight in pediatric patients with burns. *J Burn Care Rehabil.* 1990;11:405–409.

16. Curreri PW, Richmond D, Marvin J, Baxter CR. Dietary requirements of patients with major burns. *J Am Diet Assoc.* 1974;65:415–417.

17. Soroff HS, Pearson E, Artz CP. An estimation of the nitrogen requirements for equilibrium in burned patients. *Surg Gynecol Obstet.* 1961;112:159–172.

18. Day T, Dean P, Adams MC, Luterman A, et al. Nutritional requirements of the burned child: the Curreri junior formula. *Proc Am Burn Assoc.* 1986;18:86.

19. Adams MR, Kelley CH, Luterman A, Curreri PW. Nutritional requirements of the burned senior citizen: the Curreri senior formula. *Proc Am Burn Assoc.* 1987;19:83.

20. Davies JWL, Liljedahl SL. Metabolic consequences of an extensive burn. In: Polk HC, Stone HH, eds. *Contemporary Burn Management.* Boston: Little Brown & Co; 1971:151–169.

21. Long CL. Energy expenditure of major burns. *J Trauma.* 1979;19:904–906.

22. Hildreth MA, Herndon DN, Desai MH, Duke MA. Caloric needs of adolescent patients with burns. *J Burn Care Rehabil.* 1989;10:523–526.

23. Hildreth MA, Carvajal HF. Caloric requirements in burned children: a simple formula to estimate daily caloric requirements. *J Burn Care Rehabil.* 1982;3:78–80.

24. Sutherland AB. Nitrogen balance and nutritional requirements in the burn patient: a reappraisal. *Burns.* 1976;2:238–244.

25. Molnar JA, Bell SJ, Goodenough RD, Burke JF. Enteral nutrition in patients with burns or trauma. In: Rombeau JL, Caldwell FT, eds. *Enteral Nutrition.* Philadelphia: WB Saunders Co; 1984:412–433.

26. Troell L, Wretlind A. Protein and calorie requirements in burns. *Acta Chir Scand.* 1961;122:15–20.

27. Wilmore DW. Nutrition and metabolism following thermal injury. *Clin Plast Surg.* 1974;1:603–619.

28. Mayes T, Gottschlich MM, Khoury J, Warden GD. Evaluation of predicted and measured energy requirements in burned children. *J Am Diet Assoc.* 1996;96:24–29.

29. Food and Nutrition Board and National Research Council. *Recommended Dietary Allowances.* 10th ed. Washington, DC: National Academy of Sciences; 1990.

30. World Health Organization. *Energy and Protein Requirements: Report of a Joint FAO/WHO/UNV Expert Consultation.* Geneva, Switzerland: World Health Organization; 1985:206. Technical Report Series.

31. Ireton CS, Turner WW, Hunt JL, Liepa GO. Evaluation of energy requirements in burn patients. *J Am Diet Assoc.* 1986;86:331–333.

32. Saffle JR, Medina E, Raymond J, Westenskow D, et al. Use of indirect calorimetry in the nutritional management of burned patients. *J Trauma.* 1985;25:32–39.

33. Williamson J. Actual burn nutrition care practices: a national survey (Part II). *J Burn Care Rehabil.* 1989;10:278–284.

34. Gottschlich M, Alexander JW, Bower RH. Enteral nutrition in patients with burns or trauma. In: Rombeau JL, Caldwell FT, eds. *Enteral and Tube Feedings.* Philadelphia: WB Saunders Co; 1990:306–324.

35. Kagan RJ, Gottschlich MM, Mayes T, Warden GD. Estimation of calorie needs in the thermally injured child. *Proc Am Burn Assoc.* 1995;27:283.

36. Saffle JR, Medina E, Raymond J, Westenskow D, et al. Use of indirect calorimetry in the nutritional management of burned patients. *J Trauma.* 1985;25:32–39.

37. Elwyn DH, Kinney JM, Jeevanandam M, Gump FE, et al. Influence of increasing carbohydrate intake on glucose kinetics in injured patients. *Ann Surg.* 1979;190:117–127.

38. Alexander JW, MacMillen BG, Stinnett JP, Ogle CK, et al. Beneficial effects of aggressive protein feeding in severely burned children. *Ann Surg.* 1980;192:505–517.

39. Dominioni L, Trocki O, Fang CH, Alexander JW. Nitrogen balance and liver changes in burned guinea pigs undergoing prolonged high protein enteral feeding. *Surg Forum.* 1983;34:99–101.

40. Hustler D. Nutritional monitoring of a pediatric burn patient. *Nutr Clin Pract.* 1991;6:11–17.

41. O'Neil CE, Hustler D, Hildreth MA. Basic nutritional guidelines for pediatric burn patients. *J Burn Care Rehabil.* 1989;10:278–283.

42. Cunningham JJ, Lydon MK, Russell WE. Calorie and protein provision for recovery from severe burns in infants and young children. *Am J Clin Nutr.* 1990;51:553–557.

43. Cunningham JJ, Harris LJ, Briggs SE. Nutritional support of the severely burned infant. *Nutr Clin Pract.* 1988;3:69–73.

44. Pui YML, Fischer H. Factorial supplementation with arginine and glycine on nitrogen retention and body weight gain in the traumatized rat. *J Nutr.* 1979;109:240–246.

45. Minuskin ML, Lavine ME, Ulman EA, Fischer H. Nitrogen retention, muscle creatinine and orotic acid excretion in traumatized rats fed arginine and glycine enriched diets. *J Nutr.* 1981;111:1265–1274.

46. Barbul A, Fishel RS, Shimazu S, Wasserkrug HL, et al. Intravenous hyperalimentation with high arginine levels improves wound healing and immune function. *J Surg Res.* 1985;38:328–334.

47. Barbul A, Rettura G, Levonson SM, Seifter E. Arginine: a thymotrophic and wound-healing promoting agent. *Surg Forum.* 1977;28:101–103.

48. Daly JM, Reynolds J, Thom A, Kinsley L, et al. Immune and metabolic effects of arginine in the surgical patient. *Ann Surg.* 1988;208:512–521.

49. Gottschlich MM, Jenkins ME, Warden GD, Baumer T, et al. Differential effects of three enteral dietary regimens on selected outcome variables in burn patients. *J Parenter Enter Nutr.* 1990;14:225–236.

50. Saito H, Trocki O, Wang S, Gonce SJ, et al. Metabolic and immune effects of dietary arginine supplementation after burn. *Arch Surg.* 1987;122:784–789.

51. Merimee TJ, Lillicrap DA, Rabinowitz D. Effect of arginine on serum levels of human growth hormone. *Lancet.* 1965;2:668–670.

52. Mulloy AL, Kari FW, Visek WJ. Dietary arginine, insulin secretion, glucose tolerance and liver lipids during repletion of protein-depleted rats. *Metab Res.* 1982;14:471–475.

53. O'Dwyer ST, Smith RJ, Hwang TL, Wilmore DW. Maintenance of small bowel mucosa with glutamine-enriched parenteral nutrition. *J Parenter Enter Nutr.* 1989;13:579–585.

54. Smith RJ, Wilmore DW. Glutamine nutrition and requirements. *J Parenter Enter Nutr.* 1990;14:94S–99S.

55. O'Dwyer ST, Scott T, Smith RJ, Wilmore DW. 5-fluorouracil toxicity on small intestinal mucosa but not white blood cells is decreased by glutamine. *Clin Res.* 1987;35:369a.

56. Parry-Billings M, Evans J, Calder PC, Newsholme EA. Does glutamine contribute to immunosuppression after major burns? *Lancet.* 1990;336:523–525.

57. Tenenhaus M, Hansbrough JF, Zapata-Sirvent RL, Ohara M, et al. Supplementation of an elemental enteral diet with alanyl-glutamine decreases bacterial translocation in burned mice. *Burns.* 1990;20:220–225.

58. Mochizuki H, Trocki O, Dominioni L, Ray MB, et al. Optimal lipid content for enteral diets following thermal injury. *J Parenter Enter Nutr.* 1984;8:638–646.

59. Gottschlich MM, Alexander JW. Fat kinetics and recommended dietary intake in burns. *J Parenter Enter Nutr.* 1987;11:80–85.

60. Wolfe BM, Culebras JM, Sim AJ, Ball MR, et al. Substrate interaction in intravenous feeding: comparative effects of carbohydrate and fat on amino acid utilization in fasting man. *Ann Surg.* 1977;186:518–540.

61. Alexander JW, Saito H, Trocki O, Ogle CK. The importance of lipid type in the diet after burn injury. *Ann Surg.* 1986;204:1–8.

62. Arturson MG. Arachidonic acid metabolism and prostaglandin activity following burn injury. In: Ninnemann JL, ed. *Traumatic Injury and Infection and Other Immunologic Sequela.* Baltimore: University Park Press; 1983:57–78.

63. Barrocas A, Rodemann HP, Dinarello CA, Goldberg AL. Stimulation of muscle protein degradation and prostaglandin E2 release by leukocyte pyrogen (interleukin-1): a mechanism for the increased degradation of muscle proteins during fever. *N Engl J Med.* 1983;308:553–558.

64. Merlin J. Omega-6 and omega-3 polyunsaturates and the immune system. *Br J Clin Nutr.* 1984;31:111–114.

65. Ninnemann JL, Stockland AE. Participation of prostaglandin E in immunosuppression following thermal injury. *J Trauma.* 1984;24:201–207.

66. Moncada S. Biology and therapeutic potential of prostacyclin. *Stroke.* 1983;14:157–168.

67. Gamliel Z, DeBiasse MA, Demling RH. Essential microminerals and their response to burn injury. *J Burn Care Rehabil.* 1996;17:264–272.

68. Gottschlich MM, Warden GD. Vitamin supplementation in the patient with burns. *J Burn Care Rehabil.* 1990;11:275–279.

69. Klein G. Effects of burn injury on bone and mineral metabolism. In: Herndon D, ed. *Total Burn Care.* Philadelphia: WB Saunders Co; 1996:246–250.

70. Rodriguez DJ. Nutrition in major burns: state of the art. *Support Line.* 1995;17:1–8.

71. Waxman K, Rebello T, Pinderski L, O'Neal K, et al. Protein loss across burn wounds. *J Trauma.* 1985;25:32–39.

72. Herndon DN, Stein MD, Rutan TC, Abston S, et al. Failure of TPN supplementation to improve liver function, immunity and mortality in thermally injured patients. *J Trauma.* 1987;27:195–204.

73. Glucksman DL, Halser MA, Warren WD. Small intestinal absorption in the immediate postoperative period. *Surgery.* 1966;60:1020–1025.

74. Moore EE, Jones TN. Nutritional assessment and preliminary report on early support of the trauma patient. *J Am Coll Nutr.* 1983;2:45–54.

75. Silk DBA, Fairclough PD, Clark ML, Hegarty JE, et al. Use of peptide rather than free amino acid nitrogen source in chemically defined "elemental" diets. *J Parenter Enter Nutr.* 1980;4:548–553.

76. Mathews SM, Adibi SA. Peptide absorption. *Gastroenterology.* 1976;71:151–161.

77. Jenkins ME, Gottschlich MM, Warden GD. Enteral feeding during operative procedures in thermal injuries. *J Burn Care Rehabil.* 1994;15:199–205.

78. Buescher TM, Cioffi WG, Becker WK, McManus WF, et al. Perioperative enteral feedings. *Proc Am Burn Assoc.* 1990;22:162.

79. Gottschlich MM, Warden GD. Parenteral nutrition in the burned patient. In: Fischer JE, ed. *Total Parenteral Nutrition.* Philadelphia: WB Saunders Co; 1991:279–298.

80. Goodwin CW. Parenteral nutrition in thermal injuries. In: Rombeau JL, Caldwell MD, eds. *Clinical Nutrition: Parenteral Nutrition.* 2nd ed. Philadelphia: WB Saunders Co; 1993:566–584.

CHAPTER 17

Metabolic Stress and Immune Function

Andrea M. Hutchins and Eva Politzer Shronts

INTRODUCTION

The traditional approach to the nutrition support of hypermetabolic patients was to provide calories and protein via parenteral nutrition in order to meet the increased energy requirements and to provide for nitrogen losses known to occur in these patients. Improved knowledge of the hypermetabolic state, combined with experience and more sophisticated monitoring techniques, has taught dietitians that the traditional approach only rarely leads to nutritional gains, often exacerbates metabolic problems, and is immunologically counterproductive.

Current practice is to provide metabolic support, which includes using the gastrointestinal tract whenever possible, using calorie support to maintain nutritional status, and meeting nitrogen losses. Recent research has also examined the use of specialized nutrients to stimulate immune function and impact patient outcomes. This chapter outlines the hypermetabolic stress response, examines the nutritional implications of it, and examines currently available evidence on appropriate nutrition/metabolic support of these patients.

THE METABOLIC RESPONSE TO INJURY

The metabolic stress response is elicited in response to the presence of injured tissue and is driven by a combination of catabolic hormones and inflammatory mediators. The injury may be caused by any of a number of events—such as hypoxia, inflammation, necrosis, trauma, or infection—that result in the activation of the immune system.

The first response elicited by the immune system is a local one, modulated by the cell-mediated immune system. This system is, in turn, regulated by metabolically active cytokines, such as tumor necrosis factor (TNF) and interleukins (see Table 17–1). This local immune response is characterized by an increase in vascu-

Table 17–1 Selected Cytokines and Their Role

Cytokine	Role
Interferon	Antiviral activity
Lymphotoxin	Kills tumor cells
Tumor necrosis factor	Inhibits parasites and viruses; kills tumor cells
Interleukins	Messengers between leukocytes or white cells
B-cell growth factor	Promotes B-cell proliferation
B-cell differentiation factor	Promotes B-cell maturation

Source: Reprinted from the American Society for Parenteral and Enteral Nutrition (A.S.P.E.N.), Guidelines for the Use of Parenteral and Enteral Nutrition in Adult and Pediatric Patients. JPEN:71(4):1SA–52SA. A.S.P.E.N. does not endorse this material in any form other than its entirety. For information on ordering a complete set of guidelines, contact A.S.P.E.N., 8630 Fenton Street, Suite 412, Silver Spring, MD 20910; 301-587-6315.

lar permeability and an influx of cells, such as white blood cells, macrophages, and fibroblasts that initiate the healing process.[1,2]

If the precipitating event is severe and persists, the local immune response eventually leads to a systemic immune response. Cytokines affect organ function, elicit a macroendocrine response, activate the central nervous system, and release autonomic tone. The net effect of these changes is to increase the oxygen supply as well as the availability of substrates to the metabolically active tissues. Regardless of whether the potentiating event is sepsis, trauma, or surgery, once the systemic response is activated, the metabolic effects are the same and it becomes impossible to distinguish between the states. The systemic inflammatory response is associated with specific alterations in nutrient metabolism, body composition, and nutritional requirements.[1,2]

Impaired immunity is a major risk factor for sepsis and mortality in surgical and other critically ill patients. In preoperative patients, hypoalbuminemia and depressed delayed-type hypersensitivity responsiveness correlate with an increased risk of postoperative mortality.[3] The risk of sepsis and mortality is also increased in patients who are unable to respond to the intradermal injection of recall antigens or cytokines. Persistent anergy is associated with a mortality rate of approximately 50%. In contrast, the risk of mortality is significantly lower for patients who are initially anergic but later become reactive.[3]

Alterations in Substrates

Although comparisons may be made between metabolically stressed patients and patients diagnosed with simple starvation, nutrient metabolism differs markedly between these two states. Simple starvation is characterized by a reduction in basal energy expenditure. Once adaptation to the starved state occurs, there is limited use of glucose and an increased use of fatty acids and ketones for energy. The net effect is a partial sparing of the skeletal muscle mass (see Figure 17–1). Gluconeogenesis is present to provide the minimal amount of glucose that the body requires; however, it is very responsive to exogenous fuels. After an initial refeeding phase, the starved patient usually tolerates energy substrates well.[1,4,5]

In 1930, Cuthbertson[6] was the first to define the metabolic response to stress (including sepsis) and to describe the two phases recognized today. The *ebb phase,* occurring in the first 2 to 48 hours after injury, is distinguished by circulatory insufficiency and a normal or depressed metabolic rate. The ebb phase is followed by the *flow phase,* lasting a minimum of 7 days and is distinguished by an increase in energy expenditure (from carbohydrate, protein, and fat breakdown), high nitrogen excretion, and total body protein catabolism. Although the great demand by the body for protein to be used for host defense and wound healing (acute-phase reactants and coagulation factors) results in a net increase in hepatic protein synthesis,[1,4,6] this increase does not match total body catabolic rates.[5]

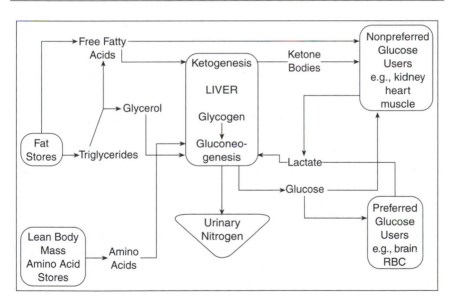

Figure 17–1 Acute Nonstressed Fasting Metabolism. The initial flow of substrate is designed to provide glucose for obligate and nonobligate glucose users. With time, ketones and fats become the main energy substrates, resulting in a reduction in daily urinary nitrogen excretion. *Source:* Reprinted with permission from F.B. Cerra et al., Metabolic Response and Nutritional Support of Patients with Severe Metabolic Stress and Trauma. A Monograph of Sandoz Nutrition, © 1984, Sandoz Nutrition.

The altered hormonal state associated with the metabolic stress response is responsible for increased substrate flow but poor utilization of the substrates. Hyperglycemia occurs as a result of increased 3-carbon glucose intermediates and increased hepatic production of glucose (gluconeogenesis and glycogenolysis), which is unresponsive to exogenous fuel sources.[1,4,7] The peripheral cellular uptake of glucose is unchanged; however, there is an increase in insulin resistance. Although the hypermetabolic patient experiences increased lipolysis and decreased lipogenesis relative to starvation, there is a marked decline in ketone production and utilization. Without the availability of ketones as an energy source, the patient with polytrauma or sepsis has a higher clearance rate and utilization of fatty acids, glycerol, and triglycerides.[1,5,7] Therefore, it seems futile to administer large amounts of substrate to provide calories to a system that is unresponsive to exogenous sources. Body fat serves primarily as a source of fuel; there is no detrimental effect in utilizing stored body fat as an energy source, provided that the patient has adequate body fat reserves.[4]

Probably the greatest metabolic change in the hypermetabolic state is seen in protein metabolism. Increased muscle protein catabolism, amino acid oxidation, gluconeogenesis, ureagenesis, and hepatic protein synthesis occur.[1,7] The overall process results in a net negative nitrogen balance, since catabolism outpaces anabolism. Skeletal muscle is broken down to gain access to the branched-chain amino acids (BCAAs) (leucine, isoleucine, and valine), which are used as energy substrates via gluconeogenesis.[1,4] However, protein is a poor source of energy. One kilogram of muscle provides only 800 calories of energy as compared to 7000 calories in 1 kilogram of fat. When body protein serves as fuel, severe wasting occurs. This results in a loss of strength in respiratory muscles and other vital muscles required for recovery.[4] The other amino acids from skeletal muscle serve as building blocks for hepatic protein production[1,4] (see Figure 17–2). Although proteolysis is unresponsive to exogenous fuels or amino acids, exogenous protein does support synthesis of proteins in the liver, wound, and the mononuclear cell mass[4,7] (see Figure 17–3).

The hypermetabolic stress response is generally self-limiting, but severe cases may progress to multiorgan failure. In multiorgan failure, substrate utilization deteriorates further. Characteristics include increased lipogenesis (manifested by a poor triglyceride clearance), decreased hepatic protein synthesis and clearance of aromatic amino acids, increased ureagenesis, and a progressive failure of gluconeogenesis eventually leading to hypoglycemia.[1]

Evaluating Nutritional Status

For metabolically stressed patients, nutrition support regimens must be tailored to meet patients' unique needs, which can rapidly change. Therefore, nutritional assessment must be a dynamic process to allow the quick identification of the changing needs of the patient. Hepatic transport protein (albumin, transferrin, thy-

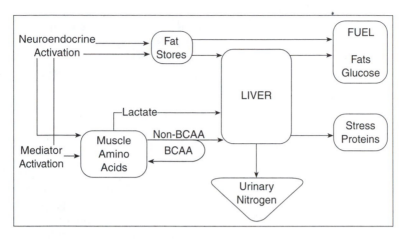

Figure 17–2 Summary of Moderate to Severe Stress Metabolism. The neuroendocrine and intrinsic mediator systems modulate the metabolic machinery to mobilize fat and amino acid stores that provide a continuous supply of fuel to meet increased energy demands and provide an increased supply of substrate for the production of stress proteins. Increased urinary nitrogen excretion is one result of the process. *Source:* Reprinted with permission from F.B. Cerra, et al. Metabolic Response and Nutritional Support of Patients with Severe Metabolic Stress and Trauma. A Monograph of Sandoz Nutrition, © 1984, Sandoz Nutrition.

roxin-binding prealbumin, and retinol-binding protein) concentrations are useful indicators of hepatic protein production and should be monitored for alterations due to hemodilution or hemoconcentration. The presence of hepatic insufficiency (eg, hepatitis, alcoholic liver disease, cirrhosis) should also be evaluated since it affects hepatic protein synthesis regardless of nutritional status. In addition, during periods of acute stress, hepatic reprioritization occurs as the liver begins producing acute-phase reactants instead of transport proteins, resulting in a decline in serum protein levels.[1,8]

During periods of acute stress, serum proteins such as prealbumin may not respond to nutrition support. Measuring C-reactive protein may be helpful in trying to interpret the unresponsiveness of prealbumin to adequate nutrition support.[9] C-reactive protein, normally not detected in the serum, is present in many acute inflammatory conditions and necrosis, often appearing within 24 to 48 hours of the onset of inflammation.[9] C-reactive protein concentrations rise as prealbumin concentrations fall in response to the inflammatory process. Once the period of acute stress begins to resolve, C-reactive protein concentrations decline and prealbumin concentrations increase in response to the continued provision of adequate nutrition support.[9] However, if the patient is being treated with salicylates and steroids, C-reactive protein disappears.[9] Measuring C-reactive protein con-

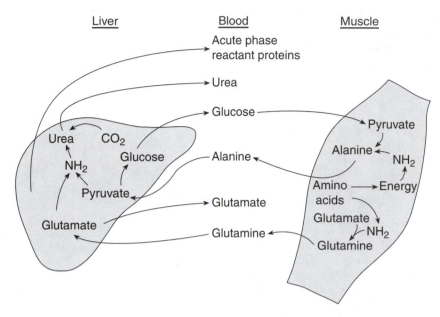

Figure 17–3 Fate of Amino Acids Generated from Muscle Catabolism. *Source:* Reprinted with permission from M.A. Bernard, D.O. Jacobs, J.L. Rombeau. Nutritional and Metabolic Support of Hospitalized Patients, p. 258, © 1986, W.B. Saunders Company.

centrations is as easy as measuring prealbumin concentrations and can often be accomplished with the same laboratory equipment. The costs of both laboratory procedures are approximately the same.[9]

Measurements of urinary creatinine and 3-methylhistidine excretion are useful indicators of skeletal muscle mass and muscle protein degradation, respectively. Nitrogen balance allows evaluation of nitrogen homeostasis and adequacy of nitrogen intake. A positive nitrogen balance of 4 to 6 g/day is assumed to reflect anabolism with an appropriate distribution of the newly synthesized protein. Because complete 24-hour urine collections are sometimes difficult to obtain, urinary creatinine excretion can be used to verify the accuracy of urine collections. Creatinine excretion varies little in the short term; therefore, once a consistent output has been determined, subsequent collections can be judged against that standard. Because all urine tests are dependent on normal renal function, the presence of renal impairment (ie, creatinine clearance <50 mL/min) rules out their use.[1,8]

Depression of the immune response, especially cell-mediated immunity, is a common accompaniment to malnutrition. Metabolic stress—including trauma, sepsis, malignancy, radiation therapy, and steroid therapy—can be associated with anergy. Therefore, anergy may not be indicative of malnutrition and should not be relied upon as an indicator of nutritional status.[1] From a prognostic standpoint, however, tests of immune function (eg, skin test reactivity and total lymphocyte count) together with serum albumin levels are predictive of postoperative morbidity and mortality.[1]

Plasma amino acid profiles or aminograms are useful for evaluating the extent of metabolic dysfunction present in metabolically stressed patients. The characteristic plasma amino acid profile associated with metabolic stress is characterized by an initial decrease in BCAAs. As multiorgan failure develops or progresses and death becomes imminent, BCAA concentrations increase.[1]

ESTIMATING NUTRITIONAL NEEDS

Energy

Although it is essential to provide adequate calories to patients with metabolic stress, excess calories should be avoided. Complications of overfeeding can affect metabolism, organ structure, and organ function. Several methods of estimating caloric requirements are available. In general, it is appropriate to use the Harris-Benedict equation to determine basal energy expenditure and then apply the appropriate stress factor (see Table 17–2). The estimated energy expenditure is usually 25 to 35 kcal/kg/day, and needs exceeding 200% of resting or basal energy expenditure are rare. In practice, daily energy intakes exceeding 2800 kcal of total energy or 2200 kcal of nonprotein energy (when nitrogen/kcal ratio is 1 g/110 kcal of nonprotein energy) are rarely needed.[1,5,10–13]

The guidelines in Table 17–2 provide an initial estimation of needs; however, continuous monitoring is essential to evaluate whether needs are being met and whether adjustments in the nutrition support regimen are needed. When available, indirect calorimetry is the preferred method of measuring energy needs as well as substrate utilization. Unfortunately, in certain clinical settings indirect calorimetry cannot be used reliably (see Chapter 7).

Protein

Protein requirements in hypermetabolic patients usually fall in the range of 1.5 to 2.0 g/kg/day. For patients with renal or hepatic insufficiency, needs should be based on individual tolerance. A nonprotein calorie (NPC) to nitrogen ratio of 100:1 or less is desirable, as this provides for the increased oxidation of protein for energy and decreased utilization of glucose.[1,5] Cerra et al[14] studied 35 hypermetabolic patients receiving enteral nutrition support. All patients received 30 to 35 kcal/kg. Of the patients, 18 received a formula with an NPC to nitrogen ratio of

Table 17–2 Categorical Classification of Stress and Associated Energy and Protein Requirements

	Stress Level and Clinical Example			
	0	*1*	*2*	*3*
Requirement	*Nonstress Starvation*	*Elective General Surgery*	*Polytrauma*	*Sepsis*
Total urinary nitrogen (g/day)	5	5–10	10–15	>15
Glucose* (mg/dL)	100 ± 20	150 ± 25	150 ± 25	250 ± 50
O₂ consumption index (mL/m²)	90 ± 10	130 ± 6	140 ± 6	160 ± 10
Insulin resistance	No	No	Yes/No	Yes
Untreated respiratory quotient	0.7	0.85	0.85	0.85 early 1.0 late
Total estimated kcal needed (kcal/kg/day)	20	25–35		
BEE multiple	1.0	1.3–1.5		
NPC:N	150:1	80–100:1		
AA (g/kg/day)	1.0	1.5–2.0		
% Total daily kcal AA	15%	20%		
CHO	60%	50%		
Fat	25%	<30%		

*In the absence of diabetes, pancreatitis, or steroid therapy.
BEE—Basal energy expenditure.
NPC—Nonprotein calories
N—Nitrogen
AA—Amino acids
CHO—Carbohydrate

Source: Adapted with permission from F.B. Cerra, *Pocket Manual of Surgical Nutrition,* pp. 43 and 60, © 1984, Mosby-Year Book, Inc.

97:1, 10 received a formula with an NPC to nitrogen ratio of 125:1, and 7 received a formula with an NPC to nitrogen ratio of 149:1. Patients with the lowest ratio had significantly greater nitrogen retention, increased plasma transferrin, and a lower respiratory quotient. The investigators concluded: "Nutrition support goals should focus on metabolic needs rather than caloric input in order to achieve the desired end points of nitrogen retention and support of visceral proteins while avoiding problems of excess nutrient administration."[14(p.622)]

Carbohydrate

Once protein requirements have been established, the remaining calories can be provided with carbohydrate and fat. A minimum of 100 g/day of carbohydrate is necessary to prime the tricarboxylic acid cycle.[1] Hypermetabolic patients exhibit glucose intolerance; therefore, the glucose provided should not exceed 5 mg/kg/minute. Excessive intravenous glucose infusion may cause hepatic infiltration that results in abnormal serum liver function tests, precipitates ventilatory failure, or impairs weaning from mechanical ventilation in patients with decreased ventilatory reserve. Metabolically, excess carbohydrate can induce hyperglycemia; increase insulin requirements; and, in extreme cases, contribute to hyperglycemic hyperosmolar nonketotic coma.[1,4,5,11] However, the insulin resistance associated with stress can resolve unpredictably, resulting in hypoglycemia if insulin has been used to maintain glucose control.[1]

Fat

Fat calories should not exceed 40% of total calories. In addition to assisting in protein sparing, fat also reduces the risk of carbohydrate overload and helps to keep total fluid volume down. In very hypermetabolic patients, fat must be provided according to patient tolerance, because hypertriglyceridemia may be present.[1] A minimum of 4% of total caloric needs should be provided as essential fatty acids to avoid deficiency. Essential fatty acid deficiency is associated with suppression of immune responses and delayed hypersensitivity responses. However, current data suggest that doses of polyunsaturated fatty acids in excess of 30% of total calories can alter immune function by depressing the response of lymphocytes to mitogens and antigens as well as decreasing bacterial clearance.[4,15]

Vitamins, Minerals, Trace Elements, and Fluids

No specific guidelines exist for dosing vitamins, minerals, and trace elements in metabolically stressed patients. In general, the Recommended Dietary Allowances can be used for enteral feedings, and the American Medical Association's Nutrition Advisory Group's guidelines can be used for parenteral nutrition[16-19] (see Table 17–3). These recommendations are not appropriate for individuals with renal failure, who should receive restricted amounts of minerals and trace elements.[1] Guidelines for these restrictions can be found in Chapter 11.

Catabolism and loss of lean body tissue increase the loss of potassium, magnesium, phosphorus, and zinc.[1] Gastrointestinal losses, sepsis, and acid-base imbalance may change the need for minerals and electrolytes. Wound healing and anabolism have been shown to increase the requirements for ascorbic acid, zinc, potassium, phosphorus, and magnesium.[1] With increased caloric intake, there may also be an increased need for B vitamins, especially thiamin and niacin.[1]

Table 17–3 Recommended Daily Maintenance Doses for Vitamins, Minerals, and Trace Elements for Adults

Vitamin, Mineral, or Trace Element	Enteral	Parenteral
Vitamin A	800–1000 µg RE	660 µg RE
Vitamin D	5–10 µg	5 µg
Vitamin E	8–10 mg TE	10 mg TE
Vitamin C	60–100 mg	100 mg
Vitamin K	70–140 µg	0.7–2 mg
Folate	200 µg	400 µg
Niacin	13–19 mg NE	40 mg NE
Riboflavin	1.2–1.6 mg	3.6 mg
Thiamin	1.0–1.5 mg	3 mg
Pyridoxine	1.8–2.2 mg	4 mg
Cyanocobalamin	2.0 µg	5.0 µg
Pantothenic Acid	4.7 mg	15 mg
Biotin	30–100 µg	60 µg
Potassium	1875–5625 mg	60–100 mEq
Sodium	1100–3300 mg	60–100 mEq
Chloride	1700–5100 mg	—
Fluoride	1.5–4.0 mg	—
Calcium	800–1200 mg	600 mg
Phosphorus	800–1200 mg	600 mg
Magnesium	300–400 mg	10–20 mEq
Iron	10–15 mg	1–7 mg
Zinc*	12–15 mg	2.5–4.0* mg
Iodine	150 µg	70–140 µg
Copper	1.5–3.0 mg	300–500 µg
Manganese	2–5 mg	0.15–0.8 mg
Chromium	0.05–0.2 mg	10–20 µg
Selenium	0.05–0.2 mg	40–80 µg
Molybdenum	75–250 µg	100–200 µg

*Additional 2 mg in acute catabolic states
NE—niacin equivalents
RE—retinol equivalents
TE—alpha-tocopheral equivalents

Source: Reprinted with permission from E.P. Shronts and J.A. Lacy, Metabolic Support, in *Nutrition Support Dietetics Core Curriculum,* 2nd ed., M.M. Gottschlich, L.E. Matarese, and E.P. Shronts, eds., p. 358, © 1993, American Society of Parenteral and Enteral Nutrition.

In critically ill patients, fluid status must be carefully monitored. High-protein nutrition support regimens produce a high renal-solute load, thereby increasing the free water requirement. A general guideline of 1 mL of water per calorie of intake in adults may be used, but other factors such as fever, gastrointestinal losses, increased ambient air temperature, and air flow may increase fluid requirements where compromised renal function or cardiovascular status may require a fluid restriction. A minimum daily intake of 400 mL/m² is generally required.[1]

ROLES OF SPECIFIC NUTRIENTS

Branched-Chain Amino Acids

In highly stressed patients, BCAA-enriched formulas have shown improved nitrogen retention, improved hepatic protein synthesis, decreased protein degradation, and less expense to reach nitrogen equilibrium.[1,5] The minimal effective dose of BCAA is 0.5 g/kg/day. To provide significant improvements in nitrogen balance, a dose of 0.8 g/kg/day is preferred.[1] Although BCAA-enriched solutions have demonstrated an impact on hepatic protein synthesis, no corresponding effects on outcome have been shown.

Glutamine

Glutamine, classically considered a nonessential amino acid, may be conditionally indispensable in critical illness. It is the most abundant free amino acid in circulation, constituting approximately 20% of the total circulating free amino acid pool. Intracellularly, it accounts for more than 50% of the intracellular free amino acid in muscle tissue. It is a precursor for synthesis of amino acids, proteins, nucleotides, and many other biologically important molecules.[10,20,21] It appears to be the preferred fuel of the gastrointestinal tract and other rapidly proliferating cells.[5,21] The major endogenous sources of glutamine are skeletal muscle and lung.[3]

Glutamine also has a number of potential regulatory functions. Under experimental conditions, it increases protein synthesis and reduces protein degradation in the skeletal muscle and stimulates glycogen synthesis in the liver.[1,10] In exercise, trauma, sepsis, and glucocorticoid treatment, glutamine requirements may exceed synthetic capacity, leading to decreased plasma glutamine concentrations and reduction of intracellular glutamine.[1,10] This may interfere with protein synthesis and influence the integrity of the intestinal mucosa as well as immune function.[10] In a study by Scheltinga et al,[22] patients receiving a glutamine-enriched total parenteral nutrition (TPN) solution exhibited significantly fewer positive microbial cultures and a significantly lower rate of clinical infection than patients receiving a standard TPN solution.

There is considerable evidence that glutamine utilization and oxidation are essential for lymphocytes. Glutamine serves dual metabolic roles for these cells. It is a primary source of energy and carbon and nitrogen precursors for nucleotide biosynthesis. Investigators have hypothesized that postinjury glutamine depletion plays a significant role in the suppression of macrophage function observed after trauma.[20] Parenteral supplementation of glutamine up to 40 g/day (0.57 g/kg) compared with an estimated normal dietary intake of only 3 to 5 g/day improved nitrogen balance and significantly reduced both infection rate and hospital stay.[13,21,22]

It has been speculated that the reduced availability of glutamine may be a factor in disruption of the gut barrier, which may result in a chronic hypermetabolic state and contribute to multiorgan failure, severe injury, and sepsis. Reduction of intracellular glutamine concentration seems to correlate with the severity of injury and sepsis. It is therefore not surprising that a low intracellular glutamine concentration in severe injury and sepsis is associated with high mortality. Researchers have suggested that repletion of glutamine pools has therapeutic value in catabolic conditions.[10]

Currently, glutamine is available in enteral formulas in the United States as either protein-bound glutamine or free glutamine, supplemented at levels of 4.0 to 14.0 g/L[21] (see Table 17–4). Although the bioavailability of protein-bound glutamine is unknown, an estimate of the glutamine content of polymeric formulas may be on the label.[21] The amount of glutamine in the formula depends on the source and amount of protein in the formula as well as the processing conditions. Because hydrolysis causes the degradation of some glutamine, the glutamine content of partially hydrolyzed formulas may be lower than expected when considering the protein source.

Glutamine-supplemented parenteral formulas are not currently available in the United States due to glutamine's limited stability in solution and concern over potential disassociation into the two toxic compounds ammonia and pyroglutamate.[21,23] However, use of more stable peptides, glycine-L-glutamine and L-alanyl-L-glutamine, appears to be a safe method of delivering glutamine parenterally.[21,24]

Although the studies performed to date have failed to demonstrate any toxicity associated with glutamine-supplemented parenteral nutrition, concern exists for patients with head injuries, hepatic encephalopathy, or renal failure since ammonia is an end-product of glutamine metabolism.[20,21,23,25] Glutamine-supplemented formulas should be used cautiously and should not exceed the recommended safe level of 0.285 to 0.571 g/kg of body weight per day.[26] Glutamine may be a preferred fuel for some tumors and has been shown to increase tumor growth in experimental models.[27] However, according to a review by Klimberg,[28] recent animal studies have failed to support this conclusion. Instead, these studies suggest that glutamine supplementation in a tumor model may be beneficial by protecting the gut from radiation enteritis; reducing morbidity; increasing natural killer cell activity, which can blunt tumor growth in the absence of therapy; and enhancing

Table 17–4 Comparison of Products Designed for Immunostimulation

Characteristics	Advera® (Ross)	Perative® (Ross)	Alitraq® (Ross)	Vivonex Plus® (Novartis)	Crucial® (Clintec)	ImmunAid® (McGaw)	Impact® (Novartis)	Impact 1.5® (Novartis)
kcal/mL	1.28	1.3	1.0	1.0	1.5	1.0	1.0	1.5
CHO								
g/1000 kcal	168.6	177.2	164	190	90	120	132	93.3
% kcal	65.5	54.5	66	76	36	48	53	38
PRO								
g/1000 kcal	46.9	66	52.6	45	62.7	80	56	53.3
% kcal	18.7	20.5	21	18	25	32	22	22
arginine								
g/1000 kcal	0	7.9	4.5	6.2	10	14	12.5	12.5
% kcal	0	2	2	2	4	5.6	5	5
glutamine								
g/1000 kcal	0	0	14.2	10	4.8	9	0	0
nucleic acid								
g/1000 kcal	0	0	0	0	0	1.0	1.2	1.2
FAT								
g/1000 kcal	17.8	37.4	15	6.7	45	22	28	46
% kcal	15.8	25	13	6	39	20	25	40
Source	Canola, MCT, sardine	Canola, MCT, corn	MCT, safflower	soy	MCT, fish, soy, lecithin	canola, MCT	structured lipid, menhaden oil	MCT, structured lipid, menhaden oil
mOsm/kg	680	385	575	650	490	460	375	550
mL to meet 100% RDA	1184	1155	1500	1800	1000	2000	1500	1250
NPC:N	108:1	97:1	120:1	115:1	67:1	~53:1	71:1	71:1
Other features	78% protein hydrolysate; soy fiber; ↑ vitamins E, C, B_6, B_{12}, folate, β-carotene	Protein hydrolysate	PRO: 42% peptide 47% free AA 11% intact whey	100% amino acids (33% BCAA)	Peptides avg length = 6 MCT:LCT = 50:50 n6:n3 = 2:1	20% of PRO = suppl BCAA	Available with guar ↑ omega-3 MCT:LCT = 27:73 n6:n3 = 1.4:1	↑ omega-3 MCT:LCT = 55:45 n6:n3 = 1:1.4

Note: Information obtained from product information and from manufacturers.

tumor cell kill from irradiation and chemotherapy. Extensive clinical trials are still needed to determine the benefit, or lack of benefit, of glutamine supplementation in patients with tumors.

Arginine

Arginine is considered a nonessential amino acid in nonstressed humans. It promotes DNA synthesis and wound healing and enhances the responsiveness of macrophages and lymphocytes to antigens. Researchers have found that arginine enhances immune functions and improves patient outcomes.[3,5,15,29,30] Thus, arginine, like glutamine, may be a conditionally indispensable amino acid in metabolically stressed patients. Arginine-supplemented enteral formulas are currently available in the United States (see Table 17–4). However, arginine supplementation has been shown to increase tumor growth in mice, using concentrations currently available in arginine-supplemented enteral formulas.[31] Whether this finding has implications for humans has yet to be demonstrated.

Arginine is also a source of nitric oxide, a highly reactive molecule resulting from the oxidation of the guanidine nitrogen of arginine, which is produced by a number of cells including macrophages and neutrophils. Nitric oxide is known to modulate hepatic protein synthesis, reduce vascular tone, mediate the vasodilating effects of endotoxin, and reduce tumor and bacterial growth. Whether any of these effects is beneficial in humans is unknown.[11,12] Nitric oxide may have some potentially negative effects as well. Nitric oxide's effect on vascular tone can lead to hypotension, especially in patients with sepsis.[11] Nitric oxide may also play a role in sepsis-related myocardial dysfunction.[11] Therefore, patients receiving arginine-supplemented enteral formulas should be monitored carefully for evidence of hypotension or myocardial dysfunction.

Cysteine

Cysteine, produced from methionine, may also be a conditionally essential amino acid in highly stressed patients. Cysteine is a precursor in glutathione synthesis. Glutathione has a role in protecting the body from free radicals, which may be related to oxidative stress and the resulting cell death and tissue damage. In a healthy adult, endogenous biosynthesis provides adequate cysteine and, therefore, adequate glutathione. However, in highly stressed patients, the conversion of methionine to cysteine may occur too slowly, resulting in an inadequate amount of cysteine and glutathione.[32] Cysteine can be found in widely varying concentrations in the protein sources commonly used for enteral formulas. However, the cysteine content of enteral formulas is not listed on most labels. Because free cysteine is unstable in solution, it is not currently supplemented in parenteral solutions. Supplementation of cysteine is not recommended, because cysteine is rapidly metabolized and excessive quantities can be toxic. Currently, most parenteral solutions and free amino acid–based enteral formulas use methionine, because it functions as a precursor to cysteine.[32]

Nucleotides

Nucleotides are precursors to DNA and RNA and provide the major energy transfer molecule adenosine triphosphate. They are formed from purines and pyrimidines, both of which are deficient in parenteral formulas and most enteral formulas. Experimental work with purines has observed that diets supplemented with yeast RNA restore delayed-type hypersensitivity, improve recovery of T-cell function, and increase resistance to infection.[3,15,28] Currently there are commercially available enteral formulas supplemented with nucleotides (Table 17–4), but no recommendations have been made regarding dosage guidelines. Adults consuming a normal diet typically ingest 1 to 2 g of nucleotides per day.[33]

Omega-6 Fatty Acids

The polyunsaturated fatty acids (PUFA) are a major component of the cell membrane. They are responsible for the structural integrity of membranes as well as eicosanoid production and release. The major PUFA constituents of membranes are of the omega-6 family. The omega-6 fatty acids increase the production of arachidonic acid, a precursor of the 2-series of prostaglandins, which have proinflammatory effects.[34] Omega-6 PUFAs are also the major component in currently available parenteral lipid emulsions.

Omega-3 Fatty Acids

There are very low levels of the omega-3 family of fatty acids in cell membranes. The omega-3 fatty acids are thought to modulate arachadonic acid metabolism, thereby affecting eicosanoid production.[1] The incorporation of omega-3 PUFA into macrophages occurs within 3 to 6 hours in cell culture and is stabilized within a few days *in vivo*. Once incorporated, membrane fluidity increases, intracellular calcium flux is reduced, macrophage cytokine release to inflammatory stimuli is altered, and T and B cell proliferative responses to specific antigen stimulation is improved. The release of TNF and interleukin-1 by the macrophages is related to the omega-6:omega-3 ratio and omega-3 and omega-6 total PUFA content of the cell membrane. The prostanoid products of eicosapentanoic acid (20:5

omega-3) are less inflammatory than those of linoleic acid (18:2 omega-6).[10,12,15] The omega-3 fatty acids are major constituents of fish oils.

Medium-Chain Triglycerides

Medium-chain-triglyceride (MCT)–containing intravenous fat emulsions have been shown to improve the utilization of lipids and are expected to be available for clinical use in the near future. Currently, several enteral formulas containing MCTs as part of their fat, as well as an MCT oil module that can be added to enteral formulas, are available (see Table 17–4). MCTs provided enterally are advantageous due to their rapid hydrolysis and absorption in the intestine as well as their rapid and complete oxidation. MCTs provided enterally or parenterally have a negligible effect on plasma lipoproteins, may circumvent the immuno-suppressive effect of omega-6 PUFAs, and have also shown an improved protein-sparing capability compared to isocaloric long-chain triglycerides (LCTs).[35] The use of parenteral MCT solutions can be limited, however, due to the potential toxicity of pure MCT solutions, which may cause metabolic acidosis in larger doses.[34] MCTs also lack essential fatty acids.

Structured Lipids

Structured lipids have the potential to provide the advantages of MCT administration while preventing the side-effects of toxicity and essential fatty acid deficiency. Structured lipids, composed of a mixture of MCTs and LCTs on a glycerol backbone, are different from physical mixtures of MCTs and LCTs. The result of hydrolyzing a mixture of MCTs and LCTs and then randomly reesterifying them on the same glycerol backbone, structured lipids offer the possibility of using different sources of lipids for specific purposes. In theory, modification of the fatty acid composition of the triglyceride or the phospholipid composition may have a variety of pharmacological effects, such as prostaglandin and leukotriene synthesis, and therefore inflammatory reactions. Structured lipids may affect the structure and property of cell membranes, pulmonary surfactant production, and atheroma formation. Presently, two enteral formulas that contain structured lipids are available in the United States. Although parenteral structured lipid solutions are not currently available in the United States, Hyltander et al[34] have demonstrated that structured LCTs and MCTs can be safely provided parenterally to metabolically stressed patients without risk of clinical or metabolic side effects. However, more studies are needed to confirm the safety and efficacy of these parenteral solutions.

Fiber

Dietary fiber has been shown to play a role in bacterial translocation and gut mucosal integrity and to stimulate mucous production in the gut, which is rich in IgA. Not all fibers have the same effect. Dietary fibers can be classified as either insoluble or soluble fiber. Insoluble fibers (eg, cellulose; some hemicelluloses; and lignins found in wheat bran, psyllium seed, and ispaghul husk) do not dissolve in water and are largely not metabolized by bacteria in the large intestine. One exception is soy polysaccharide, a common component in fiber-containing enteral formulas, which is highly fermented in the colon.[21] Insoluble fibers increase fecal mass by holding water, help prevent constipation, and help normalize bowel function in patients suffering from diarrhea.[21,36,37] Cellulose has been shown to reduce bacterial translocation, but it does not prevent the atrophy of the small intestine mucosa.[38]

Soluble fibers (eg, pectins, gums, and mucilages, which can be found in fruits and oats) either dissolve or swell in water and are fermented by bacteria in the large intestine. Soluble fibers have been reported to reduce the risk of intestinal atrophy as well as stimulate mucosal proliferation.[21,36] In the past, soluble fiber was found only in blenderized enteral formulas made from whole foods because it formed a gel when added to other enteral formulas. However, advances in fiber technology have made it possible to add soluble fibers, in particular guar, to enteral formulas (see Table 17-4).

Exact requirements for dietary fiber are unknown, but current recommendations suggest oral intakes between 20 and 35 g/day. No recommendations have been made for the amount of enteral dietary fiber intake. However, since both soluble and insoluble fibers are important in reducing bacterial translocation and maintaining the integrity of the gut mucosa, enteral formulas containing both types of fiber would be advantageous.

Antioxidants

Antioxidant therapy to prevent or reduce the damage caused by free radicals is currently under investigation. Free radicals are generated in a wide range of acute and chronic diseases (eg, acute respiratory distress syndrome and burn resuscitation), cause lipid peroxidation, and disrupt cell membranes leading to cellular death.[12,13] Although free radicals are originally generated as part of the immune response to kill invading microorganisms, the uncontrolled production of free radicals can result in more cellular injury than that caused by the original insult and can contribute to multiorgan failure. Although naturally occurring free radical scavengers exist (eg, superoxide dismutases and glutathione peroxidase), researchers have proposed supplementing nutrition support regimens with antioxidant vitamins (E and C) as a method of combating free radical damage.[12] However, studies in this area are limited and inconclusive, so it is premature to recommend the routine use of high-dose antioxidant vitamins.[12,13,15]

Multimodality Therapy

The newest enteral formulas for use in metabolically stressed patients combine several potentially immune-enhancing nutrients (glutamine, arginine, nucleotides, and omega-3 fatty acids).[39–44] Several clinical trials utilizing these new "designer" formulas have been completed to date (see Table 17–5). Studies that have compared a formula supplemented with arginine, RNA, and omega-3 fatty acids to standard enteral formulas[39,40,42–44] have reported decreased plasma concentrations of omega-6 fatty acids,[39,42] increased plasma concentrations of omega-3 fatty acids,[39,42] and decreased infectious and/or wound complications with the supplemented formula.[40,42,43] In addition, the patients who received the experimental formula also had increased T lymphocyte and helper T cell concentrations[44] and a decreased length of hospital stay.[40,42,43] Two studies[41,45] that compared a formula enriched with BCAAs, glutamine, arginine, omega-3 fatty acids, and nucleotides to elemental or standard high-protein formulas reported similar results. The patients who received the supplemented formula had fewer infectious complications[45] or abscesses[41] and increased concentrations of T lymphocytes and T-helper cells.[41] Brown et al[46] compared a formula containing partially hydrolyzed proteins and supplemented with arginine, alpha-linolenic acid, and beta-carotene to a standard enteral formula and found that patients who received the experimental formula had fewer infections and a greater change in serum concentrations of C-reactive protein. Kenler et al[47] also reported that patients had fewer infections when they received a formula supplemented with fish oil structured lipids instead of a standard enteral formula. Patients with severe burns also had reduced incidence of wound infection and length of hospital stay when they received a modular enteral feeding supplemented with omega-3 fatty acids, arginine, cysteine, histidine, vitamin A, zinc, and ascorbic acid.[48]

Two studies have examined the use of enteral formulas containing potentially immune-enhancing nutrients with patients who have human immunodeficiency virus (HIV) infection. When patients with asymptomatic HIV infection received a peptide-based formula supplemented with MCTs, sardine oil, beta-carotene, and soy polysaccharide, they maintained their body weight better and had fewer hospitalizations than patients who received standard oral supplements.[49] Patients with symptomatic HIV infection had greater weight gain and increased serum concentration of the soluble TNF receptor proteins when they received a formula supplemented with alpha-linoleic acid, arginine, and RNA instead of an isocaloric control formula.[50]

The use of formulas that combine several of the potentially immune-enhancing nutrients can result in positive patient outcomes as partially evidenced by the de-

Table 17–5 Multimodality Enteral Feeding: A Comparison of Results

Investigator	Number in Study	Study Design	Formula Comparisons	Results*
Gottschlich et al (1990)[48]	Study group (modular feeding): N = 17 Control group (Osmolite®): N = 14 Control group (Traumacal®): N = 19	In this randomized, blinded, prospective study, patients were fed enterally for 7–61 days following acute burn of greater than 10% of their body surface area.	Modular tube feeding recipe versus Osmolite® enriched with Promix® versus Traumacal®	Study group: • reduced incidence of wound infection • reduced length of hospital stay/ percent burn
Cerra et al (1991)[39]	Study group: N = 11 Control group: N = 9	In this randomized, blinded, prospective study, patients were fed via NJ for 7–10 days following trauma, surgery, or infection. Full dose of formula was achieved within 36 hours of initiation.	Impact® versus Osmolite HN®	Study group: • decreased plasma concentrations of omega-6 fatty acids • increased plasma concentrations of omega-3 fatty acids • increased plasma concentrations of arginine, glutamine, and ornithine • improved immune function as measured by *in vitro* proliferative assays
Daly et al (1992)[40]	Study group: N = 41 Control group: N = 44	In this randomized study, patients were fed via NJ or jejunostomy for 7 days postsurgery for upper GI malignancy. Full dose of formula was achieved within 4 days of initiation.	Impact® versus Osmolite HN®	Study group: • decreased infectious and wound complications • decreased length of hospital stay

continues

Table 17–5 continued

Investigator	Number in Study	Study Design	Formula Comparisons	Results*
Chlebowski et al (1993)[49]	Study group: $N = 31$ Control group: $N = 25$	In this randomized, prospective study, patients with early-stage asymptomatic HIV infection were fed orally for 6 months.	Advera® versus Ensure®	Study group: • better maintenance of body weight • more stable triceps skinfold measurements • lower blood urea nitrogen • fewer hospitalizations
Moore et al (1994)[41]	Study group: $N = 51$ Control group: $N = 47$	In this multicenter, randomized, prospective study, patients were fed via NJ or jejunostomy for 7 days posttrauma. Full dose of formula was achieved within 72 hours of initiation.	ImmunAid® versus Vivonex T.E.N.®	Study group: • increased total lymphocyte count • increased T lymphocytes • increased T-helper cells • fewer intra-abdominal abscesses • less incidence of multiple organ failure
Brown et al (1994)[46]	Study group: $N = 19$ Control group: $N = 18$	In this prospective, randomized study, patients were fed via NG, gastrostomy, or jejunostomy for 5–10 days posttrauma. Full dose of formula was achieved within 72 hours of initiation.	Perative® versus Osmolite HN® supplemented with ProMod®	Study group: • fewer infections • greater change in nitrogen balance • greater change in serum concentrations of C-reactive protein
Daly et al (1995)[42]	Study group: $N = 37$ Control group: $N = 23$	In this randomized study, patients were fed via jejunostomy for 7 days postsurgery for upper GI	Impact® versus Traumacal®	Study group: • increased plasma and cellular omega-3/omega-6 fatty acid levels • decreased PGE_2 production

	malignancy. Full dose of formula was achieved within 72 hours of initiation.		• decreased infectious and wound complications • decreased length of hospital stay
Bower et al (1995)[43]	Study group: *N* = 168 Control group: *N* = 158	In this prospective, randomized, double-blind study, patients were fed via NG, NJ, gastrostomy, or jejunostomy for 6–9 days following trauma, surgery, or sepsis. Full dose of formula was achieved within 96 hours of initiation.	Impact® versus Osmolite HN®	Study group: • increased plasma arginine and ornithine concentrations • increased serum concentrations of eicosapentaenoic and docosahexaenoic acid • decreased length of hospital stay • decreased frequency of infections
Kemen et al (1995)[44]	Study group: *N* = 21 Control group: *N* = 21	In this prospective, randomized, double-blind study, patients were fed via jejunostomy for 16 days postsurgery for upper GI malignancy. Full dose of formula was achieved within 5 days of initiation.	Impact® versus isocaloric, isonitrogenous control formula	Study group: • increased T lymphocytes and T-helper cell concentrations • increased immunoglobulin M and immunoglobulin G concentrations • increased B-lymphocyte concentrations
Kudsk et al (1996)[45]	Study group: *N* = 16 Control group: *N* = 17	In this prospective, randomized, blind study, patients with early enteral access and severe injuries received either the immune-enhancing formula or the control formula.	ImmunAid® versus Promote® with Casec®	Study group: • reduced major infectious complications • decreased length of hospital stay

continues

Table 17-5 continued

Investigator	Number in Study	Study Design	Formula Comparisons	Results*
Süttmann et al (1996)[50]	Study group: $N = 10$ Control group: $N = 10$	In this double-blind, crossover study, patients with symptomatic HIV infection who were following stable medication regimens orally consumed a control formula and a fortified formula for 4 months each.	Formula fortified with alpha-linoleic acid, arginine, and RNA versus an isocaloric control formula	Study group: • greater weight gain • increased eicosapentaenoic acid incorporated into the erythrocyte cell membranes • increased serum concentrations of the soluble tumor necrosis factor receptor proteins • increased plasma arginine concentrations
Kenler et al (1996)[47]	Study group: $N = 17$ Control group: $N = 18$	In this double-blind, prospective, randomized study, patients were fed via jejunostomy for 7 days postsurgery. Full dose of formula was achieved within 72–96 hours of initiation.	Fish oil structured lipid formula versus Osmolite HN®	Study group: • increased incorporation of eicosapentaenoic acid into plasma and erythrocyte phospholipids • decreased number of infections

*Statistically significant results ($p \leq 0.05$)

Abbreviations: NJ = nasojejunal feeding; GI = gastrointestinal; HIV = human immunodeficiency virus; NG = nasogastric creased number and frequency of infections and the decreased length of hospital stay reported by many of the studies. However, as Barton[51] has pointed out in his review of the studies on immune-enhancing enteral formulas, several of the studies had small study populations; used only a select patient population; did not use isocaloric, isonitrogenous formulas; or used an enteral formula that is not commercially available. Despite shortcomings in many of the available studies to date, Barton concludes: "It cannot be denied that the majority of the literature on the subject of immune-enhancing formulas seems to suggest that these formulas may be beneficial in selected patient populations."[51] This viewpoint is echoed by Dickerson,[52] who suggests use of this therapy in critically ill patients with an abnormal trauma index ≥25 and/or an injury severity score ≥21. Further research is needed to determine which of these nutrients are most active in producing the beneficial effects, in what doses, for what length of time, and in what specific combinations.

PROVIDING NUTRITION AND METABOLIC SUPPORT FOR PATIENTS WITH METABOLIC STRESS

During the ebb phase of metabolic stress, treatment priority is to maintain fluid and electrolyte balance. Once the flow phase of metabolic stress begins, nutrition support can be initiated. Gastrointestinal function, baseline nutritional status, and the risks associated with enteral or parenteral feeding should be considered before choosing the route for nutrition support.

Enteral versus Parenteral Nutrition Support

The early use of enteral feeding in posttraumatic patients should help maintain gut morphology and function, improve maintenance of immunologic function, and decrease risk of bacterial translocation.[1] In a study conducted by Fong et al,[53] healthy volunteers were challenged with intravenous purified *Escherichia coli* lipopolysaccharide after being fed enterally or parenterally for 7 days. The TPN group had significantly increased concentrations of glucagon, epinephrine, and TNF and a greater loss of amino acid from the extremity when compared to the group fed enterally. These responses are indicative of an increased acute-phase response and peripheral amino acid mobilization. The results led the authors to suggest that, when compared to enteral feeding, TPN may enhance postinjury metabolic alterations, including an exaggerated counterregulatory hormone response and enhanced production of cytokines. Kudsk et al[54] fed 98 patients enterally or parenterally within 24 hours of multiple trauma. When compared with the patients given TPN, the enterally fed patients had a significantly lower rate of septic complications. When the acute-phase protein levels (C-reactive protein and

α_1-acid glycoprotein) were measured in 68 of the most severely injured patients, significantly lower levels of acute-phase proteins were found in the enterally fed patients; this finding offers a possible partial explanation for this group's reduced septic morbidity.[55] These results are consistent with those reported earlier by Moore et al.[56] In a study of 75 postoperative patients, patients who received enteral nutrition had significantly lower acute-phase proteins when compared to patients who received a nutritionally matched TPN solution.[56]

Clinical studies have also reported that nitrogen retention in critically ill patients fed enterally is equal to or better than that in patients fed parenterally.[55-57] Decreased cost and risk of complications are other reasons cited for considering enteral feeding before parenteral feeding.[1]

The timing of the initiation of enteral feeding has also been shown to be important.[58-62] Most studies to date have shown that early enteral feeding (less than 36 hours following the injury or event) results in improved nutritional response (less weight loss, better nitrogen balance) and metabolic response (decreased resting metabolic expenditure and plasma catabolic hormones)[58-62] (see Table 17–6). These studies have also shown an impact on outcome with early enteral feeding, demonstrated by improved wound healing, fewer bacterial infections, and shorter median stay in the intensive care unit.[58-62] The only study in which enteral feeding did not show any benefit was by Eyer et al.[63] It is likely that the delayed initiation of the early enteral feeding (31 ± 13 hours post–intensive care unit admit) was responsible for the results in this study.

Enteral Nutrition Support

The full benefit of enteral nutrition can be realized only through correct selection of route, formula, and method of administration. In the past, enteral feeding was avoided in postinjury patients. It is now known that while stomach ileus is present for 24 to 48 hours, the small bowel has normal absorption and motility 12 to 24 hours postinjury.[1,5] Traditionally, the return of bowel sounds and the passage of flatus or stools have been used as markers to determine the resolution of small-bowel ileus. However, since bowel sounds merely represent the passage of air, they may be a poor indicator of small-bowel motility. For the many patients who receive nasogastric suctioning postoperatively, little air reaches the small intestine; this results in decreased bowel sounds with normal motility. Passage of flatus or stool indicates the return of colonic function but is a poor indicator of small bowel function. If necessary, low-residue, elemental or semielemental formulas can be utilized until adequate colonic function returns.[5] Placement of the feeding tube distal to the pylorus and slow administration (10 to 20 cc/hour) by 24-hour

Table 17–6 Early versus Delayed Enteral Feeding: A Comparison of Results

Investigator	Study Design	Results*
Chiarelli et al 1990[59] (humans)	Study: fed on admit 4.4 ± 0.49 hours after trauma (N = 10) Control: fed 48 hours after admit, 57.7 ± 2.61 hours (N = 10)	Study group: • reduced urinary catecholamines and plasma glucagon • improved nitrogen balance
Mochizuki et al 1984[60] (guinea pigs)	Group A (N = 19): 175 kcal, 2 hours postburn Group B (N = 20): 175 kcal, after 72 hours Group C (N = 18): 200 kcal, after 72 hours	Group A: • lowest RME • decreased glucagon and cortisol • increased jejunal mucosal weight
Grahm et al 1989[58] (humans)	Study: NJ fed within 36 hours of injury (N = 17) Control: NG fed after day 3 or when bowel sounds (N = 15)	Study group: • decreased bacterial infections • decreased median length of stay in ICU • improved calorie intake, nitrogen intake and balance (Days 2–4)
Schroeder et al 1991[61] (humans)	Study: immediate postop NJ with gastric decompression (N = 16) Control: routine postop NG, fluids, oral feeding when tolerated (N = 16)	Study group: • increased hydroxyproline accumulation in wounds • improved calorie intake first 4 days
Zaloga et al 1992[62] (rats)	Study: immediate postop (N = 8) Control: 72 hours after surgery (N = 9)	Study group: • twice the wound strength (bursting pressure) • less weight loss
Eyer et al 1993[63] (humans)	Study: goal-feed <24 hours of ICU admit (N = 19) Control: goal-feed >72 hours of ICU admit (N = 19)	• no benefit of early feeding demonstrated • time from ICU admit to feeding early 31 ± 13 hours, late 82 ± 11 hours • time from injury to feeding early 39 ± 12 hours, late 90 ± 12 hours

*Statistically significant results ($p \leq 0.05$)

Abbreviations: RME = resting metabolic expenditure; NJ = nasojejunal feeding; NG = nasogastric feeding; ICU = intensive care unit

Source: Reprinted with permission from E.P. Stronts, Clinical Update Review: Enteral vs. Parenteral Nutrition: A Review, *Minnesota Chapter of Enteral and Parenteral Nutrition Bulletin,* Vol. 7, p. 4, © 1995, American Society of Parenteral and Enteral Nutrition.

continuous infusion minimize gastrointestinal complications. The feedings can be progressed as tolerated every 12 hours.

The desired intake can usually be achieved within 2 to 3 days. Formula selection should be based on nutritional needs and intestinal digestive and absorptive capacity. An elemental or semielemental formula can also be used in conditions of decreased absorption; however, a minimum of 3 to 4 feet of functional small bowel is necessary to absorb even a hydrolyzed diet adequately.[1] With many modular components available, formula composition is no longer a reason to select parenteral over enteral feeding.

Parenteral Nutrition Support

Although enteral nutrition has many benefits, some conditions warrant the use of parenteral nutrition over enteral nutrition (eg, gastrointestinal obstruction, high-output gastrointestinal fistulas). Parenteral nutrition may also be used in conjunction with enteral nutrition. For example, peripheral parenteral nutrition can supplement enteral nutrition while progressing to goal tube feeding intake (eg, with malabsorption, chronic diarrhea, chronic vomiting, burns, hypermetabolism).[1] The choice of peripheral or central parenteral nutrition should be based on nutritional requirements, amount of calories and protein to be administered via parenteral nutrition, length of therapy, fluid restrictions, and viability of peripheral veins.[1] With the use of fat emulsion, peripheral parenteral nutrition can provide 30% to 60% of required calories for 5 to 7 days until gastrointestinal function returns. This method is particularly useful in patients who were malnourished preinjury and have poor nutrient stores.[1] Although there are risks involved with a central line, central parenteral nutrition has the benefit of providing more concentrated nutrients and less fluid. This is particularly helpful in patients with congestive heart failure and renal or hepatic insufficiency.[1]

Due to the glucose intolerance usually seen in metabolically stressed patients, parenteral dextrose administration should not exceed 5 mg/kg/min. Administration of the parenteral lipid emulsions currently available should not exceed 1.0 g/kg/day of fat due to immunosuppressive effects of high-dose linoleic acid.[1]

MONITORING AND PREVENTING COMPLICATIONS

In the hypermetabolic patient, progress to a lower stress level or to multiorgan failure can mean alterations in nutritional requirements. Therefore, stress level, metabolic status, and nutritional indexes must be evaluated continuously to judge the effectiveness of therapy.

The most clinically useful and available indexes for evaluating stress level are serum glucose, urinary nitrogen excretion, the oxygen consumption index, and presence of a fever and leukocytosis.[1] Metabolic indicators of substrate tolerance include serum glucose, urinary glucose/ketones, and expired gas analysis (CO_2) for carbohydrate; lipemia and serum triglycerides for fat; and blood urea nitrogen for protein. Other useful parameters are liver function tests, serum electrolytes, and intake and output. As most of the parameters are affected by other factors, serial measurements to assess trends are most useful. Weight, calorie/protein intake, nitrogen balance, and hepatic transport proteins offer a reasonably complete picture of nutritional status. If specific vitamin, mineral, or trace element deficits are suspected based on clinical or other evidence, appropriate biochemical data should be obtained prior to supplementation.

In patients with organ failure or multiple organ failure, monitoring may include such tests as expired gas analysis, plasma amino acid profiles, and creatinine excretion. In renal failure, where albumin metabolism is altered and urine output is diminished, urea kinetics is a useful means of assessing nitrogen balance.[1]

CONCLUSIONS

Metabolic stress has significant effects on nutrient metabolism, nutritional assessment, and nutritional requirements. Patients experiencing metabolic stress must undergo a careful initial evaluation. Whenever possible, the gastrointestinal tract should be used to provide nutrition to patients who are unable to eat. In the sickest patients, the use of specialized nutrients has shown great promise in improving clinical outcomes. The ultimate success of nutrition/metabolic support within a given patient depends on a thorough initial patient assessment, provision of the optimal nutrition support regimen, and ongoing monitoring. Monitoring facilitates identification of potential complications as well as the need to adjust in nutrition support based on the patient's changing needs.

REFERENCES

1. Shronts EP, Lacy JA. Metabolic support. In: Gottschlich MM, Matarese LE, Shronts EP, eds. *Nutrition Support Dietetics Core Curriculum.* Silver Spring, MD: A.S.P.E.N.; 1993:351–366.

2. Myrvik QN. Immunology and nutrition. In: Shils ME, Olson JA, Shike M, eds. *Modern Nutrition in Health and Disease.* 8th ed. Philadelphia: Lea & Febiger; 1994:623–662.

3. Borlase BC, Babineau TJ, Forse RA, Bell SJ, et al. Enteral nutrition support. In: Rippe JM, Irwin RS, Alpert JS, Fink MP, eds. *Intensive Care Medicine.* 2nd ed. Boston: Little Brown & Co; 1991:1669–1674.

4. Fish J, Shronts EP. A case for nitrogen balance vs. caloric balance in critically ill patients. *Nutr Immunol Digest.* 1993;2:1–5.

5. Charney P, Martindale R. Early enteral nutrition support in metabolic stress. *RD.* 1994;14:1,4–6,8–9.

6. Cuthbertson CP. The disturbance of metabolism produced by bony and non-bony injury, with notes on certain abnormal condition of bone. *Biochem J.* 1930;24:1245–1263.

7. Kinney JM. Metabolic response to starvation, injury and sepsis. In: Payne-James J, Grimble G, Silk D, eds. *Artificial Nutrition Support in Clinical Practice.* London: Edward Arnold/Hodder Headline Group; 1995:1–11.

8. Shronts EP. Nutritional assessment of adults with end-stage hepatic failure. *Nutr Clin Pract.* 1988;3:133–199.

9. Oltermann M. Inquire here: what is the relationship of C-reactive protein levels and nutrition assessment? *Support Line.* 1996;18:14.

10. Takala J, Pitkänen O. Nutrition support in trauma and sepsis. In: Payne-James J, Grimble G, Silk D, eds. *Artificial Nutrition Support in Clinical Practice.* London: Edward Arnold/Hodder Headline Group; 1995:403–413.

11. Heard SO, Fink MP, Cerra FB. The multiple organ dysfunction syndrome. In: Rippe JM, Irwin RS, Fink MP, Cerra FB, eds. *Intensive Care Medicine.* 3rd ed. Boston: Little Brown & Co; 1996:2137–2162.

12. Barton RG. Nutrition support in critical illness. *Nutr Clin Pract.* 1994;9:127–139.

13. Elia M. Changing concepts of nutrient requirements in disease: implications for artificial nutritional support. *Lancet.* 1995;345:1279–1284.

14. Cerra F, Shronts E, Raup S, Konstantinides N, et al. Enteral nutrition in hypermetabolic surgical patients. *Crit Care Med.* 1989;17:619–622.

15. Cerra FB. Nutritional support. In: Parillo JE, Krie RC, eds. *Critical Care Medicine: Principles of Diagnosis and Management.* St. Louis, MO: Mosby-Year Book; 1995:1363–1370.

16. American Medical Association. Guidelines for essential trace element preparations for parenteral use: a statement by the Nutrition Advisory Group. *J Parenter Enter Nutr.* 1979;3:263–267.

17. American Medical Association Department of Foods and Nutrition. Guidelines for essential trace element preparations for parenteral use. *JAMA.* 1979;241:2051–2054.

18. Gallagher-Allred C. Vitamin and mineral requirements. In: Krey SJ, Murray RL, eds. *Dynamics of Nutrition Support.* New York: Appleton-Century-Crofts; 1986.

19. Food and Nutrition Board, National Academy of Sciences, National Research Council. *Recommended Dietary Allowances.* 10th ed. National Academy Press, Washington, DC; 1989.

20. Pastores SM, Kvetan V, Katz DP. Immunomodulatory effects and therapeutic potential of glutamine in the critically ill surgical patient. *Nutrition.* 1994;10:385–391.

21. Evans ME, Shronts EP. Intestinal fuels: glutamine, short-chain fatty acids and dietary fiber. *J Am Diet Assoc.* 1992;92:1239–1246, 1249.

22. Scheltinga MR, Young LS, Benfell K, Bye RL, et al. Glutamine-enriched intravenous feedings attenuate extracellular fluid expansion after a standard stress. *Ann Surg.* 1991;214:385–395.

23. Wernerman J. Nutrition support for the intensive care unit. In: Payne-James J, Grimble G, Silk D, eds. *Artificial Nutrition Support in Clinical Practice.* London: Edward Arnold/Hodder Headline Group; 1995:469–478.

24. Burke DJ, Alverdy JC, Aoys E, Moss GS. Glutamine-supplemented total parenteral nutrition improves gut immune function. *Arch Surg.* 1989;124:1396–1399.

25. Heatley RV. The immune system and nutrition support. In: Payne-James J, Grimble G, Silk D, eds. *Artificial Nutrition Support in Clinical Practice.* London: Edward Arnold/Hodder Headline Group; 1995:99–113.

26. Stralovich A. Gastrointestinal and pancreatic disease. In: Gottschlich MM, Matarese LE, Shronts EP, eds. *Nutritional Support Dietetics Core Curriculum.* Silver Spring, MD: A.S.P.E.N.; 1993:275–310.

27. Fischer JE, Chance WT. Total parenteral nutrition, glutamine and tumor growth. *J Parenter Enter Nutr.* 1990;14:86S–89S.

28. Klimberg VS. The role of glutamine in modulating tumor growth and host response. *J Crit Care Nutr.* 1996;3:19–25.

29. Cerra FB. Modulating the inflammatory response and its associated immune dysfunction. In: Rippe JM, Irwin RS, Fink MP, Cerra FB, eds. *Intensive Care Medicine.* 3rd ed. Boston: Little Brown & Co; 1996:2204–2208.

30. Lacy JA. Immune function and nutrition support. *RD.* 1993;13:1,8–11.

31. Edwards P, Topping D, Kontaridis M, Moldawer LL, et al. Arginine-enhanced enteral nutrition augments the growth of a nitric oxide-producing tumor. *J Parenter Enter Nutr.* 1996;20:20S. Abstract.

32. Borum PR. *The Effect of Dietary Cysteine on Glutathione Synthesis.* Deerfield, IL: Clintec Nutrition Co; 1994.

33. Ziegler TR, Young LS. Therapeutic effects of specific nutrients. In: Rombeau JL, Rolandelli RH, eds. *Clinical Nutrition: Enteral and Tube Feeding.* Philadelphia: WB Saunders Co; 1997:112–137.

34. Hyltander A, Sandström R, Lundholm K. Metabolic effects of structured triglycerides in humans. *Nutr Clin Pract.* 1995;10:91–97.

35. Dahn MS. Structured lipids: an alternative energy source. *Nutr Clin Pract.* 1995;10:89–90. Editorial.

36. Palacia JC, Rombeau JL. Dietary fiber: a brief review and potential application to enteral nutrition. *Nutr Clin Prac.* 1990;5:99–106.

37. Scheppach W, Burghardt W, Bartram P, Kasper H, et al. Addition of dietary fiber to liquid formula diets: the pros and cons. *J Parenter Enter Nutr.* 1990;14:204–209.

38. Mainous MA, Deitch EA. The gut barrier. In: Zaloga GA, ed. *Nutrition in Critical Care.* St. Louis, MO: Mosby-Year Book; 1994:557–568.

39. Cerra FB, Lehmann S, Konstantinides N, Dzik J, et al. Improvement in immune function in ICU patients by enteral nutrition supplemented with arginine, RNA, and menhaden oil is independent of nitrogen balance. *Nutrition.* 1991;7:193–199.

40. Daly JM, Lieberman MD, Goldfine J, Shou J, et al. Enteral nutrition with supplemental arginine, RNA, and omega-3 fatty acids in patients after operation: immunologic, metabolic, and clinical outcome. *Surgery.* 1992;112:56–67.

41. Moore FA, Moore EE, Kudsk KA, Brown RO, et al. Clinical benefits of an immune-enhancing diet for early postinjury enteral feeding. *J Trauma.* 1994;37:607–615.

42. Daly JM, Weintraub FN, Shou J, Rosato EF, et al. Enteral nutrition during multimodality therapy in upper gastrointestinal cancer patients. *Ann Surg.* 1995;221:327–338.

43. Bower RH, Cerra FB, Bershadsky B, Licari JJ, et al. Early enteral administration of a formula (Impact®) supplemented with arginine, nucleotides, and fish oil in intensive care unit patients: results of a multicenter, prospective, randomized, clinical trial. *Crit Care Med.* 1995;23:436–449.

44. Kemen M, Senkal M, Homann H-H, Plumme A, et al. Early postoperative enteral nutrition with arginine-ω-3 fatty acids and ribonucleic acid-supplemented diet versus placebo in cancer patients: an immunologic evaluation of Impact®. *Crit Care Med.* 1995;23:652–659.

45. Kudsk KA, Minard G, Croce MA, Brown RO, et al. A randomized trial of isonitrogenous enteral diets after severe trauma. *Ann Surg.* 1996;224:531–543.

46. Brown RO, Hunt H, Mowatt-Larssen CA, Wojtysiak SL, et al. Comparison of specialized and standard enteral formulas in trauma patients. *Pharmacotherapy.* 1994;14:314–320.

47. Kenler AS, Swails WS, Driscoll DF, DeMichele SJ, et al. Early enteral feeding in postsurgical cancer patients: fish oil structured lipid-based polymeric formula. *Ann Surg.* 1996;223:316–333.

48. Gottschlich MM, Jenkins M, Warden GD, Baumer T, et al. Differential effects of three enteral dietary regimens on selected outcome variables in burn patients. *J Parenter Enter Nutr.* 1990;14:225–236.

49. Chlebowski RT, Beall G, Grosvenor M, Lillington L, et al. Long-term effects of early nutritional support with new enterotropic peptide-based formula vs. standard enteral formula in HIV-infected patients: randomized prospective trial. *Nutrition.* 1993;9:507–512.

50. Süttmann U, Ockenga J, Schneider H, Selberg O, et al. Weight gain and increased concentrations of receptor proteins for tumor necrosis factor after patients with symptomatic HIV infection received fortified nutrition support. *J Am Diet Assoc.* 1996;96:565–569.

51. Barton RG. Immune-enhancing enteral formulas: are they beneficial in critically ill patients? *Nutr Clin Pract.* 1997;12:51–62.

52. Dickerson RN. Immune-enhancing formulas in critically ill patients. *Nutr Clin Pract.* 1997;12:49–50. Editorial.

53. Fong Y, Marano MA, Barber A, He W, et al. Total parenteral nutrition and bowel rest modify the metabolic response to endotoxin in humans. *Ann Surg.* 1989;210:449–457.

54. Kudsk KA, Croce MA, Fabian TC, Minard G, et al. Enteral versus parenteral feeding: effects on septic morbidity after blunt and penetrating abdominal trauma. *Ann Surg.* 1992;215:503–513.

55. Kudsk KA, Minard G, Wojtysiak SL, Croce M, et al. Visceral protein response to enteral versus parenteral nutrition and sepsis in patients with trauma. *Surgery.* 1994;116:516–523.

56. Moore EE, Moore FA. Immediate enteral nutrition following multisystem trauma: a decade perspective. *J Am Coll Nutr.* 1991;10:633–648.

57. Kudsk KA. Gut mucosal nutritional support—enteral nutrition as primary therapy after multiple system trauma. *Gut.* 1994;35(suppl 1):S52–S54.

58. Grahm TW, Zandrozny DB, Harrington T. The benefits of early jejunal hyperalimentation in the head-injured patient. *Neurosurgery.* 1989;25:729–739.

59. Chiarelli A, Enzi G, Casadei A, Baggio B, et al. Very early nutrition supplementation in burned patients. *Am J Clin Nutr.* 1990;51:1035–1039.

60. Mochizuki H, Trocki O, Dominioni L, Brackett KA, et al. Mechanism of prevention of postburn hypermetabolism and catabolism by early enteral feeding. *Ann Surg.* 1984;200:297–310.

61. Schroeder D, Gillanders L, Mahr K, Hill GL, et al. Effects of immediate post-operative enteral nutrition on body composition, muscle function, and wound healing. *J Parenter Enter Nutr.* 1991;15:376–383.

62. Zaloga GP, Bortenschlager L, Black KW, Prielipp R, et al. Immediate post-operative enteral feeding decreases weight loss and improves wound healing after abdominal surgery in rats. *Crit Care Med.* 1992;20:115–118.

63. Eyer SD, Micon LT, Konstantinides FN, Edlund DA, et al. Early enteral feeding does not attenuate metabolic response after blunt trauma. *J Trauma.* 1993;34:639–644.

CHAPTER 18

Surgery and Wound Healing

Marion F. Winkler

INTRODUCTION

Surgical morbidity correlates best with the extent of the primary disease and with the nature of the procedure performed. Reports in the literature for well over 50 years have identified severe protein calorie malnutrition as a factor contributing to increased postoperative morbidity and mortality.[1,2] Infectious complications are increased with malnutrition, and hypoalbuminemia is frequently associated with higher surgical morbidity and mortality.[3-6] Underweight patients may lack the pulmonary reserve to tolerate a stressful event such as surgery; in the presence of undernutrition, patients may be predisposed to respiratory failure and are less likely to be weaned from ventilatory support.[7-9] Hypercatabolism that occurs following multiple trauma, shock, sepsis, and burns rapidly leads to severe lean body mass wasting, impairment of organ function, and diminution in reparative and immune processes even in previously healthy individuals.[10]

The metabolic response to trauma, illness, and sepsis characteristically involves the ebb and flow phases.[11] The *ebb phase* occurs immediately following injury and is associated with hypovolemia, shock, and tissue hypoxia. Shock results from inadequate blood volume due to hemorrhage, crushing injury, burn, or peritonitis. It can also be septic in origin or cardiogenic resulting from inadequate pump function of the myocardium. Clinically, this phase is manifested by decreased cardiac output, oxygen consumption, and body temperature. The *flow phase*—characterized by an increase in cardiac output, oxygen consumption, body temperature, and basal metabolic rate—follows fluid resuscitation and restoration of oxygen transport. Metabolically, there is a marked increase in glucose production, free fatty acid release, circulating levels of insulin, catecholamines, glucagon, cortisol, and insulin resistance. This phase is often prolonged and can be associated with postshock syndromes such as reperfusion syndrome, adult respiratory distress syndrome, acute tubular necrosis, stress bleeding from the gastrointestinal (GI) tract, hepatic dysfunction, and gut mucosal function abnormality thought to lead to translocation of bacteria from the GI tract into the bloodstream and mesenteric lymph nodes.[12,13] The condition of multiple organ dysfunction syndrome occurs when more than one of these syndromes are present. The magnitude of the hypermetabolic response appears to be associated with severity of the injury.

NUTRITIONAL ASSESSMENT AND MONITORING OF CRITICALLY ILL PATIENTS

Recognition of the severity of the patient's illness and postoperative recovery is important in the overall nutritional evaluation of the patient. Standard nutritional assessment techniques are usually unreliable in the critically ill patient. Anthropometric measurements are not sensitive to acute changes; biochemical parameters are affected by infection, stress, and hemodynamic instability; and weight may be more reflective of alterations in total body water than lean body mass or fat. Assessment of the surgical or critically ill patient should include a determination of the patient's preoperative or preinjury nutritional status; evaluation of the extent of disease, injury, or surgery and its effects on digestion, absorption, and utilization or excretion of nutrients; and evaluation of the appearance of the wound. It is also important to assess organ function; evaluate potential enteral and intravenous (IV) access; measure energy expenditure; and monitor vital signs, fluid balance, and the presence of drainage tubes and volume, appearance, and composition of the GI secretions (see Table 18–1). An understanding of the surgical care and management of the critically ill patient helps the dietetic practitioner to determine nutritional risk and establish the nutritional care plan.

Initial management following trauma is first directed toward resuscitation of the patient. This requires establishing an airway, controlling bleeding and circulation, correcting altered cardiac and thoracic physiology, establishing intravenous access, covering the wound, splinting fractures, inserting the urinary catheter, and conducting the history and physical exam.[14] Surgical intervention is often necessary to control life-threatening hemorrhage (thoracotomy, laparotomy, repair of aortic rupture), stabilize fractures, or decompress intracranial bleeding.

A number of scoring systems are used for patient management, triage, quality assurance, prediction of outcome, and stratification in clinical research trials. Dietetic practitioners may also use these scores to screen for nutritional risk. The Glasgow Coma Scale (GCS) is a quantitative measure that objectively assesses the degree of neurologic insult and level of consciousness.[14] The scale evaluates eye opening, motor, and verbal response. A GCS less than 8 is associated with a comatose state and severe head injury. Patients with minor head injury have scores of 13 to 15; those with moderate head injury have scores of 9 to 13. The GCS has

Table 18–1 Composition of Gastrointestinal Secretions

Type of Secretion	Volume (mL/24 hr)	Na (mEq/L)	K (mEq/L)	Cl (mEq/L)	HCO₃ (mEq/L)
Saliva	1500	10	26	10	30
	(500–1000)	(2–10)	(20–30)	(8–18)	
Stomach	1500	60	10	130	—
	(100–4000)	(9–116)	(0–32)	(8–154)	
Duodenum	100–2000	140	5	80	—
Ileum	3000	140	5	104	30
	(100–9000)	(80–150)	(2–8)	(43–137)	
Colon	—	60	30	40	—
Pancreas	100–800	140	5	75	115
		(113–185)	(3–7)	(54–95)	
Bile	50–800	145	5	100	35
		(131–164)	(3–12)	(89–180)	

Source: Reprinted with permission from G.T. Shires, G.T. Shires III, S.F. Lowry. Fluid, Electrolyte and Nutritional Management of the Surgical Patient, in S.I. Schwartz, G.T. Shires, F.C. Spencer, eds. *Principles of Surgery*, 6th ed., p. 65, © 1994, The McGraw-Hill Companies.

been correlated with energy expenditure. Trauma patients with acute head injury (GCS of 4 to 5) resulting from motor vehicle accident, gunshot wounds, and falls had an average measured energy expenditure 26% above predicted.[15] The medical management of head injury often involves barbiturate therapy; in patients with similar injuries receiving barbiturate therapy, energy expenditure was 14% below predicted.[15] The Revised Trauma Score includes physiologic and neurologic evaluation. Scores range from 0 to 12 and include the GCS, respiratory rate, and systolic blood pressure. The Injury Severity Score is a predictor of mortality following vehicular accidents. This scoring system uses the abbreviated injury score and assigns points based on the severity of each injured organ.

Monitoring of critically ill patients involves invasive and noninvasive technology to obtain and interpret physiologic data. An arterial line is used for continuous blood pressure measurement and provides access for repeated measurements of arterial blood gasses. A Swan Ganz pulmonary artery catheter is used to measure central venous pressure, right atrial pressure, right ventricle pressure, pulmonary artery pressure, and cardiac output (see Figure 18–1). Data obtained from these measures can also be used to estimate energy expenditure by the Fick equation.[16] Fluid resuscitation is based on the patient's individual condition, data obtained from invasive monitoring, and urinary output measurements. IV fluids are given to replace volume using crystalloid (Ringer's lactate, normal saline, hypertonic

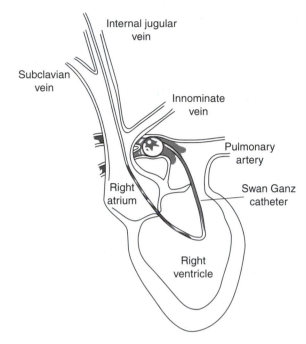

Figure 18–1 Pulmonary Artery Catheter (Swan Ganz) in Position with Balloon Inflated ("Wedged"). *Source:* From M.D. Pasquale, F.B. Cerra. Critical care. In: H.C. Polk, B. Gardner, H.H. Stone, eds, *Basic Surgery*. 4th edition, p. 794, © 1993, St. Louis, MO: Quality Medical Publishing, Inc.

saline solutions) or colloid (albumin, dextran, hespan) solutions, and/or to replenish oxygen-carrying capacity (packed red blood cells and other blood products). A patient with adequate tissue perfusion has normal mental status and pulse rate, adequate urine output (≥ 0.5 mL/kg/hr), warm pink skin, no core/extremity temperature gradient, normal systemic vascular resistance and oxygen extraction ratio, and no lactic acidosis.[14]

FEEDING THE SURGICAL PATIENT

Clinical judgment should play a major role in deciding when to initiate nutrition support. The clinician's ability to predict the clinical course and the resumption of adequate oral food intake are key elements in the decision-making process.[17] Eating is one example of return to physiologic normalcy following surgery, illness, or injury.[18] Depending on the type and severity of the surgical procedure and the organ system requiring treatment, bowel function may return within 1 to 3 days or may be delayed.

Prophylactic, postoperative nasogastric decompression following elective GI or other abdominal operations may not always be necessary. Criteria for removing nasogastric tubes typically are based on the presence of normal bowel sounds, decreased nasogastric output, and/or passage of flatus or movement of bowels in the absence of abdominal distention. Traditionally, patients resume oral feedings with a progression over 2 to 3 days from clear to full liquids and then to solids. One study of patients following surgery to the upper or lower GI tract found that resuming an oral solid diet immediately after removal of the nasogastric tube was not associated with an increased number of complications or with the need for tube reinsertion.[19] The traditional progression of withholding feedings after colonic or bowel resection until the postoperative ileus resolves is based on the assumption that oral feeding (liquids or solids) may not be tolerated in the presence of an ileus and that early feeding may predispose the intestinal anastomosis to risk or increase the potential for pulmonary complications secondary to aspiration. In a study that challenged this dictum, patients tolerated a gradual advancement from liquids to solids without complications, on the average within 2.6 days of surgery and 1.2 days before their ileus resolved.[20] Patients whose oral diet was withheld until their ileus resolved did not advance to a regular diet until postoperative day 5. Rapid dietary progression could lead to earlier discharge, lower hospital costs, and to a greater sense of well-being by patients. Dietetic practitioners may be able to facilitate dietary advancement and/or prevent unnecessary extended periods of NPO or clear-liquid diets by routinely monitoring postoperative surgical patients.

It is not uncommon to find critically ill or postoperative patients with an adynamic or paralytic ileus. An ileus occurs when the bowel loses its peristaltic and propulsive action. Symptoms generally include absence of bowel sounds and flatus, nausea, vomiting, and abdominal distention. An ileus is diagnosed by abdominal exam and X-ray in which images usually show a significant amount of air in the small and large intestine. An ileus may be neurogenic in origin resulting from trauma, myocardial infarction, painful illness, or a consequence of the postoperative state; it may be metabolic in origin; secondary to potassium deficiency, diabetic ketoacidosis, or renal failure; or it may be vascular in origin, caused by cerebrovascular accident.[18] Pharmacologic use of sedatives and paralytic agents including general anesthesia can also result in ileus.

Whenever oral intake is inadequate and the GI tract is functional, enteral nutrition should be utilized. Obstruction is the only absolute contraindication to enteral feeding.[21] When the stomach fails to empty because of atony or obstruction, or if there is predisposition to aspiration, enteric tubes should be placed distal to the ligament of Treitz. Nasoduodenally placed tubes are one option; however, these tubes frequently flip back into the stomach and require continuous monitoring and evaluation of proper position. Gaining access to the duodenum or jejunum can be accomplished at the bedside or via fluoroscopy, endoscopy, or surgery. Jejunostomy feeding tubes should be considered at the time of original operation in patients undergoing a major operative procedure of the upper-GI tract or early in the course of treatment following a significant trauma requiring surgical exploration.[18,21] Prescription of a diet or a tube-feeding regimen does not necessarily guarantee its delivery or the patient's tolerance. Combinations of enteral and parenteral nutrition may be required to meet nutritional needs in some patients. The use of parenteral nutrition in surgical or critically ill patients should complement instead of compete with the use of early enteral nutrition.[17]

Every nutritional care plan should include goals for nutritional intervention. The goals of nutrition support for the injured or stressed patient include the minimization of starvation, the prevention or correction of specific nutrient deficiencies, the provision of sufficient calories to meet energy needs, and the provision of fluid and electrolytes to maintain adequate urine output and normal serum electrolytes. Care should be taken to avoid the complications of overfeeding such as hyperglycemia (which may lead to an osmotic diuresis) and excess carbon dioxide production (which can impact the ability to wean a patient from ventilatory support). It is important to recognize that nutrition support alone cannot abolish the ongoing protein catabolism and lean body mass wasting seen in acute injury or illness, and that the bedridden septic or injured patient cannot be expected to increase or even maintain lean body mass until the source of hypermetabolism resolves and physical therapy or ambulation is initiated.[10]

Nutrition support can be supportive, adjunctive, or definitive. Examples of *supportive* therapy are the initiation of nutrition support to prevent nutritional deterioration in an adequately nourished patient who is anticipated to have a prolonged postoperative course and the use of nutrition support to rehabilitate a depleted patient who is undergoing surgical treatment. *Adjunctive* nutrition support is used as part of the therapeutic plan (for example, in the case of a patient who has acute pancreatitis or an exacerbation of Crohn's disease and requires prolonged bowel rest and monitoring). *Definitive* nutrition support is nutrition therapy that is required for the patient's existence such as in a patient with short-bowel syndrome.

THE ROLE OF PREOPERATIVE AND POSTOPERATIVE NUTRITION SUPPORT

The practice of delaying surgery to permit a period of preoperative parenteral nutrition support was relatively common in the early 1980s, as surgeons believed it would reduce postoperative mortality. Several reports even suggested a benefit from preoperative total parenteral nutrition (TPN) in patients with varying degrees of malnutrition.[22] Today the role of preoperative parenteral nutrition support is debated. When subjected to meta-analysis, studies have not permitted accurate evaluation of the efficacy of preoperative TPN because of flaws in design, randomization, patient selection, and definition of complications and clinical end points.[23,24] The Veterans Affairs Cooperative Study did find benefit for preoperative nutrition support in severely malnourished patients but, because of a high incidence of infectious complications, use of preoperative TPN in minimally malnourished individuals was not recommended.[25] Improvement in wound healing has been demonstrated in patients who maintain normal preoperative food intake, regardless of the degree of malnutrition.[26,27]

Reports of the use of postoperative nutrition support have also been mixed. For example, some studies fail to demonstrate a significant improvement in the rehabilitative phase,[28] while others have shown improvement in specific surgical populations such as esophagogastrectomy[29] and radical cystectomy.[30] Enteral nutrition support initiated early in the postoperative period has been associated with reduced septic morbidity rates in high-risk surgical patients and is preferred to TPN when the GI tract is functional.[31,32]

Consensus guidelines on the use of pre- and postoperative nutrition support have recently been published by the American Society for Parenteral and Enteral Nutrition. These guidelines state that preoperative nutrition support should be provided to malnourished patients who require a major operation but cannot undergo immediate surgery and are expected to undergo a substantial period of preoperative starvation.[33] Severely malnourished patients should have nutrition support instituted within 1 to 3 days after hospitalization and be given adequate amounts of nutrition support for 7 to 10 days.[33] Postoperative TPN should also be considered when oral or enteral feeding is not anticipated within 7 to 10 days in well nourished individuals or within 5 to 7 days in previously malnourished or critically ill patients.[34]

SURGICAL ANATOMY

The decision to use oral, enteral, or parenteral nutrition in the surgical patient is based not only on assessment of nutritional risk and preinjury/preillness nutritional status, but also on the functional capacity of the GI tract. Surgery of the GI tract is performed for many conditions, the results of which may potentially impact a person's ability to eat or drink, or alter GI physiology and affect secretory and absorptive functions (see Figures 18–2 and 18–3). These conditions include congenital malformation of the GI tract (atresia, malrotation, tracheoesophageal fistula, and gastroschisis); mechanical or functional obstruction from adhesions, volvulus, herniation, stones, or ulceration; neoplasia; infection or inflammation (inflammatory bowel disease and colitis); vascular insult (bleeding and infarction); and trauma. Surgery to alter GI physiology in the treatment of disease may include fundoplasty for reflux esophagitis; reduction of acid secretion by vago-

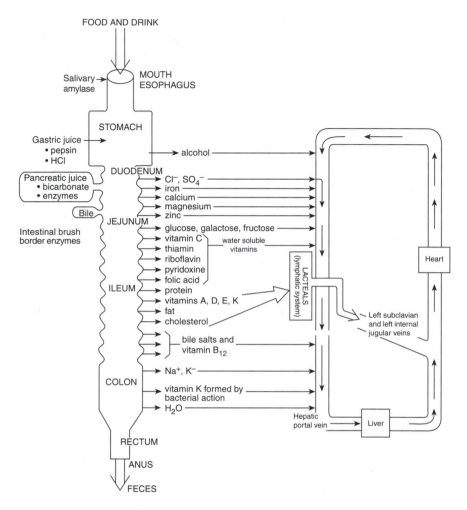

Figure 18–2 Sites of Secretion and Absorption in the Gastrointestinal Tract. *Source:* Reprinted with permission from L.K. Mahan and S. Escott-Stump, *S. Krause's Food, Nutrition, and Diet Therapy.* 9th edition, p. 13, © 1996, W.B. Saunders Company.

tomy, pyloroplasty, or antral resection; or removal of the target organ (eg, total gastrectomy). Diagnostic surgical or drainage procedures may also be performed. Often, these procedures are conducted via endoscopy (a technique that permits visual inspection of the esophagus, stomach, small or large intestine, and pancreatic or cystic ducts) or by laparoscopy (which requires an incision in the fold of the umbilicus that permits direct visualization of abdominal viscera).

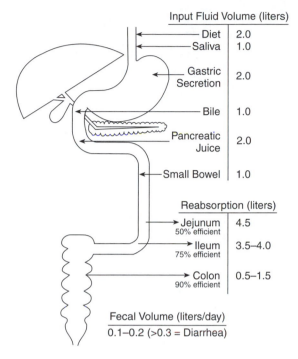

Input Fluid Volume (liters)

Diet	2.0
Saliva	1.0
Gastric Secretion	2.0
Bile	1.0
Pancreatic Juice	2.0
Small Bowel	1.0

Reabsorption (liters)

Jejunum 50% efficient	4.5
Ileum 75% efficient	3.5–4.0
Colon 90% efficient	0.5–1.5

Fecal Volume (liters/day)
0.1–0.2 (>0.3 = Diarrhea)

Figure 18–3 Intestinal Fluid Flux. *Source:* Reprinted with permission from E.C. James, et al. The small intestine. In: E.C. James, R.J. Corry, R.F. Perry, Jr., eds. *Principles of Basic Surgical Practice,* p. 274, © 1987, Hanley & Belfus.

Dietetic practitioners should have knowledge of surgical anatomy and be able to visualize the GI tract when reading the medical record or operative report. Illustrations of the GI tract are shown in Figures 18–4 through 18–7. The GI tract includes the mouth, pharynx, esophagus, stomach (fundus, body, antrum), small intestine (duodenum, jejunum, ileum), large intestine (cecum, ascending colon, transverse colon, descending colon, sigmoid colon, rectum), and anus.

The small intestine begins at the pylorus and ends at the ileocecal valve. The duodenum is approximately 10 inches in length, the jejunum is 7½ feet, and the ileum is approximately 10½ feet long. The common bile duct and main pancreatic duct enter the second portion of the duodenum at the ampulla of Vater. The head of the pancreas lies in a cavity of the first, second, and third portion of the duodenal curve. The ligament of Treitz, an important surgical landmark, stabilizes the duodenojejunal flexure. The large intestine begins at the ileocecal valve and terminates at the anus. The large intestine is divided into the cecum, colon, and rec-

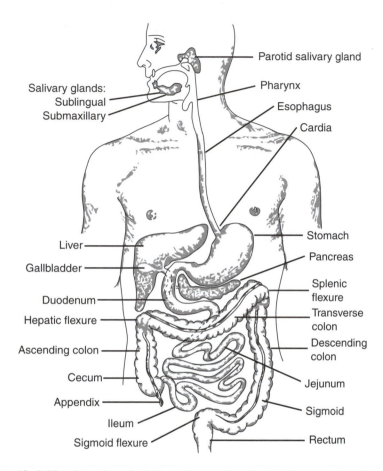

Figure 18–4 The Gastrointestinal Tract. *Source:* Reprinted with permission from L.R. Petty, Gastrointestinal surgery. In: M.H. Meeker and J.C. Rothrock, eds. *Alexander's Care of the Patient in Surgery,* 10th edition, p. 255, © 1995, Mosby-Year Book, Inc.

tum. The cecum forms a blind pouch from which the appendix projects. The ascending colon is approximately 6 inches long and extends from the ileocecal valve to the hepatic flexure. The ascending colon, which is retroperitoneal, lies behind the right lobe of the liver and in front of the kidney. The transverse colon is intraperitoneal and begins at the hepatic flexure and ends at the splenic flexure. The length of the transverse colon is 20 inches, and it lies below the stomach. The descending colon, also retroperitoneal, is 7 inches long and extends downward from the splenic flexure to just below the iliac crest. The sigmoid colon lies partly

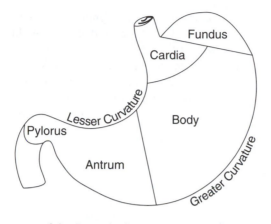

Figure 18–5 Anatomy of the Stomach. *Source:* From D.T. Dempsey, W.P. Ritchie. Gastroduodenal physiology and peptic ulcer disease. In: H.C. Polk, B. Gardner, H.H. Stone, eds. *Basic Surgery.* 4th edition, p. 196, © 1993, St. Louis, MO: Quality Medical Publishing, Inc.

in the abdomen and partly in the pelvis and extends to the rectosigmoid junction. The rectum is connected to the anus.

The liver is in the right upper quadrant of the abdominal cavity beneath the diaphragm and lateral to the stomach. The gallbladder lies on the undersurface of the right lobe of the liver and terminates in the cystic duct (see Figure 18–8). The cystic duct empties into the common bile duct and creates the outlet for hepatic secretions. The pancreas is a fixed, retroperitoneal structure lying transversely behind the stomach in the upper abdomen. The head of the pancreas is fixed to the curve of the duodenum, and the tail extends to the spleen. The pancreatic duct joins with the common bile duct at the ampulla of Vater to enter the duodenum below the pylorus.

Esophagus[35]

Swallowing disorders manifest as dysphagia, heartburn, and/or regurgitation. Dysphagia, defined as difficulty in swallowing or a problem of esophageal transit, is commonly associated with esophageal carcinoma, hiatal hernia, and achalasia. Dysphagia for liquids and solids at onset is typical of motility disorders (esophageal spasm, achalasia); dysphagia of solid foods progressing to liquids typically occurs with structural obstruction (carcinoma). Foreign materials (eg, ingestion of lye) can also result in mechanical obstruction and esophageal stenosis. Physical symptoms resulting from swallowing disorders may include cough, chest pain, weight loss, anemia, and aspiration pneumonia. These symptoms usually progress rapidly over weeks to months. The nutrition history should include questions that determine whether certain foods aggravate the symptoms, how long symptoms of dysphagia have been present, and over what period of time weight loss, if any, has occurred. For patients able to tolerate a liquid diet, use of nutrient-dense beverages and oral nutritional meal replacements is indicated. Patients who have experienced dramatic weight loss and who are unable to eat adequate quantities of food benefit from placement of a nasoenteric or percutaneously placed feeding tube prior to operative management. Unless contraindicated by obstruction or severity

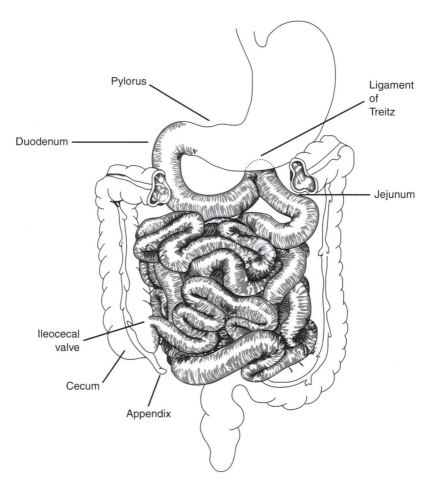

Figure 18–6 Anatomy of the Small Bowel. *Source:* Reprinted with permission from J.C. Thompson, *Atlas of Surgery of the Stomach, Duodenum, and Small Bowel,* p. 258, © 1992, Mosby-Year Book, Inc.

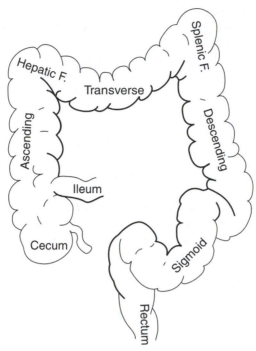

Figure 18–7 Anatomy of the Large Intestine. F = Flexure. *Source:* Reprinted with permission from L.R. Petty, Gastrointestinal surgery. In: M.H. Meeker and J.C. Rothrock, eds. *Alexander's Care of the Patient in Surgery,* 10th edition, p. 263, © 1995, Mosby-Year Book, Inc.

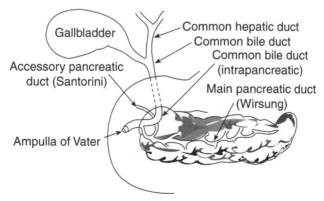

Figure 18–8 Anatomy of the Biliary Tract and Pancreas. *Source:* From B. Gardner, H.H. Stone. Acute abdominal pain. In: H.C. Polk, B. Gardner, and H.H. Stone, eds. *Basic Surgery.* 4th edition, p. 430, © 1993, St. Louis, MO: Quality Medical Publishing.

of inflammation or disease, a feeding tube can be placed at the time of diagnostic upper endoscopy. If operative management occurs, placement of a feeding jejunostomy is recommended.[36]

Hiatal hernia and reflux esophagitis are typically treated with alleviation of factors that predispose the patient to increased intraabdominal pressure such as elimination of tight-fitting clothing, reduction of weight, elevation of the head of the bed while sleeping, remaining upright after eating or drinking, and dietary restriction to decrease gastric distention and acid secretion. Nutrition management generally includes abstinence from acid stimulants such as alcohol, coffee, tobacco, chocolate, and carbonated beverages. Patients may obtain relief with fractionated meals that are dry and bland. Antacids, H_2 blockers, or proton pump inhibitors are usually prescribed.

The objectives of esophageal surgery include correction of anatomic disorders, alleviation of obstruction, and/or alteration of the esophagogastric and fundal anatomy to control reflux of gastric acid into the duodenum. A number of procedures may be performed.[37-40] An esophagectomy removes the diseased portion of the esophagus resulting from stricture, ulcer, or tumor; the procedure establishes an esophago-esophago anastomosis or an anastomosis between the esophagus and stomach (esophagogastrectomy), jejunum (esophagojejunostomy), or colon (colon interposition). Excision of diverticula may also be performed. This involves removal of a weakening in the wall of the esophagus that collects food and often causes a sensation of fullness in the neck. Hiatal herniorrhaphy is performed to restore the cardioesophageal junction and to correct gastroesophageal reflux.

A number of antireflux procedures, commonly known as fundoplication, have been described.[41] In these procedures, the esophagus, proximal stomach, and fundus are mobilized, and the posterior wall of the stomach is then brought up around the distal esophagus. The stomach walls are wrapped and sutured around the intraabdominal esophagus to create a valvular mechanism to control the reflux of gastric acid into the lower esophagus (see Figure 18–9). A vagotomy and/or pyloroplasty may also be performed. A jejunal interposition may be the procedure of choice for patients who have failed previous esophageal operations. In this procedure, the esophagus is resected and an esophagojejunostomy is created. The distal end of the jejunum is anastomosed to the stomach to serve as an esophageal replacement. Following esophagoplasty, patients need to be fed enterally while the anastomosis heals. Oral feedings are initiated after a dye study demonstrates an intact anastomosis. This testing is usually conducted around postoperative day 7.

Stomach[37]

The stomach is the primary digestive center of the GI tract. Although most digestion actually takes place in the small intestine, the stomach collects swallowed food,

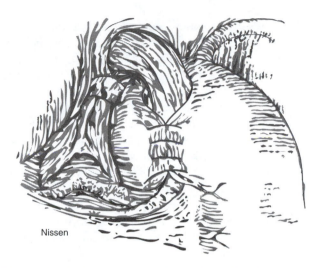

Nissen

Figure 18–9 Nissen Fundoplication. *Source:* From H.C. Polk. Difficulties in swallowing. In: H.C. Polk, B. Gardner, H.H. Stone, eds. *Basic Surgery.* 4th edition, p. 298, © 1993, St. Louis, MO: Quality Medical Publishing, Inc.

contributes to the digestion of proteins via pepsin and hydrochloric acid, mixes the chewed food particles together with digestive enzymes to make chyme, and packages it into small boluses to be further digested and absorbed in the small intestine. Many factors control digestion—the production of acid and the emptying of the stomach. Gastric acid production is influenced by visual and olfactory sensations, the autonomic neuropeptides, and neurotransmitters. Gastric emptying is controlled by the type and amount of food in the stomach, hormonal stimulation, and the autonomic nervous system. The vagus nerve plays a major role in gastric emptying. Most pathology results from alterations of the normal gastric anatomy and physiology.

Gastric ulcers, defects in the wall of the stomach, usually are the result of alterations in the homeostasis of gastric acid, mucus and alkaline secretions, the gastric epithelial cell layer, submucosal buffers, and gastric mucosal blood flow.[36] Gastric ulcers usually present with symptoms of dull epigastric pain, dyspepsia, weight loss, and nausea and vomiting. Diagnostic studies are completed to diagnose ulcers and rule out malignancy. Dietary manipulation, such as the avoidance of caffeine, pepper, alcohol, fried or fatty foods, and heavily seasoned foods is usually suggested. Nonoperative or medical management usually involves reducing acid production with H_2 blockers, antacids, and antibiotic treatment of *Helicobacter pylori,* a common bacteria that can cause ulcer recurrence.[42] The indications for surgery include bleeding, perforation, obstruction, intractable pain, the inability to rule out malignancy, and failure to heal the ulcer with standard medical treatment.[38,43]

There are several types of vagotomy procedures.[38,43] A truncal vagotomy interrupts the parasympathetic innervation of the distal esophagus and reduces gastric acid secretion in patients with ulcers. This procedure also affects the parasympathetic nerve supply to the stomach, liver, gallbladder, pancreas, and small and large intestines. Significant postvagotomy diarrhea often results. A selective vagotomy denervates the entire stomach but preserves the nerve supply to the other organs. A highly selective or parietal cell vagotomy denervates only the parietal cell area of the stomach. Gastric emptying remains relatively intact. It is not uncommon for a vagotomy to be performed in conjunction with antrectomy or pyloroplasty. Pyloroplasty forms a large passageway between the prepyloric region of the stomach and the first or second portion of the duodenum and permits rapid emptying of the stomach.

Gastrectomy involves resection of the distal portion of the stomach with an anastomosis created between the stomach and duodenum (Billroth I) or the stomach and the jejunum (Billroth II gastrojejunostomy) (see Figures 18–10 and 18–11). A partial gastrectomy may be performed to remove a benign or malignant lesion in the pylorus or upper half of the stomach; a gastrojejunostomy may also be done as a palliative surgery for an inoperable lesion. A total gastrectomy pro-

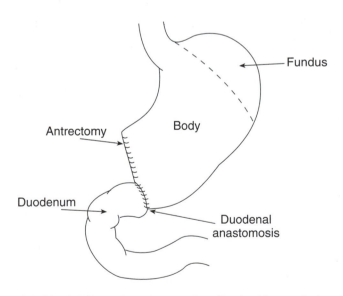

Figure 18–10 Billroth I Procedure. *Source:* Reprinted with permission from S.C. Smeltzer, B.G. Bare, eds. *Brunner and Suddarth's Textbook of Medical-Surgical Nursing,* 8th ed., p. 893, © 1996, Lippincott-Raven Publishers.

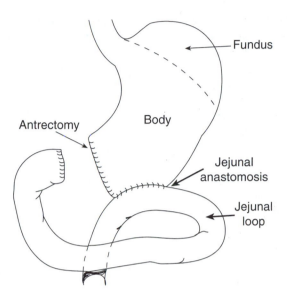

Figure 18–11 Billroth II Procedure. *Source:* Reprinted with permission from S.C. Smeltzer, B.G. Bare, eds. *Brunner and Suddarth's Textbook of Medical-Surgical Nursing,* 8th ed., p. 893, © 1996, Lippincott-Raven Publishers.

vides complete removal of the stomach and establishment of an anastomosis between the esophagus and the jejunum. Food intake is typically reduced because of loss of the stomach as a reservoir. Patients may experience pain and dysphagia following this procedure because of reflux of food and bile into the esophagus. In patients who are already nutritionally compromised, it may be prudent to place a jejunostomy for feeding at the time of gastrectomy.

Postgastrectomy syndromes have significant nutritional consequences. Patients generally report early satiety and dumping, characterized by upper abdominal bloating, reflux, cramping, nausea, vomiting, weakness, palpitations, syncope, flushing, sweating, and diarrhea.[44,45] Symptoms can occur within 15 to 30 minutes of a meal and up to 1 hour after eating. Dumping syndrome occurs from ingested food being inadequately diluted in the stomach and rapidly emptying into the jejunum. The hyperosmolarity of the food causes hypermotility of fluid into the jejunum, resulting in distention. Nutrition therapy includes fractionated meals that are low in simple sugars and high in complex carbohydrates, and separation of solids and liquids. Patients are instructed to remain in an upright position after eating if reflux is a problem. In severe cases of dumping syndrome, postprandial hypoglycemia can occur secondary to rapid absorption of carbohydrates. Malabsorption, particularly of fat (steatorrhea), may be present secondary to bacterial overgrowth and alterations in the proximal mucosa of the jejunum. Anemia, secondary to achlorhydria, results in poor iron absorption and loss of intrinsic factor. Nutrition management of severe dumping syndrome may require placement of a feeding jejunostomy coupled with intensive dietary manipulation to ensure adequate nutrient delivery.

A gastrostomy is a temporary or permanent channel from the gastric lumen to the skin. The procedure can be part of a major abdominal procedure or performed for feeding access alone. Creation of a gastrostomy permits retrograde dilatation of an esophageal stricture, decompression or postoperative drainage of the stomach, or continuous gastric drainage because of impaired gastric emptying or obstruction of the small bowel by advanced tumor. Tubes that are no longer needed for drainage can be later used for feeding. Gastrostomy tubes have provided convenient adjuncts and palliation to the postoperative care of gynecologic oncology patients who are dying of bowel obstruction.[46] When patients who are unable to swallow or eat enough food require prolonged tube feeding (longer than 30 days), a gastrostomy may be created for purposes of enteral nutrition support.[21] Contraindications for gastrostomy feeding include tracheal aspiration, reflux esophagitis, gastroparesis, and insufficient stomach from previous resection. In these situations, a tube placed into the jejunum either surgically or percutaneously is desirable.

Small Intestine[38,47,48]

Disorders of the small intestine that may require surgery include ulceration, obstruction, inflammation, perforation, or neoplasia. Resection of the small intestine involves excision of the diseased segment and bowel re-anastomosis. Since the small bowel is the site of digestion and absorption, nutritional disorders or deficiencies can occur depending on the severity of the disease and the extent of resection. When the jejunum is resected, the remaining small bowel can undergo adaptive hyperplasia and assume absorptive functions normally performed by the resected section.[49] Resections of less than 50% of small bowel typically require few dietary restrictions; however, patients with as little as 15 cm of ileal resection may need to reduce the amount of dietary fat and supplement intake with vitamin B_{12}, since the ileum is the site of B_{12} and bile salt absorption. When the distal small bowel including the ileocecal valve has been resected, patients often experience rapid intestinal transit and resulting malabsorption and diarrhea. Short-bowel syndrome occurs when less than 100 cm of small bowel remains. Patients typically require long-term home parenteral nutrition. Many patients are able to resume some oral or enteral nutrition, but frequently require intravenous solutions to maintain body weight, fluid, and electrolyte status.[50]

An ileostomy may be a temporary or permanent opening into the ileum that is performed when colonic diversion is necessary or the patient has undergone large-bowel resection. Nutrition management guidelines for patients with an ileostomy typically involve a low-residue, low-fiber diet with avoidance of gassy foods, nuts and seeds, and heavily seasoned foods.[51] A condition of desalting dehydration can occur when patients experience a remarkably high ileostomy output (greater than 1.5 to 2 liters). Patients complaining of excessive thirst who attempt to quench this thirst with extraordinary amounts of hypotonic fluids such as water, carbonated beverages, juices, and ice are at risk for this condition. A detailed nutrition history is essential, and practitioners should focus specifically on fluid intake. Strict monitoring of intake and urine and ileostomy output in the hospital setting can assist in determining fluid balance. It is important to subtract oral intake from the ileostomy output to determine the net negative fluid loss. Intensive dietary management and use of fluid replacement such as Gatorade®; Pedialyte®; or a solution of glucose, electrolytes, and water may correct this condition. Some patients who have persistent high ileostomy output have been treated with periods of IV fluid therapy and home parenteral nutrition.

Large Intestine and Rectum

Disorders of the colon due to diverticular or inflammatory disease, obstruction, or carcinoma often present with changes in bowel habits such as constipation and diarrhea, rectal bleeding, abdominal pain, and bloating. Surgical management is based on the extent of disease and site of colonic involvement. A right hemicolectomy and ileocolostomy involve resection of the right half of the colon—including the transverse and ascending colon, the cecum, and a segment of terminal ileum—when there are malignant lesions or inflammatory changes.[38] The anastomosis that is created may be end-to-end, side-to-side, or end-to-side.

Total proctocolectomy with permanent ileostomy is performed as curative treatment of ulcerative colitis and familial adenomatous polyposis. In this procedure, the entire colon and rectum are removed. Although the majority of patients adapt well to handling an abdominal stoma, it creates limitations with lifestyle habits, interpersonal relations, and self-image. A continent-preserving procedure developed in 1969 has offered patients improved quality of life.[52] Known as a Kock pouch, this procedure involves creation of a reservoir out of the terminal 50 cm of the ileum with a nipple-valve brought to the skin. Patients who have a continent ileostomy intubate the pouch several times a day to eliminate stool. More recently an alternative procedure known as an ileal pouch anal anastomosis has been successfully performed.[53] This procedure creates an ileal reservoir that is applied to the anal sphincter and allows for maintenance of natural continence. The ileal pouch can be created in a J-fashion by folding two adjacent loops of small bowel or as an S- or W-pouch by aligning the distal ileum in an S- or W-configuration (Figure 18–12). Postoperative functional results are generally acceptable with patients reporting daytime stool frequency of 4 to 6 times/day, little nighttime fecal incontinence, and improvement in lifestyle.[53–55]

Following creation of an ileal reservoir, patients are generally able to progress from a low-residue, low-fiber diet to one that includes a modest amount of fiber. Patients are usually instructed to avoid foods with seeds, hard-to-digest kernels, skin, cellulose, nuts, coconut, beans, gassy vegetables, or highly seasoned and spicy foods.[56,57] A recent study conducted among 65 patients who have undergone ileal pouch anal anastomosis at Rhode Island Hospital found that the following foods are not likely to be tolerated: lettuce, salad, nuts, beans and lentils, corn, spinach, broccoli, cauliflower and cabbage, oranges, chocolate, tomatoes, berries, mushrooms, Chinese foods, and spices.[58] In addition to dietary manipulation, patients also use psyllium mucilage and pectin preparations to maintain adequate bowel function.

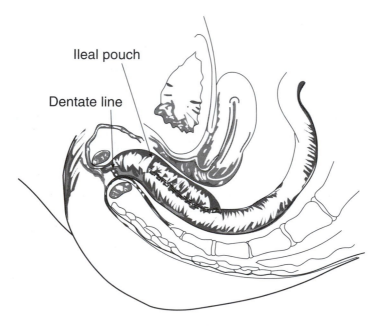

Figure 18–12 Ileal Pouch Anal Anastomosis. *Source:* Reprinted with permission of the publisher from Anal Sphincter-Saving Operations for Chronic Ulcerative Colitis, K.A. Kelly, *American Journal of Surgery,* Vol. 163, pp. 5–11, Copyright 1992 by Excerpta Medica Inc.

An anterior resection and rectosigmoidostomy are performed to remove the lower sigmoid colon and rectosigmoid portion of the rectum to treat lesions in this part of the colon. An end-to-end anastomosis is typically created. An abdominoperineal resection is performed for malignant lesions and inflammatory diseases involving the lower sigmoid colon, rectum, and anus. Abdominoperineal resection provides mobilization and diversion of the diseased segment of the lower bowel. In this procedure, the proximal end of the bowel is exteriorized as a colostomy. A colostomy may also be created in the transverse or sigmoid colon to treat an obstruction, inflammation, or trauma that has caused distention in the proximal portion of the colon[47] (see Figure 18–13). When used to decompress the bowel or allow the bowel to rest, the colostomy may be temporary; continuity is often reestablished within 3 to 12 months.

Biliary Tract[59-61]

The gallbladder is a sac-like organ located on the inferior surface of the liver. Its primary function is to store and concentrate bile, a solution of specialized enzymes that assist in the digestion of fats. The makeup of bile is a delicate balance of bile salts, cholesterol, and the phospholipid lecithin. Gallstones are abnormal concretions of cholesterol that precipitate from bile. Gallstones are most often asymptomatic, but in certain predisposed individuals (middle-aged, overweight individuals or child-bearing women) they can obstruct the cystic duct and cause inflammation or cholecystitis. Obstruction of the cystic duct, common bile duct, or ampulla of Vater by stricture or cancer can also cause cholecystitis. Symptoms usually include right upper quadrant abdominal pain, nausea, vomiting, and fever. Jaundice, a yellow discoloration of the skin and mucous membranes (sclera, conjunctiva, palate), may result from retention of abnormally large amounts of bile in body fluids. Stools are often pale in color and the urine is dark. Jaundice is clinically evident when the serum bilirubin exceeds 2 mg/dL. Hyperbilirubinemia occurs with increased hemolysis and hepatic disease that results in incomplete uptake, transport, conjugation, or excretion of bile or extra hepatic biliary tract obstruction. Diagnostic studies include sonography to examine the gallbladder and the bile ducts and radioactive scans to delineate the extra hepatic biliary tree and gallbladder. Initial treatment of cholecystitis involves a period of NPO to avoid gallbladder stimulation and nasogastric suction if the patient is vomiting. Chronic cholecystitis may be nonsurgically managed with a low-fat diet, anticholinergic drugs, and weight loss.

A cholecystectomy—removal of the gallbladder—is performed to treat cholecystitis, to treat cholelithiasis (stones), or to remove polyps or carcinoma (see Figure 18–14). Cholecystectomy can be accomplished via laparoscopy or as an open procedure (laparotomy). An intraoperative cholangiogram may be performed in

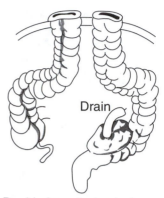

Double-barrelled colostomy
(perforation)

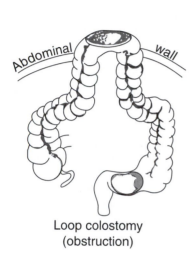

Loop colostomy
(obstruction)

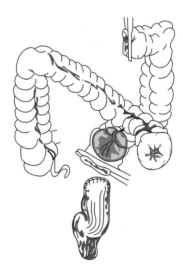

Resection with end colostomy
(Hartmann)

Figure 18–13 Loop Colostomy. *Source:* From B. Gardner, H.H. Stone. Acute abdominal pain. In: H.C. Polk, B. Gardner, H.H. Stone, eds. *Basic Surgery.* 4th edition, p. 445, © 1993, St. Louis, MO: Quality Medical Publishing, Inc.

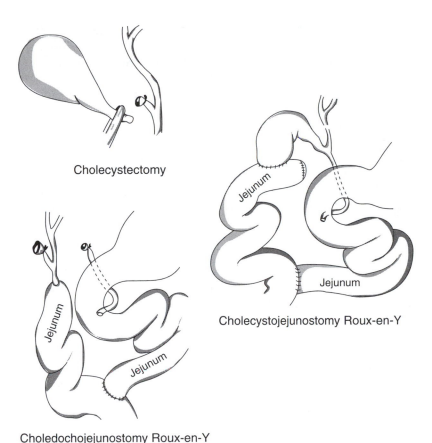

Cholecystectomy

Cholecystojejunostomy Roux-en-Y

Choledochojejunostomy Roux-en-Y

Figure 18–14 Common Operations of the Biliary Tract. *Source:* From B. Gardner, H.H. Stone. Acute abdominal pain. In: H.C. Polk, B. Gardner, H.H. Stone, eds. *Basic Surgery.* 4th edition, p. 434, © 1993, St. Louis, MO: Quality Medical Publishing, Inc.

conjunction with a cholecystectomy to visualize the common bile duct and extra- and intrahepatic ducts. A cholecystostomy establishes an opening into the gallbladder to permit drainage of the gallbladder and removal of stones. Choledochotomy and choledochostomy establish an opening into the common bile duct with the placement of a drainage T-tube in the treatment of choledocholithiasis or to relieve obstructive jaundice caused by stones in the common bile duct.

A cholecystoduodenostomy and cholecystojejunostomy create an anastomosis between the gallbladder and the duodenum or the jejunum to relieve obstruction in the distal end of the common bile duct. Biliary system obstructions may be caused by tumor in the ducts involving the head of the pancreas or the ampulla of Vater, or the presence of an inflammatory lesion, stricture, or stones in the common bile duct.

Patients who have altered flow of bile may malabsorb fat, fat-soluble vitamins, and calcium. A low-fat diet and supplementation of these nutrients are required. If large amounts of bile are being drained via T-tubes or other biliary drains or fistula, the bile can be collected and reinstilled via a gastrostomy or enterostomy feeding tube. This technique often helps with tube feeding digestion/absorption and correction of electrolyte imbalances that occur with biliary drainage.

The etiology of pancreatitis is related in the majority of cases to biliary tract disease (gallstones) or to excessive alcohol use.[62] Other causes include hypercalcemia, ischemia, ductal obstruction, trauma, or drugs. The clinical presentation varies from a mild, self-limiting disease to a severe condition associated with hypovolemia, shock, and sepsis. The predominant clinical feature is abdominal pain. Jaundice is unusual but, when present, may reflect gallstone-associated pancreatitis. The diagnosis of pancreatitis is made using a combination of the clinical presentation, laboratory tests (including serum amylase), and radiographic findings. Ultrasound may detect pancreatic swelling, edema and acute peripancreatic fluid collections, or cholelithiasis. Computerized tomography findings may demonstrate pancreatic enlargement, edema, necrosis, peripancreatic changes, fluid collections, abscess, or pseudocyst. Endoscopic retrograde cholangiopancreatography (ERCP) is useful in recurrent attacks of pancreatitis and may identify pancreatic divisum, stenosis, or duct obstruction.

Nonsurgical management of pancreatitis typically involves intravenous fluids, electrolyte replacement, and analgesics. Patients with severe attacks may also receive antibiotics and TPN. Oral intake is resumed when pain, abdominal tenderness, and ileus resolve, and serum amylase levels are normalizing. If oral intake is delayed secondary to persistent pain, tenderness, ileus, abscess, or phlegmon, patients should be started on TPN. Surgery is performed to treat secondary pancreatic infections, to correct associated biliary tract disease, or to treat progressive clinical deterioration despite optimal supportive care.[62] The surgical procedure typically involves an exploratory laparotomy with drainage and debridement as indicated. Patients with systemic toxicity and gross evidence of severe pancreatitis associated with large amounts of peritoneal exudate may be candidates for postoperative peritoneal lavage.

Surgery may also be performed for pancreatic or periampullary cancer. A total pancreatectomy removes the entire pancreas along with the spleen. A jejunostomy tube is frequently placed for postoperative feedings. Following total pancreatectomy, patients can develop significant exocrine pancreatic insufficiency resulting in diabetes and malabsorption. Achieving adequate glucose control involves coordination with insulin and dietary treatment. Malabsorption can be treated with a low-fat diet and pancreatic enzyme replacement. Patients receiving long-term enteral feedings also benefit from pancreatic enzyme replacement, and at least one study has demonstrated a marked improvement in fat and nitrogen absorption with the addition of pancreatic enzymes to both elemental and polymeric diets.[63]

A pancreaticoduodenectomy removes the head of the pancreas, the entire duodenum, a portion of the jejunum, the distal third of the stomach, gallbladder, and the lower half of the common bile duct, with reestablishment of the biliary, pancreatic, and GI systems (see Figure 18–15). The body and tail of the pancreas are preserved. More commonly known as a Whipple procedure, this radical excision is performed for carcinoma of the head of the pancreas or lesions confined to the ampulla, duodenum, or lower end of the common bile duct. Because of the nature and progression of pancreatic carcinoma, patients undergoing the Whipple procedure often benefit from placement of a feeding jejunostomy.[60]

Liver

Hepatic resection procedures depend on the lobe and segment of the liver involved.[47,60,61] Procedures include wedge biopsy or resection, excision of tumor, or major lobectomy. Patients with advanced cirrhosis and variceal bleeding may require

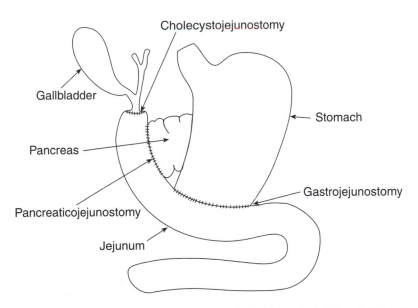

Figure 18–15 Whipple Procedure. *Source:* Reprinted with permission from S.C. Smeltzer, B.G. Bare, eds. *Brunner and Suddarth's Textbook of Medical-Surgical Nursing,* 8th ed., p. 1118, © 1996, Lippincott-Raven Publishers.

alteration of hepatic blood flow via an operative procedure that creates a portocaval shunt. The pressure in the portal system is higher than that of the systemic veins; in cirrhosis, a portal systemic venous anastomosis creates a significant shunt from the portal to systemic veins, resulting in decreased perfusion to the hepatic cells.[47] Patients often have severe hepatic dysfunction and may become encephalopathic. Nutrition management often includes protein restriction. The results of two studies suggest that the use of parenteral branched-chain amino acids may be beneficial for patients with hepatic encephalopathy in advanced liver disease.[64,65]

WOUND HEALING

An important aspect of surgical management is wound healing. A wound is defined as any physical break in tissue continuity. Wounds differ depending on the type, severity, mechanism of wounding, location, and desired outcome.[66] An elective surgical incision such as plastic surgery of the face, for example, differs significantly from a burn injury accompanied by infection, shock, and sepsis. The goals for adequate healing for an eyelid laceration may differ from the goals for healing an abdominal surgical wound, long bone fracture, or GI anastomosis. Wound healing alterations result in impaired (dehiscence, anastomotic failure, fistula) or delayed healing. Impaired wound healing often occurs in the face of concurrent injury or infection (as in a patient who has diabetes or has received radiation therapy) and almost always leads to a poor wound outcome. The process of delayed healing is best illustrated in an experimental wound model where the wound can be evaluated at specific time intervals. A poorly healing wound may have decreased tensile strength or low collagen accumulation, depending on when the wound is evaluated but may eventually heal to normal.

Pressure ulcers, lesions caused by unrelieved pressure that results in damage to underlying tissue, are wounds that are more easily prevented than treated. The National Pressure Ulcer Advisory Panel uses a staging system to characterize ulcers.[67] A stage I pressure ulcer presents as nonblanchable erythema of intact skin. Stage II ulcers have partial-thickness skin loss and usually present clinically as an abrasion, blister, or shallow crater. A stage III ulcer clinically presents as a deep crater; it is a full-thickness skin loss involving damage or necrosis of the subcutaneous tissue that may extend down to, but not through, the underlying fascia. A stage IV ulcer is a full-thickness skin loss with extensive destruction, necrosis, or damage to muscle, bone, or supporting structures.

Malnutrition is only one of the many factors that influence wound healing. Surgical technique (including the skill of the surgeon, length of operating time, and control of infection with aseptic technique and prophylactic antibiotics) and local wound care (including adequate circulation, proper positioning, topical antibiotics, and wound dressings) are extraordinarily important in promoting healing.[68-70]

Restoration and maintenance of blood volume and adequate oxygenation and tissue perfusion are essential for adequate wound healing. Certain treatments such as steroids may slow the rate of epithelialization and neovascularization and decrease collagen deposition and ultimately the tensile strength of the wound.[71] Chemotherapy can affect wound healing by inhibiting the early phases of inflammation and by interfering with protein synthesis and cell division.[71] Direct ulceration by radiation therapy can injure peripheral tissue, and neutropenia following these treatments can predispose the patient to wound infection.[71]

As early as 1959, Francis Moore described the early wound as having a high biological priority in which wound healing occurs through endocrine and metabolic control often at the expense of other tissues.[72] Most surgical wounds heal in the presence of significant preinjury weight loss and even in short-term postoperative starvation. The cachectic cancer patient who undergoes successful placement of a surgical gastrostomy tube illustrates this concept well. In the presence of complex injuries involving different tissues and organs, infection or sepsis, major burns, or severe malnutrition, the postoperative state is characterized by energy and protein demands that are substantially above normal; in these circumstances, impaired healing may occur.

A frequently asked question is, what is the role for nutrition therapy in the regulation of wound healing? It is well accepted that malnutrition is associated with an increased risk of wound-related complications, but it is unclear whether nutritional intervention can improve or accelerate the wound-healing response.[65] To date, most knowledge has been derived from animal studies where a relationship between protein depletion and delayed wound healing has been described.[73–76] Protein-depleted animals have a measurable delay in wound healing compared to normally nourished control animals. Whether this delay is present only after there have been large losses of body protein and fat stores or whether the delay occurs soon after the onset of starvation has not been effectively determined.[76] Animals who are fed protein-deficient diets have markedly reduced food intakes that lead to substantial loss of body weight. It is unclear whether the alteration in wound healing is due to decreased protein intake or malnutrition associated with substantial weight loss.

The delay in wound healing that is associated with protein depletion in animals is present in humans, and the impairment appears to occur quite early in the course of malnutrition before changes in anthropometric measurements can be detected.[30,77,78] Haydock and Hill reported significant differences in wound healing (measured by hydroxyproline accumulation in subcutaneously implanted Gore-Tex tubes) in moderately to severely malnourished patients compared to individuals with normal nutritional status.[77] Similarly, the presence of normal serum albumin and total lymphocyte counts predicted successful healing of lower extremity amputations with a 75% sensitivity and a 90% specificity; hypoalbuminemia and abnormal total lymphocyte counts were more often predictive of failure or associated with local or systemic postoperative complications.[79,80] Experimental studies have demonstrated that patients who receive adequate pre- or postoperative nutrition support (oral, enteral, or IV nutrition) have a better wound-healing response than individuals who receive inadequate dietary intake or hypocaloric feedings.[29,30,81,82]

Studies of nutritional status and pressure ulcer incidence also contribute evidence to the role of malnutrition and poor outcomes. In a study of 232 nursing home patients in the greater Chicago area, patients with pressure ulcers were all severely malnourished; yet no patient who had mild or moderate malnutrition developed a pressure ulcer.[83] Breslow found a direct relationship between pressure ulcer size and calorie intake in nursing home patients on tube feeding and an inverse relationship with body mass index, suggesting that the thinnest individuals with the largest pressure ulcers require the greatest nutritional intervention.[84] A recent review of patients in extended-care facilities reported that the presence of a stage II, III, or IV pressure ulcer plus unintentional weight loss (defined as more than 10% in 6 months or more than 5% in 1 month) was associated with hypoalbuminemia 77% of the time, and with reduced functional ability or chewing problems two thirds of the time.[85] The incidence of pressure ulcers and hypoalbuminemia and weight loss of more than 5 kg have also been correlated with a significantly greater length of hospitalization.[86]

ROLE OF SPECIFIC NUTRIENTS

All of the steps involved in wound healing require energy. Carbohydrate and fat provide sources of cellular energy. Protein and amino acids are essential for synthesis and cellular multiplication. Structurally, protein serves as part of the ground substance of the wound in the form of proteoglycans and glycoproteins. All electrolytes and other minerals are essential for normal cellular function, and many vitamins and minerals serve as enzymatic cofactors in steps of the wound healing process.

Ascorbic acid plays an important role in wound healing. Vitamin C functions as a cofactor in the hydroxylation of proline in collagen. Ascorbic acid has also been shown to enhance the cellular and humoral response to stress. In vitro studies suggest that there is an increased utilization of vitamin C during phagocytosis, and vitamin C may increase the activation of leukocytes and macrophages to the injured site.[87,88] The administration of vitamin C rapidly restores healing. Although the exact amount of supplementation remains controversial, Dickerson reports dosages of 500 to 1000 mg per day.[89] Standard enteral nutrition products contain 100 to 200 mg vitamin C per 1000 calories; several wound-healing formulas provide 240 to 340 mg vitamin C per 1000 calories. Multivitamin preparations used in TPN contain vitamins in amounts recommended for IV use by the American Medical Association Nutrition Advisory Group. Ascorbic acid is provided as a

100 mg dose in standard preparations. Although reports of clinical scurvy are few and far between, there appears to be a biochemical deficiency following injury and a high proportion of depressed plasma and leukocyte ascorbic acid levels in smokers, elderly patients, and in individuals with liver disease or cancer.[89–91] Winkler and Albina reported a surprisingly high percentage of TPN patients (40%) starting out with subnormal baseline values of vitamin C.[92] Since vitamin C is not stored in the body, depressed serum levels probably reflect recent intake; however, the combination of injury and surgery with low vitamin C levels may be of clinical relevance.

Vitamin A has been shown to enhance fibroplasia and collagen accumulation in wounds, thus hastening the healing process and enhancing the tensile strength of the wound.[93] Studies during deficiency states report that vitamin A is important in maintaining the normal humoral defense mechanism and in limiting complications associated with wound infections. Supplementation of vitamin A has been used to counteract the catabolic effect that glucocorticoids have on wound healing by reducing wound dehiscence.[94,95] Administration of 25,000 international units (IU) daily to patients receiving steroids for a period of 7 to 10 days pre- and postsurgery is prudent. Most standard enteral diets contain 2000 to 3000 IU of vitamin A per liter of formula. The wound-healing formulas contain 4000 to 8000 IU. Parenteral nutrition vitamin preparations typically provide 1 mg vitamin A as retinol, which is equal to 3300 USP units.

Minerals and trace elements are also important in wound healing. Calcium is needed for the calcium-dependent collagenases. Iron is necessary for the hydroxylation of lysine and proline in the formation of collagen, and copper is a component of many enzyme systems including lysyl oxidase, which catalyzes an important step in the cross-linking of collagen. Zinc serves as a cofactor for the enzymes responsible for cellular proliferation and is needed for the transcription of RNA, cellular replication, and collagen formulation. Zinc deficiency impairs wound healing by reducing the rate of epithelialization, reducing wound strength, and diminishing collagen synthesis. Most investigators agree that impaired wound healing that occurs in zinc deficiency can be corrected by restoring zinc levels to normal.[96,97] What is still unknown is whether supplemental zinc accelerates wound healing to an above-normal rate. Among patients receiving TPN, zinc deficiency is prevalent; one study reported low serum levels in over 30% of patients receiving TPN.[98] Zinc losses occur through the GI tract, so patients with diarrhea or high-output fistula or ostomy drainage may be at risk for zinc deficiency. Patients with burns or other wound exudates also lose zinc. Serum zinc does not necessarily correlate with whole body zinc status. Because zinc is bound to serum albumin, hyperzincuria may occur secondary to hypoalbuminemia. Dietary intake of zinc is also of concern. Because zinc is found in animal protein, it is likely that dietary zinc may be limited for the growing number of people who are following very-low-fat diets. Furthermore zinc absorption is relatively poor. Physical signs of zinc deficiency include oral, nasal, or anal dermatitis that is immediately reversible with supplemental zinc. Typical oral supplementation is 220 mg zinc sulfate (50 mg elemental zinc).[89] Most standard enteral nutrition products contain 10 mg zinc per liter. The wound-healing formulations contain between 18 and 36 mg zinc per liter. The recommended intravenous dosage for stable adults receiving TPN is 2.5 to 4 mg zinc per day. Additional zinc can be added for patients with significant small-bowel losses.

The Agency for Health Care Policy and Research publishes recommendations for the treatment of pressure ulcers that are applicable for patients who are nutritionally compromised and have wounds to heal.[67] These guidelines recommend that the practitioner (1) ensure adequate dietary intake to prevent malnutrition to the extent that this is compatible with the individual's wishes; (2) perform a nutritional assessment at least every 3 months for individuals at risk for malnutrition and for those patients who are unable to take food by mouth or who have experienced involuntary changes in weight; (3) encourage dietary intake or supplementation and use tube feeding if dietary intake is inadequate, impractical, or impossible; (4) provide 30 to 35 calories/kg/day and 1.25 to 1.5 grams of protein/kg/day; and (5) give vitamin and mineral supplements if deficiencies are confirmed or suspected.

CONCLUSIONS

Optimal nutritional care for all patients avoids the potential threats to recovery from surgery and wound healing. Knowledge of the metabolic response to surgery, stress, and trauma and the clinical effects on body composition and nutrient utilization are important for patient assessment and establishment of the nutritional care plan. Likewise, nutritional consequences of maldigestion and malabsorption that are directly related to GI surgery should be an integral part of the patient's evaluation. Dramatic degrees of protein-calorie malnutrition or clinically evident specific nutrient deficiencies are likely to impact recovery from surgery and may interfere with wound healing by delaying the healing response. The use of pre- and postoperative nutrition support and pharmacological doses of nutrients such as zinc and vitamins A and C may result in fewer postoperative and wound complications. While it is possible that a wound can heal without food, it is common sense that patients cannot recover unless they are adequately nourished or nutritionally supported.

REFERENCES

1. Mullen JL, Gertner MH, Buzby GP, Goodhart GL, et al. Implications of malnutrition in the surgical patient. *Arch Surg.* 1979;114:121–125.

2. Studley HO. Percentage of weight loss: a basic indicator of surgical risk in patients with chronic peptic ulcer. *JAMA.* 1936;106:458–460.

3. Cannon PR, Wissler RW, Woolridge RL, Benditt EP. The relationship of protein deficiency to surgical infection. *Ann Surg.* 1944;120:514–525.

4. Ching M, Grossi CE, Angers J, Zurawinsky HS, et al. The outcome of surgical treatment as related to the response of the serum albumin level to nutritional support. *Surg Gynecol Obstet.* 1980;151:199–202.

5. Reinhardt GF, Myscofski JW, Wilkens DB, Dobrin PB, et al. Incidence and mortality of hypoalbuminemic patients in hospitalized veterans. *J Parenter Enter Nutr.* 1980;4:357–359.

6. Chandra RK. Nutrition, immunity and infection: present knowledge and future direction. *Lancet.* 1983;1:688–691.

7. Windsor JA. Underweight patients and the risks of major surgery. *World J Surg.* 1993;17:165–172.

8. Larca L, Greenbaum DM. Effectiveness of intensive nutritional regimes in patients who fail to wean from mechanical ventilation. *Crit Care Med.* 1982;10:297–300.

9. Bassili HR, Deitel M. Effect of nutrition support on weaning patients off mechanical ventilators. *J Parenter Enter Nutr.* 1981;5:161–163.

10. Barton RG. Nutrition support in critical illness. *Nutr Clin Pract.* 1994;9:127–139.

11. Cuthbertson DP. The metabolic response to injury and its nutritional implications: retrospect and prospect. *J Parenter Enter Nutr.* 1979;3:108–129.

12. Wilmore DW, Smith RJ, O'Dwyer ST, Jacobs DO, et al. The gut: a central organ after surgical stress. *Surgery.* 1988;104:917–923.

13. Deitch EA, Bridges RM. Effect of stress and trauma on bacterial translocation from the gut. *J Surg Res.* 1987;42:536–542.

14. Machiedo GW. Shock. In: Polk HC, Gardner B, Stone HH, eds. *Basic Surgery.* St. Louis, MO: Quality Medical Publishing, Inc; 1993:757–772.

15. Dempsey DT, Guenter P, Mullen JL, Fairman R, et al. Energy expenditure in acute trauma to the head with and without barbiturate therapy. *Surg Gynecol Obstet.* 1985;160:128–134.

16. Liggett SB, St John RE, Lefrak SS. Determination of resting energy expenditure utilizing the thermodilution pulmonary artery catheter. *Chest.* 1987;91:562–566.

17. Pomp A, Albina JE. Parenteral nutrition in adults. In: Rakel RE, ed. *Conn's Current Therapy.* Philadelphia: WB Saunders Co; 1997;590–596.

18. Polk HC. The approach to the postoperative patient. In: Polk HC, Gardner B, Stone HH, eds. *Basic Surgery.* St. Louis, MO: Quality Medical Publishing Inc; 1993:735–744.

19. Bickel A, Shtamler B, Mizrahi S. Early oral feeding following removal of nasogastric tube in gastrointestinal operations: a randomized prospective study. *Arch Surg.* 1992;127:287–289.

20. Reissman P, Teoh TA, Cohen SM, Weiss EG, et al. Is early oral feeding safe after elective colorectal surgery? A prospective randomized trial. *Ann Surg.* 1995;222:73–77.

21. Kirby DF, DeLegge MH, Fleming CR. American Gastroenterological Association technical review on tube feeding for enteral nutrition. *Gastroenterology.* 1995;108:1282–1301.

22. Buzby GP. Overview of randomized clinical trials of total parenteral nutrition for malnourished surgical patients. *World J Surg.* 1993;17:173–177.

23. Buzby GP, Williford WO, Peterson OL, Crosby LO, et al. A randomized clinical trial of total parenteral nutrition in malnourished surgical patients: the rationale and impact of previous clinical trials and pilot study on protocol design. *Am J Clin Nutr.* 1988;47:357–365.

24. Detsky AS, Baker JP, O'Rourke K, Goel V, et al. Perioperative parenteral nutrition: a meta-analysis. *Ann Intern Med.* 1987;107:195–203.

25. Buzby GP, Veterans Affairs TPN Cooperative Study Group. Perioperative total parenteral nutrition in surgical patients. *N Engl J Med.* 1991;325:525–532.

26. Windsor JA, Knight GS, Hill GL. Wound healing response in surgical patients: recent food intake is more important than nutritional status. *Br J Surg.* 1988;75:135–140.

27. Haydock DA, Hill GL. Improved wound healing response in surgical patients receiving intravenous nutrition. *Br J Surg.* 1987;4:320–323.

28. Abel RA, Fischer JE, Buckley MJ, Barnett O, et al. Malnutrition in cardiac surgery patients. *Arch Surg.* 1976;111:45–50.

29. Moghissi K, Hornshaw J, Teasdale PR, Dawes EA. Parenteral nutrition in carcinoma of the oesophagus treated by surgery: nitrogen balance and clinical studies. *Br J Surg.* 1977;64:125–128.

30. Askanazi J, Hensle TW, Starker PM, Lockhart SH, et al. Effect of immediate postoperative nutritional support on length of hospitalization. *Ann Surg.* 1986;203:236–239.

31. Kudsk KA, Croce MA, Fabian TC, Minard G, et al. Enteral versus parenteral feeding: effects on septic morbidity after blunt and penetrating abdominal trauma. *Ann Surg.* 1992;215:503–511.

32. Moore FA, Feliciano DV, Andrassy RJ, McArdle AH, et al. Early enteral feeding, compared with parenteral, reduces post-operative septic complications: the results of a meta-analysis. *Ann Surg.* 1992;216:172–183.

33. ASPEN Board of Directors. Guidelines for the use of parenteral and enteral nutrition in adults and pediatrics. *J Parenter Enter Nutr.* 1993;17(suppl):21-22SA.

34. Mullen JL, Buzby GP, Waldman MT, Gertner MH, et al. Prediction of operative morbidity and mortality by preoperative nutritional assessment. *Surg Forum.* 1979;30:80–82.

35. Polk HC. Difficulties in swallowing. In: Polk HC, Gardner B, Stone HH, eds. *Basic Surgery.* St. Louis, MO: Quality Medical Publishing Inc; 1993:289–301.

36. Wakefield SE, Mansell NJ, Baigrie RJ, Dowling BL. Use of a feeding jejunostomy after oesophagogastric surgery. *Br J Surg.* 1995;82:811–813.

37. Moody FG, Miller TA. Stomach. In: Schwartz SI, Shires GT, Spencer FC, eds. *Principles of Surgery.* 6th ed. New York: McGraw-Hill Inc; 1994:1123–1152.

38. Petty LR. Gastrointestinal surgery. In: Meeker MH, Rothrock JC, eds. *Alexander's Care of the Patient in Surgery.* 10th ed. St. Louis, MO: Mosby; 1995:251–319.

39. Mathisen DJ, Wilkins EW. Techniques of esophageal reconstruction. In: Zuidema GD, ed. *Shackelford's Surgery of the Alimentary Tract.* Philadelphia: WB Saunders Co; 1996:389–413.

40. Polk HC. The Nissen fundoplication: operative technique and clinical experience. In: Zuidema GD, ed. *Shackelford's Surgery of the Alimentary Tract.* Philadelphia: WB Saunders Co; 1996:214–221.

41. Bjerkeset T, Edna TH, Fjosne U. Long term results after "floppy" Nissen/Rossetti fundoplication for gastroesophageal reflux disease. *Scand J Gastroenterol.* 1992;27:707–710.

42. Spechler SJ, Department of Veterans Affairs Gastroesophageal Reflux Disease Study Group. Comparison of medical and surgical therapy for complicated gastroesophageal reflux disease in veterans. *N Engl J Med.* 1992;326:786–792.

43. Dempsey DT, Ritchie WP. Gastroduodenal physiology and peptic ulcer disease. In: Polk HC, Gardner B, Stone HH, eds. *Basic Surgery.* St. Louis, MO: Quality Medical Publishing Inc; 1993:196–219.

44. Bradley EL, Isaacs J, Hersh T, Davison ED, et al. Nutritional consequences of total gastrectomy. *Ann Surg.* 1975:182:415–429.

45. Grant JP, Chapman G, Russell MK. Malabsorption associated with surgical procedures and its treatment. *Nutr Clin Pract.* 1996;11:43–52.

46. Gleeson NC, Hoffman MS, Fiorica JV, Roberts WS, et al. Gastrostomy tubes after gynecologic oncologic surgery. *Gynecol Oncol.* 1994;54:19–22.

47. Richardson JD, Gardner B. Gastrointestinal bleeding. In: Polk HC, Gardner B, Stone HH, eds. *Basic Surgery.* St. Louis, MO: Quality Medical Publishing Inc; 1993:403–421.

48. Gardner B, Stone HH. Acute abdominal pain. In: Polk HC, Gardner B, Stone HH, eds. *Basic Surgery.* St. Louis, MO: Quality Medical Publishing Inc; 1993:422–459.

49. Williamson RCN, Chir M. Intestinal adaptation. *N Engl J Med.* 1978;298:1393–1402,1444–1450.

50. Shanbhogue LK, Molenaar JC. Short bowel syndrome: metabolic and surgical management. *Br J Surg.* 1994;81:486–489.

51. Price A. Bowel control for colostomy and ileostomy. *Ostomy Q.* 1988;266:76–77.

52. Kock NJ. Intra-abdominal "reservoir" in patients with permanent ileostomy: preliminary observations on a procedure resulting in fecal "continence" in five ileostomy patients. *Arch Surg.* 1969;99:223–231.

53. Pricolo VE. Ileal pouch-anal anastomosis: the "ideal" operation for ulcerative colitis and adenomatous polyposis coli? *RI Med.* 1994;77:382–384.

54. Weinryb, RM, Gustavsson JP, Liljeqvist, L, Poppen B, et al. A prospective study of the quality of life after pelvic pouch operation. *J Am Coll Surg.* 1995;180:589–595.

55. Kohler LW, Pemberton JH, Zinsmeister AR, Kelly KA. Quality of life after proctocolectomy: a comparison of Brooke ileostomy, Kock pouch, and ileal pouch-anal anastomosis. *Gastroenterology.* 1991;101:679–684.

56. Raymond JL, Becker JM. Ileoanal pull-through: a new surgical alternative to ileostomy and a new challenge in diet therapy. *J Am Diet Assoc.* 1986;86:663–665.

57. Tyus FJ, Austhof SI, Chima CS, Keating C. Diet tolerance and stool frequency in patients with ileoanal reservoirs. *J Am Diet Assoc.* 1992;92:861–863.

58. Winkler MF, Jackson J, Green G, Pricolo V. Dietary intervention in patients following ileal pouch anal anastomosis; 1997. Unpublished data submitted to *Am J Gastroenterol.*

59. Roslyn JJ, Zinner MF. Gallbladder and extrahepatic biliary system. In: Schwartz SI, Shires GT, Spencer FC, eds. *Principles of Surgery.* 6th ed. New York: McGraw-Hill; 1994:1367–1399.

60. Petty LR. Surgery of the liver, biliary tract, pancreas, and spleen. In: Meeker MH, Rothrock JC, eds. *Alexander's Care of the Patient in Surgery.* 10th ed. St. Louis, MO: Mosby; 1995:320–365.

61. Moossa AR, Deakin M. Jaundice. In: Polk HC, Gardner B, Stone HH, eds. *Basic Surgery.* St. Louis, MO: Quality Medical Publishing Inc; 1993:460–480.

62. Yeo CJ, Cameron JL. Acute pancreatitis. In: Zuidema GD, ed. *Shackleford's Surgery of the Alimentary Tract.* 4th ed. Philadelphia: WB Saunders Co; 1996:18–37.

63. Caliari S, Benini L, Bonfante F, Brentegani MT, et al. Pancreatic extracts are necessary for the absorption of elemental and polymeric enteral diets in severe pancreatic insufficiency. *Scand J Gastroenterol.* 1993;28:749–752.

64. Cerra FB, Cheung NK, Fischer JE, Kaplowitz N, et al. Disease specific amino acid infusion (FO80) in hepatic encephalopathy: a prospective, randomized, double blind controlled trial. *J Parenter Enter Nutr.* 1985;9:288–295.

65. Freund H, Dienstag J, Lehrich J, Yoshimura N, et al. Infusion of branched-chain enriched amino acid solution in patients with hepatic encephalopathy. *Ann Surg.* 1982;196:209–220.

66. Albina JE. Nutrition and wound healing. *J Parenter Enter Nutr.* 1994;18:367–376.

67. US Department of Health and Human Services. *Treatment of Pressure Ulcers.* Rockville, MD: Agency for Health Care Policy and Research, Public Health Service; 1994.

68. Hochberg J, Murray GF. Principles of operative surgery: antisepsis, technique, sutures, and drains. In: Sabiston DC Jr, ed. *Textbook of Surgery: The Biological Basis of Modern Surgical Practice.* Philadelphia: WB Saunders Co; 1991:210–220.

69. LaVan FB, Hunt TK. Oxygen and wound healing. *Clin Plast Surg.* 1990;17:463–471.

70. Robson MC, Stenberg BD, Heggers JP. Wound healing alterations caused by infection. *Clin Plast Surg.* 1990;17:485–492.

71. Carrico TJ, Mehrhof AI, Cohen IK. Biology of wound healing. *Surg Clin North Am.* 1984;64:721–733.

72. Moore FD. *Metabolic Care of the Surgical Patient.* Philadelphia: WB Saunders Co; 1959.

73. Kobak MW, Steffe CH. The relationship of protein deficiency to experimental wound healing. *Surg Gynecol Obstet.* 1947;85:751–756.

74. Daly MN, Vars HM, Dudrick SJ. Effects of protein depletion on strength of colonic anastomoses. *Surg Gynecol Obstet.* 1972;134:15–21.

75. Irvin TT. Effects of malnutrition and hyperalimentation on wound healing. *Surg Gynecol Obstet.* 1978;146:33–37.

76. Delany HM, Demetriou AA, Teh E, Levenson SM. Effect of early postoperative nutritional support on skin wound and colon anastomosis healing. *J Parenter Enter Nutr.* 1990;14:357–361.

77. Haydock DA, Hill GL. Impaired wound healing in surgical patients with varying degrees of malnutrition. *J Parenter Enter Nutr.* 1986;10:550–554.

78. Temple WJ, Voitk AJ, Snelling CFT, Crispin JS. Effects of nutrition, diet and suture material on long term wound healing. *Ann Surg.* 1975;182:93–97.

79. Dickhaut SC, DeLee JC, Page CP. Nutrition status: importance in predicting wound-healing after amputation. *J Bone Joint Surg.* 1984;66A:71–75.

80. Kay SP, Moreland JR, Schmitter E. Nutritional status and wound healing in lower extremity amputations. *Clin Orthop.* 1987;217:253–256.

81. Bozzetti F, Temo G, Longoni C. Parenteral hyperalimentation and wound healing. *Surg Gynecol Obstet.* 1975;141:712–714.

82. Schroeder D, Gillanders L, Mahr K, Hill GL. Effects of immediate postoperative enteral nutrition on body composition, muscle function, and wound healing. *J Parenter Enter Nutr.* 1991;15:376–383.

83. Pinchcofsky-Devin GD, Kaminski MV. Correlation of pressure sores and nutritional status. *J Am Geriatric Soc.* 1986;34:435–440.

84. Breslow RA, Hallfrisch J, Goldberg AP. Malnutrition in tube fed nursing home patients with pressure sores. *J Parenter Enter Nutr.* 1991;15:663–668.

85. Gilmore SA, Robinson G, Posthauer ME, Raymond J. Clinical indicators associated with unintentional weight loss and pressure ulcers in nursing facilities. *J Am Diet Assoc.* 1995;95:984–992.

86. Samour PQ, St. Peter MJ, Harrity MR, Bistrian B. Continuous quality improvement: an implementation model for patients with pressure ulcers. *Top Clin Nutr.* 1994;10:79–85.

87. Leibovitz B, Seigel BV. Ascorbic acid, neutrophil function and the immune response. *Int J Vitam Nutr Res.* 1978;48:159–164.

88. Shilotry PG. Phagocytosis and leukocyte enzymes in ascorbic acid deficient guinea pigs. *J Nutr.* 1977;107:1513–1516.

89. Dickerson JWT. Ascorbic acid, zinc and wound healing. *J Wound Care.* 1993;2:350–353.

90. Irvin TT, Chattopadhyay DK, Smythe A. Ascorbic acid requirements in postoperative patients. *Surg Gynecol Obstet.* 1978;147:49–55.

91. Mason M, Matyk PW, Doolan SA. Urinary ascorbic acid excretion in postoperative patients. *Am J Surg.* 1971;122:808–811.

92. Winkler MF, Albina JE. Vitamin status of TPN patients. *J Parenter Enter Nutr.* 1990;14:16S.

93. Demetriou AA, Levenson SM, Rettura G, Seifter E. Vitamin A and retinoic acid: induced fibroblast differentiation in vitro. *Surgery.* 1985;98:931–934.

94. Ehrlich HP, Hunt TK. Effect of cortisone and vitamin A on wound healing. *Ann Surg.* 1968;167:324–328.

95. Hunt TK, Ehrlich HP, Garcia JA, Dunphy JE. Effect of vitamin A on reversing the inhibitor effect of cortisone on healing of wounds in animal and man. *Ann Surg.* 1969;170:633–641.

96. Chvapil M. Zinc and other factors of the pharmacology of wound healing. In: Hunt TK, ed. *Theory and Surgical Practice.* New York: Appleton-Century-Croft; 1980.

97. Liszewski RI. The effect of zinc on wound healing: a collective review. *J Am Osteopath Assoc.* 1981;81:104–106.

98. Winkler MF, Watkins CK, Ricci R, Albina JE. A nutritional support service quality improvement plan. Presented at 18th Clinical Congress of American Society for Parenteral and Enteral Nutrition; January, 1994; San Antonio, TX.

CHAPTER 19

Short-Bowel Syndrome

Peter L. Beyer

DEFINITION AND DESCRIPTION

Short-bowel syndrome has been described by the length of intestine resected, the symptoms associated with compromised digestion and absorption, or the percentage of intestine remaining. Resections of 200 to 300 centimeters or 30% to 40% of the small bowel are usually sufficient to produce, at least temporarily, the characteristic features of weight loss, large and frequent bowel movements, rapid transit rate, steatorrhea, dehydration, and various forms of malnutrition. Because the length of the small intestine differs among individuals and measures of the length of resected bowel are highly variable, the preferred descriptors are the length and nature of intestine *remaining*.[1–5]

The minimum length of small intestine required to maintain reasonable health on a long-term basis without enteral or parenteral nutrition is about 100 centimeters. A number of variables, however, affect the amount of gut required for satisfactory health. Variables that affect need for and duration of specialized nutrition support include amount of small intestine resected; whether the segment resected included jejunum, proximal ileum, or distal ileum; whether the colon or part of the colon remains; presence or lack of ileocecal valve; age of the individual; reason for intestinal resection; health of the remaining gastrointestinal (GI) tract; concurrent or past use of chemotherapy or irradiation; and numerous dietary factors.[3–6] A more detailed discussion of the impact of these factors is provided later in this chapter. Maintaining acceptable long-term nutritional status with less than 200 cm intestine is difficult, especially if the ileum has been resected. Some studies describe patient survival with less than 150 cm of GI tract.[1,2,6,7] A better measure of success, especially for patients without enteral or parenteral nutrition support, might be several years of reasonable quality of life without significant malabsorption or malnutrition.

The primary problem in short-bowel syndrome is the inability to absorb sufficient food and nutrients. In more severe cases, the problem includes the inability to absorb sufficient oral fluids and reabsorb endogenous GI secretions. Digestion may be compromised somewhat by rapid transit and poor timing between substrate presentation and hormone/enzyme secretion. But most secretory and digestive functions remain intact. Resection of the colon may contribute to problems associated with short-bowel syndrome, but short bowel really refers to insufficient length of *small* bowel. Even total colectomy does not significantly compromise nutrient absorption.

In adults, thrombosis or embolus involving mesenteric vessels, Crohn's disease, and strangulated hernias are the most common reasons for major intestinal resections.[1–6] In children, the most common causes of short-bowel syndrome include volvulus, necrotizing enterocolitis, and intestinal atresia.[7,8] Short-bowel syndrome as a consequence of trauma, neoplasms, or radiation enteritis occur less frequently, but each factor can result in special nutritional problems.

NUTRITIONAL IMPLICATIONS

Effective nutrition management of short-bowel syndrome involves all aspects of clinical nutrition practice, from appropriate assessment and nutrition therapy to careful patient diet counseling. The practitioner must have sufficient understanding of the functions of the resected and remaining intestine in secretion, digestion, and absorption. The practitioner must also have working knowledge of composition and value of specialty foods as well as enteral and parenteral products. Consideration of psychosocial issues and knowledge and skill in nutrition counseling are also involved.

Nutritional consequences of short-bowel syndrome may include macro- and micronutrient deficiencies, as well as excessive fluid and electrolyte losses. Understanding the usual role of the GI tract and its capacity for digestion and absorption can help the practitioner to (1) predict the problems likely to be encountered, (2) predict the nature and duration of nutrition therapies required, (3) prevent unnecessary additional nutritional and medical burdens, and (4) explain the rationale and mechanics of nutrition therapies to all involved. Patients typically have a poor understanding of digestive and absorptive processes and often have little understanding of the results or implications of intestinal resection.

In addition to potential macronutrient and micronutrient deficiencies, persons with short-bowel syndrome may suffer from renal, biliary, hepatic, or metabolic problems, which may be at least partly prevented by appropriate dietary management. In patients with significant resections, the pattern and type of foods consumed may make a major difference in symptoms; requirement for parenteral support; and, in some cases, survival.[3,6–12]

NORMAL GASTROINTESTINAL SECRETION, DIGESTION, AND ABSORPTION

Powerful digestive enzymes from the stomach, pancreas, and brush border of the proximal small intestine normally provide for effective digestion, even after ingestion of significant amounts of food.[13–15] Normally, digestion of most foodstuffs is completed within about the first 100 cm of small intestine. The primary exceptions are incomplete digestion of dietary fibers; resistant starch; and, in some individuals, lactose. When consumed in excess, alcohol sugars and fructose also escape digestion and pass into the colon.[15–17]

Normally, part of the dietary fiber (especially soluble fiber) and most of the maldigested starches and sugars are fermented in the colon to short-chain fatty acids and gasses. The gasses include hydrogen; carbon dioxide; and, in varying amounts, methane. Short-chain fatty acids are rapidly absorbed and, when produced in normal amounts, facilitate the transport of salts and water. Short-chain fatty acids also serve as substrates for colonocytes and are considered trophic to the colonic mucosa. The fermentation serves to salvage malabsorbed carbohydrate and decrease the potential for accumulation of osmolar substrates. Increased osmolar concentration in the lumen of the colon would decrease fluid absorption or produce net secretion. When larger amounts of carbohydrate or fiber are malabsorbed, osmolality of colonic contents and increased production of short-chain fatty acids and gasses may exceed the capacity for absorption. The result may include abdominal distention, cramping, acidification of colonic contents, decreased fluid and electrolyte absorption, and/or diarrhea. Varying degrees of the symptoms may commonly be seen in healthy persons after excessive consumption of fiber, resistant starch, fructose, or sorbitol.

Digestion of starch to oligosaccharides is primarily the result of pancreatic amylase. Enzymes from the brush border of small intestine enterocytes reduce oligosaccharides and disaccharides to monosaccharides before absorption. Except when very large amounts are consumed, only a few grams of starch, sucrose, or glucose are undigested and malabsorbed.[15–18]

Protein digestion begins in the stomach with hydrochloric acid and pepsin and continues with enzymes secreted from the pancreas and brush border. Digestion and absorption of protein, especially for animal sources, is very efficient. Reserve capacity is ample, and both digestion and absorption are essentially complete in the first one third to one half of the small intestine. Protein is usually absorbed in the form of individual amino acids and small peptides. In healthy individuals, the net efficiency of nitrogen utilization from food and amino acid and peptide formulas depends on a number of factors. Presence of fiber, carbohydrate, lipids, and the relative composition of amino acids and peptides in the protein sources are factors

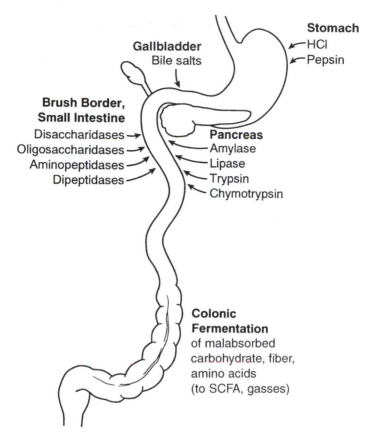

Figure 19–1 Normal Digestion.

that affect nutritional efficiency of proteins. Normally, significant amounts of proteins from GI secretions and sloughed cells are recycled.[13,14,19]

Digestion and absorption of lipid require adequate secretion of bile salts and pancreatic lipase and sufficient length of small intestine. Bile salts secreted into the intestine from the biliary tract are normally effectively reabsorbed (approximately 95%) in the distal ileum. The ileum must be intact for adequate supply of bile salts, because *de novo* hepatic synthesis is not adequate to meet requirements for effective surfactant action and micelle formation. Without an adequate supply of bile salts, absorption of lipid and fat-soluble nutrients is compromised. With usual ingestion of 60 to 100 g of dietary lipid daily, the amount of fat remaining in

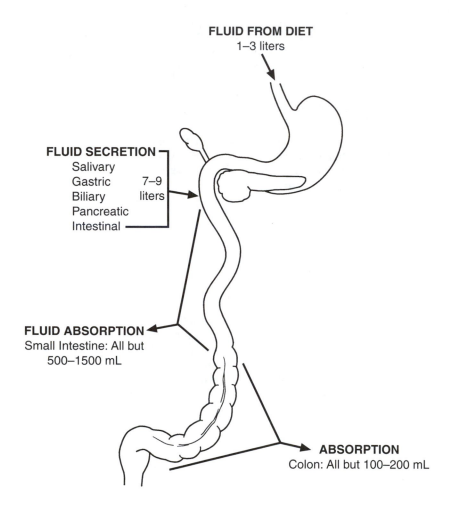

Figure 19–2 Normal Fluid Secretion and Absorption.

the stool is only about 3 to 4 g. The upper limit for fat remaining in the stool after adequate intake of fat is only about 7 g. In short-bowel syndrome, fecal fat may exceed 30 g.[14,20,21]

Secretion and Absorption of Fluids

Under normal circumstances, approximately 7 to 9 liters of fluid are secreted into the GI tract daily. In addition, 1 to 3 liters of fluid are usually consumed from food and beverages. Almost all of the fluid is secreted in the proximal GI tract, and most of the fluid is absorbed before reaching the colon (see Figure 19–2). The significant role of the ileum and distal jejunum in fluid absorption is probably underappreciated, perhaps, until after major resection of distal small bowel. Of the 8 to 10 liters of fluids ingested and secreted daily, only about 1 liter normally enters the colon and only about 100 mL water remains in the stool.[13,22] In short-bowel syndrome, most secretory and digestive mechanisms are intact. The primary problems are related to inability to absorb nutrients and fluid, partly related to lack of absorptive surface area, rapid transit, and lack of normal physiologic and anatomic controls.

Micronutrient Absorption

Most absorption of micronutrients is completed midway through the jejunum. The ileum is capable of absorbing micronutrients but normally provides a "re-

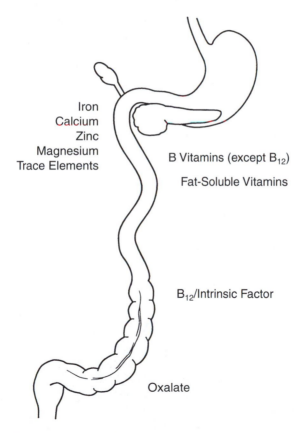

Figure 19–3 Micronutrient Absorption.

serve" function for vitamin-mineral absorption. Vitamin B12, however, is absorbed only in the terminal ileum.[13,22]

NUTRITIONAL ASSESSMENT

Because patients with short-bowel syndrome often have prior histories of nutrition problems and are at significant nutritional risk, a thorough nutritional assessment is indicated. The assessment should include a thorough diet history, weight history, measures of somatic and visceral protein status, medical and surgical history, estimate of nutrient requirements, and evaluation of appropriate socioeconomic factors.

Knowledge of the amount and nature of the remaining intestine is critical in the patient's outcome.[4-6,8-12,23] For example, even when all of the jejunum is resected, sufficient adaptation eventually occurs in the ileum to enable the patient to live a relatively normal life without specialized nutrition support and without extreme alterations in dietary habits. On the other hand, the patient who has only 150 cm of distal ileum and has lost the ileocecal valve is likely to require a prolonged period of parenteral support and considerable attention to a long list of potential nutritional problems to maintain satisfactory health and well-being. The checklist for nutritional assessment in Exhibit 19–1 can serve as the basis for nutrition decisions and predictors for nutritional care requirements.

Practitioners may encounter some difficulty when attempting to evaluate the amount and location of functional intestine. Incomplete or missing records, hazy

---

Exhibit 19–1 Checklist for Nutritional Assessment

- length of small intestine remaining
- nature of small bowel remaining (jejunum, ileum, etc)
- function of remaining GI tract, including small and large intestine, liver, gallbladder, pancreas, and stomach
- reason for original surgery
- nutritional problems prior to surgery
- current and past nutrient intake/diet therapy
- duration of time since the resection(s)
- net fluid and electrolyte balance (intake minus urine and stool output)
- laboratory and clinical measures of absorptive function
- nutritional status including vitamin and mineral levels
- pertinent prescription and over-the-counter medications
- psychosocial circumstances

Exhibit 19–2 Indicators of Significant Maldigestion/Malabsorption

---

- continued weight loss despite adequate intake
- difficulty maintaining adequate hydration
- average fecal output greater than 2 liters
- presence of steatorrhea (or fecal fat >15 g after 75–100 g fat/day)
- serum cholesterol <120, carotene <50
- presence of intact carbohydrate in stool (eg, rice/pasta)
- B_{12} deficiency (due to ileal malabsorption)
- hypomagnesemia and/or hypokalemia

---

or inaccurate patient recall, lack of clear-cut descriptions of the resected or remaining bowel, and individual complications make determining the remaining GI function difficult. The average "textbook" (postmortem) length of the small bowel is approximately 700 cm, but the range varies in unusually small or large individuals.[23] The duodenum is only about a foot in length (about 20 to 30 cm), the jejunum about 8 feet (200 to 300 cm), and the ileum approximately 12 feet (300 to 400 cm). However, *in vivo* lengths, which are more typical of those described in operative reports, are about half those of postmortem descriptions (350 cm or about 11 feet).[9]

When considering or predicting a patient's requirements for immediate and long-term nutritional care, the practitioner must consider the normal functions of the resected intestine and the degree to which the remaining segments are able to maintain homeostasis. Exhibit 19–2 provides several indicators that may help in determining when the patient has significant problems with digestion and absorption. The reason(s) for the patient's bowel resection, measures of small bowel and GI transit time, and endoscopy and/or radiologic examination may all help in characterizing the remaining GI tract.

GENERAL CONSIDERATIONS WITH MAJOR BOWEL RESECTION

Almost all patients with short bowel will initially need parenteral and/or enteral nutrition support. Volumes of parenteral fluid may be considerably greater than normal, especially in the first weeks after surgery. Parenteral solutions may need to compensate for the loss of endogenous GI fluids and electrolytes normally secreted into the GI tract. Approximately 3 to 5 liters of water and 200 milliequivalents of sodium may be required per day to keep the patient in balance. Protein and calories are adjusted to meet the patient's needs considering oral intake and GI losses. If the patient was markedly depleted before the surgery, appropriate caution is advised to avoid refeeding syndrome.

The duration of specialized nutrition support depends a great deal on the patient's nutritional status prior to surgery, the status of the remaining GI tract, and how well the patient's enteral/oral nutrition is managed after the operation. Malnutrition or prolonged periods without enteral nutrition result in decreased gut mass, surface area, and function, and require more caution with the weaning and adaptation processes. Adaptation refers to the epithelial hypertrophy and hyperplasia in the remaining bowel; increased villous height and thickness; and, to a lesser degree, increased length.[3,6,24,26] The adaptation process may continue to occur over several months to about a year, depending on the amount of bowel resected and the health of the remaining GI tract.

Epithelial hyperplasia begins almost immediately after operation, even to some degree in the absence of luminal stimulation.[27] Maximal stimulation, however, occurs when nutrients are supplied by way of the GI tract, soon after the operative procedure, and in frequent or continuous doses. Patients are usually provided with enough nutrition parenterally to meet most nutrient needs and enteral nutrition is gradually increased. To enhance the adaptation process, oral replacement fluids might be administered initially, followed by continuous feeding of isotonic (or more dilute) enteral formulas. In general, food is trophic to the GI tract; however, specific nutrients have been shown to enhance the adaptation process. Glutamine, nucleotides, short-chain fatty acids (eg, from colonic fermentation of soluble fiber), other amino acids, and sugars all have been found to be trophic.[26-33]

Young and healthy patients have better adaptive responses than, for example, an elderly individual whose original reason for bowel resection was radiation enteritis or small-bowel infarct. The adaptation that occurs after surgery typically improves the patient's condition but rarely absolves the patient of all features of short-bowel syndrome or the precarious nutritional status associated with it.

One complication that often retards progress with oral/enteral feeding is gastric acid hypersecretion. The hypersecretion occurs immediately after surgery and is usually proportional in amount and duration to the extent of intestinal resection. Excess acid entering the small intestine reduces the effectiveness of pancreatic and brush border enzymes. Hypersecretion of acid is normally determined by comparing fasting gastric acid secretion to normal basal levels, which are approximately 1.2 to 2.0 mmol/hr.[34] Hypersecretion does not preclude oral/enteral feeding but makes it less likely to serve as the only means of nutrition support.[4-9]

Deliberate attempts to overfeed the patient with short-bowel syndrome (ie, have the patient eat two to three times normal volume to compensate for diminished absorptive efficiency) often result in patient frustration and excessive fluid and electrolyte losses, especially in patients who have had major ileal resections. When patients eat normal or larger than normal amounts of foods, they often report a cycle of bloating and massive outputs followed by ravenous hunger and thirst, which again encourage overconsumption. Small, frequent feedings typically work best. Some patients require supplemental parenteral nutrition, primarily to replace fluid and electrolyte losses resulting from the inability to regulate their diet.

When only 100 cm of proximal small bowel remains, parenteral nutrition must be provided for prolonged periods to maintain adequate nutrition and hydration. Continuous enteral feeding is often used simultaneously to provide maximum GI stimulation, shorten recovery time, and improve hydration. As the patient progresses, frequent, small feedings of isotonic liquids and solid foods are usually recommended. Parenteral support can usually be reduced to intermittent feedings that provide supplemental fluids, electrolytes, and calories. In rare cases, parenteral support can be discontinued entirely. Nutritional assessment should be performed, if possible, prior to surgery and at appropriate intervals thereafter. Consequences of short bowel (eg, protein, vitamin, and mineral deficiency; growth failure; and dehydration) should be prevented whenever possible.

CONSIDERATIONS FOR SPECIFIC TYPES OF RESECTION

Resection Involving the Duodenum

Duodenal resections are usually associated with operative procedures involving the stomach and pancreas (eg, Billroth I and II or Whipple procedure). The duodenum is only a few inches long, and duodenal resection does not result in short-bowel syndrome. The consequences of duodenal resection depend on the number and amount of digestive and absorptive functions lost with the operative procedure. Lactose intolerance, poor tolerance to concentrated sugars, and decreased absorption of iron and calcium are typical problems.

Jejunal Resection

Jejunal resections are less common than more distal bowel resections, but this procedure may be performed to treat patients who experience trauma, adhesions, Crohn's disease, volvulus, or necrotizing enterocolitis. The length of the jejunum varies from one individual to another; it is approximately 200 to 300 cm or 40% of the small bowel. The duodenum and jejunum combined are extremely active in digestive and absorptive processes. The absorption of most minerals (especially iron, calcium, and zinc) and vitamins occurs in the upper jejunum. Only small amounts of protein and fat normally escape absorption, and about 5% to 20% of carbohydrate from a normal mixed meal remains unabsorbed by the time food enters the ileum. Like other disaccharides, lactose is normally digested and absorbed high in the jejunum. No significant degree of fiber digestion occurs, however, until fiber is subjected to bacterial fermentation in the very distal small bowel and colon.

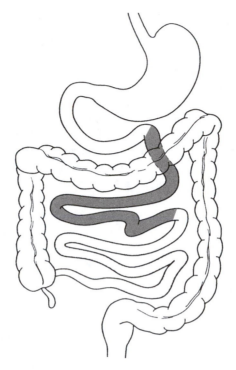

Figure 19–4 Jejunal Resection.

Under normal conditions, the ileum plays primarily a backup role in the absorption of major foodstuffs. After jejunal resection, the ileum is able to take over most of the functions of the jejunum; however, until sufficient hypertrophy and hyperplasia occur in the remaining gut, the patient may not efficiently absorb concentrated foodstuffs. After jejunal resection, large quantities of lactose and high concentrations of sugars may not be sufficiently digested or absorbed in the ileum because of rapid transit and decreased absorptive surface. Significant amounts of sugars may enter the colon, resulting in osmotic secretion of fluid; fermentation of large amounts of carbohydrate; and the classic symptoms of bloating, abdominal cramping, and diarrhea similar to that seen in dumping syndrome. If the same foods are taken in small quantities spread throughout the day, fewer problems are likely to occur. Mild fat and nitrogen malabsorption may also occur initially but improve with adaptation of the remaining gut.

Gastric hypersecretion may occur after jejunal resection, which may cause small intestine mucosal damage and compromise proximal digestive functions. Large amounts of gastric acid emptying into the duodenum may inhibit brush border and pancreatic enzymes, resulting in compromised digestive efficiency. Hypersecretion may be treated medically, and it typically becomes less of a problem after a few weeks. If the colon is intact, hyperoxaluria may occur especially with high dietary intake of oxalate. Increased absorption of oxalate is probably the result of unabsorbed free fatty acids binding with calcium, which allows dietary oxalate to be absorbed in the colon more efficiently than usual.[3,12] Moderate restriction of oxalate to approximately 100 to 300 mg per day and supplementation with 400 to 800 milligrams of calcium daily and/or high fluid intake usually prevents hyperoxaluria from occurring.

Maximal adaptation after significant jejunal resection may take several months, depending on the length of bowel resected and the nutrition therapy provided. The patient is generally advised to use a moderately low-fiber, low-lactose diet and to eat five to seven small meals. A standard multivitamin and a multimineral product is recommended. After a satisfactory recovery and adaptation period, the patient may no longer need to be as careful with diet. The long-term recommendation might be to limit large amounts of lactose, avoid extremes in simple sugar intake, and avoid foods containing significant quantities of alcohol sugars. Sorbitol, xylitol, and mannitol are alcohol sugars (as noted by the ol in the name) and are to be avoided. Prunes, pears, and certain berries are notably high in sorbitol. Apple juice, while not especially concentrated in alcohol sugars, is often consumed in large enough quantities to be associated with clinical symptoms. Because intake of several nutrients in the Western diet is already marginal, a high-quality diet is encouraged and a balanced multivitamin, multimineral supplement might be appropriate. Long-term outpatient evaluation should include a general review of nutrient intake, routine laboratory data, and weight history.

Ileal Resection

Because most digestive and absorptive functions are normally completed in the jejunum and the only unique role of the ileum is absorption of vitamin B_{12} and bile acids, some people may think that ileal resection has little consequence. However, due to the combination of more rapid transit time and the loss of the site for absorption of bile acid, vitamin B_{12}, and intrinsic factor, ileal resection can result in the nutrition-related problems discussed below.[3,4,6,9]

Normally greater than 90% of bile acids are absorbed in the terminal ileum and are recycled after a meal. With significant ileal resection, bile acid reabsorption may be greatly reduced, creating a cascade of nutrition-related problems. *De novo* hepatic synthesis of bile salts may not be sufficient to provide adequate emulsification and surfactant activity for normal fat digestion. Pancreatic lipase is less efficient due to ineffective reduction in lipid droplet size. Micelle formation occurs less readily, and net absorption of fat and fat-soluble nutrients is reduced.[21]

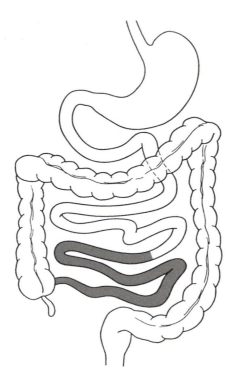

Figure 19–5 Ileal Resection.

The fraction of unabsorbed fat in stools is normally less than 7%, but in short-bowel syndrome involving complete ileal resections, malabsorbed fat may increase to greater than 30%. Unconjugated bile acids passed into the colon are potent secretagogues and can increase net luminal fluid volume and result in diarrhea. Unabsorbed fatty acids and fatty acids hydroxylated by colonic bacteria can also reduce colonic absorption of water and ions.[3,21,34] Because of more rapid transit, efficiency and capacity of digestion in the proximal gut are further reduced.

Decreased absorptive capacity may result in an excess of substrates delivered to the colon. Bacterial fermentation normally allows salvage of malabsorbed carbohydrate, fiber, and nitrogenous compounds, but the amount of substrate the colon can handle may be exceeded. Unusual loads of malabsorbed substrate—especially carbohydrate—result in gas, bloating, acidic and watery stools, and frank malabsorption.

Rapid transit of nutrients through the upper GI tract decreases absorption of most nutrients. Absorption of divalent cations (eg, calcium, iron, zinc, and magnesium) and fat-soluble vitamins is often reduced and may require long-term monitoring. In theory, if significant fatty acid malabsorption occurs, divalent cations may bind more than usual with fatty acids and leave insoluble fatty acid mineral-soaps. In short-bowel syndrome, sufficient amounts of free fatty acids may bind with calcium and other divalent cations to free dietary oxalate. Osteoporosis or osteomalacia are common consequences of long-term short-bowel syndrome, and magnesium adequacy is particularly troublesome.[9,10,36] Oxalate is normally bound to calcium and other minerals and is not as readily absorbed. Oxalate kidney stones are a significant problem in short-bowel syndrome, especially involving ileal resections.[21,35-38] If the ileocecal valve is removed in the surgery, transit time through the GI tract is shorter, malabsorption is more likely, and risk of bacterial overgrowth in the remaining small bowel is increased.

Most whole fruits and vegetables are poorly digested and generally provide little caloric value in patients with short-bowel syndrome. Foods with small amounts of finely divided fiber (eg, potato, breads, tomato-based sauces, or vegetable juices) need not be totally restricted and may actually enhance the adaptive process. Some fibers can be fermented to short-chain fatty acids and used as an energy substrate for colonocytes, and to a lesser degree, for the patient. In patients with remaining colon, production of short-chain fatty acids from small amounts of fermentable fiber may facilitate absorption of water and electrolytes.[17,27,31] If the patient is able to maintain nutritional stability with oral foods, fibrous foods may add variety to the diet. Vitamin B_{12} is absorbed only in the distal ileum and must be replaced in parenteral formulas or by injection. Normal stores are considered to be sufficient for 2 to 4 years, but some patients may not have had adequate vitamin B_{12} stores prior to surgery.

Resections of Both the Ileum and Colon

With resection of both the ileum and colon, primary problems include rapid GI transit, macro- and micronutrient malabsorption, and dehydration. Colonic "salvage" of carbohydrates is lost, and the capacity for fluids and electrolyte absorption is further reduced. Without the colon, malabsorbed fatty acids and bile acids do not produce the adverse effects on colonic mucosa; however, some of the dietary lipid is hydrolyzed to free fatty acids, which still bind with divalent cations like zinc, magnesium, and calcium. The combination of rapid transit, malabsorption of lipid, and malabsorption of fluids and electrolytes make this problem worthy of concern. Enhanced oxalate absorption, which is a problem in ileal resection with retained colon, is not a problem with resection of both the ileum and the colon.

After ileal resections of greater than 100 cm, parenteral nutrition is usually required to nourish and maintain the patient during the postsurgical weaning and adaptation process.[4,6,9] The initial diet should be provided in frequent, small feedings. Nourishment should be relatively low in fiber and based primarily on starch, animal protein, and small amounts of fats. Only small amounts of lactose

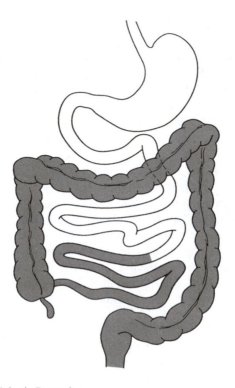

Figure 19–6 Ileal-Colonic Resection.

are likely to be tolerated. Taking a few grams of lactose with other foods usually causes little problem. Caffeinated beverages may increase net GI secretion. Hyperosmolar formulas and concentrated sugars are likely to be inefficiently absorbed and increase fluid secretion into the distal gut. If such foods are introduced in one fourth to one third of normal portion size, or taken in bits throughout the day, fewer problems are likely to be encountered.

The amount of fat tolerated depends largely on the presence of colon and length of remaining ileum. As discussed above, more generous amounts of fat are usually better tolerated by patients who have also had the colon resected. For patients with a small jejunal remnant attached to the ascending or transverse colon, normal dietary fats should be limited to 40 to 60 g. In both situations, increasing dietary fat may further decrease malabsorption of metals.

Because medium-chain triglycerides (MCTs) are readily solubilized, easily hydrolyzed, and absorbed, they can serve as a calorie source and a vehicle to enhance absorption of lipid-soluble nutrients. Special beverages and foods made with MCTs (margarines, salad dressings, etc) can make fat restriction less of a problem. Caution is advised with the use of MCTs. Typically, patients tolerate about 30 g MCT oil per day, especially when it is incorporated into foods or as part of nutrient supplements. Greater quantities, especially taken as a bolus, may cause loose stools.

MASSIVE SMALL-BOWEL RESECTION

Massive resection usually refers to procedures that leave small intestine remnants of 100 cm or less. After massive resections, long-term survival without at least supplemental total parenteral nutrition (TPN) is rare unless the ileocecal valve and/or a significant length of colon remains.[4,11,32,39] Immediately after massive resection, gastric hypersecretion occurs. The hypersecretion may last weeks to months after the initial surgery and may postpone the use of the remaining GI tract for a major route for nutrition support. The excess acid produced with hyper-

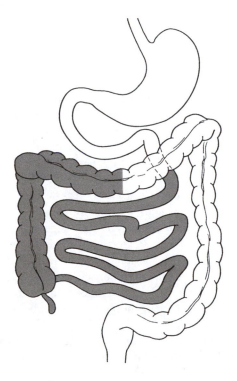

Figure 19–7 Massive Resection.

secretion decreases the effectiveness of pancreatic and remaining small-bowel enzymes and may produce peptic ulcer disease.

With massive resection, care must be taken to prevent overfeeding by oral or enteral routes before significant adaptation occurs. One of the most common reasons for dehydration and subsequent requirement for fluid and electrolyte replacement is the overconsumption or overinfusion of foods and liquids—especially if the foods are hypertonic. Consumption of normal amounts of desserts and soft drinks in some patients may result in significant fluid losses. Patients not only have to restore usual urinary and evaporative water losses but must also replace the large amount of oral and endogenous fluid lost from the remaining GI tract. Even after adaptation has occurred, the patient may not be able to maintain adequate nutrient, fluid, and electrolyte balance without at least intermittent parenteral support.

In addition to nutrition therapy, several other approaches are being evaluated for management of short-bowel syndrome including reversal of the remaining intestinal segment and intestinal lengthening, neovascularization, and transplantation. To improve adaptive responses after surgery, trophic agents such as insulin-like growth factor, recombinant human growth hormone, and interleukin-1 are being investigated.[40–44]

Some bowel resections can only be considered catastrophic. After mesenteric infarct, for example, the patient is often left with only a segment of duodenum anastomosed to the midcolon. In such extreme cases of short-bowel syndrome, patient survival depends on TPN. Adaptation sufficient to enable the patient to rely totally on enteral nutrition cannot be expected. Initially, patients usually suffer from gastric hypersecretion and, when oral feedings are attempted, patients have difficulty with fluid and electrolyte losses. The goal is to provide up to (but not greater than) one fourth to one third of the calories orally. Isotonic, low-fat, relatively low-fiber foods are likely to be the best tolerated.[27,37]

With extreme short bowel, transit rate is so rapid that large quantities of foods appear in the stool (or ostomy bag) almost as soon as they leave the stomach. Only small amounts of sugars, amino acids, and electrolytes are absorbed in the small-bowel remnant. If the colon remains, malabsorbed sugars can produce an osmotic diarrhea resulting in net fluid loss. Bacteria can ferment very small amounts of carbohydrate and fiber to short-chain fatty acids, which are readily absorbed by the colonic mucosa. In limited amounts, short-chain fatty acids may serve as fuel for the colonic flora and the colonic mucosal cells. In the intact colon, however, only about 5% to 10% of the human energy supply can be provided through colonic salvage of carbohydrates.

After massive resection, usually only enough surface area exists for digestion and absorption of small quantities of protein and carbohydrate and very little fat. Allowing patients to eat as desired often resulted in excess fluid and electrolyte losses and dehydration. Patients may at times have difficulty absorbing their own secretions in response to meals. Parenteral nutrition is usually required to meet at least half their needs for energy and almost all their needs for micronutrients.

PATIENT EDUCATION

After major surgical resection, patients may not be prepared to make the recommended changes in eating habits. They may first have to deal with the medical and surgical problems they have encountered and accept that their lives may not be normal thereafter. They may also, at least at first, be encumbered with parenteral or enteral formulas, pumps, special tests, and procedures. Before dietary counseling, functions and capacities of the remaining GI tract should be explained as clearly and objectively as possible so the rationale for nutrition therapy also becomes clear. Options for nutrition support and associated consequences should be discussed with the patient and family. Repetition, consistency, and appreciation for the patient's desire to eat "normally" are appropriate considerations in counseling.

Because food habits, tastes, and taste perceptions are slow to change, every effort should be made to guide and communicate with the patient and the patient's family. Frequent checks of the patient's (and family's) feelings and understanding should be made. The mechanics of diet and nutrition support should be outlined and, where possible, quantitative guidelines and examples (rather than just dos and don'ts) should be provided. Information should be provided in short bursts, and previous guidelines should be summarized before presenting new material.

Typically, nutrition counseling and education cannot be completed in the hospital setting. The most important concepts should be emphasized, along with a few simple examples in writing. Patients are usually ready for more information or explanations after they have been involved in activities related to shopping, meal planning, preparation, and eating in different settings. Follow-up nutrition counseling should be scheduled to allow an opportunity to review information, ask and answer question, and adjust therapies or goals as needed.

REFERENCES

1. Haymond HE. Massive resection of the small intestine. *Surg Gynecol Obstet.* 1935;61:693–705.

2. Simons BE, Jordan GL. Massive bowel resection. *Am J Surg.* 1969;118:953–959.

3. Trier JS. The short bowel syndrome. In: Sleisenger MH, Fordtran JS, eds. *Gastrointestinal Disease: Pathology, Diagnosis, Management.* 3rd ed. Philadelphia: WB Saunders Co; 1983:873–879.

4. Gouttebel MC, Saint-Aubert B, Astre C, Joueux H. Total parenteral nutrition needs in different types of short bowel syndrome. *Dig Dis Sci.* 1986;31:718–723.

5. Nightingale JM, Leannard-Jones JE. Adult patients with short bowel due to Crohn's disease often start with a short normal bowel. *Eur J Gastroenterol Hepatol.* 1995;7:989–991.

6. Weser E. The management of patients after small bowel resection. *Gastroenterology.* 1976; 71:146–150.

7. Grosfeld JL, Rescorla FJ, West K. Short bowel syndrome in infancy and childhood. *Am J Surg.* 1986;151:41–46.

8. Liefaard G, Heineman E, Molenaar JC, Tibboel D. Prospective evaluation of the capacity of the bowel after major and minor resections in the neonate. *J Pediatr Surg.* 1995;30:388–391.

9. Rombeau JL, Rolandelli RH. Enteral and parenteral nutrition in patients with enteric fistulas and short bowel syndrome. *Surg Clin North Am.* 1987;67:551–571.

10. Ladefoged K, Nicolaidou P, Jarnum S. Calcium, phosphorus, magnesium, zinc, and nitrogen balance in patients with severe short bowel syndrome. *Am J Clin Nutr.* 1980;33:2137–2144.

11. Nightengale JM. The short bowel syndrome. *Eur J Gastroenterol Hepatol.* 1995;7:514–520.

12. Vanderhoof JA. The short bowel syndrome in children. *Curr Opin Pediatr.* 1995;7:560–568.

13. Davenport HD. *Physiology of the Digestive Tract.* 5th ed. Chicago: Year Book Medical Publishers; 1984.

14. Caspary WF. Physiology and pathophysiology of intestinal absorption. *Am J Clin Nutr.* 1992;55:299S–308S.

15. Levin RJ. Digestion and absorption of carbohydrates—from molecules and membranes to humans. *Am J Clin Nutr.* 1994;59:690S–698S.

16. Rumessen JJ, Gudmand-Hoyer E. Functional bowel disease: malabsorption and abdominal distress after ingestion of fructose, sorbitol and fructose-sucrose, and fructose-sorbitol mixtures. *Gastroenterology.* 1988;95:694–700.

17. Cummings JH, Englyst HN. Fermentation in the human large intestine and the available substrates. *Am J Clin Nutr.* 1987;45:1243–1255.

18. Cummings JH, Englyst HN, Wiggins HS. The role of carbohydrates in lower gut function. *Nutr Rev.* 1986;44:50–54.

19. Grimble GK, Silk DBA. The nitrogen source of elemental diets—an unresolved issue? *Nutr Clin Pract.* 1990;5:227–230.

20. Thompson AB, Schoeller C, Keelan M, Smith L, et al. Lipid absorption: passing through the unstirred layers, brush border membrane and beyond. *Can J Physiol Pharmacol.* 1993;71:531–555.

21. Riley JW, Glickman RM. Fat malabsorption—advances in our understanding. *Am J Med.* 1979;67:980–988.

22. Cashman MD. Principles of digestive physiology for clinical nutrition. *Nutr Clin Pract.* 1986;1:241–249.

23. Carbonnel F, Cosnes J, Chevret S, et al. The role of anatomic factors in nutritional autonomy after extensive small bowel resection. *J Parenter Enter Nutr.* 1996;20:275–280.

24. Hollinshead WH, Rosse C. *Textbook of Anatomy.* 4th ed. Philadelphia: Harper & Row; 1985.

25. Roediger WEW. Metabolic basis of starvation diarrhea: implications for treatment. *Lancet.* 1986;8489:1082–1083.

26. Gracey MS. Nutrition bacteria and the gut. *Br Med Bull.* 1981;37:71–75.

27. Sacks AI, Warwick GJ, Barnard JA. Early proliferative events following intestinal resection in the rat. *J Pediatr Gastroenterol Nutr.* 1995;21:158–164.

28. Byrne TA, Persinger RL, Young LS, Zeigler TR, et al. A new treatment for patients with short-bowel syndrome. *Ann Surg.* 1995;222:243–255.

29. Hines OJ, Bilchik AJ, Whang EE, Zinner MJ, et al. Amino acids mediate postprandial proabsorption. *J Surg Res.* 1995;58:81–85.

30. Sales MG, de-Freitas O, Zucoloto S, Okano N, et al. *Am J Clin Nutr.* 1995;62:87–92.

31. Ortega MA, Nunez MC, Gil A, Sanchez-Pozo A. Dietary nucleotides accelerate intestinal recovery after food deprivation in old rats. *J Nutr.* 1995;125:1413–1418.

32. Reilly KJ, Frankel WL, Bain AM, Rombeau JL. Colonic short chain fatty acids mediate jejunal growth by increasing gastrin. *Gut.* 1995;37:81–86.

33. Levy E, Frileux P, Sandrucci S, Ollivier JM, et al. Continuous enteral nutrition during the early adaptive stages of the short bowel syndrome. *Br J Surg.* 1988;75:549–553.

34. McGuigan JE. Peptic ulcer and gastritis. In *Harrison's Principles of Internal Medicine.* 12th ed. New York: McGraw-Hill; 1991:1229–1233.

35. Papazian A, Minaire Y, Descos L, Andre C, et al. Relationship between the extent of ileal lesion of resection and vitamin B_{12}, bile salt and fat absorption. *Hepato Gastroenterol.* 1981;28:106–109.

36. Compstom JE, Horton LWI, Ayers AB, Tighe JR, et al. Osteomalacia after small intestinal resection. *Lancet.* 1978;8054:9–12.

37. Bosaeus I, Carlsson NG, Anderson H. Low-fat versus medium fat enteral diets: effects on bile salt excretion in jejunostomy patients. *Scan J Gastroenterol.* 1986;21:891–896.

38. Anderson H, Bosaeus I, Hellberg R, Hulten L. Effects of a low-fat diet and antidiarrhoeal agents on bowel habits after excisional surgery for classical Crohn's disease. *Acta Chir Scand.* 1982;149:285–290.

39. Beyer PL, Frankenfield D. Enteral nutrition in extreme short bowel. *Nutr Clin Pract.* 1987;2:60–64.

40. Panis Y, Messing B, Rivet P, Coffin B, et al. Segmental reversal of the small bowel as an alternative to intestinal transplantation in patients with short bowel syndrome. *Ann Surg.* 1997;225:401–407.

41. Figueroa CR, Harris PR, Birdsong E, Franklin FA, et al. Impact of intestinal lengthening on the nutritional outcome for children with short bowel syndrome. *J Pediatr Surg.* 1996;31:912–916.

42. Williams JK, Carlson GW, Austin GE, Austin ED, et al. Short gut syndrome: treatment by neovascularization of the small intestine. *Ann Plast Surg.* 1996;37:84–89.

43. Inaba T, Saito H, Fukushima R, Hashiguchi Y, et al. Effects of growth hormone and insulin-like growth factor 1 treatments on the nitrogen metabolism and hepatic IGF-1-messinger RNA expression in postoperative parenterally fed rats. *J Parenter Enter Nutr.* 1996;20:325–331.

44. Liu Q, Du XX, Schindel DT, Yang ZX, et al. Trophic effects of interleukin 11 in rats with experimental short bowel syndrome. *J Pediatr Surg.* 1996:1047–1050.

PART III

The Delivery of Nutrients

CHAPTER 20

Enteral Nutrition

Annalynn Skipper and Natalie B. Ratz

INTRODUCTION

Enteral feeding includes oral ingestion of solids and liquids as well as introduction of nutrients directly into the gastrointestinal tract using a feeding tube. Due to advances in equipment, formulas, and techniques, enteral feeding has steadily gained popularity over the last 20 years. More recently, growth in the numbers of enterally fed patients has been fueled by recognition that enteral feeding enhances gastrointestinal immunity[1] and is usually more economical than parenteral feeding.[2,3]

ENTERAL VERSUS PARENTERAL NUTRITION

Since Alexander's 1980 study of enteral feeding in burned children,[4] there has been interest in the effect of enteral feeding on outcome. In a subsequent study, patients receiving parenteral nutrition were found to have an increased rate of septic complications (6.4% versus 14.1%, $p = .01$) when compared to those receiving enteral feeding alone.[5] A meta-analysis of eight different studies found that patients who tolerated enteral feedings following surgery had significantly fewer total complications (38% versus 59%, $p = .007$) and fewer septic complications (17% versus 44%, $p = .0001$) than those receiving parenteral nutrition.[6]

Given a functioning gastrointestinal tract, enteral feeding has been successfully used to meet the nutrient needs of patients with cancer,[7] acquired immune deficiency syndrome,[8] liver disease,[9] respiratory failure,[10] inflammatory bowel disease,[11] trauma,[12] burns,[13] neurologic impairment,[14] or following surgery.[15] Enteral feedings have been used throughout the life cycle, including neonatal,[16] pediatric,[17] obstetric,[18] and geriatric patients.[19]

Contraindications to enteral feeding include diffuse peritonitis, intestinal obstruction, intractable vomiting, paralytic ileus, severe diarrhea, gastrointestinal ischemia, short-bowel syndrome, pancreatitis, and high-output enterocutaneous fistulae.[20]

PATIENT SELECTION

The ultimate indication for enteral feeding is a functioning gastrointestinal tract. Successful enteral feeding is dependent upon a bowel of sufficient length and condition for adequate nutrient absorption. The minimum amount of small intestine needed for absorption of enteral nutrients is approximately 100 centimeters. (There are reports of patients with less functioning bowel tolerating enteral feeding following hypertrophic treatment with growth hormone and glutamine.) Additionally, an intact ileocecal valve enhances nutrient absorption by delaying intestinal transit time. Adequate gastrointestinal motility is necessary to avoid stasis of feeding and subsequent abdominal distention or vomiting. Adequate airway protection is necessary to minimize the risk of aspiration.

ENTERAL FORMULAS

Feedings with mixtures of milk, eggs, wine, dried beef, or other substances have been mentioned in the literature since about 1600.[21] As gastrostomy and jejunostomy tubes became available at the turn of the 20th century, standardized recipes for liquid feedings were developed. Goodhart and Whol[22] recommended 2500 to 3000 cc of a diet made from homogenized milk, skim milk powder, eggs, and sucrose. With the advent of the blender, foods served on a general tray were liquified and dispensed in large-volume containers. In some institutions, recipes were developed for mixtures of different baby foods with milk, juice, and oil. These hyperosmolar, high-protein concoctions may have been a major factor in the development of tube-feeding syndrome.[23,24] In addition, these products were labor-intensive to prepare, and formulas were prone to contamination and inconsistent texture. In response to these problems, commercial blenderized diets were developed. These diets are occasionally promoted as a source of potentially undiscovered nutrients that might not be present in newer, synthetic diets. However, randomized trials have not been performed to document this potential advantage, and commercial blenderized diets are obsolete.

Development of Commercial Formulas

The first commercial enteral formula was developed for infants in the 1920s.[25] Powdered, milk-based formulas for adults were introduced in the 1950s. During the same period, experiments with formulas containing hydrolyzed protein and glucose were conducted. By 1960, a commercial, chemically defined formula diet containing a small amount of fat was available.[26] However, commercial enteral products were not widely used until isotonic enteral formulas became available in the 1970s. In the mid-1970s, crystalline amino acids were combined in modified amino acid patterns to meet the needs of patients with liver or renal failure. Since that time, the number of enteral products has grown steadily. Today, almost 100 of these products are now available (see Appendixes 20–A and 20–B for a list of enteral and modular formulas).

Enteral Formula Selection

A primary role of the clinician caring for enterally fed patients is the selection of an appropriate enteral formula. Nutrient composition, nutrient density, cost, and viscosity are important considerations in enteral formula selection.

NUTRIENT COMPOSITION

Protein

The majority of enteral formulas contain protein from soy or casein. Originally based on the protein requirements for healthy individuals, the protein content of these formulas has steadily increased. Therefore the amount of protein in enteral formulas varies widely (8% to 25%).

Formulas containing crystalline amino acids are also available. Products containing crystalline amino acids do not require enzymatic action for digestion and absorption, making them suitable for patients with documented protein malabsorption. In addition, they may be combined to form unique amino acid profiles. They have been used to develop formulas with specialized amino acid profiles for renal failure, hepatic failure, stress, and inborn errors of metabolism. Disadvantages of these products include poor patient acceptability due to their bitter taste. Also, crystalline amino acids increase the number of particles in solution when compared with whole protein, resulting in a hyperosmolar, poorly tolerated formula. Therefore, crystalline amino acids offer little advantage in enteral formulas unless specialized amino acid profiles are needed.

For over two decades it has been known that peptides are as effectively absorbed by the gut as free amino acids.[27,28] Therefore, peptide-containing products that have been hydrolyzed from casein or soy have effectively replaced the more expensive crystalline amino acid diets.

Patients with decompensated cirrhosis and hepatic encephalopathy have decreased serum levels of the branched-chain amino acids (leucine, isoleucine, and valine). They also have elevated levels of aromatic amino acids (phenylalanine, tyrosine, and tryptophan). Branched-chain amino acids are thought to inhibit aromatic amino acids from crossing the blood-brain barrier and acting as false neurotransmitters. Casein is approximately 23% branched-chain amino acids, and a higher branched-chain enteral formula (containing 35% branched-chain amino acids) was developed. This formula also contained lowered levels of aromatic amino acids.

During trauma or sepsis, branched-chain amino acids are metabolized by skeletal muscle. Therefore, formulas containing branched-chain amino acids are thought to enhance nitrogen balance in severely stressed patients. Today, these formulas typically contain approximately 45% to 50% of amino acids from branched chains.

Further modifications in the amino acid profiles of enteral protein sources have been made based on knowledge of amino acid utilization in stress. Researchers have identified glutamine as the preferred fuel for the enterocyte; this finding increased interest in glutamine-supplemented formulas. The optimum amount of glutamine is unknown, but 25% of protein from glutamine has been recommended.[29] There is presently no evidence that free glutamine is better utilized than glutamine from other sources; however, the addition of free glutamine is necessary to increase the glutamine content of enteral formulas beyond the 9% to 10% found in typical proteins.

Carbohydrate

The carbohydrate sources for enteral formulas are large molecules such as glucose oligosaccharides, dextrins, and maltodextrins, which have the advantage of decreasing osmolality. The optimum amount of carbohydrate in enteral feedings is unknown and fluctuates widely as other macronutrients are modified. Carbohydrate in enteral formulas can vary from a low of 27% to 30% in formulas designed for diabetes to a high of 76% to 91% in low-fat, monomeric formulas.

Fat

A minimum of about 15 to 25 grams of fat per day is needed for fat-soluble vitamin absorption. Another minimum for fat intake is approximately 4% to 5% of calories from linoleic acid in order to prevent essential fatty acid deficiency. Because fat is a concentrated energy source, the fat content of enteral formulas is frequently much higher than the minimum requirements. More recently, the role of lipids in hemodynamics, oxygenation, inflammation, and immunocompetence has been illuminated and the type and amount of lipids in enteral formulas have received wide attention.

Lipids are categorized based on the carbon chain length into short-chain (C2 to C4), medium-chain (C6 to C12), and long-chain (C14 to C24) fatty acids. Depending upon the location of the first double bond from the terminal methyl end of the carbon chain, the polyunsaturates may be subdivided into omega-3, omega-6, omega-7, and omega-9 fatty acids.[30]

Traditionally, high linoleic acid, polyunsaturated fat sources such as corn, safflower, sunflower, or soybean oil were used for enteral feedings. Recent revelations concerning the negative effect of linoleic acid on immunity have led to reconsideration of enteral fat sources. An increased use of linolenic acid, which is an omega-3 fatty acid, is expected as sources become more available. Fish oils have been included in several newer enteral products. However, due to high cost and poor palatability, they have not been widely accepted.

Medium-chain triglycerides are made from fractionated coconut oil and contain 8.3 kcal/g. They do not require hydrolysis by bile salts and pancreatic lipase. They are absorbed unchanged into the enterocyte and do not require carnitine for transport into the mitochondria. Although medium-chain triglycerides are a useful calorie source for patients with impaired fat absorption, they do not contain essential fatty acids. Thus, they should not be used as the sole fat source for long periods of time.

Fiber

Early commercial tube feedings were designed to be low in residue and, thus, fiber free. However, as other formula modifications failed to reduce the incidence of diarrhea, attempts were made to add fiber to commercial enteral formulas as a means of increasing stool bulk.[31] These attempts were hampered by the hydrophilic properties of fiber, which cause formula to thicken during processing and storage.

A commercial formula containing soy polysaccharide (95% insoluble and 5% soluble fiber) was first marketed in 1984. Similar formulas are now manufactured by most major enteral formula companies. Initially, these formulas were promoted as a means to reduce diarrhea, but results with formulas containing insoluble fiber have been inconclusive.[32–34] Because fiber is a necessary nutrient, it may be appropriate to use fiber containing enteral formulas for long-term tube feedings. However, the short-term advantages of formulas containing insoluble fiber are unclear.

Results with soluble fibers such as guar gum or pectin to retard diarrhea have been more promising. In a study controlled for antibiotics and other medications with gastrointestinal side effects, a significant reduction in diarrhea was noted when subjects were given 20 g (2% wt/volume) of partially hydrolyzed guar gum.[35] In another study, Zimmaro et al[36] found that pectin would reverse liquid stool in normal subjects fed a standard tube feeding. Commercial formulas containing pectin are not currently available. However, pectin has been successfully added to enteral formulas just prior to administration in amounts of 1% to 2% weight per volume.[37] Another source of pectin is banana flakes, which can be administered in a dose of 1 to 3 tablespoons every 8 hours.[38]

A promising area of research is the study of short-chain fatty acids, which are produced from soluble fiber by endogenous bacterial degradation in the colon. Acetate, propionate, and butyrate are produced in a 60:20:20 molar ratio. Their biologic functions include maintaining the integrity of the colonic epithelium, stimulating mucosal proliferation, and enhancing water and electrolyte absorption. They are avidly absorbed by the colon and are thought to be the primary fuel for the colonocyte, supplying up to 4.4 calories per gram.[39] Short-chain fatty acids infused into the colon have been found to reverse colonic fluid secretion induced by enteral feeding.[40]

Vitamins and Minerals

Most enteral formulas have extra amounts of vitamins and minerals added to allow for wound healing and stress. Many formulas also contain molybdenum, selenium, and carnitine. The amount of formula needed to meet patients' needs varies among products. Therefore, vitamin and mineral supplementation may be required for some patients using one of the liquid vitamin and mineral preparations mentioned in Chapter 5.

Nutrient Density

The nutrient density of enteral feedings is a function of the fluid content. Enteral formulas range in caloric density from 0.5 to 2.0 kcal/mL. The fluid content of these formulas is found in Appendix 20–A. Formula selection is based on calorie and fluid needs.

Osmolality

Osmolality refers to the number of osmotically active particles per kilogram of water. Attempts have been made to keep enteral formulas near 300 mOsm/kg water, which is the osmolality of human serum. Osmolarity refers to the number of osmotically active particles per liter of solution. This figure is generally lower than the osmolality, especially for more concentrated solutions. Osmolality is the more commonly used term.

Enteral feedings with an osmolality less than 200 mOsm slow gastric emptying. The effect of high-osmolality formulas on gastric emptying is unclear. Although high-osmolality formulas have been implicated in delayed gastric emptying, it has also been suggested that high-osmolality formulas play a role in dumping syndrome and the resulting diarrhea. Keohane et al[41] found no demonstrable difference in side effects when patients were given hypotonic, isotonic, or hypertonic feedings. However, to avoid controversy, many clinicians prefer to use formulas of moderate osmolality (300–450 mOsm/kg).

REGULATION OF FORMULA MANUFACTURE

The manufacture and labeling of enteral formulas is regulated by the Food and Drug Administration (FDA). These products are considered to be "medical foods"—a subcategory of foods for special dietary use. According to the FDA, medical foods that are required for special, infrequently occurring medical conditions have a defined composition that must be ensured by manufacturing methods. They are currently subject to regulation for quality control, labeling, nutrient content, formula recall, notification for new products, and exempt products.[42] Efficacy studies are required for drugs or parenteral products, but not for enteral products. Therefore, marketing claims made for specific products should be viewed in that context.

THE ENTERAL FORMULARY

Because few institutions have the resources to stock all enteral products that are available on the market, many institutions have adapted the drug formulary[43] system for enteral products. Goals of an enteral formulary are threefold: (1) to provide an appropriate choice of products to allow clinicians to effectively manage nutrition problems of the patients served; (2) to contain costs by taking advantage of volume-purchasing discounts[44]; and (3) to reduce the need for storage space.

In most institutions, the formulary is established by a group of clinicians and administrators who contribute according to their expertise. Dietitians generally coordinate the formulary process, test products for patient acceptability, and compare formulas for nutrient composition. Physicians and nurses are usually included to assist with needs assessment and to lend support to the process. Administrators may be needed to negotiate contracts with formulary companies and to advise concerning the existence of purchasing agreements within the institution or hospital system.

Usually the formulary can be limited to less than 10 products. Requests for nonformulary products may be honored, or a generic substitution policy may be developed to control costs. New products on the market can be reviewed and added as needed, while old or little-used products can be deleted.

GENERIC FORMULAS

As enteral formulas have been perfected, the market for them continues to grow. Thus, generic enteral formulas are now available. Major drug chains offer "house brands" of nutritional supplements, food manufacturers are potentially expanding into the marketplace, and generic specialty products are available at much lower prices than comparable brands. Individuals who oppose generic products suggest that reduced profit margins hinder research, development, and product innovation. Those who favor generic products believe that any type of competition improves the marketplace. In any case, it is essential that quality of generic formulas is maintained. In the future, dietitians will need to be familiar with quality-control aspects of the manufacturing process as well as the indications for product usage.

INITIATION OF ENTERAL FEEDING

Researchers believe that initiation of enteral feeding as early as possible following injury offers many advantages.[45] In trauma patients, investigators found reduced septic complications when enteral feeding was compared with 5% dextrose[15] or parenteral nutrition.[46,47] In animals, enteral nutrition has been shown to preserve gut mass[48,49] and to stimulate IgA production.[50] Early enteral feeding may attenuate the stress response to injury.[51] In surgery patients, early enteral feeding may prevent gastric or intestinal stasis. Gastric feedings may also offer stress ulcer prophylaxis by increasing gastric pH.[52]

Enteral feeding access may be obtained as soon as the patient is hemodynamically stable enough to tolerate the procedure. Because dietitians are sometimes responsible for feeding tube placement, the procedure is included in Exhibit 20–1. Generally, nasogastric, nasoenteric, or percutaneously placed tubes may be used as soon as placement is confirmed and patency is established.[53] Enteral feeding tube placement is confirmed by a variety of methods. Radiographic confirmation of tube placement is the safest method, but auscultation of the abdomen while air is injected into the feeding tube with a syringe is used when radiography is impractical. Fluoroscopic placement and direct vision are also used.

Surgically placed jejunostomy tubes may be used within 24 hours of placement. In a recent review of the topic, Minard and Kudsk[45] concluded that enteral feeding should begin within the first 48 hours after injury and possibly within 24 hours after injury. These numbers may require review in light of recent reports of enteral feedings continuing during surgery in individuals undergoing burn debridement.[54] Further studies may prove the value of continuing enteral feeding in other surgical procedures not involving the gastrointestinal tract.

Although early enteral feedings offer many advantages, caveats do exist. There is a metabolic cost to enteral feeding.[55] In critically ill patients, hemodynamic stability is a prerequisite for initiation of enteral feeding. In one study,[56] a 55% incidence of complications with feeding jejunostomies was attributed to bowel ischemia, and the authors cautioned against early initiation of enteral feeding in patients at risk for low mesenteric blood flow. Rombeau[57] suggested feeding critically ill patients if they meet the following criteria: (1) fewer than two failing

Exhibit 20–1 Procedure for Nasoduodenal Feeding Tube Placement

Contraindications

Ensure that no contraindications to feeding tube placement are present. Contraindications to nasoduodenal tube placement are:

- recent esophageal or gastric surgery
- absence of gag reflex

Equipment Needed

- small-caliber feeding tube with weighted tip
- guidewire
- water-soluble lubricant
- cup of water with straw
- stethoscope
- catheter tip syringe
- tape

Positioning

Sitting or supine

Procedure

1. Measure the tube from mouth to earlobe and down to anterior abdomen so that the tip of the tube is 6 cm below the xiphoid process. Mark this distance on the tube. This is the amount of tube that should be inserted.
2. Most tubes designed for enteral feeding are self-lubricating when moistened. If necessary, apply water-soluble lubricant liberally to the tube.
3. Ask the patient to flex his/her neck and gently insert the tube into a patent naris.
4. Advance the tube into the pharynx aiming posteriorly. Ask the patient to swallow if he/she is able to cooperate.
5. Once the tube has been swallowed, confirm that the patient can speak clearly and breathe without difficulty, and gently advance the tube to the appropriate length. If the patient is able, instruct him/her to drink water through a straw. As the patient is swallowing, gently advance the tube.
6. Confirm correct placement into the stomach by injecting approximately 20 mL of air with a catheter tip syringe while auscultating the epigastric area.
7. Remove the guidewire from the tube. Postpyloric tube passage may be aided by asking the patient to lie in the right decubitus position for 1 to 2 hours. An abdominal radiograph at this point may confirm the presence of the tip in the duodenum or that the tube is coiled in the stomach and may need to be withdrawn for some distance. The tube should not be fixed to the nose.
8. The patient should first lie in a supine position for 1 to 2 hours and then in the left decubitus position for 1 to 2 hours to facilitate passage of the tube into the duodenum.
9. At this point, position of the tube should be confirmed by chest or abdominal X-ray. If the tube has not passed beyond the stomach by this time, placement

continues

Exhibit 20–1 continued

> of the tip may be necessary through the pylorus by flexible upper endoscopy or under fluoroscopy.
> 10. Once the tube is in the duodenum, carefully tape the tube to the patient's nose ensuring that the pressure is not applied by the tube against the naris. Tape the tube out of line of the patient's vision. Use tape and a safety pin to secure the tube to the patient's gown.
>
> *Source:* Reprinted with permission from J.A. Sands, Incidence of Pulmonary Aspiration in Intubated Patients Receiving Enteral Nutrition Through Wide and Narrow Bore Nasogastric Feeding Tubes, *Heart and Lung,* vol. 20, pp. 75–80. © 1991, Mosby-Year Book, Inc.

organ systems; (2) a cardiac index of more than $2L/m^2$ with a mean arterial blood pressure of more than 70 mmHg, without the need for alpha-sympathetic stimulation; and (3) arterial oxygen saturation of more than 95% on inspired concentrations of oxygen less than 60% and with less than 5 cm of positive end-expiratory pressure. Minard and Kudsk[45] suggest correcting severe tachycardia, hypotension, and volume deficits before initiating enteral feeding. They also suggest that use of vasopressors other than renal dose dopamine is a relative contraindication to enteral feeding. In head-injured patients, poor tolerance of enteral feeding has been documented due to inhibited gastric motility associated with increased intracranial pressure.[58] These criteria remain largely untested and, no doubt, exceptions exist. Therefore, careful patient selection based on sound clinical judgment and clear, consistent communication with the medical team is appropriate to enhance the success of early enteral feeding.

FORMULA ADMINISTRATION

Once the decision is made to implement enteral feeding, the method of formula administration is considered. Several methods for feeding have been used. *Bolus feedings* involve the rapid administration of 250 to 500 mL of formula several times daily. A syringe is used to inject feedings into the feeding tube. *Intermittent feedings* are also administered several times daily, but over at least a half hour. Gravity may be used to allow formula to flow slowly into the feeding tube, or a pump may be used to control the flow rate. *Continuous feedings* are administered over 10 to 24 hours daily.[59] They may be administered by gravity, but a pump is most often used. Continuous feedings with a pump are usually preferred in institutional settings. Other methods may be used in outpatient settings.

Several research studies have attempted to determine the superiority of one feeding method over another. Bolus feedings lower esophageal sphincter pressure to incompetent levels,[60] which documents the potential for increased aspiration risk with bolus feeding. Based on these findings, bolus feedings should be avoided unless the patient is able to recognize and communicate that aspiration is occurring.

In another study, no difference was found in the incidence of aspiration when continuous and intermittent feedings were compared.[61] It seems that continuous feedings are used more efficiently[62] and enable quicker achievement of the caloric goal.[63] Feedings over 16 hours rather than 24 hours may result in more rapid protein repletion[64] and lowered energy expenditure, but neither method seems to impact nutrient absorption.[65] Continuous administration of nutrients is usually recommended for intestinal feedings but, when patient convenience or reimbursement practices dictate, gastric feedings may be given using continuous or intermittent methods.

Once the method of feeding is established, the initial rate and feeding concentration is determined. Formerly, elaborate regimens for initiating feedings were recommended. One group of investigators[66] found significant nutrient deficits as a result of using these "starter regimens." Several prospective trials have shown that polymeric and monomeric formulas may be initiated full strength at rates of 50 to 87 mL/hr[66-68] with no disadvantages in tolerance. Others have reported successful initiation of full-strength monomeric feedings in critically ill, elderly, hypoalbuminemic patients.[69] One practice that has worked well is to initiate full-strength formula at 20 to 40 mL per hour. Increases of 10 to 20 mL per hour may be made several times daily if the formula is tolerated. The progression is continued until the goal is reached. Borlase et al[69] suggested a slower initial rate (10 mL/hr) but a quicker progression (a 10 mL increase per 8 hours) for their intensive care unit patients. This protocol has merit, but it may be difficult to implement unless feeding tolerance can be assessed and the rate of feeding increased on each nursing shift.

The maximum rate for enteral feeding is dependent on the condition of the gastrointestinal tract. In normal individuals, tolerance of enteral feeding at rates up to 720 mL per hour without adverse effects has been noted.[70] With patients, however, a more conservative approach may be needed. Recently, Riachi and colleagues suggested that enteral formulas could be administered at rates up to 2.1 kcal per minute without complaint.[71] At least one study suggested that administration of more than 2 kcal per minute may inhibit biliopancreatic secretions.[72] For critically ill, mechanically ventilated patients, decreased duodenal motor tolerance has been reported, and a more conservative approach may be needed in this patient population.[73]

MONITORING

Monitoring enteral feedings consists of regular attention to nutritional status, fluid status, and gastrointestinal tolerance. In addition, monitoring should include regular assessment of the presence or absence of complications. Monitoring parameters vary according to patient acuity, duration of feeding, and institutional practice. If electrolyte changes are necessary, then daily monitoring may be needed until the patient is stable. For critically ill patients, daily monitoring is usually required. In nutritionally stable patients who are receiving goal formula, monitoring may occur weekly or as indicated. For patients who are discharged home or to long-term care, the complexity and frequency of nutrition monitoring may be decreased but never discontinued entirely. A suggested protocol for monitoring each of these patient groups is presented in Table 20–1.

Nutritional Status

Nutrition monitoring begins with a comparison of nutrient intake to nutrient requirements. During the first few days of enteral feedings, nutrient intake may be less than optimal because of formula progression or poor tolerance. Later, patient activities or medical treatment may also interfere with feeding. Compensatory increases in the enteral feeding prescription may be required to meet caloric goals.

Laboratory monitoring of patients receiving enteral feeding is based on underlying disease state, organ function, and duration of feeding. Appropriate use of laboratory monitoring is discussed in Chapter 1, as well as in the chapters on specific disease states.

Fluid Status

In stable patients, serum levels of sodium, blood urea nitrogen, hemoglobin, and albumin are indicators of fluid status. Generally hemoconcentration indicates

---

Table 20–1 Suggested Monitoring of Enteral Feedings

Parameter	Critically Ill Patients or Feeding Initiation	Nutritionally Stable Patients
Albumin	Weekly	Weekly
Prealbumin	Weekly	Weekly
Electrolytes, BUN, creatinine	Daily, then 3 × week	3 × week
Magnesium, phosphorus, calcium	Daily, then 3 × week	Weekly
Liver function tests	1–2 × week	Weekly
Nitrogen balance	1–2 × week	Weekly
Weight	Daily	1–2 × week
Intake and output	Daily	Daily
Bowel function	Daily	Daily
Urine or blood glucose	2 × daily	Monthly

underhydration and hemodilution indicates overhydration. For critically ill patients, hydration may be monitored using data from thermodilution catheters. For hospitalized patients, fluid intake and output should be recorded daily while enteral feeding continues. Fluid intake should exceed output (including losses from wound exudate, fistulas, and drains) by an amount adequate to cover insensible losses (eg, lungs, skin). For long-term patients, clinical signs of hydration—including skin turgor, presence of axillary sweat, condition of the mucous membranes, and presence or absence of edema—provide insight into fluid status. While critically ill patients are usually overhydrated, stable patients more often suffer from underhydration.

The water content of tube feedings is a part of the total fluid intake. Adjustments in water intake may involve changing intravenous fluids, the concentration of the enteral feeding, or the amount of water given to flush the feeding tube.

Gastrointestinal Tolerance

During the initial stage of tube feeding, the presence of bowel sounds, nausea, distention, and vomiting are assessed daily. Stool frequency and consistency are also assessed on a daily basis. For gastric feedings, particularly during the initial period, gastric residuals are measured several times daily. Because elevated residuals indicate delayed gastric emptying and potentially increased risk for aspiration, feedings are advanced only when gastric residuals are within acceptable limits (150 to 200 mL).[74]

As soft, small-bore feeding tubes tend to collapse on withdrawal of fluid using a syringe, measurement of residuals cannot be accomplished if tubes less than 10-French are used.[75] Residuals are not anticipated with intestinal feedings where there is no place for feedings to collect. They are unnecessary in stable, alert patients whose tolerance to feedings is well established.

COMPLICATIONS OF ENTERAL FEEDING

The safety, economy, and simplicity of enteral feeding are widely touted. However, enteral feeding may result in significant complications in untrained hands or in the absence of appropriate monitoring. The complexities of gastrointestinal tolerance superimposed on intercurrent fluid, electrolyte, hormonal, nutritional, and disease processes often render enteral nutrition more challenging to manage than parenteral nutrition.

Clogged Tubes

Nutrient delivery is impeded by a clogged tube; therefore, ongoing monitoring of tube patency is appropriate to ensure optimal nutrient intake. Most feeding pumps have occlusion alarms, which automate this process. For gravity feedings, administering the tap water flush before the feeding and observing how well it flows through the tube provides an assessment of tube patency.

Factors that may affect the incidence of clogged tubes are tube size and material, administration of medications through the tube, and formula viscosity. In one study, silicone tubes were found to clog less often than polyurethane ones.[76] In other studies, tubes clogged more often when continuous feedings were given[61] and when gastric residuals were aspirated.[77] Tube feedings coagulate with decreased pH. Therefore, exposure to gastric acid with gastric tube placement may increase the incidence of clogged tubes. Marcuard et al[78] reported a significantly higher incidence of clogged nasogastric than nasointestinal tubes.

Increased formula viscosity has been proposed as a cause of clogged tubes. Therefore, larger lumen tubes have been suggested for concentrated, blenderized, or fiber-containing formulas. However, Collier and colleagues[79] found that fiber-containing formulas could successfully be administered through a 5-French needle catheter jejunostomy with strict adherence to a protocol that included flushing the tube every 6 hours with water (10 mL normal saline) and avoiding administration of medications through the tube.

Probably the most frequent cause of clogging is medications administered via the feeding tube. For patients who are able to swallow, oral administration of medications is ideal. The incidence of clogged tubes is minimized by flushing the tube once every 6 to 8 hours and after every interruption of the feeding.

If patency is compromised, it may usually be restored by instilling warm water, capping the tube, allowing a few minutes to pass, and then instilling air into the tube via a syringe. Flushing the tube with cranberry juice is often recommended, but this practice has been shown to increase the incidence of clogged tubes when compared to flushing tubes with distilled water.[80] Viokase®, Pancrease®, Pancreatin®, papain, bromelain, chymotrypsin, meat tenderizer, and cola or other carbonated beverages have been suggested as tube-declogging agents, but comparisons have also shown that these fluids have little advantage over distilled water.[76,81]

A 72% success rate with unclogging feeding tubes has been found using the following procedure. Remove liquid formula proximal to the tube obstruction with a syringe. Irrigate with water. If the feeding tube is not clear, prepare a solution by crushing one Viokase tablet with one sodium bicarbonate tablet and diluting it in 5 mL of water. Inject it into the catheter. Clamp the tube and wait 5 minutes. Irrigate the tube with 50 mL of tap water.[82]

Despite design innovations, the potential exists for a stylet to perforate the gastrointestinal tract if reinserted into the feeding tube. Therefore, this practice should never be considered as a means to restore patency to a clogged tube. Another potential danger exists when small syringes are used to irrigate tubes. Syringes with a volume less than 20 mL can generate enough pressure to rupture small-bore tubes. Therefore, irrigation of the tube with larger syringes is recommended.

Aspiration

Pharyngeal aspiration has been documented in 45% of normal, sleeping adults and in 70% of patients with a depressed level of consciousness,[83] but pulmonary infections in these individuals are rare. However, aspiration of bacteria-laden fluids into the lower respiratory tract may result in pneumonia. Mortality rates of 17% to 62% have been reported for patients who develop aspiration pneumonia.[84] For patients receiving enteral feedings, the reported incidence of aspiration ranges from 0.8% to 95%.[85,86] Because aspiration pneumonia is a potentially lethal complication of tube feeding, significant attention should be paid to its prevention.

An active gag reflex or a strong reflexive cough act as barriers to pulmonary aspiration of gastrointestinal contents. However, many candidates for enteral feeding do not have an intact gag reflex. Gag reflex may be disrupted after stroke, head injury, or other neurologic impairment. Head and/or neck surgery may damage gag reflex, leaving the patient with a permanently indefensible airway. Mechanical ventilation disrupts the cough and gag reflex as well. Patients with a depressed level of consciousness may not recognize aspiration when it happens and fail to clear secretions from the lung.

Enteral feeding may be a predisposing factor to aspiration as the presence of a feeding tube probably compromises the lower esophageal sphincter. For example, a review of 720 autopsies revealed that the presence of a nasogastric tube was associated with a sixfold increase in pulmonary aspiration.[87] In a prospective study of 70 patients who were orotracheally intubated, Ibanez and colleagues[88] found over twice the incidence of gastrointestinal reflux in patients with a nasogastric tube compared to patients without one. In a retrospective review of patients with percutaneous gastrostomy tubes or nasogastric tubes, the incidence of aspiration was significantly greater in patients with nasogastric tubes (6% versus 24%, $p = 0.09$).[88] Mittal and others[89] demonstrated that a tube in the pharynx was associated with more frequent spontaneous relaxation of lower esophageal pressure, again suggesting that the presence of the tube predisposes to aspiration.

Traditionally, small-bore feeding tubes have been suggested as a means to reduce the risk of aspiration. However, two small studies of this topic do not support this idea. Sands[90,91] found no difference in the incidence of aspiration when patients received feedings via small-bore, soft feeding tubes (10-French or less) versus larger, stiff feeding tubes. Another study of 11 subjects found no difference in aspiration rates between those fed with an 8-French tube and a 14-French tube.[92]

Another popular suggestion to avoid aspiration of enteral feedings is to use postpyloric feedings, which are thought to be less likely to reflux into the airway. However, reflux of duodenally administered solutions into the stomach has been demonstrated[93] as has tube migration into the stomach following confirmation of transpyloric placement.[94] While one study noted a lowered incidence of pneumonia in critically ill patients receiving jejunal versus gastric feedings,[95] Kocan and

Hickisch[96] reported greater aspiration rates from gastrostomy (6.5%) and jejunostomy (5.6%) than from nasoenteric (3.8%) tubes. In a recent report, Strong et al[97] found equal aspiration rates in patients fed intragastrically and postpylorically. This finding was borne out by the prospective study of Coben et al,[60] who found no significant difference in lower esophageal sphincter pressure between patients who had percutaneous gastrostomy tubes and those who had no feeding tubes. Thus, the practice of postpyloric feeding, while theoretically attractive, does not eliminate the need for other precautions against aspiration.

Protocols to prevent aspiration include (1) confirmation of feeding tube placement radiographically or with pH measurements prior to initiating feeding; (2) monitoring gastrointestinal residual volume; and (3) elevating the head of the bed 30 to 45 degrees during and 30 to 60 minutes after feeding.[98] Use of intermittent or continuous rather than bolus feedings, and jejunal access for those with persistent aspiration of tube feedings has also been suggested.[99]

Monitoring for aspiration may be enhanced by adding methylene blue dye (1 mL/500 mL) to feeding. This popular practice enables detection of pulmonary aspiration of enteral formula upon observation of pulmonary secretions. Monitoring the glucose content of tracheobronchical secretions has also been suggested as a means to detect aspiration.[100] However, because tracheobronchial secretions normally contain glucose, this practice is probably not a valid indicator of aspiration.[101]

Diarrhea

Despite innovative formula and delivery system modifications, diarrhea remains the primary gastrointestinal complication of enteral feeding. The reported incidence of tube-feeding diarrhea varies from 2.3% to 68%.[75,85] The wide variation in the reported incidence of diarrhea points to the fact that there is no clear definition of the term. One standard gastroenterology text states that diarrhea is an abnormal looseness of stool with increased liquidity or decreased consistency and output in excess of 235 g/day.[102] However, a variety of definitions of diarrhea have been used for study purposes.[103] Ongoing confusion on this issue is highlighted by the work of Benya et al[104]; these investigators documented a 43% incidence of diarrhea subjectively reported by patients and nurses, while none of the patients had stool in excess of 250 g/day.

The most frequent assumption is that diarrhea in enterally fed patients is related to enteral feeding. However, diarrhea is also a well-known side effect of many commonly used antibiotics and has been associated with administration of hyperosmolar medications via the feeding tube. Diarrhea has also been attributed to malnutrition,[105] hypoalbuminemia,[106] cimetidine,[107] and magnesium-containing antacids.[108] Sorbitol added to medications has been implicated as a cause of diarrhea; however, identification of these medications is complicated by the fact that sorbitol may not be listed on the drug label.[109] It has also been suggested that large volumes of tube-feeding formula contain cathartic doses of magnesium.[110]

Diarrhea and Method of Formula Administration

The method of tube-feeding administration has been cited as a causative factor in tube-feeding diarrhea. Jones et al have suggested continuous feedings using pumps to reduce the incidence of diarrhea.[111] However, two studies did not document significant difference in diarrheal incidence between patients receiving continuous feedings and patients receiving intermittent feedings.[96,112]

Initiation of formula at a diluted concentration and slow rate has been recommended to reduce the incidence of diarrhea. However, full-strength monomeric and elemental diets with osmolality up to 630 mmol/L can be initiated at rates greater than 80 mL/hr without adverse effects[65,66] in patients with normal bowel function, inflammatory bowel disease, or short-bowel syndrome.

Diarrhea and Formula Composition

Tube-feeding diarrhea has been attributed to various formula components. Because lactose intolerance is found in a large number of adults, lactose-containing feedings were initially identified as a cause of diarrhea.[113] As a result, the majority of commercial enteral formulas are now lactose-free and, thus, of moderate osmolality. In other countries, milk-based formulas are still used, and controlled trials of hyperosmolar formulas containing lactose have shown acceptable tolerance.[65,66,68]

While fiber is a necessary nutrient, formulas containing soy polysaccharide have not been shown to reduce the incidence of diarrhea significantly in enterally fed patients.[32,114] Results of formulas with the soluble fibers pectin and guar gum have been more encouraging, but enteral feedings that contain soluble fiber are not commercially available.

Diarrhea and Hypoalbuminemia

Because diarrhea has been observed near the end of life in those dying of starvation,[115] hypoalbuminemia has been proposed as a cause of diarrhea in enterally fed patients. However, in a retrospective review, Patterson et al[116] found no difference in the incidence of diarrhea between hypoalbuminemic and normoalbuminemic patients. In a study of 68 patients, Pesola et al[117,118] observed that intensive care unit patients who developed diarrhea had slightly higher mean serum albumin levels than did those without diarrhea. Benya et al[119] found no difference in nutrient absorption in normo- and hypoalbuminemic patients. Borlase et al[69] successfully fed hypoalbuminemic patients with full-strength feedings given at a slow initial rate. Thus, hypoalbuminemia is probably not a factor in tube-feeding tolerance.

Management of Diarrhea

Management of tube-feeding diarrhea is often not coordinated with concurrent manipulation of the enteral formula and medications. Patients' understandable impatience with symptoms frequently leads to cessation of the tube feeding before treatment is given time to work. While formula modifications (such as decreasing the strength of the feeding or changing to an elemental or peptide diet) are often suggested as a means of managing diarrhea, they rarely solve the problem. A more effective approach is to review the medical record for temporal relationships between initiation of tube feeding and the onset of diarrhea, as well as to review the medication profile for the presence of prokinetic agents, laxatives, magnesium- or sorbitol-containing medications, or drugs such as antibiotics and chemotherapeutic agents known to cause diarrhea. Occasionally tube malposition is identified as a cause of diarrhea.

If an obvious cause of diarrhea is not identified, the tube feeding may be held for 24 hours, and the presence of diarrhea noted. If diarrhea continues, a workup is indicated.[120] Edes et al[109] suggested the following diarrhea workup: (1) perform digital rectal examination for impacted stool; (2) in the absence of impaction, obtain stool guaiac and determine fecal leucocytes, sodium, potassium, and osmolality; (3) calculate stool osmotic gap (stool osmolality − 2 [stool sodium-stool potassium]); (4) osmotic diarrhea is suggested by osmotic gap greater than 100 mmol/L; (5) where indicated, stool and parasites. *C. difficile,* ova, and assayed for may be cultured.

Control of diarrhea has been obtained with a variety of medications. Opium, paregoric, codeine, and the synthetic antidiarrheals diphenoxylate hydrochloride with atropine sulfate (Lomotil) and loperamide hydrochloride (Imodium) increase smooth muscle tone, subsequently slowing gastrointestinal motility. These drugs are contraindicated in hepatic encephalopathy, where diarrhea is desired to prevent retention of nitrogenous wastes; in the presence of *C. difficile,* where diarrhea is desired to prevent accumulation of toxins; and in the presence of ulcerative colitis, where decreased intestinal motility may result in toxic megacolon. The opiates, as well as Lomotil, may cause somnolence, which can mask changes in central nervous system function. Therefore, another antidiarrheal medication is often selected for neurologically impaired patients. In tube-fed patients whose diarrhea is associated with extensive small-bowel resection or diabetes mellitus, cholestyramine has been used successfully to retard diarrhea.[121]

Infection

Tube-feeding formulas are an excellent medium for bacterial growth. Contaminated feedings may present significant risk for immunocompromised patients. This risk is compounded in patients whose gastric pH is increased as the result of H_2 receptor antagonists[122] or patients who are receiving hypomotility agents.[123]

Commercial enteral formulas are sterile until opened, but there are many opportunities for contamination to occur once the original package is penetrated. Traditional enteral feeding involves emptying canned or reconstituted formula into containers and administering the feeding using a pump. Touch contamination may occur at many different points during this process. In addition, prolonged exposure to room temperature during storage, transportation or administration, and reuse of containers or administration sets may offer opportunities for contamination.

Contaminated enteral feedings have been identified as a source of infection in hospitalized patients.[124,125] It has been reported in enteral formulas requiring reconstitution or manipulation[126-128] as well as in a closed system.[129,130] Formula preparation under a laminar flow hood has been used to reduce the incidence of bacterial contamination,[131] but this option may not be practical. Therefore, many institutions avoid formulas that require reconstitution.

Another option to reduce the potential for contamination is to limit formula hang time and change bags and tubing frequently. As enteral feeding containers are kept at room temperature, the question of how long to hang them arises. The optimum hang time has not been defined, and many hospitals change bags and tubing every 24 hours. Although changing enteral feeding bags and tubing every 48 hours would reduce costs, one study found unacceptable levels of contamination in enteral feedings exposed to room temperature for 48 hours.[132]

Based on the attractive theory that reduced container manipulation may lessen the potential for contamination, prepackaged, closed-system feedings have been developed.[133] In a study using a closed delivery system and a peptide diet, Wagner et al[134] found significantly less bacterial growth when the closed system ($p <$ 0.001) was compared with canned formula emptied into bags or with formula mixed from powder. In a simulated study in a nursing home, Dentinger et al[135] found safe levels of bacteria in prefilled 1500-mL containers hung at room temperature for 36 hours. As retrograde contamination has been reported,[129,136] closed systems do not eliminate concerns about bacterial contamination.

In addition, there are concerns about the ability to modify formulas in closed systems with additives. More than 40% more waste was reported for a closed system when compared with a traditional system.[134] While bacterial contamination of formula should be avoided, the increased costs of closed-system feedings may make them prohibitively expensive.

CONCLUSIONS

The formulas, equipment, and protocols for administration of tube feeding have improved substantially over the last two decades. Intensive research into enteral feeding methods has provided a scientific basis for enteral feeding practice. Further research into enteral formulas is needed as the effect of nutrients on the disease process is elucidated. Increased regulation of enteral formulas is anticipated as efficacy studies are needed to support product claims. New tests of gastrointestinal function will improve practitioners' ability to identify appropriate candidates for enteral feeding, and improved tolerance will result.

REFERENCES

1. Alverdy JC, Chi HS, Sheldon GF. The effect of parenteral nutrition on gastrointestinal immunity: the importance of enteral stimulation. *Ann Surg.* 1985;202:681–684.

2. Schwartz DB. Enhanced enteral and parenteral nutrition practice and outcomes in an intensive care unit with a hospital-wide performance improvement process. *J Am Diet Assoc.* 1996;96:484–489.

3. Szeluga DJ, Stuart RK, Brookmeyer R, Utermohlen V, et al. Nutritional support of bone marrow transplant recipients: a prospective, randomized clinical trial comparing total parenteral nutrition to an enteral feeding program. *Cancer Res.* 1987;47:3309–3316.

4. Alexander JW, McMillan BG, Stinnett JD, Osle CK, et al. Beneficial effects of aggressive protein feeding in severely burned children. *Ann Surg.* 1980;192:505–517.

5. The Veterans Affairs Total Parenteral Nutrition Cooperative Study Group. Perioperative total parenteral nutrition in surgical patients. *N Engl J Med.* 1991;325:525–532.

6. Moore FA, Feliciano DV, Andrassy RJ. Early enteral feeding, compared with parenteral, reduces postoperative septic complications: the result of a meta-analysis. *Ann Surg.* 1992;216:172–183.

7. Burt ME, Gorschboth CM, Brennan MF. A controlled, prospective, randomized trial evaluating the metabolic effects of enteral and parenteral nutrition in the cancer patient. *Cancer.* 1982;49:1092–1105.

8. Kotler D, Tierney A, Ferraro R, Cuff P, et al. Effect of enteral alimentation and repletion of body cell mass in malnourished patients with acquired immunodeficiency syndrome. *Am J Clin Nutr.* 1991;3:149–154.

9. Kearnes PJ, Young H, Garcia G, Blaschke T, et al. Accelerated improvement of alcoholic liver disease with enteral nutrition. *Gastroenterology.* 1992;102:200–205.

10. Mowatt-Larson CA, Brown RO. Specialized nutritional support in respiratory disease. *Clin Pharm.* 1993;12:276–292.

11. Giaffer MH, North G, Holdsworth CD. Controlled trial of polymeric versus elemental diet in the treatment of active Crohn's disease. *Lancet.* 1990;335:816–819.

12. Kudsk KA, Minard G, Croce MA, Brown RO, et al. A randomized trial of isonitrogenous enteral diets after severe trauma. An immune enhancing diet reduces septic complications. *Ann Surg.* 1996;224:531–540.

13. Gottschlich MM, Jenkins M, Warden GD, Baumer T, et al. Differential effects of three enteral dietary regimens on selected outcome variables in burn patients. *J Parenter Enter Nutr.* 1990;14:225–236.

14. Kirby DF, Clifton GL, Turner H, Marion DW, et al. Early enteral nutrition after brain injury by percutaneous endoscopic gastrojejunostomy. *J Parenter Enter Nutr.* 1991;15:298–302.

15. Moore EE, Jones TN. Benefits of immediate jejunostomy feeding after major abdominal trauma—a prospective, randomized study. *J Trauma.* 1986;26:874–881.

16. Macdonald DD, Skesch CH, Carse H, Dryburgh F, et al. Randomized trial of continuous nasogastric, bolus nasogastric, and transpyloric feeding in infants of birth weight under 1400 grams. *Arch Dis Child.* 1992;67:429–431.

17. Chellis MJ, Sanders SV, Webster H, Dean JM, et al. Early enteral feeding in the pediatric intensive care unit. *J Parenter Enter Nutr.* 1996;1:71–73.

18. Barclay BA. Experience with enteral nutrition in the treatment of hyperemesis gravidarum. *Nutr Clin Pract.* 1990:5:153–155.

19. Ciocon JO, Silverstone PA, Graver LM, Foley CJ, et al. Tube feeding in elderly patients: indications, benefits and complications. *Arch Intern Med.* 1988;148:429–433.

20. ASPEN Board of Directors. Guidelines for the use of parenteral and enteral nutrition in adult and pediatric patients. *J Parenter Enter Nutr.* 1993;17:1SA–51SA.

21. Randall HT. Enteral nutrition: tube feeding in acute and chronic illness. *J Parenter Enter Nutr.* 1984;8:113–136.

22. Goodhart RS, Whol MG. *Modern Nutrition in Health and Disease.* Philadelphia: Lea & Febiger; 1964:22.

23. Gault MH, Dixon ME, Doyle M, Cohen WM, et al. Hypernatremia, azotemia, and dehydration due to high-protein tube feeding. *Ann Intern Med.* 1968;68:778–791.

24. Telfer N, Persoff M. The effect of tube feeding on the hydration of elderly patients. *J Gerontol.* 1965;20:536–543.

25. Anderson SA, Chginn MI, Fisher KD. History and current status of infant formulas. *Am J Clin Nutr.* 1982;35:381–397.

26. Greenstein JP, Otey MC, Birnbaum SM, Winitz M, et al. Quantitative nutritional studies with water soluble, chemically defined diets. X: Formulation of a nutritionally complete liquid diet. *J Nat Cancer Inst.* 1960;24:211–219.

27. Adibi SA. Intestinal transport of dipeptides in man: relative importance of hydrolysis and intact absorption. *J Clin Invest.* 1971;50:2266–2275.

28. Silk DBA, Fairclough PD, Clark ML, Hegarty JE, et al. Use of a peptide rather than free amino acid nitrogen source in chemically defined "elemental" diets. *J Parenter Enter Nutr.* 1980;4:548–553.

29. Smith RJ, Wilmore DW. Glutamine nutrition and requirements. *J Parenter Enter Nutr.* 1990;14:94S–99S.

30. Gottschlich MM. Selection of optimal lipid sources in enteral and parenteral nutrition. *Nutr Clin Pract.* 1992;7:152–165.

31. Frank HA, Green LC. Successful use of a bulk laxative to control the diarrhea of tube feeding. *Scand J Plast Reconstr Surg.* 1979;13:193–194.

32. Dobb GJ, Towler SC. Diarrhea during enteral feeding in the critically ill: a comparison of feeds with and without fibre. *Intensive Care Med.* 1990;16:252–255.

33. Frankenfield DC, Beyer PL. Dietary fiber and bowel function in tube fed patients. *J Am Diet Assoc.* 1991;91:590–596.

34. Hart GK, Dobb GJ. Effect of a fecal bulking agent on diarrhea during enteral feeding in the critically ill. *J Parenter Enter Nutr.* 1988;12:465–468.

35. Homann HH, Kemen M, Fussenich C, Senkal M, et al. Reduction in diarrhea incidence by soluble fiber in patients receiving total or supplemental enteral nutrition. *J Parenter Enter Nutr.* 1994;18:486–490.

36. Zimmaro DM, Rolandelli RH, Koruda MJ, Settle RG, et al. Isotonic tube feeding formula induces liquid stool in normal subjects: reversal by pectin. *J Parenter Enter Nutr.* 1989;13:117–123.

37. Sinkler S, Reitmeier CA, Mills L. Addition of pectin and temperature influence the viscosity of some tube-feeding formulas. *J Am Diet Assoc.* 1994;94:85–86.

38. Emery EA, Ahmad S, Koethe JD, Skipper A, et al. Low dose pectin from banana flakes controls diarrhea in patients on enteral feeding. *Nutr Clin Pract.* 1997;12:72–75.

39. Campos ACL, Meguid MM. Short-chain fatty acids: present prospect—future alternative? *J Parenter Enter Nutr.* 1988;12:98S–101S.

40. Bowling TE, Raimundo AH, Grimble GK, Silk DBA. Reversal by short-chain fatty acids of colonic fluid secretion induced by enteral feeding. *Lancet.* 1993;342:1266–1268.

41. Keohane PP, Attrill H, Love M, Frost P, et al. Relation between osmolality of diet and gastrointestinal side effects in enteral nutrition. *Br J Med.* 1984;288:678–680.

42. Mueller C, Nestle M. Regulation of medical foods: toward a rational policy. *Nutr Clin Pract.* 1995;10:8–15.

43. American Society of Hospital Pharmacists. ASHP guidelines on formulary system management. *Am J Hosp Pharm.* 1992;49:648–652.

44. Durfee DD, Skinner-Domen VM. Cost effectiveness of an enteral products formulary. *Am J Hosp Pharm.* 1984;41:2352–2354.

45. Minard G, Kudsk KA. Is early feeding beneficial? How early is early. *New Horiz.* 1994;2:156–163.

46. Moore FA, Moore EE, Jones TN, McCroskey BL. TEN vs TPN following major abdominal trauma—reduced septic morbidity. *J Trauma.* 1989;29:916–923.

47. Kudsk KA, Croce MA, Fabian TC, Minord G, et al. Enteral vs. parenteral feeding: effects on septic morbidity following blunt and penetrating trauma. *Ann Surg.* 1992;215:503–513.

48. Kudsk KA, Stone JM, Carpenter G, Sheldon GF. Effects of enteral and parenteral feeding of malnourished rats on body composition. *J Trauma.* 1982;22:904–906.

49. Popp MB, Wagner SC. Nearly identical oral and intravenous nutritional support in the rat: effects on growth and body composition. *Am J Clin Nutr.* 1984;40:107–115.

50. Burk DJ, Alverdy JC, Aoys E, Moss GS. Glutamine supplemented rats total parenteral nutrition improves gut immune function. *Arch Surg.* 1989;124:1396–1399.

51. Jenkins M, Gottschlich M, Alexander JW, Warden GD. Effect of immediate enteral feeding on the hypermetabolic response following severe burn injury. *J Parenter Enter Nutr.* 1989;13:12S.

52. Solem LD, Strae RG, Fischer RP. Antacid therapy and nutritional supplementation in the prevention of Curling's ulcers. *Surg Gynecol Obstet.* 1979;148:367–370.

53. Starkey JF, Jefferson PA, Kirby DF. Taking care of percutaneous endoscopic gastrostomy. *Am J Nurs.* 1988;88:42–45.

54. Jenkins ME, Gottschlich MM, Warden GD. Enteral feeding during operative procedures in thermal injuries. *J Burn Care Rehab.* 1994;15:199–205.

55. Heymsfield SB, Erbland M, Casper K, Grossman G, et al. Enteral nutritional support: metabolic, cardiovascular, and pulmonary interrelations. *Clin Chest Med.* 1986;7:41–67.

56. Smith-Choban P, Max MH. Feeding jejunostomy: a small bowel stress test? *Am J Surg.* 1988;155:112–117.

57. Rombeau JL. Enteral nutrition in critical illness. In: Borlase BC, Blackburn GL, Forse RA, eds. *Enteral Nutrition.* New York: Chapman & Hall; 1994:25–36.

58. Norton JA, Ott LG, McClain CJ, Adams L, et al. Intolerance to enteral feeding in the brain injured patient. *J Neurosurg.* 1988;68:62–66.

59. Heymsfield SB, Erbland M, Casper K, Grossman G, et al. Enteral nutritional support: metabolic, cardiovascular, and pulmonary interrelations. *Clin Chest Med.* 1986;7:41–67.

60. Coben RM, Weintraub A, DiMarino AJ, Cohen S. Gastroesophageal reflux during gastrostomy feeding. *Gastroenterology.* 1994;106:13–18.

61. Ciocon JO, Galindo-Ciocon DJ, Tiessen C. Continuous compared with intermittent tube feeding in the elderly. *J Parenter Enter Nutr.* 1992;16:525–528.

62. Heymsfield SB, Casper C, Grossman GD. Bioenergetic and metabolic response to continuous versus intermittent feeding. *Metabolism.* 1987;36:570–575.

63. Heibert JM, Brown A, Anderson RG, Halfacre S, et al. Comparison of continuous versus intermittent tube feedings in adult burn patients. *J Parenter Enter Nutr.* 1981;5:73–75.

64. Pinchofsky-Devin GD, Kaminski MV. Visceral protein increase associated with interrupted versus continuous enteral hyperalimentation. *J Parenter Enter Nutr.* 1985;18:333–337.

65. Keohane PP, Attrill H, Love M, Frost P, et al. Relation between osmolality of diet and gastrointestinal side effects in enteral nutrition. *Br Med J.* 1984;288:678–680.

66. Rees RGP, Keohane PP, Grimble GK, Frost PG, et al. Tolerance of elemental diet administered without starter regimen. *Br Med J.* 1985;290:1869–1870.

67. Rees RGP, Keohane PP, Grimble GK, Frost PG, et al. Elemental diet administered nasogastrically without starter regimens to patients with inflammatory bowel disease. *J Parenter Enter Nutr.* 1986;10:258–262.

68. Nyulasi IB, Metz G. Methods of introducing nasoenteric feeding. *Med J Australia.* 1984;141:496–498.

69. Borlase BC, Bell SJ, Lewis EJ, Swails W, et al. Tolerance to enteral feeding diets in hypoalbuminemic critically ill geriatric patients: a prospective randomized trial. *Surg Gynecol Obstet.* 1992;174:181–183.

70. Zarling EJ, Parmar JR, Mobrahan S, Clapper BS. Effects of enteral formula infusion rate, osmolality, and chemical composition upon clinical tolerance and carbohydrate absorption in normal subjects. *J Parenter Enter Nutr.* 1986;11:588–590.

71. Riachi G, Ducrotte P, Guedon C, Bouteloup C, et al. Duodenojejunal motility after oral and enteral nutrition in humans: a comparative study. *J Parenter Enter Nutr.* 1996;20:150–155.

72. Vidon N, Sogni P, Chaussade S, et al. Gastrointestinal and biliopancreatic response to continuous nasogastric feeding in man: effect of increasing nutrient infusion rate. *Clin Nutr.* 1994;13:307–313.

73. Dive A, Miesse C, Jamart J, et al. Duodenal motor response to continuous enteral feeding is impaired in mechanically ventilated critically ill patients. *Clin Nutr.* 1994;13:302–306.

74. McClave SA, Snider HL, Lowen CC, McLaughlin AJ, et al. Use of residual volume as a marker for enteral feeding intolerance: prospective blinded comparison with physical examination and radiographic findings. *J Parenter Enter Nutr.* 1992;16:99–105.

75. Kelly TWJ, Patrick MR, Hillman KM. Study of diarrhea in critically ill patients. *Crit Care Med.* 1983;11:7–9.

76. Metheny N, Eisenberg P, McSweeney M. Effect of feeding tube properties and three irrigants on clogging rates. *Nurs Res.* 1988;37:165–169.

77. Powell KS, Marcuard SP, Farrior ES, Gallagher ML. Aspirating gastric residuals causes occlusion of small-bore feeding tubes. *J Parenter Enter Nutr.* 1993;17:243–246.

78. Marcuard SP, Stegall KL, Trogdon S. Clearing obstructed feeding tubes. *J Parenter Enter Nutr.* 1989;13:81–83.

79. Collier P, Kudsk K, Glezer J, Brown RO. Fiber containing formula and needle catheter jejunostomies: a clinical evaluation. *Nutr Clin Pract.* 1994;8:101–103.

80. Wilson M, Haynes-Johnson V. Cranberry juice or water? a comparison of feeding tube irrigants. *Nutr Supp Serv.* 1987;7:23–24.

81. Nicholson LJ. Declogging small-bore feeding tubes. *J Parenter Enter Nutr.* 1987;11:594–597.

82. Marcuard SP, Stegall KS. Unclogging feeding tubes with pancreatic enzyme. *J Parenter Enter Nutr.* 1990;14:198–200.

83. Huxley EJ, Viroslav J, Gray WR, Pierce AK. Pharyngeal aspiration in normal adults and patients with depressed consciousness. *Am J Med.* 1978;64:564–568.

84. Cameron JL, Mitchell WH, Zuidema GD. Aspiration pneumonia: clinical outcome following documented aspiration. *Arch Surg.* 173;16:160–164.

85. Cataldi-Betcher EL, Seltzer MH, Slocum BA, Jones KW. Complications occurring during enteral nutrition support: a prospective study. *J Parenter Enter Nutr.* 1983;7:546–552.

86. Winterbauer RH, Durning RB, Barron E, McFadden MC. Aspirated nasogastric feeding solution detected by glucose strips. *Ann Intern Med.* 1986;95:647–688.

87. Olivares L, Segovia A, Revuelta R. Tube feeding and lethal aspiration in neurological patients: a review of 720 autopsy cases. *Stroke.* 1974;5:654–657.

88. Ibanez J, Penafiel A, Raurich JM, Marse P, et al. Gastroesophageal reflux in intubated patients receiving enteral nutrition: effect of supine and semirecumbent positions. *J Parenter Enter Nutr.* 1992;16:419–422.

89. Mittal RK, Stewart WR, Schimmer BD. Effect of a catheter in the pharynx on the frequency of transient lower esophageal sphincter relaxations. *Gastroenterology.* 1992;103:1236–1240.

90. Sands JA. Incidence of pulmonary aspiration in intubated patients receiving enteral nutrition through wide- and narrow-bore nasogastric feeding tubes. *Heart Lung.* 1991;20:75–80.

91. Sands JA. Letter to the editor. *Heart Lung.* 1991;20:427.

92. Dotson RG, Robinson RG, Pingleton SK. Gastroesophageal reflux with nasogastric tubes: effect of nasogastric tube size. *Am J Resp Crit Care Med.* 1994;149:1659–1662.

93. Gustke RF, Vara RR, Soergel KH. Gastric reflux during perfusion of the proximal small bowel. *Gastroenterology.* 1970;59:890–895.

94. Treolar DM, Stechmiller J. Pulmonary aspiration in tube-fed patients with artificial airways. *Heart Lung.* 1984;13:667–671.

95. Montecalvo MA, Steger KA, Faber HSW, Smith BF, et al. Nutritional outcome and pneumonia in critical care patients randomized to gastric versus jejunal feedings. *Crit Care Med.* 1992;20:1377–1387.

96. Kocan MJ, Hickisch SM. A comparison of continuous and intermittent enteral nutrition in NICU patients. *J Neurosci Nurs.* 1986;18:333–337.

97. Strong RM, Condon SC, Solinger MR, Namihas N, et al. Equal aspiration rates from postpyloric and intragastric-placed small-bore nasoenteric feeding tubes: a randomized, prospective study. *J Parenter Enter Nutr.* 1992;16:59–63.

98. Metheny N. Minimizing respiratory complications of nasoenteric tube feedings: state of the science. *Heart Lung.* 1993;22:213–223.

99. American Gastroenterological Association technical review on tube feeding for enteral nutrition. *Gastroenterology.* 1995;108:1282–1301.

100. Kinsey GC, Murray MJ, Swensen SJ, Miles JM. Glucose content of tracheal aspirates: implications for the detection of tube feeding aspiration. *Crit Care Med.* 1994;22:1557–1562.

101. Elpern E. Pulmonary aspiration in hospitalized adults. *Nutr Clin Pract.* 1997;12:5–13.

102. Fine RD, Krejs GJ, Fordtran JS. Diarrhea. In: Schlesinger MH, Fordtran JS, eds. *Gastrointestinal Disease: Pathophysiology, Diagnosis and Management.* Philadelphia: WB Saunders Co; 1993:1043–1072.

103. Bliss DZ, Guenter PA, Settle RG. Defining and reporting diarrhea in tube-fed patients—what a mess! *Am J Clin Nutr.* 1992;55:753–759.

104. Benya R, Layden TJ, Mobrahan S. Diarrhea associated with tube feeding: the importance of using objective criteria. *J Clin Gastroenterol.* 1991;13:167–172.

105. Roediger WE. The metabolic basis of starvation: implications for treatment. *Lancet.* 1986;1:1082–1084.

106. Brinson RR, Kolts BE. Hypoalbuminemia as an indicator of diarrheal disease in the critically ill patient. *Crit Care Med.* 1987;15:506–509.

107. Guenter PA, Settle R, Perlmutter S, Marino PL, et al. Tube feeding-related diarrhea in acutely ill patients. *J Parenter Enter Nutr.* 1991;15:277–280.

108. Kohn CL, Keithley JK. Techniques for evaluating and managing diarrhea in the tube-fed patient. *Nutr Clin Pract.* 1987;2:250–257.

109. Edes TE, Walk BE, Austin JL. Diarrhea in tube-fed patients: feeding formula not necessarily the cause. *Am J Med.* 1990;88:91–93.

110. Kandil HE, Opper FH, Switzer BR, Heizer WD. Marked resistance of normal subjects to tube feeding-induced diarrhea: the role of magnesium. *Am J Clin Nutr.* 1993;57:73–80.

111. Jones BJM, Payne S, Silk DBA. Indications for pump-assisted enteral feeding. *Lancet.* 1980;1:1057–1058.

112. Taylor TT. A comparison of two methods of nasogastric tube feedings. *J Neurosurg Nurs.* 1982;14:49–55.

113. Walike BC, Walike JW. Relative lactose intolerance: a clinical study of tube-fed patients. *JAMA.* 1977;238:948–951.

114. Frankenfield DC, Beyer PL. Soy-polysaccharide effect on diarrhea in tube-fed, head-injured patients. *Am J Clin Nutr.* 1989;50:533–558.

115. Anonymous. Hunger disease. Reprinted in *Nutrition.* 1994;10:365–380.

116. Patterson ML, Dominguez JM, Lyman B, Cuddy PG, et al. Enteral feeding in the hypoalbuminemic patient. *J Parenter Enter Nutr.* 1990;14:362–365.

117. Pesola GE, Hogg JE, Yonnios T, McConnell RE, et al. Isotonic nasogastric tube feedings: do they cause diarrhea? *Crit Care Med.* 1989;17:1151–1155.

118. Pesola GR, Hogg JE, Eissa N, Matthews DE, et al. Hypertonic nasogastric tube feedings: do they cause diarrhea? *Crit Care Med.* 1990;18:1378–1382.

119. Benya R, Zarling EJ, Monteagudo J, Mobarhan S. Protein and carbohydrate absorptive efficiency of chronically malnourished and well nourished patients during enteral feeding initiation. *J Am Coll Nutr.* 1991;10:50–56.

120. Heimburger DC. Diarrhea with enteral feeding: will the real cause please stand up? *Am J Med.* 1990;88:89–90.

121. Pietrusko RG. Drug therapy reviews: pharmacotherapy of diarrhea. *Am J Hosp Pharm.* 1979;36:757–767.

122. Garvey BM, McCambley JA, Tuxen DV. Effects of gastric alkalinization on bacterial colonization in critically ill patients. *Crit Care Med.* 1989;17:211–216.

123. Vantrappen G, Janssens J, Hellemans J, Ghoos Y. The interdigestive motor complex of normal subjects and patients with bacterial overgrowth of the small intestine. *J Clin Invest.* 1977;59:1158–1166.

124. Casewell MW, Cooper JE, Webster M. Enteral feeds contaminated with *Enterobacter cloacae* as a cause of septicemia. *Br J Med.* 1981;282:973.

125. Keighley MRB, Mogg B, Bentley S, Allen C. "Home Brew" compared with commercial preparation for enteral feeding. *Br J Med.* 1982;248:163.

126. Anderson KR, Norris DJ, Godfrey LB, Avent CK, et al. Bacterial contamination of tube feeding formulas. *J Parenter Enter Nutr.* 1984;8:673–678.

127. Fagerman KE. Limiting bacterial contamination of enteral nutrient solutions: 6-year history with reduction of contamination at two institutions. *Nutr Clin Pract.* 1992;7:31–36.

128. Thurn J, Crossley K, Gerdts A, Maki M, et al. Enteral hyperalimentation as a source of nosocomial infection. *J Hosp Infect.* 1990;15:203–217.

129. Donius MA. Contamination of a prefilled ready-to-use enteral feeding system compared with a refillable bag. *J Parenter Enter Nutr.* 1993;17:461–464.

130. Schreiner RL, Eitzen H, Gfell MA, Kress S, et al. Environmental contamination of continuous drip feedings. *Pediatrics.* 1979;63:232–237.

131. White WT, Acuff TE, Sykes TR, et al. Bacterial contamination of enteral nutrient solution: a preliminary report. *J Parenter Enter Nutr.* 1979;3:459–461.

132. Kohn CL. The relationship between enteral formula contamination and length of enteral delivery set usage. *J Parenter Enter Nutr.* 1991;15:567–571.

133. Vaughn LA, Manore M, Winston D. Bacterial safety of a closed administration system for enteral nutrition solutions. *J Am Diet Assoc.* 1988;88:35–38.

134. Wagner DR, Elmore MF, Knoll DM. Evaluation of "closed" vs "open" systems for the delivery of peptide-based enteral diets. *J Parenter Enter Nutr.* 1994;18:453–457.

135. Dentinger B, Faucher KJ, Ostrom SM, Schmidl MK. Controlling bacterial contamination of an enteral formula through the use of a unique closed system: contamination, enteral formulas, closed system. *Nutrition.* 1995;11:747–750.

136. Payne-James JJ, Rana SK, Bray MJ, McSwiggan DA, et al. Retrograde (ascending) bacterial contamination of enteral diet administration systems. *J Parenter Enter Nutr.* 1992;16:369–373.

Appendix 20–A

Enteral Formulas

Formula	kcal/cc	Carbohydrate Source	CHO g/L (% kcal)	Protein Source	PRO g/L (% kcal)	Fat Source	Fat (% kcal)	Fiber Source	Fiber g/L	Volume to Meet RDA	% Water	mOsm/ kg	Comments	Manufacturer
0.5–0.9 kcal/mL														
Ensure High Protein	0.94	Sucrose, Maltodextrine	128.3 (54.7)	Sodium & calcium caseinates, Soy protein isolate	50 (21.3)	Safflower oil, Canola oil, Soy oil	25 (24)			1000 cc	84.7	610		R
Entrition 0.5	0.5	Maltodextrine	68 (54.5)	Sodium & calcium caseinates	17.5 (14)	Corn oil, Soy lecithin	17.5 (31.5)			4000 cc	92.6	120	Closed system only	N
Introlite	0.53	Hydrolyzed cornstarch	70.5 (53.3)	Sodium & calcium caseinates, Soy protein isolate	22.2 (16.7)	MCT oil, Corn oil	18.4 (30)			1321 cc	92	220		R
1.0–1.4 kcal/mL														
Ensure	1.06	Corn syrup, Maltodextrine, Sucrose	169 (63.9)	Sodium & calcium caseinates, Soy protein isolate, Whey protein concentrate	37.2 (14.1)	Safflower oil, Canola oil, Corn oil	25.8 (22)			1887 cc	84.5	555		R
Entrition HN	1	Maltodextrin	114 (45.6)	Sodium & calcium caseinates, Soy protein isolate	44 (17.6)	Corn oil, Soy lecithin	41 (36.8)			1300 cc	84	300	Closed system only	N
Isocal	1.06	Maltodextrin	135 (50)	Sodium & calcium caseinates, Soy protein isolate	34 (13)	Soy oil, MCT oil	44 (37)			1890 cc	84	270		MJ
Isocal HN	1.06	Maltodextrin	123 (46)	Sodium & calcium caseinates, Soy protein isolate	44 (17)	Soy oil, MCT oil	45 (37)			1180 cc	84	270		MJ
Isosource HN	1.2	Hydrolyzed cornstarch	160 (52)	Sodium & calcium caseinates, Soy protein isolate	53 (18)	MCT oil, Canola oil	41 (30)			1500 cc	81.9	330		No

Product		Carbohydrate source		Protein source		Fat source		Fiber source		Volume	%	mOsm	Comments	
Isosource Standard	1.2	Hydrolyzed cornstarch	170 (56)	Sodium & calcium caseinates, Soy protein isolate	43 (14)	MCT oil, Canola oil	41 (30)			1500 cc	81.9	360		No
Isosource VHN	1	Hydrolyzed cornstarch	130 (50)	Sodium & calcium caseinates	62 (25)	MCT oil, Canola oil	29 (25)	Soy fiber, Guar gum	10	1250 cc	84.7	300		No
Nutren 1.0	1	Maltodextrin, Corn syrup solids	127 (51)	Calcium-potassium caseinate	40 (16)	Canola oil, MCT oil, Corn oil, Soy lecithin	38 (33)			1500 cc	85.2	300		N
Osmolite	1.06	Maltodextrin	151.1 (57)	Sodium & calcium caseinates, Soy protein isolate	37.1 (14)	Safflower oil, Canola oil, MCT oil	34.7 (29)			1887 cc	84.1	300		R
Osmolite HN	1.06	Maltodextrin	143.9 (54.3)	Sodium & calcium caseinates, Soy protein isolate	44.3 (16.7)	Safflower oil, Canola oil, MCT oil	34.7 (29)			1321 cc	84.2	300		R
Osmolite HN Plus	1.2	Maltodextrin	157.5 (52.5)	Sodium & calcium caseinates	55.5 (18.5)	Safflower oil, Canola oil, MCT oil	39.3 (29)			1000 cc	82	360		R
Perative	1.3	Maltodextrin	177.2 (54.5)	Sodium caseinate, Lactalbumin hydrolysate, L-arginine	66.6 (20.5)	Canola oil, MCT oil, Corn oil	37.4 (20.5)			1155 cc	78.9	385		R
ProBalance	1.2	Maltodextrin	156 (52)	Calcium-potassium caseinate	54 (18)	Canola oil, MCT oil, Corn oil, Soy lecithin	40.6 (30)	Soy poly-saccharides, Gum arabic	10	1000 cc	81.9	450	Geriatric formula	N
Promote	1	Hydrolyzed cornstarch, Sucrose	130 (52)	Sodium & calcium caseinates, Soy protein isolate	62.5 (25)	Safflower oil, Canola oil, MCT oil	26 (23)			1250 cc	83.7	340		R
Replete	1	Maltodextrin, Corn syrup solids	113 (45)	Calcium-potassium caseinate	62.5 (25)	Canola oil, MCT oil, Soy lecithin	34 (30)			1000 cc	84.4	350		N

continues

Formula	kcal/cc	Carbohydrate Source	CHO g/L (% kcal)	Protein Source	PRO g/L (% kcal)	Fat Source	Fat (% kcal)	Fiber Source	Fiber g/L	Volume to Meet RDA	% Water	mOsm/ kg	Comments	Manufacturer
Sustacal Liquid	1.01	Sugar, Corn syrup	139 (55)	Sodium & calcium caseinates, Soy protein isolate	61 (24)	Soy oil	23 (21)			1060 cc	85	650		MJ
Sustacal Basic	1.06	Corn syrup, Sucrose	148 (56)	Casein, Soy protein isolate	37 (14)	Soy oil	35 (30)			1890 cc	85	500		MJ
1.5–2.0 kcal/mL														
Comply	1.5	Maltodextrin	180 (48)	Sodium & calcium caseinates	60 (16)	Canola oil, Sunflower oil, MCT oil, Corn oil	61 (36)			830 cc	77	440		MJ
Deliver 2.0	2	Corn syrup	200 (40)	Sodium & calcium caseinates	75 (15)	Soy oil, MCT oil	102 (45)			1000 cc	71	640		MJ
Ensure Plus	1.5	Corn syrup, Maltodextrin, Sucrose	200 (53.3)	Sodium & calcium caseinates, Soy protein isolate	54.9 (14.7)	Corn oil	53.3 (32)			1420 cc	76.9	690		R
Ensure Plus HN	1.5	Maltodextrin, Sucrose	199.9 (53.3)	Sodium & calcium caseinates, Soy protein isolate	62.6 (16.7)	Corn oil	50 (30)			974 cc	76.9	650		R
Impact 1.5	1.5	Hydrolyzed cornstarch	140 (38)	Sodium & calcium caseinates, L-arginine	80 (22)	MCT oil, Palm kernel oil, Sunflower oil, Menhaden oil	69 (40)			1250 cc	78	550		No
Isosource 1.5 Cal	1.5	Hydrolyzed cornstarch, Sugar, Soy fiber, Guar gum	170 (44)	Sodium & calcium caseinates	68 (18)	Canola oil, MCT oil, Soybeam oil	65 (38)			933 cc	77.8	650		No

Product														
Nutren 1.5	1.5	Maltodextrin	169.2 (45)	Calcium-potassium caseinate	60 (16)	MCT oil, Canola oil, Corn oil, Soy lecithin	67.6 (39)			1000 cc	77.6	430		Ne
Nutren 2.0	2	Corn syrup, Maltodextrin, Sucrose	196 (39)	Calcium-potassium caseinate	80 (16)	MCT oil, Canola oil, Corn oil, Soy lecithin	106 (45)			750 cc	70	720		Ne
Sustacal Plus	1.52	Corn syrup solids, Sugar	190 (50)	Sodium & calcium caseinates	61 (16)	Corn oil	57 (34)			1180 cc	78	630		MJ
Two Cal HN	2	Maltodextrin, Sucrose	217.3 (43.2)	Sodium & calcium caseinates	83.7 (16.7)	Corn oil, MCT oil	90.9 (40.1)			947 cc	71.2	690		R
Fiber														
Ensure with Fiber	1.1	Maltodextrin, Sucrose	162 (55)	Sodium & calcium caseinates, Soy protein isolate		Corn oil	37.2 (30.5)	Soy fiber	14.4	1420 cc	82.9	480		R
Fibersource	1.2	Hydrolyzed cornstarch	170 (56)	Sodium & calcium caseinates	43 (14)	MCT oil, Canola oil	41 (30)	Soy fiber	10	1500 cc	82.3	390		No
Fibersource HN	1.2	Hydrolyzed cornstarch	160 (52)	Sodium & calcium caseinates	53 (18)	MCT oil, Canola oil	41 (30)	Soy fiber	6.8	1500 cc	82.1	390		No
Impact with Fiber	1	Hydrolyzed cornstarch	140 (53)	Sodium & calcium caseinates, L-arginine	56 (22)	Palm kernel oil, Sunflower oil, Menhaden oil	28 (25)	Soy fiber, Guar gum	10	1500 cc	86.8	375		No
Jevity	1.06	Maltodextrin, Corn syrup	154.4 (54.3)	Sodium & calcium caseinates	44.3 (16.7)	Safflower oil, Canola oil, MCT oil	34.7 (29)	Soy fiber	14.4	1321 cc	83.5	300		R

continues

Formula	kcal/cc	Carbohydrate Source	CHO g/L (% kcal)	Protein Source	PRO g/L (% kcal)	Fat Source	Fat (% kcal)	Fiber Source	Fiber g/L	Volume to Meet RDA	% Water	mOsm/ kg	Comments	Manufacturer
Jevity Plus	1.2	Corn syrup, Maltodextrin, Fructooligo-saccharides	174.6 (52.5)	Sodium & calcium caseinates	55.5 (18.5)	Safflower oil, Canola oil, MCT oil, Soy lecithin	39.3 (29)	Oat fiber, soy fiber, Gum arabic	12	1000 cc	81	450		R
Nutren 1.0 with Fiber	1	Maltodextrin, Corn syrup solids	127 (51)	Calcium-potassium caseinate	40 (16)	Canola oil, MCT oil, Corn oil, Soy lecithin	38 (33)	Soy poly-saccharides	14	1500 cc	84	310		Ne
Promote with Fiber	1	Hydrolyzed cornstarch, Sucrose	139.4 (50)	Sodium & calcium caseinates	62.5 (25)	Safflower oil, Canola oil, MCT oil	28.2 (25)	Oat fiber, soy fiber	14.4	1000 cc	83	370		R
Replete with Fiber	1	Maltodextrin, Corn syrup solids	113 (45)	Calcium-potassium caseinate	62.5 (25)	Canola oil, MCT oil, Soy lecithin	34 (30)	Soy poly-saccharides	14	1000 cc	83.6	390		Ne
Sustacal with Fiber	1.06	Maltodextrin, Sugar	139 (53)	Sodium & calcium caseinates, Soy protein isolate	46 (17)	Corn oil	35 (30)	Soy fiber, Carrageenan	10.6	1420 cc	85	480		MJ
Ultracal	1.06	Maltodextrin	123 (46)	Sodium & calcium caseinates	44 (17)	Canola oil, MCT oil	45 (37)	Oat fiber, Soy fiber, Carrageenan	14.4	1180 cc	85	310		MJ
Elemental/ Hydrolyzed Protein														
Alitraq	1	D malto-dextrin, Sucrose, Fructose	165 (66)	Soy hydrolysate, Whey protein concentrate, Lactal-bumin hydrolysate free amino acids	52.5 (21)	MCT oil, Safflower oil	15.5 (13)			1500 cc	84.6	575	Supplemental glutamine	R

											MJ
Criticare HN	1.06	Maltodextrin, Modified cornstarch	220 (81.5)	Hydrolyzed casein, Amino acids	38 (14)	Safflower oil, Emulsifiers	5.3 (4.5)	1890 cc	83	650		
Crucial	1.5	Maltodextrin, Cornstarch	33.75 (36)	Hydrolyzed casein, L-arginine	23.5 (25)	MCT oil, Fish oil, Soy oil, Soy lecithin	16.9 (39)	1500 cc	76.8	490		Ne
L-Emental	1	Maltodextrin	205.6 (82.2)	Free amino acids	38.2 (15.3)	Safflower oil	2.8 (2.5)	2000 cc	85.3	630		NM
L-Emental Plus	1	Maltodextrin	190 (76)	Free amino acids	45 (18)	Soybean oil	6.7 (6)	1800 cc	83.3	650		NM
Peptamen	1	Maltodextrin, Cornstarch	127 (51)	Hydrolyzed whey protein	40 (16)	MCT oil, Sunflower oil, Soy lecithin	39 (33)	1500 cc	85	270		Ne
Peptamen VHP	1	Maltodextrin, Cornstarch, Guar gum	104.5 (42)	Hydrolyzed whey protein	62.5 (25)	MCT oil, Soybean oil, Soy lecithin	39 (33)	1500 cc	84.1	300		Ne
Pro-Peptide	1	Maltodextrin, Starch	127.2 (51)	Hydrolyzed whey protein	40 (16)	MCT oil, Sunflower oil	39.2 (33)	1500 cc	88	270	Peptide-based	NM
Pro-Peptide Vanilla	1	Maltodextrin, Starch	127.2 (51)	Hydrolyzed whey protein	40 (16)	MCT oil, Sunflower oil	39.2 (33)	1500 cc	88	380	Peptide-based	NM
Pro-Peptide VHN	1	Maltodextrin, Starch	104.4 (42)	Hydrolyzed whey protein	62.4 (25)	MCT oil, Soybean oil, Soy lecithin	39.2 (33)	1500 cc	84.4	300	Peptide-based	NM
Reabilan	1	Maltodextrin, Tapioca starch	131.5 (52.5)	Casein peptides, Whey peptides	31.5 (12.5)	MCT oil, Soy oil, Canola oil, Soy lecithin	40.5 (35)	2000 cc	85	350	Small peptide formula	Ne
Reabilan HN	1.33	Maltodextrin, Tapioca starch	158 (47.5)	Casein peptides, Whey peptides	58.2 (17.5)	MCT oil, Soy oil, Canola oil, Soy lecithin	54 (35)	1500 cc	81	490	Small peptide formula	Ne

continues

Formula	kcal/cc	Carbohydrate Source	CHO g/L (% kcal)	Protein Source	PRO g/L (% kcal)	Fat Source	Fat (% kcal)	Fiber Source	Fiber g/L	Volume to Meet RDA	% Water	mOsm/ kg	Comments	Manufacturer
SandoSource Peptide	1	Hydrolyzed cornstarch	160 (65)	Casein hydrolysate, Free amino acids	50 (20)	MCT oil, Soybean oil, Hydroxylated lecithin	17 (15)			1750 cc	84	490		No
Travasorb HN	1	Glucose oligo-saccharides	175 (70)	Hydrolyzed lactalbumin	45 (18)	MCT oil, Sunflower oil	13.5 (12)			2000 cc	85.5	560		Ne
Travasorb MCT	1	Corn syrup solids	122.8 (50)	Lactalbumin, Sodium & potassium caseinates	49.6 (20)	MCT oil, Sunflower oil	33 (30)			2000 cc	86.3	250		Ne
Travasorb STD	1	Glucose oligo-saccharides	190 (76)	Lactalbumin	30 (12)	MCT oil, Sunflower oil	13.5 (12)			2000 cc	85.5	560		Ne
Tolerex	1	Maltodextrin	230 (91)	Free amino acids	21 (8)	Safflower oil	1.5 (1)			3160 cc	86.4	550		S
Vital High Nitrogen	1	Hydrolyzed cornstarch, Sucrose	185 (73.9)	Partially hydrolyzed Whey, Meant, & Soy	41.7 (16.7)	Safflower oil, MCT oil	10.8 (9.4)			1500 cc	86.7	500		R
Vivonex Plus	1	Maltodextrin, Modified starch	190 (76)	Free amino acids	45 (18)	Soybean oil	6.7 (6)			1800 cc	85	650		No
Vivonex T.E.N.	1	Maltodextrin, Modified starch	210 (82)	Free amino acids	38 (15)	Safflower oil	2.8 (3)			2000 cc	85.3	630		No
Disease Specific														
Advera	1.28	Maltodextrin, Sucrose	215.8 (65.5)	Soy protein hydrolsate, Sodium caseinate	60 (18.7)	Canola oil, MCT oil	22.8 (15.8)	Soy fiber		1184 cc	80.2		HIV/AIDS formula	R
Choice dm	1.06	Maltodextrin, Sugar	106 (40)	Milk protein concentrate	45 (17)	Vegetable oil, Soy lecithin	51 (43)	Microcrystalline cellulose, Soy fiber	14.4	1000 cc	85		Glucose intolerance	MJ

Product	kcal/mL	Carbohydrate source	Protein (g)	Protein source	Fat (g)	Fat source	Fiber	Free water	Volume	% water	mOsm	Indication	Notes
DiabetiSource	1	Maltodextrin, Fructose, Vegetables, Fruits	90 (36)	Calcium caseinate, Beef	50 (20)	Sunflower oil, Canola oil, Beef	49 (44)		4.4	1500 cc	84.9	360	Glucose intolerance	No
Glucerna	1	Maltodextrin, Fructose	95.8 (34.3)	Sodium & calcium caseinate	41.8 (16.7)	Safflower oil, Canola oil, Soy lecithin	54.4 (49)	Soy fiber	15	1422 cc	85.3	355	Glucose intolerance	R
Glytrol	1	Maltodextrin, Modified cornstarch, Fructose	100 (40)	Calcium-potassium caseinates	45 (18)	Canola oil, Safflower oil, MCT oil	47.5 (42)	Gum arabic, Soy poly-saccharides, Pectin	15	1400 cc	85.5	380	Glucose intolerance	Ne
Hepatic-Aid II	1.2	Maltodextrin, Sugar	57.3 (57.3)	Amino acids	15 (15)	Soybean oil, Lecithin, Mono- & di-glycerides	12.3 (27.7)				82.4	560	Hepatic formula	McG
Immun-Aid	1	Maltodextrin	120 (48)	Lactalbumin, Free amino acids	37 (32)	Canola oil, MCT oil, Soy lecithin	22 (20)			2000 cc	82	460	Immuno-compromised	McG
Impact	1	Hydrolyzed cornstarch	130 (53)	Sodium & calcium caseinates, L-arginine	56 (22)	Palm kernel oil, Sunflower oil, Menhaden oil	28 (25)			1500 cc	85.5	375		No
L-Emental Hepatic	1.2	Maltodextrin, Sugars	168.5 (57.3)	Free amino acids	44.1 (15)	Soybean oil, Lecithin, Mono- & di-glycerides	36.2 (27.7)					560	Hepatic formula	NM
Lipisorb Liquid	1.35	Corn syrup solids, Sucrose	161 (48)	Sodium caseinate	57 (17)	MCT oil, Corn oil	57 (35)			1180 cc	80	630	AIDS/Fat malabsorption	NM

continues

Formula	kcal/cc	Carbohydrate Source	CHO g/L (% kcal)	Protein Source	PRO g/L (% kcal)	Fat Source	Fat (% kcal)	Fiber Source	Fiber g/L	Volume to Meet RDA	% Water	mOsm/ kg	Comments	Manufacturer
Lipisorb Powder	1	Corn syrup solids, Sucrose	117 (46)	Sodium caseinate	35 (14)	MCT oil, Corn oil	47.9 (40)			2000 cc	83.3	320	AIDS/Fat malabsorption	NM
Magnacal Renal	2	Maltodextrin, Sugar	200 (40)	Calcium & sodium caseinate	75 (15)	Canola oil, Sunflower oil, MCT oil, Corn oil, Soy lecithin	101 (45)			1000 cc	71	570	Dialysis	NM
Nepro	2	Corn syrup	215.2 (43)	Calcium, magnesium & sodium caseinates	69.9 (14)	Safflower oil, Soy oil, Soy lecithin	95.6 (43)			947 cc	70.3	635	Renal failure	R
NutriHep	1.5	Maltodextrin, Modified cornstarch	290 (77)	Crystalline L-amino acids, Whey protein concentrate	40 (11)	MCT oil, Canola oil	21.2 (12)			1000 cc	76	690	Hepatic formula	Ne
NutriVent	1.5	Maltodextrin	100 (27)	Calcium-potassium caseinate	67.5 (18)	Canola oil, MCT oil, Corn oil, Soy lecithin	94 (55)			1000 cc	78.1	450	Pulmonary formula	Ne
Portagen	0.676	Corn syrup solids, Sucrose	76.7 (46)	Sodium caseinate	23.3 (14)	MCT oil, Corn oil	32 (40)				89.4	230		MJ
Protain XL	1	Maltodextrin	129 (52)	Sodium & calcium caseinates	57 (22)	Sunflower oil, MCT oil, Corn oil	30 (27)	Soy fiber	8	1250 cc	83	340		MJ
Pulmocare	1.5	Sucrose, Maltodextrin	105.7 (28.2)	Sodium & calcium caseinates	62.6 (16.7)	Canola oil, MCT oil, Safflower oil	93.3 (55.1)			947 cc	78.5	475	Pulmonary formula	R
Renalcal Diet	2	Maltodextrin, Modified cornstarch	290.4 (58.1)	Whey protein concentrate, Free amino acids	34.4 (6.9)	MCT oil, Canola oil, Corn oil, Soy lecithin	82.4 (35)			1000 cc	70.4	600	Renal failure	Ne

Respalor	1.52	Corn syrup solids, Sugar	148 (39)	Sodium & calcium caseinates	76 (20)	Canola oil, MCT oil	71 (41)		1420 cc	77	580	Pulmonary formula	MJ
Suplena	2	Maltodextrin, Sucrose	255.2 (51)	Sodium & calcium caseinates	30 (6)	Safflower oil, Soy oil, Soy lecithin	95.6 (43)		947 cc	71.2	600	Predialysis formula	R
TraumaCal	1.5	Corn syrup, Sugar	142 (38)	Sodium & calcium caseinates	82 (22)	Soy oil, MCT oil	68 (4)		2000 cc	78	490		MJ
Blenderized													
Compleat Modified	1.07	Maltodextrin, Vegetables, Fruits	140 (53)	Beef, Calcium caseinate	43 (16)	Canola oil	37 (31)	4.4	1500 cc	83.7	300		No
Compleat Regular	1.07	Maltodextrin, Vegetables, Fruits, Nonfat milk	130 (48)	Beef, Nonfat milk	43 (16)	Corn oil	43 (36)	4.4	1500 cc	84.3	450		No
Pediatric													
Kindercal	1.06	Maltodextrin, Sugar	135 (50)	Calcium & sodium caseinate, Milk protein concentrate	34 (13)	MCT oil, Corn oil, Sunflower oil	44 (37)	Soy fiber 6.3	1–10 yrs– 950 cc	85			MJ
L-Emental Pediatric	0.8	Maltodextrin, Modified starch	130 (63)	Free amino acids	24 (12)	MCT oil, Soybean oil	24 (25)				360		NM
NeoCate One +	1	Corn syrup solids	146 (58)	Free amino acids	25 (10)	Coconut oil, Canola oil, Safflower oil	35 (32)			85	610		SHS
Pediasure	1	Hydrolyzed cornstarch, Sucrose	109.7 (43.9)	Sodium caseinate, Whey protein concentrate	30 (12)	Safflower oil, Soy oil, MCT oil	49.7 (44.1)			84.4	345		R

continues

Formula	kcal/cc	Carbohydrate Source	CHO g/L (% kcal)	Protein Source	PRO g/L (% kcal)	Fat Source	Fat (% kcal)	Fiber Source	Fiber g/L	Volume to Meet RDA	% Water	mOsm/ kg	Comments	Manufacturer
Pediasure with Fiber	1	Hydrolyzed cornstarch, Sucrose	113.5 (43.9)	Sodium caseinate, Whey protein concentrate	30 (12)	Safflower oil, Soy oil, MCT oil	49.7 (44.1)	Soy fiber	5		84.4	345		R
Peptamen Junior	1	Maltodextrin, Cornstarch, Guar gum	137.5 (55)	Hydrolyzed whey protein	30 (12)	MCT oil, Soybean oil, Canola oil, Soy lecithin	38.5 (33)			1000 cc	85	260		Ne
Resource-Just for Kids	1	Hydrolyzed cornstarch, Sucrose	110 (44)	Sodium & calcium caseinates, Whey protein concentrate	30 (12)	Sunflower oil, Soybean oil, MCT oil	50 (44)			1000 cc		390		No
Vivonex Pediatric	0.8	Maltodextrin, Modified starch	130 (63)	Free amino acids	24 (12)	MCT oil, Soybean oil	24 (25)				89.3	360		No

MJ = Mead Johnson
Ne = Nestle Clinical Nutrition
NM = Nutrition Medical
No = Novartis Nutrition
R = Ross Laboratories Division/Abbott Laboratories
SHS = SHS North America

Modular Formulas

Formula	kcal	Carbohydrate Source	CHO Content	PRO Source	PRO Content	Fat Source	Fat g (% kcal)
Casec	370 kcal/100 g			Calcium caseinate	88 g PRO/100 g		
Elementra	25 kcal/6.6 g			Hydrolyzed whey	5.22 g PRO/6.6 g		
MCT Oil	8.3 kcal/g					MCT oil	
Microlipid	4.5 kcal/cc					Safflower oil, Polyglycerol esters of fatty acids, Soy lecithin	7.5 g Fat/15 cc
Moducal	30 kcal/8 g	Maltodextrin					
Polycose Powder	23 kcal/6 g	Glucose polymers	94 g/100 g powder				
Polycose Liquid	2 kcal/1 cc	Glucose polymers	50 g/100 cc liquid				
ProMod	28 kcal/6.6 g		0.67 g CHO/6.6 g	D-Whey protein	5 g PRO/6.6 g	Soy lecithin	0.6 g Fat/6.6 g
Propac Plus	9.3 kcal/2.5 g			Milk protein	2.2 g PRO/2.5 g	Lecithin	<0.05 g Fat/2.5 g
Sumacal	19.3 kcal/5 g	Maltodextrin	4.75 g CHO/5 g				

CHO = carbohydrate; PRO = protein

CHAPTER 21

Management of Total Parenteral Nutrition

Polly Lenssen

INDICATIONS FOR TOTAL PARENTERAL NUTRITION

The appropriate use of total parenteral nutrition (TPN) remains a controversial issue in the field of nutrition support. The expense of TPN, the risks inherent in central venous access, the potential complications of substrate- and electrolyte-rich fluid administration, and the apparent adverse physiologic consequences of bypassing the gut have yielded to the wisdom of using enteral nutrition as the standard of care whenever access to a functioning gastrointestinal tract permits. TPN may carry more risk than benefit in several patient populations, including those undergoing chemotherapy[1] and major surgery.[2–5] In these patient groups, TPN is only recommended for patients with severe malnutrition.[3,4,6] Indications for TPN in other patient groups rely primarily on expert opinion in the absence of definitive clinical efficacy trials.[7] The nature of the patient's gastrointestinal dysfunction, the severity of malnutrition, the degree of hypercatabolism, the anticipated length of therapy, the medical prognosis, and the patient's advance directives deserve collective consideration before initiation of TPN.

Nonfunctional Gastrointestinal Tract

Primary Therapy

Small-Bowel Resection. Patients with a residual jejunal length of less than 60 to 100 cm usually require long-term TPN; if the colon has been preserved, only patients with a jejunal length less than 30 to 50 cm may need long-term TPN.[8–11] Periodic reevaluation of bowel adaptation distinguishes patients who are able to tolerate oral or enteral feedings from those who are truly dependent on TPN for long-term survival.[12,13] Prior malnutrition or postsurgical complications delaying enteral intake may result in the need for TPN in those patients with less severe resections.

Refractory Inflammatory Bowel Diseases. TPN in refractory Crohn's disease results in a high rate but variable length of clinical remission.[14,15] Randomized trials, however, have failed to show that TPN and bowel rest are superior to elemental diets.[16,18] In general, TPN is reserved for Crohn's patients who have high-output fistulas or bowel obstruction or in whom enteral therapy fails to ameliorate gastrointestinal symptoms or improve nutritional status, including growth failure in children.[7,19]

TPN in ulcerative colitis is rarely indicated, as its success rate as primary therapy is poor.[15,19] Furthermore, enteral nutrition appears equivalent in terms of remission rate and need for surgical intervention and has the advantages of less cost and complications.[20] Thus, TPN is generally limited in ulcerative colitis to preoperative patients with malnutrition and in whom enteral nutrition is not possible.[7,19]

Enterocutaneous Fistula. High-output fistulas of the upper gastrointestinal tract (gastroduodenum, pancreas, and jejunoileal region) that cannot be managed with enteral feeding are more likely to close spontaneously with TPN; in many cases, they do not require surgery when TPN is provided.[21]

Chronic Intestinal Pseudo-Obstruction. Patients with clinically active pseudo-obstruction require TPN; in patients with recurring attacks, TPN may become permanent therapy.[7]

Adjunctive Therapy

Severe Gastrointestinal Toxicities Associated with Chemotherapy and Radiation. TPN provided during prolonged esophagitis and stomatitis or nausea and vomiting prevents malnutrition and, during bone marrow transplantation, improves survival.[22] It further avoids the potential complications of enteral techniques during bone marrow depression, including aspiration pneumonia and erosive gastrointestinal bleeding.

Severe Diarrhea. TPN presents the only alternative for diarrhea refractory to medications and aggravated by enteral feeding, as can occur in a variety of diseases including radiation enteritis, infectious diarrhea, and chronic protracted diarrhea of infancy.[7,23] In patients who have severe diarrhea associated with acquired immune deficiency syndrome, controlled clinical trials are lacking as to whether TPN improves survival time and decreases morbidity; individual cases should be evaluated with respect to prognosis and potential for increased independence with TPN.[7]

Concurrent Severe Malnutrition. When severe malnutrition exists in any malabsorptive syndrome or otherwise nonfunctional gastrointestinal tract, early

TPN should be considered to restore nutritional status and minimize morbidity related to malnutrition.[3,7]

Concurrent Severe Catabolism. The results of several studies suggest that the provision of enteral nutrition rather than TPN results in far fewer infections in patients with trauma and critical illness.[24,25] However, when severe catabolism accelerates loss of lean body mass during an injury or illness in which the gastrointestinal tract is nonfunctional or the provision of enteral nutrients is inadequate, TPN may be necessary. The critical level of lean tissue loss associated with impaired immune response, poor wound healing, and respiratory muscle deterioration begins when body weight loss exceeds 10% to 15%.[26] Patients with extensive burns, trauma, or complicated sepsis may fall in this category.

Organ Failure

Pancreatitis

TPN appears to have no effect on clinical outcome or complications associated with mild pancreatitis.[27] TPN, however, suppresses pancreatic secretions and is considered an important therapeutic adjunct in patients with severe pancreatitis if bowel rest is needed beyond 1 week.[7,28,29] Contraindications to use of the gastrointestinal tract include the presence of abdominal pain, ascites, elevated serum amylase, or pancreatic fistulas.

Hepatic Failure

In patients with alcohol-induced cirrhosis, TPN formulas enriched in branched-chain amino acids and reduced in aromatic amino acids result in the delivery of more protein as well as in an equal or more rapid recovery from encephalopathy than the use of neomycin, lactulose, or standard amino acid solutions.[30] Whether enteral formulas with the same amino acid modifications are as efficacious as hepatic TPN solutions has not been studied. If nutrition support is undertaken in patients with alcoholic liver failure, the functional status of the gastrointestinal tract and the risk of aspiration due to alteration in mental status should determine the route of feeding.

The nutrition support of patients with hepatitis or cirrhosis from other causes has not been systematically studied. Candidates for liver transplantation, however, should be provided TPN if they are malnourished and do not tolerate enteral nutrition because of gastrointestinal dysfunction or aspiration risk.[31] Guidelines for the use of a specialty amino acid solution for liver failure include patients with grade 2 or higher encepholapathy, abnormal plasma amino acid profiles, or encephalopathy associated with standard amino acid solutions.[32]

Renal Failure

Acute renal failure as a complication of surgery or sepsis is associated with marked protein catabolism and a high mortality rate. Clinical studies have not conclusively demonstrated a benefit of TPN on survival or recovery of renal function.[33] Initiation guidelines for TPN should consider degree of catabolism, gastrointestinal function, and anticipated length of renal failure.

Multisystem Organ Failure

Encephalopathy due to poor oxygenation, sepsis, or liver disease may necessitate TPN in patients with multiple organ failure.

Other Indications

Perioperative Patients

Surgical patients are candidates for TPN only if the gastrointestinal tract cannot be safely accessed. The use of preoperative TPN additionally requires the presence of severe malnutrition to demonstrate any benefit.[3] In the postoperative period, it is recommended to wait 7 to 10 days without nutrient intake before initiating TPN in well-nourished patients for whom enteral access is not possible, patients who develop obstruction, or patients who fail to tolerate adequate amounts of enteral feeding.[2,7]

Hyperemesis Gravidarum

Numerous case reports have described successful pregnancy outcome when TPN was provided for intractable nausea and vomiting.[34–37] In these cases, TPN offers the benefit of optimal fetal growth and development when attempts at enteral feeding have failed.

Anorexia Nervosa

Patients with anorexia nervosa who are severely malnourished and demonstrate an unfavorable psychiatric assessment are the least likely to respond to conventional therapy and oral refeeding. This subset, ranging from an estimated 1% to 10% of anorexia patients requiring hospital admission, may benefit from TPN when enteral nutrition is contraindicated for physical or emotional reasons.[7,38]

Neonatal Conditions

The negligible energy stores in premature infants and the negative consequences of malnutrition on brain growth and development mandate the immediate use of TPN in neonates who are unable to tolerate enteral nutrition. Specific indications for neonatal TPN include congenital malformation of the gastrointestinal tract, gastroschisis, meconium ileus, short-bowel syndrome, necrotizing enterocolitis, substrate transport defects, paralytic ileus, malabsorption syndromes, chylothorax, lymphangiectasia, and extreme prematurity.[7]

PRESCRIPTION OF TOTAL PARENTERAL NUTRITION

General Considerations

The TPN prescription begins with calculation of energy, protein, fluid, electrolyte, and micronutrient needs. How energy is distributed between dextrose, lipids, and protein in the prescription depends on a variety of factors, including the age, nutritional status, and clinical condition of the patient as well as institutional factors. The younger the patient, the higher the energy needs are relative to protein requirements. The energy and protein content is further determined by the therapeutic goal to maintain or replete the patient or to provide for increased needs during stress. For example, it may be inappropriate to provide extra energy to replete a malnourished patient during an acute event such as sepsis; however, after clinical resolution of the infection, a higher energy level may be targeted. A relative contraindication to a macronutrient affects the substrate distribution (eg, dextrose with diabetes, protein in renal insufficency, or fluid with congestive heart failure or pulmonary edema).

Finally, institutional factors such as the cost of solutions, formulary available, and type of delivery system exert a major influence on the TPN prescription. A two-in-one delivery system (dextrose-amino acid combination with separate infusion of lipids) requires two pumps; lipids may be infused continuously or intermittently (on a daily or less frequent schedule). A three-in-one or total nutrient admixture (dextrose, amino acid, and lipids in a single container) requires only one pump and results in the continuous infusion of lipids. In addition, some institutions have the ability to compound stock solutions in only a limited number of concentrations, while some have an automated compounding system capable of highly individualized substrate prescriptions.

It is beyond the scope of this chapter to provide specific guidelines for prescribing TPN given the diversity of practice situations. The health care team responsible for TPN at any institution that provides nutrition support is obligated to develop in a multidisciplinary fashion a safe, clinically appropriate, and cost-conscious formulary, delivery system, and protocol (including standing physician orders) for determining TPN prescriptions. General guidelines on appropriate dose ranges for macronutrients as well as electrolyte, vitamin, and trace element requirements are described in Table 21–1. Exhibit 21–1 provides examples of TPN calculations using both two-in-one and three-in-one systems.

Some practical questions recur in the calculation and prescription of TPN. Should protein kcal be included in total energy calculations?[39] The example pro-

Table 21–1 Daily Maintenance Nutrient Needs during TPN

Nutrient	Adults	Adolescents	Children
Protein (g/kg) *Available as crystalline amino acids in 3.5%–15% solutions; 4 kcal/g protein*			
Maintenance	1.0	1.0	7–10 years: 1.2 4–6 years: 1.5 1–3 years: 1.8
Stress	1.5–2.0	2.0	7–10 years: 2.4 1–6 years: 3.0
Energy (kcal/kg)			
Maintenance 1.2–1.3 × basal needs	30	40–50	7–10 years: 50–60 4–6 years: 60–70 1–3 years: 70–85
Rehabilitation/stress 1.5 × basal needs	40–45	45–65	7–10 years: 65–75 4–6 years: 75–90 1–3 years: 90–100
Carbohydrate (mg/kg/min)[a] *Available as dextrose monohydrate in 2.5%–70% solutions; 3.4 kcal/g dextrose*	< 5	< 7–10	< 10–15
Lipid *Available as long-chain triglycerides derived from soybean or safflower oil, glycerol, egg-yolk phospholipid in 10% (1.1 kcal/mL), 20% (2 kcal/ mL) and 30% (3 kcal/mL) solutions. Lower phospholipid content per kcal of 20% and 30% solutions favors their use over 10% solutions*	% of total kcal: Minimum 6–8% Maximum 60%	% of total kcal: Minimum 6–8% Maximum 60%	1–4 g/kg

	1500 mL/m²	1500 mL/m²	100 mL/kg up to 10 kg + 50 mL/kg for each kg 11–20 kg + 20 mL/kg for each kg 21–40 kg
Maintenance fluid See Table 21–5 for fluid and sodium imbalances during TPN			
Potassium[b] *Available as phosphate, chloride, and acetate salts*	60–120 mEq	60–120 mEq	2–3 mEq/kg
Sodium[b] *Available as chloride, acetate, or phosphate salts*	50–100 mEq	50–100 mEq	2–4 mEq/kg
Calcium *Available as gluconate salt*	10–25 mEq	0.25–0.5 mEq/kg	10–30 mEq
Phosphorus *Available as potassium or sodium salts*	10–20 mmol	0.5–1.0 mmol/kg	1–2 mmol/kg
Magnesium *Available as sulfate salt*	16–32 mEq	16–32 mEq	0.25–0.5 mEq/kg
Zinc *Available as chloride or sulfate salt in single entity or combination preparation*	2.5–4.0 mg	2.5–4.0 mg	100 µg/kg[c]
Copper *Available as sulfate salt in single entity or combination preparation*	0.5–1.5 mg	0.5–1.5 mg	20 µg/kg[c]
Manganese *Available as chloride salt in single entity or combination preparation*	150–800 µg	150–800 µg	2–10 µg/kg[c]
Chromium *Available as chloride salt in single entity or combination preparation*	10–15 µg	10–15 µg	0.2 µg/kg[c]
Selenium *Available as selenious acid in single entity or combination preparation*	40–80 µg	40–80 µg	3 µg/kg
Molybdenum *Available as ammonium molybdate as single entity*	20–120 µg[d]	20–120 µg[d]	0.25 µg/kg

continues

Table 21–1 continued

Nutrient	Adults	Adolescents	Children
Vitamins *Available as adult and pediatric multivitamin combinations of water- and fat-soluble vitamins or single infusions of cobalamin, folate, thiamine, pantothenic acid, pyridoxine, ascorbic acid, and vitamin K*			
A	3300 IU (990 RE)	3300 IU (990 RE)	2300 IU (690 RE)
D	200 IU (5 RE)	200 IU (5 RE)	400 IU (10 RE)
E	10 IU (6.7 RE)	10 IU (6.7 RE)	IU (7 RE)
B$_1$ (thiamine)	3.0 mg	3.0 mg	1.2 mg
B$_2$ (riboflavin)	3.6 mg	3.6 mg	1.4 mg
Niacin	40 mg	40 mg	17 mg
Folic acid	400 µg	400 µg	140 µg
B$_6$ (pyridoxine)	4 mg	4 mg	1.1 mg
Panthothenic Acid	15 mg	15 mg	5.0 mg
Biotin^e	60 µg	60 µg	20 µg
B$_{12}$ (cobalamin)	5 µg	5 µg	1.0 µg
C	100 mg	100 mg	80 mg
Vitamin K *Available as a component of pediatric but not adult multivitamin combinations to avoid interference with anticoagulants*	1–2 mg (or 10 mg once weekly)		200 µg (as part of multivitamin combination)

| **Iron** *Available as iron-dextran* | Only indicated in patients on long-term TPN with no other sources of iron | Only indicated in patients on long-term TPN with no other sources of iron | Only indicated in patients on long-term TPN with no other sources of iron |

Recommended daily trace element supplementation for adults from: American Medical Association. Guidelines for essential trace element preparations for parenteral use. American Medical Association Department of Food and Nutrition. *JAMA.* 1979;241:2051–2054.

Recommended daily vitamin supplementation for adults and adolescents from: Multivitamin preparations for parenteral use: a statement by the nutrition advisory group. *J Parenter Enter Nutr.* 1979;3:258–262.

Recommended daily vitamin, mineral, and trace element supplementation for children from: Greene HL, Hambridge KN, Schanler R, et al. Guidelines for the use of vitamins, trace elements, calcium, magnesium, and phosphorus in infants and children receiving total parenteral nutrition: Report of the Subcommittee on Pediatric Parenteral Nutrient Requirements from the Committee on Clinical Practice Issues of the American Society for Clinical Nutrition. *Am J Clin Nutr.* 1988;48:1324–1342.

[a] To calculate carbohydrate dose, divide total mg dextrose per day by 1440 min/day/wt in kg. For example, 1700 mL 25% dextrose in a 70 kg patient = 425 g dextrose × 1000 mg/g ÷ 1440 min/day/70 kg = 4.2 mg/kg/min dextrose.

[b] After determining phosphate needs, remainder provided primarily as chloride salt (except in presence of metabolic acidosis) to meet chloride needs.

[c] Up to 5 years; older than 5 years, use guidelines for adolescent and adult.

[d] Manufacturer's recommendation.

[e] Currently available multivitamin combinations do not contain biotin.

Exhibit 21–1 Sample TPN Prescriptions

Patient. 35-year-old woman undergoing allogeneic bone marrow transplantation for non-Hodgkins lymphoma with severe mucositis and fever of unknown origin. Serum chemistries are all normal.

Ht = 178 cm; Wt = 66 kg; Body surface area = 1.8 m²; Estimated needs = 2140 kcal (1.5 × basal), 95 g protein (1.5 g/kg), 2700 mL fluid.

Example 1. Two-in-one system using stock solutions

Twice weekly: 500 mL 20% lipids

Daily:

> 1800 mL 25% dextrose/5% amino acids
>
> Multivitamin injection (if no folate or cobalamin, these must be added)
>
> Trace element package (if no selenium, this must be added)
>
> Vitamin K 1 mg (may be added weekly as 10 mg)

Per 1000 mL:

> 30 mEq sodium chloride
>
> 25 mEq potassium chloride
>
> 15 mEq potassium phosphate
>
> 8 mEq calcium gluconate
>
> 16 mEq magnesium sulfate

Provides average daily: 2175 kcal, 13% kcal as fat, 90 g protein, 4.7 mg/kg/min CHO, 1940 mL fluid

1. Determine volume of standard 25% dextrose/5% amino acid concentration to meet protein needs:

$$95 \text{ g protein} \div 50 \text{ g/L protein} = 1.9 \text{ L}$$

2. Calculate total kcal
   a. Lipid: 500 mL 20% lipid × 2 kcal/mL × 2 days = 2000 kcal; divide by 7 days/wk ≅ 285 kcal/day
   b. CHO: 1.9 L × 250 g/L CHO × 3.4 kcal/g CHO = 1615 kcal
   c. Protein: 95 g protein × 4 kcal/g = 380 kcal
   d. Total kcal: 2380; this overfeeds the patient by 140 kcal/day

3. Adjust kcal by decreasing 25% dextrose/5% amino acid solution to 1.8 L (compromising protein support to 90 g):
   a. Lipid: Same lipid dose ≅ 285 kcal
   b. CHO: 1.8 L × 250 g/L CHO × 3.4 kcal/g CHO = 1530 kcal plus
   c. Protein: L × 50 g/L protein × 4 kcal/g = 360 kcal plus
   d. Total kcal = 2175

4. Verify carbohydrate load is < 5.0 mg/kg/min:

> (1.8 L × 250 g/L CHO × 1000 mg/g) ÷ 66 kg ÷ 1440 min = 4.7 mg/kg/min

continues

Exhibit 21–1 continued

5. Calculate fluid from TPN:
   1800 mL 25% dextrose/5% amino acids +
   (500 mL 20% lipids × 2 days ÷ 7 days/week) = 1940 mL
   There are likely other sources of fluid (medications, blood products) in this patient to meet the remainder of maintenance fluid needs.

Example 2. Three-in-one system compounded from 10% amino acid, 70% dextrose, and 20% lipid solutions
Daily:
   1724 mL 5.5% amino acid, 2.5% lipid, 22.7% dextrose
   Multivitamin injection (if no folate or cobalamin, these must be added)
   Trace element package (if no selenium, this must be added)
   Vitamin K 1 mg (may be added weekly as 10 mg)
   60 mEq sodium chloride
   45 mEq potassium chloride
   30 mEq potassium phosphate
   16 mEq calcium gluconate
   24 mEq magnesium sulfate

Provides 2140 kcal, 20% kcal as fat, 95 g protein, 4.1 mg/kg/min CHO, 1724 mL fluid

1. Calculate volume of 10% amino acid to provide 95 g protein:
   95 g protein ÷ 100 g/L = 950 mL
2. Determine % fat kcal goal (in this example 20%) and calculate volume of 20% lipid:
   20% kcal as fat × 2140 kcal = 428 fat kcal or 42.8 g fat;
   428 fat kcal ÷ 2 kcal/mL = 214 mL
3. Calculate g CHO to provide remaining kcal and volume of 70% dextrose:
   2140 kcal - 380 protein kcal - 428 fat kcal = 1332 CHO kcal
   1332 kcal ÷ 3.4 kcal/g CHO = 392 g CHO
   392 g CHO ÷ 700 g/L = 560 mL
4. Verify carbohydrate load is < 5.0 mg/kg/min
   (392 g CHO × 1000 mg/g) ÷ 66 kg ÷ 1440 min = 4.1 mg/kg/min
5. Total fluid = 1724 mL; calculate final substrate concentration if desired
   a. % amino acid = 95 g ÷ 1724 mL = 5.5%
   b. % lipid = 42.8 g ÷ 1724 mL $\cong$ 2.5%
   c. % CHO = 392 g ÷ 1724 mL = 22.7%
6. If more fluid is desired, sterile water can be added.

vided in Exhibit 21–1 does include protein as part of total energy. In two-in-one systems, is it safe to infuse lipid emulsions beyond 12 hours? The Centers for Disease Control and Prevention recommended 12-hour hang times for separate lipid emulsions[40]; more recent data suggest that longer hang times may be safe and metabolically more advantageous in patients at risk for impaired fat clearance.[41]

Solutions Available

Table 21–2 lists the composition of lipid emulsions in the 20% concentration. Table 21–3 details the composition of adult and pediatric amino acid formulas in the 10% concentration and hepatic amino acid formulas. Other specialty formulas (renal and trauma) have been omitted because of the lack of data to support their clinical efficacy.

MONITORING

The implementation of standing physicians' orders, clinical practice guidelines, and protocols or care pathways that detail nutrition and metabolic monitoring is essential in minimizing TPN-associated complications.[42] The parameters and minimum measurement frequencies required to deliver TPN safely and effica-ciously vary among patient populations and clinical conditions. General recom-mendations for TPN monitoring are summarized in Table 21–4.

Table 21–2 Composition of 20% Lipid Emulsions

	Intralipid® 20%[1] (Clintec)	Liposyn®II 20%[2] (Abbott)	Liposyn®III 20%[2] (Abbott)
Fat content (g/100 mL)			
Safflower oil	—	10	—
Sunflower oil	20	10	20
Fatty acids (%)			
Linoleic acid	50%	65.8%	54.5%
Oleic acid	26%	17.7%	22.4%
Palmitic acid	10%	6.6%	10.5%
Stearic acid	3.5%	3.4%	4.2%
Linolenic acid	9%	4.2%	8.3%
mOsm/L	260	258	292

Note: All formulas are 2 kcal/mL and contain 1.2 g/100 mL egg phosphatides and 2.25 g/100 mL glycerin.
[1]Intralipid® also available in 10% and 30% concentration.
[2]Liposyn®II and III also available in 10% concentration.

Source: Adapted with permission from AHFS Drug Information, © 1997, American Society of Health-System Pharmacists.

Table 21–3 Composition of Selected Amino Acid Solutions

	Standard 10% Solutions			Pediatric Solutions		Hepatic Failure 8% Solutions	
	Aminosyn®II (Abbott)	FreAmine®III (McGaw)	Travasol® (Baxter)	Aminosyn®PF 7% (Abbott)	TrophAmine®10% (McGaw)	Aminosyn®HF (Abbott)	HepatAmine® (McGaw)
Nitrogen (g/100 mL)	1.53	1.53	1.65	1.07	1.55	1.2	1.2
Essential Amino Acids (mg/100 mL)							
Isoleucine	660	690	600	534	820	900	900
Leucine	1000	910	730	831	1400	1100	1100
Lysine	1050	730	580	475	820	610	610
Methionine	172	530	400	125	340	100	100
Phenylalanine	298	560	560	300	480	100	100
Threonine	400	400	420	360	420	450	450
Tryptophan	200	150	180	125	200	66	66
Valine	500	660	580	452	780	840	840
Nonessential Amino Acids (mg/100 mL)							
Alanine	993	710	2070	490	540	770	770
Arginine	1018	950	1150	861	1200	600	600
Proline	722	1120	680	570	680	800	800
Serine	530	590	500	347	380	500	500
Taurine	—	—	—	50	25		
Histidine[1]	300	280	480	220	480	240	240
Tyrosine[1]	270	—	40	44	240	—	—
Glycine	500	1400	1030	270	360	900	900
Cysteine	—	< 20	—	—	< 16	< 20	< 20

continues

Table 21-3 continued

	Standard 10% Solutions			Pediatric Solutions		Hepatic Failure 8% Solutions	
	Aminosyn®II (Abbott)	FreAmine®III (McGaw)	Travasol® (Baxter)	Aminosyn®PF 7% (Abbott)	TrophAmine®10% (McGaw)	Aminosyn®HF (Abbott)	HepatAmine® (McGaw)
Glutamic acid	738	—	—	576	500	—	—
Aspartic acid	700	—	—	370	320	—	—
Electrolytes (mEq/L)							
Sodium	45.3	10	—	3.4	5	10	10
Chloride	—	<3	—	—	<3	<3	<3
Acetate	71.8	89	87	32.5	97	62	62
Phosphate (mmol/L)	—	10	—	—	—	10	—
mOsm/L	873	950	1000	586	875	768–785	768–785
pH	5-6.5	6-7	6	6.4	5-6	6-6.8	6-7

[1]Histidine and tyrosine are considered essential in infants.

Source: Adapted with permission from AHFS Drug Information, © 1997, American Society of Health-System Pharmacists; Aminosyn®HF from product literature.

Table 21–4 General Recommendations for TPN Monitoring

Baseline	*Routine*	*As Clinically Indicated*
Weight, height, body surface area	**Every 8 hours**	**Fluid disorders**
Body composition (arm fat and muscle areas, bioelectrical imped-	Vital signs	Urine sodium or fractional sodium excretion
	Temperature	Serum osmolality
	Urine fractionals	Urine specific gravity
ance, subjective or	**Daily**	**Protein status**
functional measures)	Weight	Nitrogen balance, serum
Serum electrolytes,	Fluid intake and	prealbumin
glucose, creatinine,	output	**Lipid disorders**
blood urea nitrogen	Serum electrolytes,	Serum triglyceride or lipid
Serum magnesium,	glucose, creatinine,	clearance test
calcium, phosphorus	blood urea nitrogen	Respiratory quotient
Serum triglyceride and	until stable; then	Essential fatty acids (if fat-
cholesterol	twice weekly	free TPN is necessary)
Liver function tests	**Weekly**	**Hepatic encephalopathy**
Serum albumin or	Serum magnesium,	Plasma amino acids
prealbumin	calcium, phospho-	**Gastrointestinal losses**
Complete blood count	rus, albumin	Serum trace elements
Energy (estimated or	Liver function tests	Stool electrolytes
measured), protein,	Complete blood count	**Respiratory compromise**
fluid, and micronutri-	Review of actual oral,	Pa_{CO_2}
ent needs	enteral, and TPN	Indirect calorimetry,
	intake	respiratory quotient
		Acid-base disorders
		Blood pH
		Anion gap
		Long-term TPN
		Body composition measures
		Serum trace elements, vitamins

Nutritional Parameters

Energy Intake versus Needs

Documentation of Delivery. The prescription of TPN does not always equate with the delivery of the prescribed volume, especially in patients with multipurpose venous catheters for whom other intravenous products may have medical priority. The use of double- and triple-lumen catheters and placement of catheters strictly for nutrition have helped to resolve this problem.[43] Nevertheless, the following circumstances may interfere with the desired infusion volume: (1) disconnect time from the infusion pump for ambulation, baths, and tests or treatments performed away from the bedside; (2) intravenous medications requiring continuous infusion; and (3) inappropriate infusion rates. Daily or periodic documentation from the medical record of the actual TPN infused is the most desirable method to assess the adequacy of the TPN delivered. Adjustments in infusion rates or volumes frequently remedy situations in which the actual intake deviates from the prescription.

Change in Clinical Status. Whether initial energy needs are estimated by an equation or measured by indirect calorimetry, patients require periodic reassessment to avoid the complications of over- or underfeeding. Clinical situations that may trigger a review of energy needs include changes in (1) fever or infection status, (2) major organ function, (3) wound healing status, (4) weight (nonfluid gain or loss), and (5) activity level. Daily manipulation of TPN energy is impractical and without clinical merit; however, a periodic review of overall clinical status in relation to the appropriateness of the TPN prescription and actual delivery, combined with any available nutritional assessment indexes, will help prevent iatrogenic feeding problems.

Protein Status

Nitrogen Balance. Data on nitrogen balance reflect total body protein flux without regard to the functional implications of changes in protein balance in the individual organs or tissues. However, with reliable collections and relatively little cost, an estimation of balance from urinary urea nitrogen, or more accurately from total urinary nitrogen by pyrochemiluminescence, helps the clinician determine if the patient is anabolic (positive balance) or catabolic (negative balance).[44-46] If body weight or blood urea nitrogen (BUN) change during the period of observation, nitrogen balance should be corrected for changes in the body urea pool by subtracting from the balance:

Change in body urea N (g) =

$$(BUN_f - BUN_i \text{ in g/L}) \times BW_i \text{ (kg)} \times 0.60 \text{ (L/kg)} + (BW_f - BW_i \text{ in kg}) \times BUN_f \text{ (g/L)} \times 1.0 \text{ (L/kg)}$$

where i and f are the initial and final values of the measurement period, BW is body weight, and the fraction of body weight assumed to be water is 60%.[47]

Visceral Proteins. Serum albumin is useful as an index of visceral protein mass in only a small proportion of clinically stable patients on TPN. In patients with acute illness, serum values are largely affected by nonnutritional parameters, especially in clinical settings of altered vascular permeability and fluid imbalance.[48]

An albumin measurement is necessary for the evaluation of calcium status, since 50% of total calcium is protein bound (see discussion of phosphorus and calcium imbalances below).

Among the serum proteins with shorter half-lives, including transferrin, prealbumin (transthyretin), and retinol-binding protein, prealbumin has been advocated as the most practical serum protein for determining visceral protein status and monitoring response to nutrition support therapies. Patients with a value <110 mg/L warrant consideration for nutrition support intervention.[49] Changes in prealbumin status have been correlated with nitrogen balance in patients on TPN; thus, this easily measured, inexpensive analyte may substitute for more labor-intensive balance studies in evaluating whether a patient is anabolic or catabolic.[50] Because inflammatory states and hepatic and renal dysfunction depress all serum proteins,[51] serial monitoring of prealbumin may best indicate changes in metabolic stress that alter overall TPN management, not just protein support.

Lymphocyte Counts, Skin Test Antigens, and Other Immunological Parameters. There are no data to support the use of tests of immune function in monitoring the progress of patients on TPN, although researchers are currently investigating how the components of TPN may be altered to modulate the immune response.

Body Composition

Anthropometry. Small changes in body composition that occur over short time periods in patients on TPN are not accurately described by anthropometric measures of muscle and fat volumes derived from upper arm skinfold thickness and circumference.[52] Measurements are distorted by the increase in total body water as a fraction of the fat-free mass, especially during the administration of sodium-containing intravenous fluids or in patients with congestive heart failure, liver disease, and other conditions that alter fluid balance.[53] Prior to TPN intervention, however, the easily obtained upper arm measurements help assess baseline nutritional status. Serial measurements provide more reliable information about changes in fat (energy) and muscle (protein) stores when the period of nutritional intervention extends over months and when changes in body composition are large, and thus may best be reserved for patient populations in whom long-term nutrition monitoring is anticipated. Interpretation of serial data should be tempered by the knowledge that skinfold measurements are related in a nonlinear fashion to total body fat and, when relying on a single site, that fat accumulates at different rates between skinfold sites.[53]

Urinary Creatinine. Urinary creatinine is an inexpensive assay associated with fat-free mass when renal function is normal. Muscle catabolism does not significantly alter its excretion.[54] However, intraindividual variability makes three successive collections desirable for valid interpretation.[55] Age-corrected values for creatinine expressed relative to height have been published.[54]

Bioelectrical Impedance. Bioelectical impedance is a noninvasive, relatively inexpensive tool that has been used to detect changes in body composition during TPN.[56,57] Multifrequency (rather than single-frequency) measurements appear to account for shifts in abnormal water or electrolyte distribution.[58]

Other Clinical Methods. No objective technique can replace observation at the bedside. In addition to palpating muscle groups, Hill and Windsor describe simple methods to assess grip strength (ask the patient to squeeze strongly the clinician's index and middle fingers for at least 10 seconds) and respiratory muscle function (ask the patient to blow hard a strip of paper held 10 cm from the patient's lips).[52] Based on extensive body composition studies in critically ill patients, Hill has determined that physiologic functions are significantly impaired when body protein loss exceeds 20%; ill patients cross into this high-risk zone when they have lost 10% to 15% of body weight.[26]

Metabolic Parameters

Fluid, Electrolyte, and Mineral Status

Fluid Balance and Hydration Status. Most patients on TPN require strict daily monitoring of fluid intake and output and hydration status. Hydration status assessment includes body weight, vital signs, clinical signs and symptoms (such as skin turgor and neck vein distention), urine specific gravity, serum sodium, glucose, and BUN. The degree to which a patient is susceptible to dehydration or the adverse sequelae of fluid overload (such as pulmonary edema) is related to the severity of the patient's illness and underlying major organ function. Critically ill patients, particularly young children, may require assessment of hydration status several times daily.

An accurate weight obtained at the same time daily is a simple means of monitoring overall fluid balance. A change in 24 hours of 2% or more reflects a fluid shift. Serum sodium provides some guide to intravascular volume status by approximating serum osmolality when multiplied by a factor of two. Because hyperglycemia and azotemia can significantly increase serum osmolality, a better estimation can be made with the following equation:

$$(2 \times \text{serum sodium in mEq/L}) + (\text{glucose in mg/dl} \div 20) +$$
$$(\text{BUN in mg/dl} \div 2.8)$$

Values greater than 300 mOsm/L suggest dehydration, and values less than 280 mOsm/L suggest overhydration. Similarly, urine specific gravity less than 1.010 indicates overhydration and greater than 1.030 suggests dehydration.

Serum and Urine Electrolytes. Serum electrolytes are determined daily until the levels stabilize within normal ranges. If fluid balance is also stable, then monitoring every 2 to 3 days may suffice. Calcium, phosphorus, and magnesium require weekly assessment. Patients in highly anabolic states need more frequent monitoring of phosphorus and magnesium; these minerals are utilized during active protein synthesis and may abruptly drop to dangerously low levels. Patients on drug therapies associated with electrolyte wasting (eg, amphotericin, diuretics, foscarnet, cyclosporine) also need more frequent electrolyte monitoring, as do patients with decreased renal excretion. Urine sodium may be required to assess sodium needs, since serum sodium is indicative of total body water status more than sodium status. A preferred method for determining the patient's ability to excrete sodium is the fractional sodium excretion (or FE_{NA}),[59] which calculates the sodium excreted as a percentage of sodium filtered with normal values being greater than 1%.

Fractional sodium excretion = (urine sodium × serum creatinine) ÷ (serum sodium × urine creatinine)

Serum Trace Elements. Trace element assays may not be readily available and add cost to TPN monitoring. When trace elements are appropriately supplemented, they do not require routine monitoring. Monitoring should be reserved for (1) severely malnourished patients as part of baseline assessment to determine replacement requirements, (2) neonates and infants, (3) patients with significant gastrointestinal losses, and (4) patients on long-term TPN.[60] Empirical management based on clinical signs and symptoms is addressed in the discussion of micronutrient metabolism.

Acid-Base Balance

Acid-base disorders often require modification of TPN electrolyte additives. Acidosis may be offset with substituting sodium and/or potassium acetate for the chloride salt equivalent, and vice versa with alkalosis. Often acid-base status can be adequately assessed with information from the history and/or clinical course; physical examination; and routine electrolyte assessment, particularly serum bicarbonate. Determination of blood pH and P_{CO_2} levels depends on the need to confirm clinical impressions. Chapter 6 discusses the diagnosis of acid-base disorders.

Organ Function

Renal. Serum creatinine and BUN are measured prior to initiation of TPN to establish baseline kidney function, and daily after initiation until the patient is stable. Thereafter, the frequency depends on other clinical circumstances affecting renal function.

Liver. Liver function tests, serum glutamic-oxaloacetic transaminase, total and indirect bilirubin, and alkaline phosphatase require weekly assessment because of the known association of TPN with altered liver function. Any evolving liver process, regardless of etiology, necessitates close monitoring during TPN as alterations in substrate metabolism and electrolyte distribution may occur.

Respiratory. Available blood gasses may be observed in patients with respiratory compromise for the possible effects of excess intravenous substrates on CO_2 production. If indirect calorimetry is available, calculation of the respiratory quotient helps determine the appropriateness of the total energy prescription and substrate distribution[61–63] (see Chapter 7).

Gastrointestinal. Return of gastrointestinal function signals time to initiate weaning to enteral tube or oral feeding. Assessment of bowel function is discussed in detail in Chapter 8.

Substrate Tolerance

Glucose. Glucosuria (urine glucose of 2+ or more) usually precedes serum glucose elevations. Urine glucose should be checked every 6–8 hours after initiation of TPN. Daily serum glucose monitoring is indicated until values are consistently < 200 mg/dL.

Lipid. Baseline serum triglyceride and cholesterol identify any preexisting hyperlipidemia. Intravenous lipids may be restricted to a dose providing essential fatty acids (4% to 8% of total energy as lipid) only if the fasting serum triglyceride exceeds 400 to 500 mg/dL prior to starting TPN; they are avoided altogether if the fasting level exceeds 1000 to 2000 mg/dL.

Serum triglyceride concentrations respond dramatically to the infusion rate of lipid emulsions; thus, it is important to monitor periodically the plasma clearance of lipid emulsions to adjust administration rates and total lipid dose according to the individual patient's tolerance.[64] Clearance of lipid emulsions is most commonly assessed by plasma triglyceride concentration several hours following cessation of fat infusion. Visual turbidity is an unreliable index because it may not always reveal a fat layer in the presence of an elevated triglyceride concentration, nor does it provide quantitative information.[65] Upper limits for triglyceride are not well established in the literature. For pediatrics, levels have been suggested at 250 mg/dL during a continuous infusion[65]; for adults 300 to 350 mg/dL 6 hours postinfusion has been suggested.[66] A more direct method is to measure the clearance of the actual lipid emulsion particles during infusion by nephrolometric techniques, which are often available in hospital laboratories.[67]

Infectious Parameters

The risk of catheter sepsis necessitates daily monitoring of temperature and catheter site and periodic determinations of a complete blood count. Complications of infection are discussed elsewhere in this volume.

COMPLICATIONS OF PARENTERAL NUTRITION

Fluid, Electrolyte, and Mineral Imbalances

Fluid and Sodium Imbalances

TPN management requires a sound knowledge and application of the principles of fluid and electrolyte maintenance. Fluid and ionic shifts between the major body water spaces—intracellular and extracelluar (intravascular, interstitial, and lymph)—or changes in total body water or electrolyte content may necessitate alterations in the TPN composition or volume.

Critically ill patients on TPN, who are often on intravenous antibiotics and other medications in aqueous solution, are prone to iatrogenic fluid overload. Sources of water that patients may not easily manage include (1) the oxidation of substrates, which yields approximately 500 mL water daily in a typical TPN regimen, (2) muscle catabolism, which liberates up to 500 mL daily during severe catabolism, and (3) the TPN fluid itself.[68] High sodium loads from TPN, saline hydration fluids, medications, and exogenous albumin may contribute to fluid overload, presenting as weight gain and hyponatremia, especially in patients with compromised liver or cardiac function. Conversely, increased water losses above normal renal losses (30 to 120 mL/hr) and insensible losses (800 to 1000 mL/day in the adult)—as during fever, diarrhea, vomiting, gastroenteric suction or drainage, high respiratory rates, burns, wounds, or osmotic diuresis—require fluid replacement in addition to the TPN fluid. Many of these clinical conditions are associated with sodium and other electrolyte losses. Changes in TPN should always be considered in light of total fluid and electrolyte management. Common causes and intervention strategies for disorders in fluid and sodium balance are described in Table 21–5.

Potassium Imbalances

Mild hypokalemia during TPN can occur in patients undergoing protein anabolism as potassium shifts intracellularly. Approximately 3.0 mEq potassium accompanies each gram of nitrogen retained.[69] Glucose infusion, insulin therapy, and alkalosis also result in a redistribution of potassium from the extracellular to intracellular space. Hypokalemia due to total body loss of potassium occurs with diarrhea, vomiting, intestinal fistulas, and potassium-wasting drugs such as amphotericin, thiazide diuretics, and steroids.

Hyperkalemia as a complication of TPN is uncommon and, in the presence of normal renal function, is most likely due to rapid intravenous administration of potassium. Potassium infusion rates should never exceed 20 mEq/hr in adults and 10 mEq/hr in children unless the patient is on a cardiac monitor. Hyperkalemia is more frequently observed when renal function is impaired by disease or drugs (eg,

Table 21–5 Fluid and Sodium Imbalances during TPN

Imbalance	Common Causes	Signs and Symptoms	Intervention
Fluid deficits			
Extracellular (Intravascular + Interstitial)	Fever Gastrointestinal losses Excessive use	Decreased urine output Postural hypotension Decreased central venous pressure Poor skin turgor Thirst, weakness Increased hematocrit Increased creatinine, BUN Rapid weight loss	Fluid replacement with fluid of similar composition to that lost
Intravascular to interstitial shift	"Third spacing" of fluids	Signs and symptoms of hypovolemia, except weight may increase	Colloid therapy may be indicated Maintain intravascular volume with minimum necessary fluid and sodium
Total body water	Fever Gastrointestinal losses Diabetes insipidus Prolonged artificial ventilation Inadequate water intake	Weakness, restlessness, delirium, tetany Fever, flushed skin Oliguria Serum sodium >145 mmol/L; osmolality >300 mOsm/L	Free water replacement
Fluid overload			
Extracellular	Renal dysfunction Nephrotoxic drugs Decreased renal blood flow Congestive heart failure Liver disease	Pitting edema Excessive weight gain Increased blood pressure Dyspnea Distended neck veins Decreased hematocrit in absence of bleeding Decreased urine sodium Intake > output	Diuretics Sodium and fluid restriction Use of concentrated lipid, dextrose, and amino acid solutions
Total body water	Excessive free water intake	Headache, mental confusion	Free water restriction

continues

Table 21–5 continued

Imbalance	Common Causes	Signs and Symptoms	Intervention
	Inappropriate antidiuretic hormone syndrome	Muscle twitching, seizures Increased intracranial pressure Weight gain Decreased urine output Serum sodium <130 mmol/L, osmolality <280 mOsm/L	Avoidance of rapid IV infusions
Hypernatremia (serum sodium >145 mmol/L)	Dehydration: fever, sweating, hyperventilation Osmotic diuresis Hyperglycemia Hypercalcemia Osmotic diuretics Antidiuretic hormone deficiency Head trauma Pituitary tumors	Fever Intense thirst Confusion	Free water replacement
Hyponatremia (serum sodium <135 mmol/L)	1. Sodium loss: Gastrointestinal (low urine sodium) Salt-losing nephropathy, diuretics, adrenal insufficiency (high urine sodium)	1. Hypotension Thready pulse, cold clammy skin Restlessness Oliguria	1. Isotonic or hypertonic saline Increase sodium in TPN
	2. Excess free water intake ("dilutional hyponatremia") Congestive heart failure, cirrhosis, edema, "third spacing" of fluid	2. Signs and symptoms similar to total body water excess	2. Free water restriction Use of concentrated lipids, dextrose, and amino acid solutions

Source: Adapted with permission from *Fluid, Electrolyte and Total Parenteral Nutrition Guidelines,* 5th ed., © 1985, Fred Hutchinson Cancer Research Center.

spironolactone, cyclosporine, or FK-506). Trauma-induced catabolism may aggravate hyperkalemia in this setting due to intracellular leakage of potassium.

Chloride Imbalances

Hyperchloremic acidosis is rarely observed because amino acid solutions no longer have a high chloride content. Some solutions still contain some hydrochloride salts and have been implicated in the development of metabolic acidosis.[70]

Phosphorus and Calcium Imbalances

Hypophosphatemia was among the first reported metabolic complications of TPN when phosphate-free solutions resulted in precipitous drops in serum levels, coma, decreased red blood cell 2,3-diphosphoglycerate and adenosine triphosphate, and increased affinity of hemoglobin for oxygen.[71] It was quickly recognized that nitrogen- and glucose-rich solutions caused a rapid shift of phosphorus into the intracellular space to support new tissue synthesis and participate in glycolysis for the production of high-energy phosphate intermediates. Hypophosphatemia due to TPN may be accompanied by decreased serum magnesium and potassium, glucose intolerance, and fluid shifts; these symptoms are collectively termed the *refeeding syndrome*. Signs and symptoms associated with decreased serum phosphorus include irritability and confusion, paresthesia, muscular weakness and frank rhabdomyolysis, hypoventilation, diminished leukocyte and platelet function, anorexia, nausea, and vomiting.[59] Patients with depleted levels of total body phosphorus but with normal serum levels prior to the initiation of TPN (such as those with chronic weight loss, alcohol abuse, and chronic antacid or diuretic therapy) are more likely to develop hypophosphatemia.[72] To avoid the refeeding syndrome in at-risk patients, TPN should be advanced slowly and electrolytes monitored closely. Malnourished patients in particular have high phosphorus needs up to 40 to 50 mEq per 1000 kcal.[73] Aluminum-containing medications, such as sucralfate, should also be considered as a possible source of hypophosphatemia in patients on TPN.[74] Other medications associated with phosphorus wasting include foscarnet, cyclophosphamide, and cisplatin.

Hyperphosphatemia is usually of concern only in patients with renal insufficiency. Signs and symptoms associated with elevated serum phosphorus are not well described and are generally attributable to secondary hypocalcemia.[59] To control hyperphosphatemia, parenteral phosphorus is reduced or deleted. Also, the use of 20% rather than 10% lipid emulsions is recommended because the phosphorus content per calorie delivered is less.[73]

Calcium disorders are not readily detected by serum values because of hormonal regulation of serum calcium and large skeletal reserves. Half of total calcium is protein bound; ideally, ionized calcium, which is the metabolically active component, is measured when calcium imbalance is a concern. Hypocalcemia may occur as a consequence of hypoalbuminemia, hypomagnesemia, vitamin D deficiency, or calcium-wasting drugs such as foscarnet. In states of hypoalbuminemia when only total serum calcium is available, there is a 0.8 mg/dL decline in total concentration of serum calcium for each 1.0 mg/dL decrease in albumin concentration below 4.0 g/dL.[75] Hypocalcemia may manifest clinically as paresthesia, tetany, seizures, cardiac arrhythmias, and hypotension.[59]

Hypercalciuria is common during TPN. The etiology of negative calcium balance is unknown but appears to be attenuated by higher levels of phosphate administration.[76] Limiting any periods of immobilization helps preserve total body calcium stores. In patients on long-term TPN, excessive calcium loss contributes to the frequent complication of bone disease. Howard and colleagues have summarized causes of hypercalciuria in home-TPN patients; these include high protein loads, hyperglycemia due to hypertonic dextrose solutions, high sodium loads, aluminum toxicity from additives (calcium gluconate, phosphate salts, vitamins, and trace elements), and possibly excess vitamin D.[77] Acetate may be added to solutions to minimize the release of calcium carbonate stored in the bone to buffer the acid load generated by parenteral amino acids.[77]

Hypercalcemia may be observed in patients with renal insufficiency, tumor lysis following chemotherapy, and some malignancies (breast cancer, multiple myeloma). Clinical symptoms include depression, lethargy, hypertension, nausea, vomiting, and constipation.[56] When this occurs, calcium should be reduced or deleted from the TPN solution.

Magnesium Imbalances

Magnesium deficiency can occur in patients with (1) excessive gastrointestinal losses, (2) renal losses due to a renal disorder or administration of aminoglycoside, cyclosporine, FK-506, foscarnet, diuretics, cisplatin, or (3) active tissue synthesis. Signs and symptoms of magnesium deficiency include apathy, muscular weakness, tetany, convulsions, nausea and vomiting, hypokalemia, and hypocalcemia.[59]

Hypermagnesemia is most likely to occur in patients with renal insufficiency. Symptoms of lethargy, nausea, hypotension, and arrhythmias occur only with a very high serum level.[59]

Metabolic Acidosis

TPN is a source of hydrogen ions, both as nonvolatile acids when amino acids are converted into an anion end product and as volatile acids when nutrients are oxidized to CO_2 and H_2O. Additional acid may be generated from the partial combustion of glucose and fat during states of hypoxia, poor tissue perfusion, or hypermetabolism when incomplete glycolysis or lipolysis lead to pyruvic and lactic acid or ketone body accumulation, respectively.[78]

In actual practice, metabolic acidosis associated with TPN administration is no longer a significant complication with current amino acid formulations that contain sufficient bicarbonate precursors in the form of sodium acetate. Nonetheless, metabolic acidosis presents a potentially dangerous problem in those patients receiving TPN who have conditions associated with (1) increased bicarbonate loss, such as with diarrhea, small bowel or pancreatic fistula, or proximal renal tubular acidosis; (2) decreased acid excretion, such as with acute or chronic renal failure, distal renal tubular acidosis, or amphotericin and potassium-sparing diuretic administration; and (3) lactic acid accumulation, such as in shock or sepsis.[71,78] Sodium or potassium can be provided as acetate salts to help correct acidosis.

Researchers have observed that frequent saline flushes contribute to an excessive chloride load in neonates and therefore should be considered in calculating the TPN chloride.[79] Also in neonates, cysteine chloride added to TPN solutions to enhance calcium and phosphate solubility can lead to increased need for acetate.[80]

Glucose Metabolism

Hyperglycemia

Glucose intolerance is among the most common complications of TPN. It may cause significant fluid and electrolyte shifts as well as contribute to the high rates of infection observed with TPN. Hyperglycemia may occur (1) when large glucose doses are initiated too quickly; (2) during stress, infection, steroid administration, pancreatitis, or liver or renal failure; and (3) in susceptible individuals with obesity, diabetes, or a strong family history of diabetes. Limiting total daily carbohydrate initially to 2.5 to 3.0 mg/kg/min in patients at risk for hyperglycemia and 5.0 mg/kg/min in all other adults is prudent[81]; 10.0 to 15.0 mg/kg/min is an appropriate dose in children and infants. See Table 21–1 for the calculation of total daily carbohydrate load. Insulin is added in small increments to the TPN formula to maintain serum glucose < 200 mg/dL and urine glucose < 2+. Serum and urine glucose should be monitored every 6 to 8 hours as insulin therapy is adjusted. Glucose levels between 160 and 200 mg/dL are an appropriate goal during stress.[82] Providing a greater proportion of calories as fat may be beneficial in patients with impaired insulin secretion or metabolism. In patients who are severely refractory to exogenous insulin (ie, requiring up to 100 units insulin per liter TPN), an insulin drip may achieve better glucose control. The insulin dose must be carefully titrated and all pertinent staff made acutely aware that the separate insulin and glucose infusions must not be individually interrupted. Several authors have discussed management of the diabetic patient on TPN.[83–86]

Hyperglycemic, hyperosmolar nonketotic coma is a serious complication that underscores the importance of glucose surveillance in patients on TPN. The syndrome occurs when severe hyperglycemia raises plasma osmolality and leads to a large osmotic diuresis, hypernatremia, dehydration, stupor, coma, and eventually death. The mortality rate is estimated at 40% to 50%. Diabetes, stress, and uremia aggravate hyperosmolar coma.[73] Therapy includes the immediate termination of TPN, infusion of hypotonic saline and regular insulin (10 to 20 units/hour) to lower blood glucose slowly. Metabolic acidosis is corrected with bicarbonate administration.

Hypoglycemia

The most common cause of hypoglycemia during TPN is excessive insulin administration. Patients on insulin therapy with labile glucose levels are best managed with insulin drips that are titrated frequently. Rebound hypoglycemia as a consequence of abrupt discontinuation of TPN appears to be a rare event; multiple studies have documented the safety of this practice in both adults and children over 2 years old.[87–90] Patients with labile serum glucose levels or decreasing insulin requirements (eg, those on a taper of steroid therapy), however, should be observed for this potential complication. Symptoms include headache, nausea, diaphoresis, tremors, confusion, and eventually death.

Fat Metabolism

Hyperlipidemia

Hyperlipidemia is most often associated with excess doses or administration rates relative to the individual's ability to clear lipid emulsions from the bloodstream. Critically ill patients with major organ dysfunction may exhibit less efficient clearance and thus require frequent monitoring for elevated blood lipids.[91] Reducing the dose and/or lengthening the infusion time usually lowers postinfusion serum triglyceride levels. Most ill patients tolerate an administration rate of lipids at 0.1 g/kg/hr, and stable patients on cyclic schedules tolerate 0.15 g/kg/hr.[92] Administration of 10% lipid emulsions results in a hyperlipidemia associated with an abnormal metabolite lipoprotein X, apparently due to a high phospholipid-to-triglyceride ratio.[93,94] Thus, more clinicians prefer the use of 20% lipid emulsions. Pancreatitis due to fat emulsion-induced hyperlipidemia is rare; when this occurs, as with pathological hyperlipoproteinemias, the use of intravenous lipid is contraindicated.[92]

Essential Fatty Acid Deficiency

Essential fatty acid deficiency was an early complication of TPN because of the unavailability of fat emulsions in the United States until 1975. As long as linoleic acid is provided as at least 4% of total calories in adults and 2% in infants, this syndrome is not observed except in individuals who exhibit an allergic reaction or an absolute contraindication for several weeks or longer to intravenous fat.

Stressed patients receiving fat-free TPN demonstrate biochemical evidence of essential fatty acid deficiency within a matter of weeks[95]; relatively stable patients may become deficient within 1 month.[96] Clinical manifestations include dermatitis, alopecia, thrombocytopenia, anemia, poor wound healing, increased serum liver enzymes, and fatty liver; these symptoms occur as early as 6 weeks after the initiation of fat-free TPN.[71] Cutaneous application or oral ingestion of linoleic-rich oils have alleviated biochemical deficiency.[96–98]

When intravenous fat cannot be safely given to an individual on TPN for longer than 1 to 2 months, an assay for fatty acid status is recommended. Decreased plasma levels of linoleic acid and arachidonic acid (tetraene) and an increased plasma level of eicosatrienoic acid (triene), with a triene:tetraene ratio > 0.4 is evidence of biochemical deficiency.

Acute Allergic Reaction

Immediate, adverse reactions to lipids occur in a small fraction of individuals. Allergic reactions are due to the egg component. Acute adverse reactions include hyperlipemia, dyspnea, cyanosis, flushing, sweating, dizziness, headache, back or chest pain, and nausea and vomiting.

Carnitine Deficiency

Carnitine carries fatty acids from cytoplasm to their site of oxidation in the mitochondria. Carnitine deficiency leads to fatty liver, fatty muscle, impaired ketogenesis, and neurologic symptoms. Despite the observation of hypocarnitinemia in infants and adults on TPN, alterations in fat metabolism have not been clearly demonstrated.[99] Some investigators suggest carnitine supplementation for neonates receiving TPN for more than 2 weeks.[100]

Protein Metabolism

Azotemia

When patients with normal renal function receive TPN, BUN may rise compared to pre-TPN levels but should remain within the normal laboratory range. An elevated BUN related to dehydration is corrected by appropriate fluid therapy. Prerenal azotemia can lead to osmotic diuresis and dehydration.[73]

In patients with mild to moderate renal insufficiency, determining when protein intake is excessive and requires modification is often difficult, especially when intercurrent catabolism or steroid administration stimulate nitrogen release into the bloodstream. Manipulation of the intravenous protein to levels no lower than 0.8 g/kg[91] and observation of the effect on BUN may guide therapy in the individual patient. In patients with significant azotemia, ideally dialysis therapy accompanies TPN so that full nutrition support can be provided to minimize the contribution of muscle catabolism to the urea pool.

Hyperammonemia

The incidence of hyperammonemia decreased with the advent of crystalline amino acid solution. Early protein hydrolysates contained excessive amounts of ammonia and insufficient arginine for urea cycle metabolism. Hyperammonemia, however, has been observed with amino acid solutions in children, infants, and patients with urea cycle defects, such as ornithine transcarbamylase deficiency.[101,102]

Plasma Amino Acid Imbalance

Low plasma levels of the nonessential amino acids tyrosine and cysteine have been reported in infants and cirrhotic adults receiving tyrosine- and cysteine-free TPN.[103,104] The liver enzyme system that converts phenylalanine to tyrosine and methionine to cysteine appears impaired. Low levels of plasma taurine, another nonessential amino acid, have also been observed in infants[105] and adults[106] and are implicated in experimental models as a cause of TPN-associated biliary stasis.[107,108] Pediatric amino acid solutions containing tyrosine, cysteine, and taurine normalize plasma amino acids, result in better weight gain, and appear to decrease liver complications in neonates on TPN.[109–111] Whether older infants and children as well as adults require these nonessential amino acids during TPN remains undetermined.

A deficiency of glutamine, another nonessential amino acid that is a preferential fuel for both the gastrointestinal tract and lymphocytes and is lacking in TPN solutions because of instability, has been described in patients on TPN. Glutamine-supplemented TPN appears to result in improved nitrogen balance,[112,113] maintenance of gut mucosal architecture,[114] and enhanced immunity[115,116] compared to standard TPN solutions in humans. However, glutamine failed to reduce gastrointestinal toxicity due to chemotherapy.[117] No guidelines have been developed for specific indications and doses of either intravenous or oral glutamine as a supplement to TPN. Similarly, arginine may be relatively deficient in available TPN formulations, but no minimum recommended levels have been determined.[118]

Imbalances in other plasma amino acids, which standard amino acid formulations may aggravate, have been noted in a variety of other clinical situations. The clinical benefits of solutions enriched with branched-chain amino acid in stressed and injured patients with low circulating levels of these amino acids have not been adequately demonstrated, and widespread use is not warranted.[119,120] Branched-chain enriched formulations that have reduced content of aromatic amino acids and methionine may help reverse hepatic encephalopathy, but should be reserved for patients with documented aberrations in circulating amino acid concentrations as discussed earlier in TPN indications in hepatic disease.[30,32] Hepatic encephalopathy is usually multifactorial in etiology, and amino acid imbalances are rarely the sole causative agent.[121]

Micronutrient Metabolism

Trace Elements

Deficiencies are uncommon when trace elements are appropriately supplemented such as with commercially available combination packages containing copper, zinc, manganese, chromium, and sometimes selenium and molybdenum. Copper and zinc deficits may occur in patients with excessive gastrointestinal losses; unfortunately replacement guidelines are not well described in the literature. One study in adults described zinc losses of up to 17 mg/L of stool or ileostomy output and 10 mg/L of small-bowel fistula or stoma output.[122]

Elevated manganese levels as well as associated neurologic symptoms have been described during TPN in patients with liver disease.[123-127] It is recommended to remove manganese from TPN solutions in patients with persistent hyperbilirubinemia. The biliary excretion of copper may also predispose this trace element toward toxic tissue deposition in the liver,[68] and empirical elimination may be warranted in liver disease.

Serum chromium levels have been elevated in children on long-term TPN, leading to the recommendation to delete it as a routine additive for these patients.[99] When iron dextran is deemed necessary, serum iron level, total iron-binding capacity, and percentage saturation require monitoring every 6 months to ensure adequate replacement and to prevent iron overload.[99]

Vitamins

Current adult and pediatric intravenous multivitamin preparations are formulated to prevent clinically recognizable deficiency and toxicity syndromes. A hypersensitivity reaction has been linked to the polysorbate of the multivitamin formulation.[128] If multivitamins are purposely or inadvertently withheld, the risk of potentially lethal lactic acidosis due to thiamine deficiency cannot be overemphasized.[129-134]

Patients receiving extended periods of TPN support and simultaneous folate-inhibiting drug therapy, such as dilantin, may be at risk for the hematologic manifestations of folate deficiency; serum folate can be monitored or additional folate empirically added to TPN. Both biochemical and clinical vitamin A toxicity have been reported in patients with renal failure on TPN.[135] In such patients, it is recommended to reduce administration of fat-soluble vitamins to twice weekly and provide water-soluble vitamins on a daily basis in lieu of a complete multivitamin preparation.[91] Vitamin K deficiency, manifested as bleeding, may occur in TPN patients with liver disease and low prothrombin levels. Vitamin C has been implicated in the development of hyperoxaluria and renal insufficiency[136,137] and is empirically reduced to < 250 mg/day in renal failure.[91]

Hepatobiliary and Gastrointestinal Abnormalities

Steatosis

Biochemical elevations of aminotransferase values and alkaline phosphatase often occur 1 to 2 weeks after initiation of TPN and are associated with histologic evidence of fatty infiltration within liver cells. Steatosis, or fatty liver, is the most common hepatic complication of TPN in adults, whereas cholestasis is more prevalent in children.[138] The incidence of steatosis has decreased with the more moderate provision of total energy and the substitution of dextrose kcal with 10% to 30% kcal as lipid.[138,139] Medium-chain triglycerides appear to offer a further protective effect.[140] Other pathogenic mechanisms in the development of steatosis have been implicated, including infusion of excess quantities of amino acids; high calorie-to-nitrogen ratios; and deficiencies of glutamine, essential fatty acids, carnitine, or choline.[138,141] Steatosis is a transient, reversible phenomenon in patients on short-term TPN.

Cholestasis

Intrahepatic cholestasis may be observed after 2 to 6 weeks of TPN therapy and is signaled by a rise in alkaline phosphatase, followed by elevation of bilirubin and to a lesser extent serum glutamic-oxaloacetic transaminase and serum gamma-glutamyltransferase. It may be more common than laboratory findings would suggest.[138] Etiologic factors in infants include immaturity of the biliary secretory system, absence of oral intake, sepsis, the presence of conditions that require gastrointestinal surgery, and hypoxia.[138,142] Taurine supplemented in pediatric amino acid solutions or the administration of ursodeoxycholic acid are approaches used to promote bile flow in infants.[142] Early enteral feeding is encouraged to reduce the risk and severity of cholestasis.[143] In infants with persisting cholestasis even after the cessation of TPN, the provision of exogenous cholecystokinin reversed the hepatic abnormalities.[144,145]

The exact pathogenic mechanisms of cholestasis in adults are unknown, although clinical circumstances that parallel those of neonates are proposed and include sepsis, gastrointestinal pathology (short-bowel syndrome, inflammatory bowel disease, ileal resection), lack of enteral stimulation, and increased production of lithocholate (a bile acid toxic to the liver) during conditions of intestinal bacterial overgrowth.[138] Ursodeoxycholic acid is under investigation as a therapy for cholestasis in adult patients as well.[146] Cyclic TPN, restriction of daily carbohydrate load to < 5.0 mg/kg/min, enteral stimulation (even at minimal amounts), and avoidance of overfeeding by basing energy prescription on accurate measurement of needs are all empirical recommendations to minimize the risk of cholestasis.

Progressive liver disease is rare but has been reported in premature and low-birth-weight infants and in patients on long-term TPN.[138,147,148] Researchers do not know the relative contribution of direct TPN hepatotoxicity in the evolution of chronic serious liver disease versus other causes related to the primary disease, complications such as sepsis, and drug toxicities.

Gallbladder Stasis and Cholelithiasis

Sludge in the gallbladder is a common ultrasound finding in patients on TPN longer than 4 weeks. Patients with ileal disorders (short-bowel syndrome or ileal disease)[99] or obesity[149] are particularly predisposed to gallstone formation. Impaired bile flow and gallbladder stasis during TPN may lead to cholestasis.[138] Encouraging oral intake or initiating tube feeding as early as possible to stimulate gallbladder function is the best prophylaxis for gallbladder complications. Alternatively, exogenous cholecystokinin is reported to reduce stasis.[150] Acute cholecystitis should be suspected in patients on TPN longer than 1 month who experience abdominal pain.[99]

Gastrointestinal Atrophy

Lack of luminal nutrients during TPN is associated with villous hypoplasia, colonic mucosal atrophy, decreased gastric function, impaired gastrointestinal immunity, and gut bacterial translocation in experimental models.[118,151] The relevance of these findings to humans is yet to be determined. Intestinal alterations due to TPN appear to be much less pronounced in humans than those observed in animals.[114,152,153] In a large, prospective study of surgical patients, bacterial translocation was not associated with the administration of TPN.[154] Furthermore, normal volunteers on 2 weeks of TPN failed to demonstrate any decrease in concentrations of secretory immunoglobulin A and intraepithelial cells, important components of gastrointestinal immunity.[155] Glutamine has been investigated as a conditionally essential amino acid during TPN to maintain gut function,[114,156] although its efficacy remains to be established[157,158]; in fact, it may have deleterious effects on liver enzymes when used for extended periods.[159] In general, the quantity and characteristics of enteral nutrients necessary to prevent adverse gastrointestinal sequelae in humans are unknown; the prudent clinician minimizes as much as clinically possible the length of time a patient is NPO and provides as complex an enteral diet as is tolerated.

Respiratory Abnormalities

A large carbohydrate intake increases CO_2 production,[160-163] but there is no convincing evidence that this phenomenon is clinically important in patients without preexisting pulmonary disease.[164] Excessive amino acid intakes also increase resting metabolic expenditure, O^2 consumption, and CO^2 production.[165,166] Fat emulsions at rapid infusion rates (4 to 8 hours) may impair pulmonary diffusion capacity, likely by providing precursors for eicosanoids, potent metabolites that can alter pulmonary vasomotor tone.[92,167] Slow infusion rates (18 to 24 hours) are important for patients with marginal pulmonary reserves, and clinicians should be alert to the potential impact of lipids on oxygenation.[167]

Hematological Abnormalities

Thrombocytopenia

Recurrent chronic thrombocytopenia in children on TPN longer than 3 months for short-bowel syndrome has been attributed to lipid emulsions.[168] However, in neonates no change in platelet count was observed with fat infusion.[169] Slow infusions of lipids have minimal effect on platelet aggregation and bleeding time.[170] Even preexisting thrombocytopenia is not a contraindication to the use of lipid emulsions.[171] Fat emulsions appear to depress circulating levels of tissue plasminogen activator, but the clinical significance of this phenomenon is unknown.[172]

Hemolytic Anemia

Hemolytic anemia due to the "fat overload syndrome" is a rare complication of lipid emulsions, but should be recognized as a potential consequence of hyperlipemia.[92]

Immunologic Impairment

TPN is associated with high infection rates compared to no feeding[3,22] or enteral feeding.[24,25] Some hypotheses that have been suggested for this phenomenon are overfeeding of glucose or lipid, specific nutrient deficiencies (eg, glutamine), and lack of enteral stimulation of gut immunity. Elevated serum glucose impairs neutrophil and complement function and predisposes patients to candida infections.[173,174] In infants, lipid infusion is associated with an increased risk for bacteremia, possibly by promoting bacterial growth in the central venous access line rather than a direct effect of lipids on immunity.[175] Indeed, the weight of the evidence suggests that large amounts of lipids (up to 4 g/kg) and fast infusion rates (100 to 200 mL/hr of 20% emulsions) beyond what is routinely recommended in clinical practice are required to demonstrate an adverse effect on neutrophil, phagocyte, and reticuloendothelial system function.[176] There is no evidence that lipids affect humoral immunity or the complement system, and their impact on cellular immunity (T-cell lymphocyte activities) is not clearly established.[177] The role of alternative preparations to omega-6 fatty acid–based emulsions on the inflammatory response and other immune activities is under investigation, and these alternative preparations may become pharmacologically significant components of TPN for specific patient populations at risk for altered immunocompetence.[177,178]

DETERMINATION OF AN END POINT TO THERAPY

Therapeutic Goals

The general goals of nutrition therapy are established prior to the initiation of TPN and reevaluated frequently. Minimizing the length of time on TPN to that which is medically necessary not only contains costs, but also may help prevent hepatobiliary, gastrointestinal, and infectious complications.

Repletion/Maintenance

Matarese has said that determining when to terminate nutrition support is an art more than a science.[179] There are no single laboratory or nutritional parameters that signal reconstitution of normal nutritional status. General trends may be gleaned from laboratory data, weight, and body composition measures, but more importantly from subjective assessment of stamina and physical functioning. Severely malnourished patients at the start of therapy seldom regain premorbid nutritional status during hospitalization and continue the repletion process in the home setting.[179] The patient's clinical condition and ability to resume and progressively increase enteral intake, whether by tube or mouth, provide signposts for the end of therapy, especially in patients with relatively intact lean body stores.

Discharge Planning

Ideally, discharge planning should be considered when the therapeutic goals are established. If it is anticipated that the patient will be discharged without TPN, the health care team should plan for a period of transition to an oral diet or tube feeding. If TPN is required after discharge, the health care team must ensure that safe, effective therapy can be delivered and appropriately monitored at home either in a hospital-based program or by a carefully selected vendor. If an extended-care facility will be providing further medical care, it may or may not be willing to accept TPN patients.

Prognosis

When to discontinue TPN in a patient with a known terminal illness or extremely poor prognosis is usually a difficult ethical decision. To guide such decisions, it has been recommended that facilities develop and periodically review written protocols for the provision and termination of nutrition support with the help of legal and ethical counsel.[180] The patient's wishes should be considered foremost, but other factors may influence a decision including the medical risks of continuing therapy and, if the patient may otherwise be discharged from the hospital, the financial and/or medical feasibility to continue TPN at home or in another health care facility.

Transitional Feeding Techniques

Resumption of adequate oral intake to sustain nutritional status is an individualized process in patients on TPN. Variables that may affect the length of transition to an oral diet include the length of time the patient is NPO; the severity of gastrointestinal disturbances; ongoing medication therapy; the flexibility of the hospital food system; and the patient's subjective food preferences, motivation, and social/financial support system. Separating psychologic, disease-related, and TPN-related variables that adversely affect oral intake is often difficult, as parenteral solutions appear to have an independent physiologic effect as well. In experimental models, high concentrations of glucose and amino acids in the blood decrease appetite,[181] and when disease pathology has been eliminated as a variable, appetite remains suppressed 1 to 2 weeks following complete cessation of TPN.[182] One double-blinded clinical trial involving patients undergoing marrow transplantation and on TPN demonstrated that patients who were randomized to receive only intravenous hydration at hospital discharge resumed adequate oral intake significantly earlier than those randomized to continue TPN; there were no apparent adverse consequences (as measured by weight status and hospital readmission rate) from terminating TPN at hospital discharge, even in patients with low oral energy intakes.[183] Transition to enteral tube feeding is often less difficult because of the control the clinician exerts in the formula, method, and rate of enteral nutrition provided.

Gastrointestinal Function

It is recommended that patients demonstrate adequate gastrointestinal function prior to tapering TPN. If at the initiation of enteral intake, gastrointestinal function is suboptimal with signs of delayed gastric emptying, diarrhea, nausea, or vomiting, a conservative approach to refeeding is indicated. If gastrointestinal symptoms become aggravated by oral or tube feeding, attempts should be discontinued or modified by decreasing the rate of the tube feeding, using an elemental or semielemental formula, or limiting the amount and the complexity of the oral diet.

Tapering Methods

Ideally TPN is tapered as enteral tube or oral intake increases such that intravenous and enteral intake together meet estimated nutrient requirements. Documentation of actual oral intake, including fluids, is important. Cyclic TPN provided during the evening and night over 10 to 16 hours, depending on the patient's nutritional status and nutrient needs, frees the patient from the physiologic effects of a continuous infusion. In some patients who have no ongoing gastrointestinal disturbances and are otherwise clinically stable, a trial off TPN may be successful.[183]

CONCLUSIONS

TPN may be a lifesaving modality for patients whose illnesses do not permit adequate nourishment via the gastrointestinal tract. Because serious complications may arise from the use of TPN, it should be reserved for indicated conditions. TPN requires the skills of many disciplines to prescribe, administer, and monitor it in a safe and appropriate manner. In the future, the indications for TPN will likely be further defined. The components of TPN will also be manipulated to treat and/or better support specific clinical conditions.

REFERENCES

1. McGeer AJ, Detsky AS, O'Rourke K. Parenteral nutrition in cancer patients undergoing chemotherapy: a meta-analysis. *Nutrition.* 1990;6:233–240.

2. Detsky AS, Baker JP, O'Rourke K, Goel V. Perioperative parenteral nutrition: a meta-analysis. *Ann Intern Med.* 1987;107:195–203.

3. Veterans Affairs Total Parenteral Nutrition Cooperative Study Group. Perioperative total parenteral nutrition in surgical patients. *N Engl J Med.* 1991;325:525–532.

4. Klein S, Koretz RL. Nutrition support in patients with cancer: what do the data really show? *Nutr Clin Pract.* 1994;9:91–100.

5. Brennan MF, Pisters PW, Posner M, Quesada O, et al. A prospective randomized trial of total parenteral nutrition after major pancreatic resection for malignancy. *Ann Surg.* 1994;220:436–444.

6. Health and Public Policy Committee, American College of Physicians. Parenteral nutrition in patients receiving cancer chemotherapy. *Ann Intern Med.* 1989;110:734–736.

7. American Society of Parenteral and Enteral Nutrition Board of Directors. Guidelines for the use of parenteral and enteral nutrition in adult and pediatric patients. *J Parenter Enter Nutr.* 1993;17(suppl):1SA–52SA.

8. Nightingale JM, Lennard-Jones JE, Gertner DJ, Wood SR, et al. Colonic preservation reduces need for parenteral therapy, increases incidence of renal stones, but does not change high prevalence of gallstones in patients with a short bowel. *Gut.* 1992;33:1493–1497.

9. Nightingale JM. The short-bowel syndrome. *Eur J Gastroenterol Hepatol.* 1995;7:514–520.

10. Jeejeebhoy KN. Short bowel syndrome. In: Shils ME, Olson JA, Shike M, eds. *Modern Nutrition in Health and Disease.* 8th ed. Philadelphia: Lea & Febiger; 1994:1036–1042.

11. Klein S. Influence of nutrition support on clinical outcome in short bowel syndrome and inflammatory bowel disease. *Nutrition.* 1995;11(suppl 2):233–237.

12. Purdum PP III, Kirby DF. Short-bowel syndrome: a review of the role of nutrition support. *J Parenter Enter Nutr.* 1991;15:93–101.

13. Byrne TA, Persinger RL, Young LS, Ziegler TR, et al. A new treatment for patients with short-bowel syndrome: growth hormone, glutamine, and a modified diet. *Ann Surg.* 1995;222:243–254.

14. Lerebours E, Messing B, Chevalier B, Bories C, et al. An evaluation of total parenteral nutrition in the management of steroid-dependent and steroid-resistant patients with Crohn's disease. *J Parenter Enter Nutr.* 1986;10:274–278.

15. Sitzmann JV, Coverse RL Jr, Bayless TM. Favorable response to parenteral nutrition and medical therapy in Crohn's colitis: a report of 38 patients comparing severe Crohn's and ulcerative colitis. *Gastroenterology.* 1990;99:1647–1652.

16. Lochs H, Marosi L, Ferenci P, Hortnage H. Has total bowel rest a beneficial effect in the treatment of Crohn's disease? *Clin Nutr.* 1983;2:61–64.

17. Jones VA. Comparison of total parenteral nutrition and elemental diet in induction of remission of Crohn's disease: Long-term maintenance of remission by personalized food exclusion diets. *Dig Dis Sci.* 1987;32(suppl):100S–107S.

18. Greenberg GR, Fleming CR, Jeejeebhoy KN, Rosenberg HH, et al. Controlled trial of bowel rest and nutritional support in the management of Crohn's disease. *Gut.* 1988;29:1309–1315.

19. Afonso JJ, Rombeau JL. Parenteral nutrition for patients with inflammatory bowel disease. In: Rombeau JL, Caldwell MD, eds. *Clinical Nutrition: Parenteral Nutrition.* 2nd ed. Philadelphia: WB Saunders Co; 1993;2:427–441.

20. Gonzalez-Huiz F, Fernandez-Banares F, Esteve-Comas M, Abad-Lacruz A, et al. Enteral versus parenteral nutrition as adjunct therapy in acute ulcerative colitis. *Am J Gastroenterol.* 1993;88: 227–232.

21. Meguid MM, Campos ACL. Gastrointestinal fistulas: clinical and nutritional management. In: Rombeau JL, Caldwell MD, eds. *Clinical Nutrition: Parenteral Nutrition.* 2nd ed. Philadelphia: WB Saunders Co; 1993;2:462–497.

22. Weisdorf SA, Lysne J, Wind D, Haake RJ, et al. Positive effect of prophylactic total parenteral nutrition on long-term outcome of bone marrow transplantation. *Transplantation.* 1987;43:833–838.

23. Tanphaichitr V, Leelahagul P. Principles and practice of nutritional support in diarrhea. *Nutr Clin Pract.* 1988;3:14–18.

24. Kudsk KA, Croce MA, Fabian TC, Minard G, et al. Enteral versus parenteral feeding: effects on septic morbidity after blunt and penetrating abdominal trauma. *Ann Surg.* 1992;215:503–511.

25. Moore FA, Feliciano DV, Andrassy RJ, McArdle AH, et al. Early enteral feeding, compared with parenteral, reduces postoperative septic complications. *Ann Surg.* 1992;216:172–183.

26. Hill GL. Body composition research: implications for the practice of clinical nutrition. *J Parenter Enter Nutr.* 1992;16:197–218.

27. Sax HC, Warner BW, Talamini MA, Hamilton FN, et al. Early total parenteral nutrition in acute pancreatitis: lack of beneficial effects. *Am J Surg.* 1987;153:117–124.

28. Helton WS. Intravenous nutrition in patients with acute pancreatitis. In: Rombeau JL, Caldwell MD, eds. *Clinical Nutrition: Parenteral Nutrition.* 2nd ed. Philadelphia: WB Saunders Co; 1993;2:442–461.

29. Pisters PW, Ranson JH. Nutritional support in acute pancreatitis. *Surg Gynecol Obstet.* 1992;175:275–284.

30. Freund HR, Fischer JE. The use of branched chain amino acids (BCAA) in acute hepatic encephalopathy. *Clin Nutr.* 1986;5:135–138.

31. Driscoll DF, Palombo JD, Bistrian BR. Nutritional and metabolic considerations of the adult liver transplant candidate and organ donor. *Nutrition.* 1995;11:255–263.

32. Shronts EP, Teasley KM, Thoele SL, Cerra FB. Nutrition support of the adult liver transplant candidate. *J Am Diet Assoc.* 1987;87:441–451.

33. Feinstein EI. Total parenteral nutritional support of patients with acute renal failure. *Nutr Clin Pract.* 1988;3:9–13.

34. Kirby DF, Fiorenza V, Craig RM. Intravenous nutritional support during pregnancy. *J Parenter Enter Nutr.* 1988;12:72–80.

35. Zibell-Frisk D, Jen KL, Rick J. Use of parenteral nutrition to maintain adequate nutritional status in hyperemesis gravidarum. *J Perinatol.* 1990;10:390–395.

36. Charlin V, Borghesi L, Hasbun J, Von Mulenbrock R, et al. Parenteral nutrition in hyperemesis gravidarum. *Nutrition.* 1993;9:29–32.

37. MacBurney M, Wilmore DW. Parenteral nutrition in pregnancy. In: Rombeau JL, Caldwell MD, eds. *Clinical Nutrition: Parenteral Nutrition.* 2nd ed. Philadelphia: WB Saunders Co; 1993;2:696–715.

38. Goldbloom DS, Garfinkel PE. Anorexia nervosa and bulima. In: Jeejeebhoy KN, ed. *Current Therapy in Nutrition.* Philadelphia: BC Decker Inc; 1988:370–381.

39. Miles JM, Klein JA. Should protein be included in calorie calculations for a TPN prescription? point-counterpoint. *Nutr Clin Pract.* 1996;11:204–206.

40. CDC guidelines on infection control. *Infect Control.* 1982;3:52–72.

41. Ebbert ML, Farraj M, Hwang LT. The incidence and clinical significance of intravenous fat emulsion contamination during infusion. *J Parenter Enter Nutr.* 1987;11:42–45.

42. Lykins TC. Nutrition support clinical pathways. *Nutr Clin Pract.* 1996;11:16–20.

43. Aker SN, Cheney CL, Sanders JE, Lenssen PL, et al. Nutritional support in marrow graft recipients with single versus double lumen right atrial catheters. *Exp Hematol.* 1982;10:732–737.

44. Konstantinides FN. Nitrogen balance studies in clinical nutrition. *Nutr Clin Pract.* 1992;7:231–238.

45. Boehm KA, Helms RA, Storm MC. Assessing the validity of adjusted urinary urea nitrogen as an estimate of total urinary nitrogen in three pediatric populations. *J Parenter Enter Nutr.* 1994;18:172–176.

46. Milner EA, Cioffi WG, Mason AD Jr, McManus WF, et al. Accuracy of urinary urea nitrogen for predicting total urinary nitrogen in thermally injured patients. *J Parenter Enter Nutr.* 1993;17:414–416.

47. Kopple JD. Uses and limitations of the balance technique. *J Parenter Enter Nutr.* 1987;11(suppl 5):79–85.

48. Fleck A, Raines G, Hawker F, Trotter J, et al. Increased vascular permeability: a major cause of hypoalbuminaemia in disease and injury. *Lancet.* 1985;1:781–784.

49. Prealbumin in Nutritional Care Consensus Group. Measurement of visceral protein status in assessing protein and energy malnutrition: standard of care. *Nutrition.* 1995;11:169–171.

50. Church JM, Hill GL. Assessing the efficacy of intravenous nutrition in general surgical patients: dynamic nutritional assessment with plasma proteins. *J Parenter Enter Nutr.* 1987;11:135–139.

51. Carpentier YA, Barthel J, Bruyns J. Plasma protein concentrations in nutritional assessment. *Proc Nutr Soc.* 1982;41:405–417.

52. Hill GL, Windsor JA. Nutritional assessment in clinical practice. *Nutrition.* 1995;11(suppl 2):198–201.

53. Heymsfield SB, Casper K. Anthropometric assessment of the adult hospitalized patient. *J Parenter Enter Nutr.* 1987;11(suppl 5):36–41.

54. Walser M. Creatinine excretion as a measure of protein nutrition in adults of varying age. *J Parenter Enter Nutr.* 1987;11(suppl 5):73–78.

55. Lukaski HC. Methods for the assessment of human body composition: traditional and new. *Am J Clin Nutr.* 1987;46:537–556.

56. Robert S, Zarowitz BJ, Hyzy R, Eichenhorn M, et al. Bioelectrical impedance assessment of nutritional status in critically ill patients. *Am J Clin Nutr.* 1993;57:840–844.

57. Scheltinga MR, Young LS, Benfell K, Bye RL, et al. Glutamine-enriched intravenous feedings attenuate extracellular fluid expansion after a standard stress. *Ann Surg.* 1991;214:385–395.

58. Jacobs DO, Scheltinga MRM. Metabolic assessment. In: Rombeau JL, Caldwell MD, eds. *Clinical Nutrition: Parenteral Nutrition.* 2nd ed. Philadelphia: WB Saunders Co; 1993:245–274.

59. Cogan MG. *Fluid and Electrolytes: Physiology and Pathophysiology.* Norwalk, CT: Appleton & Lange; 1991.

60. Leung FY. Trace elements in parenteral micronutrition. *Clin Biochem.* 1995;28:561–566.

61. Kinney J. The search for clinical relevance. *Nutr Clin Pract.* 1992;7:203–206.

62. McClave SA, Snider HL. Use of indirect calorimetry in clinical nutrition. *Nutr Clin Pract.* 1992;7:207–221.

63. Porter C, Cohen NH. Indirect calorimetry in critically ill patients: role of the clinical dietitian in interpreting results. *J Am Diet Assoc.* 1996;96:49–54, 57.

64. Carpentier YA, Thonnart N. Parameters for evaluation of lipid metabolism. *J Parenter Enter Nutr.* 1987;11(suppl 5):104–108.

65. Adamkin DH, Gelke KN, Andrews BF. Fat emulsions and hypertriglyceridemia. *J Parenter Enter Nutr.* 1984;5:563–567.

66. Roesner M, Grant JP. Intravenous lipid emulsions. *Nutr Clin Pract.* 1987;2:96–107.

67. Carlson LA, Rossner RA. Methodological study of an intravenous fat tolerance test with intralipid emulsion. *Scand J Clin Lab Invest.* 1972;29:271–280.

68. Albina JE, Melnik G. Fluid, electrolytes and body composition. In: Rombeau JL, Caldwell MD, eds. *Clinical Nutrition: Parenteral Nutrition.* 2nd ed. Philadelphia: WB Saunders Co; 1993:132–149.

69. Halperin ML, Jeejeebhoy KN, Levine DZ. Acid-base, fluid and electrolyte aspects of parenteral nutrition. In: Kokko JP, Tannen RL, eds. *Fluids and Electrolytes.* Philadelphia: WB Saunders Co; 1986:817–831.

70. Klotz R. Do the crystalline amino acid formulas impact acid-base balance in the patient on parenteral nutrition? *Hosp Pharm.* 1988;23:78–82.

71. Rudman D, Williams PJ. Nutrient deficiencies during total parenteral nutrition. *Nutr Rev.* 1985;43:1–13.

72. Solomon SM, Kirby DF. The refeeding syndrome: a review. *J Parenter Enter Nutr.* 1990;14:90–97.

73. Giner M, Curtas S. Adverse metabolic consequences of nutritional support: macronutrients. *Surg Clin North Am.* 1986;66:1025–1047.

74. Miller SJ, Simpson J. Medication-nutrient interactions: hypophosphatemia associated with sucralfate in the intensive care unit. *Nutr Clin Pract.* 1991;6:199–201.

75. Pak CYC. Calcium disorders: hypercalcemia and hypocalcemia. In: Kokko JP, Tannen RL, eds. *Fluids and Electrolytes.* Philadelphia: WB Saunders Co; 1986:472–501.

76. Wood RJ, Sitrin MD, Cusson GJ, Rosenberg IH. Reduction of total parenteral nutrition-induced urinary calcium loss by increasing the phosphorus in the total parenteral nutrition prescription. *J Parenter Enter Nutr.* 1986;10:188–190.

77. Howard L, Alger S, Michalek A, Heaphey L, et al. Home parenteral nutrition in adults. In: Rombeau JL, Caldwell MD, eds. *Clinical Nutrition: Parenteral Nutrition.* 2nd ed. Philadelphia: WB Saunders Co; 1993:814–839.

78. Kushner RF. Total parenteral nutrition-associated metabolic acidosis. *J Parenter Enter Nutr.* 1986;10:306–310.

79. Groh-Wargo S, Ciaccia A, Moore J. Neonatal metabolic acidosis: effect of chloride from normal saline flushes. *J Parenter Enter Nutr.* 1988;12:159–161.

80. Laine L, Shulman RJ, Pitre D, Lifschitz CH, et al. Cysteine usage increases the need for acetate in neonates who receive total parenteral nutrition. *Am J Clin Nutr.* 1991;54:565–567.

81. Rosmarin DK, Wardlaw GM, Mirtallo J. Hyperglycemia associated with continuous infusion rates of total parenteral nutrition dextrose. *Nutr Clin Pract.* 1996;11:151–156.

82. Mizock B. Alterations in carbohydrate metabolism during stress: a review of the literature. *Am J Med.* 1995;98:75–85.

83. McMahon M, Manji N, Driscoll DF, Bistrian BR. Parenteral nutrition in patients with diabetes mellitus: theoretical and practical considerations. *J Parenter Enter Nutr.* 1989;13:545–553.

84. Sunyecz LA, Cicci AJ, Mirtallo J. Nutrition support of the diabetic patient. *J Pharm Pract.* 1992;5:290–299.

85. Ziegler TR, Smith RJ. Parenteral nutrition in patients with diabetes mellitus. In: Rombeau JL, Caldwell MD, eds. *Clinical Nutrition: Parenteral Nutrition.* 2nd ed. Philadelphia: WB Saunders Co; 1993:649–666.

86. Hongsermeier T, Bistrian BR. Evaluation of a practical technique for determining insulin requirements in diabetic patients receiving total parenteral nutrition. *J Parenter Enter Nutr.* 1993;17:16–19.

87. Wagman LD, Newsome HH, Miller KB, Thomas RB, et al. The effect of acute discontinuation of total parenteral nutrition. *Ann Surg.* 1986;204:524–529.

88. Krzywda EA, Andris DA, Whipple JK, Street CC, et al. Glucose response to abrupt initiation and discontinuance of total parenteral nutrition. *J Parenter Enter Nutr.* 1993;17:64–67.

89. Werlin SL, Wyatt D, Camitta B. Effect of abrupt discontinuation of high glucose infusions during parenteral nutrition. *J Pediatr.* 1994;124:441–444.

90. Eisenberg PG, Gianino S, Clutter WE, Fleshman JW. Abrupt discontinuation of cycled parenteral nutrition is safe. *Dis Colon Rectum.* 1995;38:933–939.

91. Druml W. Nutritional support in acute renal failure. *Clin Nutr.* 1993;12:196–207.

92. Carpentier YA, Van Gossum A, Dubois DY, Deckelbaum RJ. Lipid metabolism in parenteral nutrition. In: Rombeau JL, Caldwell MD, eds. *Clinical Nutrition: Parenteral Nutrition.* 2nd ed. Philadelphia: WB Saunders Co; 1993:35–74.

93. Tashiro T, Mashima Y, Yamamori H, Horibe K, et al. Increased lipoprotein X causes hyperlipidemia during intravenous administration of 10% fat emulsion in man. *J Parenter Enter Nutr.* 1991;15:546–550.

94. Messing B, Peynet J, Poupon J, Pfeiffer A, et al. Effect of fat-emulsion phospholipids on serum lipoprotein profile during 1 mo of cyclic parenteral nutrition. *Am J Clin Nutr.* 1990;52:1094–1100.

95. Clemans GW, Yamanaka W, Flournoy N, Aker SN, et al. Plasma fatty acid patterns of bone marrow transplant patients primarily supported by fat-free parenteral nutrition. *J Parenter Enter Nutr.* 1981;5:221–225.

96. Miller DG, Williams SK, Palombo JD, Griffin RE, et al. Cutaneous application of safflower oil in preventing essential fatty acid deficiency in patients on home parenteral nutrition. *Am J Clin Nutr.* 1987;46:419–423.

97. Richardson TJ, Sgoutas D. Essential fatty acid deficiency in four adult patients during total parenteral nutrition. *Am J Clin Nutr.* 1975;2:258–263.

98. Friedman Z, Shochat SJ, Maisels MJ, Marks KH, et al. Correction of essential fatty acid deficiency in newborn infants by cutaneous application of sunflower-seed oil. *Pediatrics.* 1976;58:650–654.

99. Moukarzel AA, Ament ME. Home parenteral nutrition in infants and children. In: Rombeau JL, Caldwell MD, eds. *Clinical Nutrition: Parenteral Nutrition.* 2nd ed. Philadelphia: WB Saunders Co; 1993:791–813.

100. Tibboel D, Delemarre FM, Przyrembel H, Bos AP, et al. Carnitine deficiency in surgical neonates receiving total parenteral nutrition. *J Pediatr Surg.* 1990;25:418–421.

101. Seashore JH, Seashore MR, Riely C. Hyperammonemia during total parenteral nutrition in children. *J Parenter Enter Nutr.* 1982;6:114–118.

102. Felig DM, Brusilow SW, Boyer JL. Hyperammonemic coma due to parenteral nutrition in a woman with heterozygous ornithine transcarbamylase deficiency. *Gastroenterology.* 1995;109:282–284.

103. Laidlaw SA, Kopple JD. New concepts of the indispensable amino acid. *Am J Clin Nutr.* 1987;46:593–605.

104. Rudman D, Kutner M, Ansley J, Jansen R, et al. Hypotyrosinemia, hypocystinemia, and failure to retain nitrogen during total parenteral nutrition of cirrhotic patients. *Gastroenterology.* 1981;81:1025–1035.

105. Zelikovic I, Chesney RW, Friedman AL, Ahlfors CE. Taurine depletion in very low birth weight infants receiving prolonged total parenteral nutrition: role of renal immaturity. *J Pediatr.* 1990;116:301–306.

106. Desai TK, Maliakkal J, Kinzie JL, Shrinpreis MN, et al. Taurine deficiency after intensive chemotherapy and/or radiation. *Am J Clin Nutr.* 1992;55:708–711.

107. Guertin F, Roy CC, LePage G, Perea A, et al. Effect of taurine on total parenteral nutrition-associated cholestasis. *J Parenter Enter Nutr.* 1991;15:247–251.

108. Belli DC. Taurine in TPN solutions? *Nutrition.* 1994;10:82–84.

109. Helms RA, Christensen ML, Mauer EC, Storm MC. Comparison of a pediatric versus standard amino acid formulation in preterm neonates requiring parenteral nutrition. *J Pediatr.* 1987;110:466–470.

110. Heird WC, Dell RB, Helms RA, Greene HL, et al. Amino acid mixture designed to maintain normal plasma amino acid patterns in infants and children requiring parenteral nutrition. *Pediatrics.* 1987;80:401–408.

111. Beck R. Use of a pediatric parenteral amino acid mixture in a population of extremely low birth weight neonates: frequency and spectrum of direct bilirubinemia. *Am J Perinatol.* 1990;7:84–86.

112. Stehle P, Zander J, Mertes N, Albers S, et al. Effect of parenteral glutamine peptide supplements on muscle glutamine loss and nitrogen balance after major surgery. *Lancet.* 1989;1:231–233.

113. Ziegler TR, Young LS, Benfall K, Scheltinga M, et al. Clinical and metabolic efficacy of glutamine-supplemented parenteral nutrition after bone marrow transplantation: a randomized, double-blind, controlled study. *Ann Intern Med.* 1992;116:821–828.

114. van der Hulst RRWJ, von Meyenfeldt MF, Arends J-W, von Kreel BK, et al. Glutamine and preservation of gut integrity. *Lancet.* 1993;341:1363–1365.

115. Ogle CK, Ogle JD, Mao JX, Simon J, et al. Effect of glutamine on phagocytosis and bacterial killing by normal and pediatric burn patient neutrophils. *J Parenter Enter Nutr.* 1994;18:128–133.

116. O'Riordain MG, Fearon KC, Ross JA, Rogers P, et al. Glutamine-supplemented total parenteral nutrition enhances T-lymphocytes in surgical patients undergoing colorectal resection. *Ann Surg.* 1994;220:212–221.

117. Van Zaanen HCT, van der Lelie H, Timmer JG, Fürst P, et al. Parenteral glutamine dipeptide supplementation does not ameliorate chemotherapy-induced toxicity. *Cancer.* 1994;74:2879–2884.

118. Dudrick PS, Souba WW. Special fuels in parenteral nutrition. In: Rombeau JL, Caldwell MD, eds. *Clinical Nutrition: Parenteral Nutrition.* 2nd ed. Philadelphia: WB Saunders Co; 1993:209–222.

119. Brennan MF, Cerra F, Daly JM, Fischer JE, et al. Report of a research workshop: branched-chain amino acids in stress and injury. *J Parenter Enter Nutr.* 1986;10:446–452.

120. Frankel WL, Evans NJ, Rombeau JL. Scientific rationale and clinical application of parenteral nutrition in critically ill patients. In: Rombeau JL, Caldwell MD, eds. *Clinical Nutrition: Parenteral Nutrition.* 2nd ed. Philadelphia: WB Saunders Co; 1993:597–616.

121. O'Keefe SJD. Parenteral nutrition in liver disease. In: Rombeau JL, Caldwell MD, eds. *Clinical Nutrition: Parenteral Nutrition.* 2nd ed. Philadelphia: WB Saunders Co; 1993:676–695.

122. Wolman SL, Anderson GH, Marliss EB, Jeejeebhoy KN. Zinc in total parenteral nutrition: requirements and metabolic effects. *Gastroenterology.* 1979;79:458–467.

123. Hambridge KM, Sokol RJ, Fidanza SJ, Goodall MA, et al. Plasma manganese concentrations in infants and children receiving parenteral nutrition. *J Parenter Enter Nutr.* 1989;13:168–171.

124. Mehta R, Reilly JJ. Manganese levels in a jaundiced long-term total parenteral nutrition patient: potentiation of haloperidol toxicity? *J Parenter Enter Nutr.* 1990;14:428–430.

125. Ejima A, Imamura T, Nakamura S, Saito H, et al. Manganese intoxication during total parenteral nutrition. *Lancet.* 1992;339:426.

126. Taylor S, Manara AR. Manganese toxicity in a patient with cholestasis receiving total parenteral nutrition. *Anaesthesia.* 1994;49:1013.

127. Fredstrom S, Rogosheske J, Gupta P, Burns LJ. Extrapyramidal symptoms in a BMT recipient with hyperintense basal ganglia and elevated manganese levels. *Bone Marrow Transplant.* 1995;15:989–992.

128. Levy M, Dupuis LL. Parenteral nutrition hypersensitivity. *J Parenter Enter Nutr.* 1990;14:213–215.

129. Deaths associated with thiamine-deficient total parenteral nutrition. *MMWR.* 1989;38:43–46.

130. Rovelli A, Bonomi M, Murano A, Locasciulli A, et al. Severe lactic acidosis due to thiamine deficiency after bone marrow transplantation in a child with acute monocytic leukemia. *Haematologica.* 1990;75:579–581. Letter.

131. Oriot D, Wood C, Gottesman R, Huault G. Severe lactic acidosis related to acute thiamine deficiency. *J Parenter Enter Nutr.* 1991;15:105–109.

132. Lange R, Erhard J, Eigler FW, Roll C. Lactic acidosis from thiamine deficiency during parenteral nutrition in a two-year-old boy. *Eur J Pediatr Surg.* 1992;2:241–244.

133. Kitamura K, Takahashi T, Tanaka H, Shimotsuma M, et al. Two cases of thiamine deficiency-induced lactic acidosis during total parenteral nutrition. *Tohoku J Exp Med.* 1993;171:129–133.

134. Barrett TG, Forsyth JM, Nathavitharana KA, Booth IW. Potentially lethal thiamine deficiency complicating parenteral nutrition in children. *Lancet.* 1993;341:901.

135. Gleghorn EE, Eisenberg LD, Hack S, Parton P, et al. Observations of vitamin A toxicity in three patients with renal failure receiving parenteral alimentation. *Am J Clin Nutr.* 1986;44:107–112.

136. Friedman AL, Chesney RW, Gilbert EF, Gilchrist KW, et al. Secondary oxalosis as a complication of parenteral alimentation in acute renal failure. *Am J Nephrol.* 1983;3:248–252.

137. Swartz RD, Wesley JR, Somermeyer MC, Lau K. Hyperoxaluria and renal insufficiency due to ascorbic acid administration during total parenteral nutrition. *Ann Intern Med.* 1984;100:530–531.

138. Quigley EMM, Marsh MN, Shaffer JL, Markin RS. Hepatobiliary complications of total parenteral nutrition. *Gastroenterology.* 1993;104:286–301.

139. Buchmiller CE, Kleinman-Wexler RL, Ephgrave KS, Booth B, et al. Liver dysfunction and energy source: results of a randomized clinical trial. *J Parenter Enter Nutr.* 1993;17:301–306.

140. Baldermann H, Wicklmayr M, Rett K, Banholzer P, et al. Changes of hepatic morphology during parenteral nutrition with lipid emulsions containing LCT or MCT/LCT quantified by ultrasound. *J Parenter Enter Nutr.* 1991;15:601–603.

141. Buchman AL, Dubin M, Jenden D, Moukarzel A, et al. Lecithin increases plasma free choline and decreases hepatic steatosis in long-term parenteral nutrition patients. *Gastroenterology.* 1992;102:1363–1370.

142. Hofmann AF. Defective biliary secretion during total parenteral nutrition: probable mechanisms and possible solutions. *J Pediatr Gastroenterol Nutr.* 1995;20:376–390.

143. Moss RL, Das JB, Raffensperger JG. Total parenteral nutrition-associated cholestasis: clinical and histopathological correlation. *J Pediatr Surg.* 1993;28:1270–1274.

144. Rintala RJ, Lindahl H, Pohjavuori M. Total parenteral nutrition-associated cholestasis in surgical neonates may be reversed by intravenous cholecystokinin: a preliminary report. *J Pediatr Surg.* 1995;30:827–830.

145. Teitelbaum DH, Han-Markey T, Schumacher RE. Treatment of parenteral-nutrition associated cholestasis with cholecystokinin-octapeptide. *J Pediatr Surg.* 1995;30:1082–1085.

146. Beau P, Labat-Labourdette J, Ingrand P, Beauchant M. Is ursodeoxycholic acid an effective therapy for total parenteral nutrition-related liver disease? *J Hepatol.* 1994;20:240–244.

147. Messing B, Zarka Y, Lemann M, Iglicki F, et al. Chronic cholestasis associated with long-term parenteral nutrition. *Transplant Proc.* 1994;26:1438–1439.

148. Colomb V, Goulet O, De Potter S, Ricour C. Liver disease associated with long-term parenteral nutrition in children. *Transplant Proc.* 1994;26:1467.

149. Tighe AP, Allison DB, Kral JG, Heymsfield SB. Nutritional support of obese patients. In: Rombeau JL, Caldwell MD, eds. *Clinical Nutrition: Parenteral Nutrition.* 2nd ed. Philadelphia: WB Saunders Co; 1993:716–736.

150. Sitzmann JV, Pitt HA, Steinborn PA, Pasha ZR, et al. Cholecystokinin prevents parenteral nutrition induced biliary sludge in humans. *Surg Gynecol Obstet.* 1990;170:25–31.

151. Spitz J, Gandhi S, Hecht G, Alverdy J. The effects of total parenteral nutrition on gastrointestinal tract function. *Clin Nutr.* 1993;12(suppl 1):S33–S37.

152. Jackson WD, Grand RJ. The human intestinal response to enteral nutrients: a review. *J Am Coll Nutr.* 1991;10:500–509.

153. Buchman AL, Moukarzel AA, Bhuta S, Belle M, et al. Parenteral nutrition is associated with intestinal morphologic and functional changes in humans. *J Parenter Enter Nutr.* 1995;19:453–460.

154. Sedman PC, Macfie J, Sagar P, Mitchell CJ, et al. The prevalence of gut translocation in humans. *Gastroenterology.* 1994;107:643–649.

155. Buchman AL, Mestecky J, Moukarzel A, Ament ME. Intestinal immune function is unaffected by parenteral nutrition in man. *J Am Coll Nutr.* 1995;14:656–661.

156. Tremel H, Kienle B, Weilemann LS, Stehle P, et al. Glutamine dipeptide supplemented TPN maintains intestinal function in critically ill. *Gastroenterology.* 1994;107:1595–1601.

157. Soeters P. Glutamine: the link between depletion and diminished gut function. *J Am Coll Nutr.* 1996;15:195–196.

158. Buchman AL. Glutamine: is it a conditionally required nutrient for the human gastrointestinal system? *J Am Coll Nutr.* 1996;15:199–205.

159. Hornsby-Lewis L, Shike M, Brown P, Klang M, et al. L-glutamine supplementation in human parenteral nutrition patients: stability, safety, and effects on intestinal absorption. *J Parenter Enter Nutr.* 1994;18:268–273.

160. Askanazi J, Rosenbaum SH, Hyman AL, Silverberg PA, et al. Respiratory changes induced by the large glucose loads of total parenteral nutrition. *JAMA.* 1980;245:1444–1447.

161. Covelli HD, Black JW, Olsen MS, Beekman JF. Respiratory failure precipitated by high carbohydrate loads. *Ann Intern Med.* 1981;95:79–81.

162. Rodriguez JL, Askanazi J, Weissman C, Hensle TW, et al. Ventilatory and metabolic effects of glucose infusions. *Chest.* 1985;88:512–518.

163. Liposky JM, Nelson LD. Ventilatory response to high caloric loads in critically ill patients. *Crit Care Med.* 1994;22:796–802.

164. Wilson DO, Rogers RM, Hoffman RM. State of the art: nutrition and chronic lung disease. *Am Rev Respir Dis.* 1985;132:1347–1365.

165. Greig PD, Elwyn DH, Askanazi J, Kinney JM. Parenteral nutrition in septic patients: effect of increasing nitrogen intake. *Am J Clin Nutr.* 1987;6:1040–1047.

166. Takala J, Askanazi J, Weissman C, Lasala PA, et al. Changes in respiratory control induced by amino acid infusions. *Crit Care Med.* 1988;16:465–469.

167. Gaare JM, Manner T, Wiese S, Askanazi J. Nutrition in pulmonary diseases. In: Rombeau JL, Caldwell MD, eds. *Clinical Nutrition: Parenteral Nutrition.* 2nd ed. Philadelphia: WB Saunders Co; 1993:631–648.

168. Goulet O, Girot R, Maier-Redelsperger M, Bougle D, et al. Hematologic disorders following prolonged use of intravenous fat emulsions in children. *J Parenter Enter Nutr.* 1986;10:284–288.

169. Spear ML, Spear M, Cohen AR, Pereira GR. Effect of fat infusions on platelet concentration in premature infants. *J Parenter Enter Nutr.* 1990;14:165–168.

170. Herson VC, Block C, Eisenfeld L, Maderazo EG, et al. Effects of intravenous fat infusion on neonatal neutrophil and platelet function. *J Parenter Enter Nutr.* 1989;13:620–622.

171. Miles JM. Intravenous fat emulsions in nutritional support. *Curr Opin Gastroenterol.* 1991;7:306–311.

172. Altomare DF, Semeraro N, Colucci M. Reduction of the plasma levels of tissue plasminogen activator after infusion of a lipid emulsion in humans. *J Parenter Enter Nutr.* 1993;17:274–276.

173. Hennessey PJ, Black T, Andrassy RJ. Nonenzymatic glycosylation of immunoglobulin G impairs complement fixation. *J Parenter Enter Nutr.* 1991;15:60–64.

174. Hotstetter HK. Handicaps to host defense: effects of hyperglycemia on C3 and Candida albicans. *Diabetes.* 1990;39:271–275.

175. Freeman J, Goldmann DA, Smith NE, Sidebottom DG, et al. Association of intravenous lipid emulsion and coagulase negative staphylococcal bacteremia in neonatal care units. *N Engl J Med.* 1990;323:301–308.

176. Palmblad J. Intravenous lipid emulsions and host defense—a critical review. *Clin Nutr.* 1991;10:303–308.

177. Gogos CA, Kalfarentzos F. Total parenteral nutrition and immune system activity: a review. *Nutrition.* 1995;11:339–344.

178. Gottshlich MM. Selection of optimal lipid sources in enteral and parenteral nutrition. *Nutr Clin Pract.* 1992;7:152–165.

179. Matarese LE. Reassessment and determining an end point of therapy. In: Krey S, Murray RL, eds. *Dynamics of Nutrition Support: Assessment, Implementation, Evaluation.* Norwalk, CT: Appleton-Century-Crofts; 1986:479–488.

180. The American Dietetic Association. Position of The American Dietetic Association: issues in feeding the terminally ill adult. *J Am Diet Assoc.* 1992;92:996–1002.

181. Hansen BW, DeSomery CH, Hagedorn PK, Kalnasy LW. Effects of enteral and parenteral nutrition on appetite in monkeys. *J Parenter Enter Nutr.* 1977;1:83–88.

182. Martyn PA, Hansen BC, Jen KC. The effects of parenteral nutrition on food intake and gastric motility. *Nurs Res.* 1984;33:336–342.

183. Charuhas PC, Fosberg K, Bruemmer B, Aker SN, et al. A double-blind, randomized trial comparing outpatient parenteral nutrition with intravenous hydration: effect on resumption of oral intake after marrow transplantation. *J Parenter Enter Nutr.* 1997;21:157–161.

CHAPTER 22

Transitional Feeding

Annalynn Skipper

INTRODUCTION

The ultimate goal of nutrition support is to progress the patient to the most nearly normal nutrient intake possible. Although the majority of patients ultimately return to oral intake, they may receive any combination of enteral, parenteral, or oral feedings during a protracted hospital course. The transitional periods during which patients change from one feeding type to another are critical to nutritional progress. According to Zibrida and Carlson: "Transitional feeding refers to a directed change in the feeding modality and bridges the gap between one feeding modality and another."[1] Careful management of transitional feeding is appropriate to maintain nutritional status and to speed recovery. Because supporting data for transitional feeding practice are limited, protocols for transitional feeding are often based on clinical experience and vary widely between institutions. Rather than present specific protocols, this chapter reviews the rationale for transitional feeding and proposes some general principles upon which to base practice.

INITIATION OF NUTRITION SUPPORT

Several basic principles of feeding initiation may be applied to oral, enteral or parenteral nutrition support. In starved patients, slow initiation of feeding is suggested to prevent adverse metabolic consequences such as refeeding syndrome or volume overload. Tolerance to the initiation and progression of feedings varies widely and should be the basis for decisions about feeding advancement. Therefore, frequent monitoring is important until goal feedings are achieved. During periods when two or more types of feedings are administered, excess caloric intake may result. Because overfeeding may result in hyperglycemia, hypercapnia, hepatic steatosis, and possibly increased incidence of infection, it should be avoided. Premature discontinuation of one type of feeding before another is tolerated may result in underfeeding, which should also be avoided.

Refeeding Syndrome

Refeeding syndrome is a constellation of symptoms that result from intracellular shifts of phosphorus, magnesium, and potassium when nutrient intake is reinitiated in starved patients.[2] In case reports, refeeding syndrome is attributed to administration of large amounts of dextrose in the absence of adequate electrolytes and vitamins.[3,4] Excess sodium exacerbates fluid retention and, if the patient is overhydrated, a weakened heart muscle is unable to pump fluid from the heart.[5] Excess carbohydrate administration contributes to hyperglycemia and requires potassium for glycogen synthesis as well as magnesium and phosphorus for synthesis of adenosine triphosphate (ATP).[6] In addition, patients given thiamine-free total parenteral nutrition (TPN) may develop beriberi.[7] Any of the previously mentioned situations may result in death if inappropriately managed.

Although the incidence of refeeding syndrome is unknown, the potential morbidity and mortality mandate careful monitoring for prevention. Inadequate or absent food intake for a prolonged period of time, alcohol abuse, anorexia nervosa, diabetes mellitus, and antacid use have been implicated as risk factors for refeeding syndrome.[2]

Refeeding syndrome usually develops over several days. Volume overload and hyperglycemia may occur within a few hours of excess fluid and carbohydrate administration. A nadir of serum phosphorus and magnesium concentrations usually appear 2 to 3 days following achievement of anabolism. Patients with severe hypophosphatemia (≤ 1.0 mg/dL) may exhibit impaired white cell function, hemolytic anemia, or neuromuscular manifestations such as weakness, numbness, paresthesias, confusion, acute reflexic paralysis, coma, or Guillain-Barré–like syndrome.[8,9] Diminished ATP production may result in respiratory muscle failure, or cardiovascular symptoms.[10] Symptoms of hypomagnesemia include hypokalemia, hypocalcemia, neuromuscular symptoms (including weakness), seizures, depression, psychosis, and cardiac arrythmia.[11]

Refeeding syndrome may be avoided by initiation of reduced amounts of carbohydrate (2–3 g/kg/day for adjusted body weight), which are increased gradually with adequate blood sugar control.[12] Repletion of serum concentrations of potassium, magnesium, and phosphorus prior to initiating nutrition support is recommended. Daily monitoring of serum electrolyte concentrations is recommended, even after goal feedings are reached. As protein and lipid do not appear to exacerbate refeeding syndrome, they may be initiated at 1.5 g/kg/day and 1 g/kg/day, respectively. Total calorie intake should not exceed 25 kcal/kg/day for the first week.

The Gastrointestinal Effects of Parenteral Nutrition

The gastrointestinal effects of starvation as well as the gastrointestinal effects of a prolonged period without oral intake while receiving adequate nutrition with TPN have been studied.[13,14] Levine et al[15] demonstrated decreased small intestinal mass and disaccharidase activity in animals given TPN. In a later study, the same researchers demonstrated that amino acids rather than dextrose were necessary to maintain gut mass.[16] Parenteral nutrition has also been associated with delayed gastric emptying.[17] More recently, parenteral nutrition has been associated with decreased gastrointestinal immunity,[18] probably the result of bacterial translocation from the gastrointestinal tract[19] rather than reduced immunoglobulin A (IgA) production.[20] It is unclear whether these effects are the result of gastrointestinal disuse, parenteral nutrition, or other factors.

DISCONTINUING TOTAL PARENTERAL NUTRITION

Although there are a number of advantages to discontinuing parenteral nutrition as quickly as possible, rapid cessation of parenteral nutrition has been considered a risk factor for rebound hypoglycemia. However, several studies reported no detrimental effects on serum insulin or glucagon levels when TPN was abruptly discontinued.[21–24] Despite these findings, many clinicians reduce the TPN rate by one half for a few hours before discontinuing it altogether. For patients who receive enteral or oral feedings, blood sugar levels should be adequately maintained; for those who will not receive oral or enteral nutrition, blood sugar levels should be monitored and carbohydrate given as indicated. For patients whose oral intake is progressing more slowly, TPN may be decreased incrementally as oral intake increases.

TPN may be used as a vehicle for supplemental electrolytes for patients with stable but extraordinary needs. When TPN is discontinued in these patients, the need for continued electrolyte supplementation should be evaluated and a plan devised for oral or enteral electrolyte administration.

If possible, monitoring to ensure adequate intake following cessation of TPN is appropriate. However, Winkler et al[22–25] noted improvement in plasma proteins following cessation of TPN and did not recommend waiting until serum proteins normalized before discontinuing TPN.

The Effect of Parenteral Nutrition on Appetite

In early reports of the psychologic effects of TPN, patients described persistent feelings of hunger.[25,27] While these authors reported that patients who complained of hunger were able to tolerate only small amounts of foods, others have reported hyperphagia in patients receiving TPN.[28]

Studies in monkeys found an incremental decrease in voluntary food intake when TPN was administered as 25% to 100% of caloric intake,[29] confirming the work of earlier investigators.[30,31] The negative effect of parenteral lipid on appetite has been observed in animals[32] but not in humans.[33] In a study of 20 healthy young men,[34] caloric intake decreased when 68% of resting energy expenditure (REE) was given as fat or glucose alone, but not when 34% of REE was given as fat or glucose alone. Oral intake was decreased when peripheral parenteral nutrition was given as 17% protein, 34% fat, and 34% glucose. These findings suggest that the amount of parenteral calories may have a greater impact on appetite than the substrate distribution of calories provided.

Appetite depression persisting for up to 2 weeks following cessation of TPN has been reported in animals.[30-32] However, Sriram et al[35] found that voluntary oral intake increased proportionally within 3 days when TPN was decreased by 50%. Clamon et al[36] found transient depression in oral intake following discontinuation of TPN in cancer patients who had received TPN for 30 days or more. Clinical experience suggests that nonnutritional factors including motivation, depression, and disease process play a role in resumption of oral intake following cessation of TPN. Therefore, an individualized approach to the achievement of oral intake is needed.

Weaning from Long-Term Total Parenteral Nutrition

The majority of patients receive TPN for a few days or weeks. However, the number of patients receiving long-term TPN has grown. Many patients manage TPN successfully, despite lifestyle restrictions and expense. For those with short-bowel syndrome, bowel transplantation has been the only alternative to permanent TPN. However, growth hormone and glutamine have been used to stimulate bowel hypertrophy, with reduction or discontinuation of TPN in approximately 85% of patients.[37]

Initiation of Oral Intake

Readiness for oral intake depends upon the length of time the patient has been NPO, the severity and duration of illness, the resultant disability, nutritional status at the time of surgery, the patient's functional level, and motivation or other psychologic factors.[38] In the absence of factors that preclude oral intake, the expression of hunger or desire for food is possibly the best indicator that the patient will eat.

The time course for reintroduction of oral intake following surgery varies. Fromm et al[39] found that most patients returned to oral intake 5.3 days following gastrojejunostomy; the time was increased to 7.8 days if a vagotomy was performed. Meguid et al[38] studied the return to oral intake in cancer patients undergoing colorectal surgery and found that approximately 50% of well-nourished patients were eating 10 days postoperatively. In contrast, only 27% of malnourished patients were eating well in 10 days.

For many patients, particularly those who have been on mechanical ventilation, a swallowing evaluation is appropriate to establish tolerance to oral feedings. In the event of poor swallowing ability, patients should be evaluated to determine the most appropriate type of oral feeding.

Following surgery, patients have traditionally progressed to clear liquids, then to full liquids, and finally to solid foods. However, full liquid diets are poorly tolerated by patients with lactose intolerance, and they probably unnecessarily delay the progression to solid food.

The initiation of a general diet following consumption of a liter of clear liquids is one protocol that has worked well. However, two studies[40,41] found similar tolerance to clear liquids and solid foods when both were given as the first postoperative meal. These authors concluded that routine use of clear liquid diets postoperatively is not indicated.

Although young, previously healthy patients often eat well following a course of enteral or parenteral nutrition, others do not. Individuals whose socioeconomic background renders them unfamiliar with foods served on a hospital diet may respond to encouragement from family members and to foods prepared outside the hospital and brought in at mealtime. Elderly patients may require assistance with menus and meals, or may have different perceptions of adequate and appropriate intake during illness. Patients with cancer may suffer appetite or taste alterations or depression, depending upon the stage of the disease. Patients with a history of gastrointestinal complaints such as inflammatory bowel disease, pancreatitis, or cholecystitis may associate eating with pain and therefore fear intake of certain foods. For some patients, appetite stimulants such as megestrol acetate may effectively increase calorie intake.[42] An individualized approach, a skillful nutrition care team, and a cooperative food service can do much to alleviate these problems and to achieve optimal oral intake during the transition to oral feeding.

REFERENCES

1. Zibrida JM, Carlson SJ. Transitional feeding. In: *Nutrition Support Dietetics Core Curriculum.* 2nd ed. Silver Spring, MD: American Society for Parenteral and Enteral Nutrition, 1993.

2. Brooks MJ, Melnik G. The refeeding syndrome: an approach to understanding its complications and preventing its occurrence. *Pharmacotherapy.* 1995;15:713–726.

3. Askanazi J, Elwyn DH, Silverburg PA, Rosenbaum SH, et al. Respiratory distress secondary to a high carbohydrate load: a case report. *Surgery.* 1980;87:596–598.

4. Covelli HD, Black JW, Olsen MS, Beekman JF. Respiratory failure precipitated by high carbohydrate loads. *Ann Intern Med.* 1981;95:579–581.

5. Guirao X, Franch G, Gil MJ, Garcia-Domingo MI, et al. Extracellular volume, nutritional status, and refeeding changes. *Nutrition.* 1994;10:558–561.

6. Solomon SM, Kirby DF. The refeeding syndrome: a review. *J Parenter Enter Nutr.* 1990;14:90–97.

7. Deaths associated with thiamine-deficient total parenteral nutrition. *MMWR.* 1989;38:43–46.

8. Knochel JP. The pathophysiology and clinical characteristics of severe hypophosphatemia. *Arch Intern Med.* 1977;137:203–220.

9. Weintraub MI. Hypophosphatemia mimicking acute Guillain-Barré syndrome. *JAMA.* 1976;235:1040–1041.

10. Lichtman MA, Miller DR, Cohen J, Waterhouse C. Reduced red cell glycolysis, 2,3-diphosphoglycerate and adenosine triphosphate concentration, and increased hemoglobin-oxygen affinity caused by hypophosphatemia. *Ann Intern Med.* 1971;74:562–568.

11. Rude RK. Magnesium metabolism and deficiency. *Endocrinol Metabol Clin North Am.* 1993;22:377–395.

12. Apovian CM, McMahon MM, Bistrian BR. Guidelines for refeeding the marasmic patient. *Crit Care Med.* 1990;18:1030–1033.

13. Anonymous. Hunger disease. Reprinted in *Nutrition.* 1994;10:365–380.

14. Guedon C, Schmitz J, Lerebours E, Metayer, et al. Decreased brush border hydrolase activities without gross morphologic changes in human intestinal mucosa after prolonged total parenteral nutrition of adults. *Gastroenterology.* 1986;90:373–378.

15. Levine GM, Deren JJ, Steiger E, Zinno R. The role of oral intake in maintenance of gut mass and disaccharide artistry. *Gastroenterology.* 1974;67:975–982.

16. Spector MH, Levine GM, Deren JJ. Direct and indirect effects of dextrose and amino acids on gut mass. *Gastroenterology.* 1977;72:706–710.

17. McGregor IL, Wiley ZD, Lavigne ME, Way LW. Slowed rate of gastric emptying of solid food in man by high caloric parenteral nutrition. *Am J Surg.* 1979;138:652–654.

18. Alverdy J, Chi HS, Sheldon GF. The effect of parenteral nutrition on gastrointestinal immunity. *Ann Surg.* 1985;202:681–684.

19. Wells CL, Maddaus MA, Simmons RL. Proposed mechanisms for the translocation of intestinal bacteria. *Rev Infect Dis.* 1988;10:958–979.

20. Buchman AL, Mestecky J, Moukarzel A, Ament ME. Intestinal immune function is unaffected by parenteral nutrition in man. *J Am Coll Nutr.* 1995;14:656–661.

21. Wagman LD, Newsome HH, Miller KB, Thomas RB, et al. The effect of acute discontinuation of total parenteral nutrition. *Ann Surg.* 1986;204:524–529.

22. Winkler MF, Pomp A, Caldwell MD, Albina JE. Transitional feeding: the relationship between nutritional intake and plasma protein concentrations. *J Am Diet Assoc.* 1989;89:969–970.

23. Perl M, Hall RCW, Dudrick SJ, Englert DM, et al. Psychological aspects of long-term home hyperalimentation. *J Parenter Enter Nutr.* 1980;4:554.

24. Jordan HA, Moses H, MacFayden BV, Dudrick SJ. Hunger and satiety in humans during parenteral hyperalimentation. *Psychosom Med.* 1974;36:144.

25. diCecco S, Nelson J, Burns J, Fleming CR. Nutritional intake of gut failure patients on home parenteral nutrition. *J Parenter Enter Nutr.* 1987;11:529–532.

26. Martyn PA, Hansen BC, Jen KC. The effects of parenteral nutrition on food intake and gastric motility. *Nurs Res.* 1984;33:336.

27. DeSomery CH, Hansen BW. Regulation of appetite during total parenteral nutrition. *Nurs Res.* 1978;27:19.

28. Hansen BW, DeSomery CH, Hagedorn PK, Kalnasy LW. Effects of enteral and parenteral nutrition on appetite in monkeys. *J Parenter Enter Nutr.* 1977;1:83.

29. Woods SC, Stein LJ, McKay D, Porte D. Suppression of food intake by intravenous nutrients and insulin in the baboon. *Am J Physiol.* 247;1984:R393.

30. Welch I, Saunders K, Read N. Effect of ileal and intravenous infusions of fat emulsions on feeding and satiety in human volunteers. *Gastroenterology.* 1985;89:1293–1297.

31. Gil KM, Skeie B, Kvetan V, Askanazi J, et al. Parenteral nutrition and oral intake: effect of glucose and fat infusions. *J Parenter Enter Nutr.* 1991;15:426–432.

32. Sriram K, Pinchofsky G, Kaminski MV. Suppression of appetite by parenteral nutrition in humans. *J Am Coll Nutr.* 1984;3:317.

33. Clamon G, Gardner L, Pee D, Strumbo P, et al. The effect of intravenous hyperalimentation on the dietary intake of patients with small cell lung cancer. *Cancer.* 1985;55:1572–1578.

34. Bryne TA, Persinger RL, Young LS, Ziegler TR, et al. A new treatment for patients with short-bowel syndrome. *Ann Surg.* 1995;222:243–255.

35. Sriram K, Pinchofsky G, Kaminski MV. Suppression of appetite by parenteral nutrition in humans. *J Am Coll Nutr.* 1984;3:317.

36. Clamon G, Gardner L, Pee D, Strumbo P, et al. The effect of intravenous hyperalimentation on the dietary intake of patients with small cell lung cancer. *Cancer.* 55:1572.

37. Bryne TA, Persinger RL, Young LS, Ziegler TR, Wilmore DW. A new treatment for patients with short-bowel syndrome. *Ann Surg.* 1995;222:243–255.

38. Meguid MM, Mughal MM, Dbonis D, Meguid V, et al. Influence of nutritional status on the resumption of adequate food intake in patients recovering from colorectal cancer operations. *Surg Clin North Am.* 1986;66:1167–1176.

39. Fromm D, Resitartis D, Kozol R. An analysis of when patients eat after gastrojejunostomy. *Ann Surg.* 1988;207:14–20.

40. Jeffery KM, Harkins B, Cresci GA, Martindale RG. The clear liquid diet is no longer a necessity in the routine postoperative management of surgical patients. *Am Surg.* 1996;62:167–170.

41. Tchekmedyian NS. Treatment of anorexia with megestrol acetate. *Nutr Clin Pract.* 1993;8:115–118.

42. Herrington AM, Herrington JD, Church CA. Pharmacologic options for the treatment of cahexia. *Nutr Clin Pract.* 1997;12:101–113.

PART IV

Organizational Considerations in Nutrition Support

CHAPTER 23

The Nutrition Support Team and the Role of the Dietitian

Annalynn Skipper

THE NUTRITION SUPPORT TEAM

Many hospitals and regulatory agencies accept the multidisciplinary nutrition support team (NST) as the standard of care for provision of enteral and parenteral feedings.[1,2] NSTs provide cost-effective therapy,[3–12] improve nutrient intake,[13–15] reduce complications,[16–20] decrease catheter sepsis,[21–28] and increase appropriate use of therapy.[29]

Several models for the organization of the NST have been proposed.[30–32] The major distinguishing features among models are organizational structure, team composition, scope of practice, and referral mechanisms. An understanding of these differences is essential to promote effective team function, determine adequate staffing, and compare productivity.

Team Organization

The traditional organizational structure for the NST is one where a free-standing department operates with its own director, clinicians, support personnel, budget, and office space. In another common model, team members retain appointments in their primary departments but collaborate on patient care and report clinically to a team director. Administrative costs are usually absorbed by supporting departments. In institutions with few patients receiving enteral or parenteral nutrition and institutions with insufficient resources for a nutrition support service, a nutrition support committee may provide oversight for practice.

The appropriate model for a nutrition support service is based on available resources, institutional structure, and patient load. There are examples of each model functioning well, and there is no clear evidence that one model is more effective than another.

Team Composition

The NST is usually composed of dietitians, nurses, pharmacists, and physicians. Social workers, respiratory therapists, metabolic cart technicians, researchers, administrators, and support personnel may also be included. The amount of time each member allocates to the team may vary but should be adequate to maintain clinical competence and to ensure patients' safety. Some teams have a volume of patients adequate to require several clinicians from each discipline; smaller teams may use members who are part-time or function as consultants.

Although many advocate a physician as team director, this is not always possible. There are relatively few board-certified nutrition support physicians, and economics often limit the time that qualified physicians can devote to nutrition support. Nurses, dietitians, and pharmacists often serve successfully as team directors. The choice of a team director should be based on leadership and administrative skills rather than clinical discipline.

Scope of Practice

The NST may function in an advisory capacity, performing a nutritional assessment and following the patient to make recommendations for nutrition management. With such a system, implementation of the recommendations is the responsibility of the referring physician, and team members usually spend a great deal of time educating and communicating with referring physicians.

In another model, the NST may actually manage patients by placing parenteral or enteral access, ordering or performing tests, implementing enteral or parenteral feedings, monitoring nutritional progress, and modifying therapy as needed. Members of this type of team also educate and communicate with referring physicians, but spend additional time with the logistics necessary to implement therapy.

Most teams have administrative responsibilities such as receiving and assigning new patients, billing, developing policies and procedures, and keeping records. The administrative load has been increased by recent regulations,[2] and NSTs may now collect data for clinical indicators,[33] critical pathways,[34] or other quality assurance programs. NSTs may also supervise the purchasing and compounding of enteral and parenteral products. In teaching hospitals, the NST may have responsibilities to medical, pharmacy nursing, or dietetics education programs, or it may have established fellowship programs. Some teams collect data for clinical research studies or maintain a research laboratory. The amount of time required for these activities may dictate practice patterns and staffing levels.

Referrals

Referral to the NST may be left to the discretion of individual physicians or may be dictated by institutional policy. Some institutions mandate NST approval before nutrition support is initiated or before specific enteral or parenteral formulas can be ordered. Health maintenance organizations may also mandate NST approval before enteral or parenteral nutrition is implemented in order to reduce costs.

ROLE OF THE DIETITIAN

Because of their unique skills and knowledge, dietitians have been included as NST members since the genesis of the concept. Dietitians possess special expertise in nutrient requirements that is necessary to provide every type of nutrition support therapy. The essential nature of dietetic services to successful nutrition support has been well established.[35] Patient care duties vary according to institutional protocol but usually center on assessing nutritional status, developing and implementing a nutrition care plan, and monitoring the results of nutrition support for patients of all ages and in all health care settings.

Assessment

It is the responsibility of the nutrition support dietitian to perform initial nutritional assessment prior to the implementation of therapy, and serial nutritional assessments throughout the course of therapy. To do this, the dietitian reviews the medical record for medical and surgical history; obtains and evaluates the patient's nutrition history; interprets laboratory data; and may perform body composition studies, indirect calorimetry, or a nutrition-focused physical examination. Based on these data, the dietitian assesses degree and type of malnutrition. The dietitian then determines requirements for macronutrients, fluid, and micronutrients.

Planning and Implementation

The dietitian may design and implement or participate in the design and implementation of nutrition therapy by selecting the most appropriate, practical, and cost-effective regimen. The plan is adapted for patients with metabolic stress, organ dysfunction, and a myriad of underlying diseases. Optimal, achievable goals for nutrition therapy are established and a plan to achieve them is developed.

Monitoring Tolerance to Therapy

Successful nutrition support is dependent on continuing assessment of the patient's tolerance to nutrition therapy. With inadequate monitoring, discontinuance of feeding and nutrition support failure often result. Serial monitoring of nutritional parameters is necessary to ensure adequacy of nutrition therapy and to allow modification of nutrition therapy as the patient's condition changes. The nutrition support dietitian collaborates with other team members to help enforce protocols for monitoring nutritional status and to suggest appropriate deviations from these protocols when necessary.

Transitional Feeding

During a complicated hospital course, critically ill patients may require oral, enteral, and parenteral nutrition. The initiation or discontinuation of any of these therapies is a critical time that requires careful coordination of nutrient intake and monitoring of feeding tolerance to maintain nutritional status. During transitional periods, the dietitian monitors nutrient intake using intake and output records and calorie counts. Tolerance to therapy is monitored by following abdominal exams and bowel function. The dietitian frequently determines initiation and progression of new feeding methods as well as discontinuance of old ones.

Patient Education and Discharge Planning

Educating patients about normal nutrition, appropriate nutritional supplements, and modified diets is a well-established role for the dietitian. The nutrition support dietitian may perform this service for patients who are followed to discharge or may refer patients to another staff member when nutrition support is completed.

For patients receiving enteral feedings, the dietitian may assume almost complete responsibility for discharge planning,[36] determining the home feeding schedule, and teaching the patient to recognize formula intolerance and to manage complications of enteral feeding. Dietitians may also teach patients to operate a feeding pump, administer the formula, flush the feeding tube, and care for the feeding tube site. The dietitian may take a similar role in teaching patients who receive parenteral feeding to monitor tolerance to feedings and to recognize complications. By definition, patients who receive home parenteral feeding should have a nonfunctioning gastrointestinal tract. However, the desire for oral gratification is so strong that most patients continue to eat. These patients require attention from the dietitian to direct them toward appropriate oral intake.

Patient Advocacy

In the complexities of patient care, nutrition is a detail to everyone but the dietitian. It is the responsibility of the dietitian to bring this detail continually to the attention of the primary caregiver and to ensure that nutrition issues are included in the overall care plan.

Administrative Duties

Administrative duties are frequently viewed negatively by clinicians whose primary focus is patient care. However, the power to improve patient care is derived from careful attention to administrative duties. For example, the data gathering that justifies additional staff or program expansion is an administrative duty. Attention to cost-effectiveness is necessary to win approval for equipment and staff. Administrative skills enable the dietitian to assume a leadership role.

Documentation of Services

The current economic climate in health care makes documentation of services an essential task. Nutrition support dietitians have the responsibility of knowing their patient population by recording the number and type of patients seen. Expression of activities in terms of patient days and percentage of time spent in various activities makes data easily understandable to those unfamiliar with nutrition support terminology.

Research

The importance of research to the profession of dietetics cannot be overstated. Research forms the basis for the advancement of practice.[37] In addition to the regular journal reading required to maintain current practice and the literature review that precedes policy development, it is also the duty of the nutrition support dietitian to research clinical issues and to conduct outcomes research.

UNIQUE ASPECTS OF NUTRITION SUPPORT PRACTICE

There are several differences between nutrition support and traditional dietetics. Most important of these is the concept of episodic versus follow-up care. The episodic model, used in traditional dietetics, involves seeing a patient once during hospitalization for evaluation, formulating a nutritional care plan, and providing nutrition education. A small number of patients are hospitalized long enough for a follow-up visit.

The patient receiving nutrition support typically has a longer hospital stay, with sometimes frequent and rapid changes in status. Revisions of the nutritional care plan are ongoing, mandating daily follow-up. Because of the complexity of care required by nutrition support patients, the nutrition support dietitian is often responsible for a smaller census than other members of the dietetic staff. This potential source of arithmetic conflict is easily resolved if comparison of workloads is based on the number of patients seen, assessments completed, or orders or notes written rather than the number of patient beds assigned to each dietitian.

PREPARATION

The role of the dietitian on the NST has not evolved without appropriate preparation. Education, experience, and credentialing are components of this preparation.

Education

A four-year degree and registered dietitian status are minimal qualifications for the nutrition support dietitian. Two surveys reported that these credentials, along with work experience, are necessary to function on an NST.[38,39] The majority of respondents to one survey agreed that an advanced degree is necessary for effective nutrition support practice.[39] Subsequent surveys document that many nutrition support dietitians have an advanced degree.[40,41] Although nutrition support dietitians with graduate education may be better suited to research or teaching positions, there are no data documenting superior patient care skills in either group.[39]

Regardless of educational background, the nutrition support dietitian must have expertise in nutritional biochemistry; pathophysiology of disease; nutritional assessment; and the composition, preparation, and delivery of parenteral, enteral, and oral nutrients. Familiarity with medical, surgical, and pharmacologic therapies and their impact on the patient's ability to ingest and absorb nutrients is essential. In addition, the nutrition support dietitian must be able to read, evaluate, and apply scientific literature. Excellent communication and team building skills are mandatory for team participation. Many nutrition support dietitians possess technical knowledge of computers, calorimeters, and other equipment. Some positions require business or research skills. Dietitians will undoubtedly acquire other skills as practice changes.

Nutrition support dietitians should ensure that their knowledge remains current by attending seminars; workshops; and state, local, and national meetings of nutrition societies; by reading the current literature; by conferring with colleagues; and through mentoring. Fellowship programs exist to provide supervised experience in nutrition support practice.[42] The dynamic nature of the field demands continuing education.

Experience

Experience in general clinical dietetics, preferably in an acute care setting, provides knowledge of the health care environment and contributes to the clinical acumen and maturity that is a prerequisite for successful nutrition support practice. The general experience also develops skills in nutrition management of endocrine, gastrointestinal, coronary, pulmonary, renal, and hepatic diseases, providing a basis for dealing with the complex management of patients receiving nutrition support.

Credentialing

According to *Webster's Seventh New Collegiate Dictionary,* the word *credential* is defined as "warranting credit or confidence."[43] Members of many professions have sought to assure consumers of their credibility through credentialing.

Because nutrition support is a distinct area of dietetic practice, certification has been available since 1988.[44] Qualified applicants may take the Certified Nutrition Support Dietitian examination offered by National Board of Nutritional Support Certification.

Several documents are available to assist in delineating the role of the nutrition support dietitian. A complete set of standards of care and a practice manual are available from the American Society for Parenteral and Enteral Nutrition (ASPEN).[45,46] A position paper published by The American Dietetic Association (ADA) has been recently updated,[35] and standards of practice have been jointly validated by ASPEN and ADA.[47] These documents serve as useful guides to practice.

ROLE EXPANSION

Since the role of the nutrition support dietitian was first described,[48] it has undergone tremendous change.[49-52] Dietitians have expanded their skills to include indirect calorimetry, body composition analysis, feeding tube insertion, and nutrition-focused physical assessment. Recent practice surveys report that dietitians are writing parenteral nutrition orders,[40] prescribing enteral feedings, and participating in decisions regarding the route of enteral feeding.[41]

A flexible approach to job role enables individuals to take advantage of opportunities for expansion. Current trends toward alternate site care, multiskilled health care workers, and increased operating efficiencies offer tremendous opportunity for creative practitioners.[53]

Committed personnel may accomplish role expansion in logical, stepwise fashion. The first step is to identify an area into which expansion is possible. Planning for this expansion is necessary, as is obtaining the support of key administrative personnel. Training may be needed to ensure competency. Performing the new role in a consistent fashion and for a sufficient length of time is necessary for it to become established. Careful recordkeeping is necessary to determine costs and to document the benefit to patients and the institution. The final step is evaluation of the new role and institution of modifications to improve performance. An example of this model appears in Exhibit 23–1.

Exhibit 23–1 Example of Role Expansion

1. Identify area into which role expansion is possible
   a. Quality improvement data indicate that enteral feedings are not being initiated promptly.
   b. The nurse who has been trained to place tubes works only three days a week.
   c. Dietitians are available six days a week, and it appears that feedings could be initiated sooner if dietitians could place the tubes.
2. Plan for role expansion
   a. Conduct a needs assessment
      How many feeding tubes are placed monthly?
      Who is currently trained to place feeding tubes?
      Are there individuals who are trained to do this task who are not currently performing the task?
      Are there problems or complications with the current system?
   b. Identify optimal staffing to meet the need
      Is the service needed seven days a week?
      Is the service needed 24 hours a day?
      How many labor hours per week are needed to perform this service?
   c. Identify training needs
      How did those currently placing tubes receive their training?
      Is a qualified teacher available?

continues

Exhibit 23–1 continued

> How much time does training take?
> Is supervised practice needed?
> Is certification or licensure needed?
> 3. Obtain administrative support
>   a. Develop a proposal including budget and revenue (benefit) projections
>   Obtain input from administration of various departments involved
>   Obtain input from key physicians (those likely to refer patients)
>   Obtain input from appropriate institutional committees
> 4. Implement the program
>   a. Develop pilot program
>   Identify time frame for a pilot program
>   Identify sample patient population
>   Identify appropriate clinical and administrative oversight
>   b. Train staff
>   c. Conduct the pilot program
> 5. Perform monitoring
>   a. Record the number of tubes placed and pertinent patient information
>   b. Record labor hours
>   c. Record supplies used
>   d. Record outcomes
>   e. Record complications
> 6. Perform evaluation
>   a. Summarize data collected during pilot phase
>   b. Obtain appropriate administrative and clinical input
>   c. Review outcomes
>   d. Make needed adjustments
> 7. Perform the new role

CONCLUSIONS

Participation in the team effort enables the dietitian to interact with professionals from other disciplines to impact significantly on patient care. Nutrition support is a dynamic field, changing constantly as new information and technology become available. The role of the dietitian on the nutrition support team is a challenging one that provides many opportunities for personal and professional growth.

REFERENCES

1. Regenstein M. Nutrition support teams—alive, well and still growing. Results of a 1991 ASPEN survey. *Nutr Clin Pract.* 1992;7:296–301.

2. Nutrition care. In: Joint Commission on Accreditation of Healthcare Organizations. *1996 Accreditation Manual for Hospitals.* Oakbrook Terrace, IL: Joint Commission on Accreditation of Healthcare Organizations; 1996;1:75–76.

3. Mutchie KD, Smith KA, MacKay MW, Marsh C, et al. Pharmacist monitoring of parenteral nutrition: clinical and cost effectiveness. *Am J Hosp Pharm.* 1979;36:785–787.

4. Shildt RA, Rose M, Stollman L, Bell B. Organization of the nutritional support service at a medical center: one year's experience. *Military Med.* 1982;147:55–58.

5. Friedman MH, Higa AM, Davis AJ. A unique team approach to optimal nutritional support with minimal cost. *Nutr Supp Serv.* 1983;3(2):27–28.

6. Weinsier RL, Heimburger DC, Samples CM, Dimick AR, et al. Cost containment: a contribution of aggressive nutritional support in burn patients. *J Burn Care Rehabil.* 1985;6:436–441.

7. O'Brien DD, Hodges RE, Day AT, Waxman KS, et al. Recommendations of nutritional support team promote cost containment. *J Parenter Enter Nutr.* 1986;10:300–302.

8. Faubion WC, Wesley JR, Kahlidi N, Silva J. Total parenteral nutrition catheter sepsis: impact of the team approach. *J Parenter Enter Nutr.* 1986;10:642–645.

9. Balet A, Cardona D. Importance of a nutrition support team to promote cost containment. *Ann Pharmacother.* 1992;26:265.

10. Roberts MF, Levine GM. Nutrition support team recommendations can reduce hospital costs. *Nutr Clin Pract.* 1995;7:227–230.

11. Gianino MS, Brunt LM, Eisenberg PG. The impact of a nutritional support team on the cost and management of multilumen central venous catheters. *J Intraven Nurs.* 1992;15:327–332.

12. Hassell JT, Games AD, Shaffer B, Harkins LE. Nutrition support team management of enterally fed patients in a community hospital is cost-beneficial. *J Am Diet Assoc.* 1994;94:993–998.

13. Traeger SM, Williams GB, Milliren G, Young DS, et al. Total parenteral nutrition by a nutrition support team: improved quality of care. *J Parenter Enter Nutr.* 1986;10:408–412.

14. Powers DA, Brown RO, Cowan GSM, Luther RW, et al. Nutritional support team vs nonteam management of enteral nutritional support in a Veterans Administration medical center teaching hospital. *J Parenter Enter Nutr.* 1986;10:635–638.

15. Gales BJ, Riley DG. Improved total parenteral nutrition therapy management by a nutritional support team. *Hosp Pharm.* 1994;29:469–470, 473–475.

16. Hickey MM, Munyer TP, Salem RB, Most RL. Parenteral nutrition utilization: evaluation of an educational protocol and consult service. *J Parenter Enter Nutr.* 1979;3:433–437.

17. Nehme AE. Nutritional support of the hospitalized patient: the team concept. *JAMA.* 1980;243:1906–1908.

18. Dalton MJ, Schepers G, Gee JP, Alberts CC, et al. Consultative total parenteral nutrition teams: the effect on the incidence of total parenteral nutrition-related complications. *J Parenter Enter Nutr.* 1984;8:146–152.

19. Brown RO, Carlson SD, Cowan GS, Powers DA, et al. Enteral nutritional support management in a university teaching hospital: team vs nonteam. *J Parenter Enter Nutr.* 1987;11:52–55.

20. Fisher GG, Opper FH. An interdisciplinary nutrition support team improves quality of care in a teaching hospital. *J Am Diet Assoc.* 1996;96:176–178.

21. Copeland EM, MacFadyen BV, Dudrick SJ. Prevention of microbial catheter contamination in patients receiving parenteral hyperalimentation. *South Med J.* 1974;67:303–306.

22. Ryan JA, Abel RM, Abbott WM, Hopkins CC, et al. Catheter complications in total parenteral nutrition: a prospective study of 200 consecutive patients. *N Engl J Med.* 1974;190:757–761.

23. Sanders RA, Sheldon GF. Septic complications of total parenteral nutrition: a five year experience. *Am J Surg.* 1976;132:214–220.

24. Padberg FT, Ruggiero J, Blackburn GL, Bistrian BR. Central venous catherization for parenteral nutrition. *Ann Surg.* 1981;193:264–270.

25. Pemberton LB, Mandal J, Lyman B, Covinsky JO. Developing a metabolic support service. *Missouri Med.* 1983;80:635–640.

26. Keohane PP, Jones BJ, Attrill H, Cribb A, et al. Effect of catheter tunneling and a nutrition nurse on catheter sepsis during total parenteral nutrition: a controlled trial. *Lancet.* 1983;2:1388–1390.

27. Byrne WJ. Documentation of the need for a nutritional support team for the supervision of central venous alimentation in a children's hospital. *Nutr Supp Serv.* 1983;3:49–50, 52.

28. Jacobs DO, Melnik G, Forlaw L, Gebhardt C, et al. Impact of a nutritional support service on VA surgical patients. *J Am Coll Nutr.* 1984;3:311–315.

29. Maurer J, Weinbaum F, Turner J, Brady T, et al. Reducing the inappropriate use of parenteral nutrition in an acute care teaching hospital. *J Parenter Enter Nutr.* 1996;20:272–274.

30. Blackburn GL, Bothe A, Lahey M. Organization and administration of a nutrition support service. *Surg Clin North Am.* 1981;61:709–719.

31. Hamaoui E, Rombeau JL. The nutrition support team. In: Rombeau JL, Caldwell MD, eds. *Parenteral Nutrition.* Philadelphia: WB Saunders Co; 1986:237–256.

32. Skipper A. Organization and administration of a nutrition support service. In: Skipper A, ed. *Nutrition Support Policies Procedures, Forms, and Formulas.* Gaithersburg, MD: Aspen Publishers Inc; 1995:13–14.

33. Skipper A. Data collection systems for clinical indicators. *Nutr Clin Pract.* 1991;6:156–158.

34. Lykins TC. Nutrition support clinical pathways. *Nutr Clin Pract.* 1996;11:16–20.

35. Position of The American Dietetics Association: the role of the registered dietitian in enteral and parenteral nutrition support. *J Am Diet Assoc.* 1997;97:302–304.

36. Skipper A, Rotman N. Survey of the role of the dietitian in preparing patients for discharge on home enteral feeding. *J Am Diet Assoc.* 1990;90:939–946.

37. Smitherman AL, Wyse BW. The backbone of our profession. *J Am Diet Assoc.* 1987;87:1394.

38. Jones MG, Bonner JL, Stitt KR. Nutrition support service: role of the clinical dietitian. *J Am Diet Assoc.* 1986;86:68–71.

39. Agriesti-Johnson C. Nutrition support team survey. In: *Training for Dietitians Working in Critical Care.* Columbus, OH: Ross Laboratories; 1985:7–12.

40. Mueller CM, Colaizzo-Anas T, Shronts EM, Gaines JA. Order writing for parenteral nutrition by registered dietitians. *J Am Diet Assoc.* 1996;96:764–767.

41. Olree K, Skipper A. The role of the nutrition support dietitian as viewed by chief clinical and nutrition support dietitians: implications for training. *J Am Diet Assoc.* 1997;97:1255–1263.

42. Skipper A. Training for nutrition support dietitians. *Nutrition.* 1996;12:730–732.

43. *Webster's Seventh New Collegiate Dictionary.* Springfield, MA: G&C Webster; 1969.

44. American Society for Parenteral and Enteral Nutrition. Committee reports: dietitian's committee. *Nutr Clin Pract.* 1988;3:86.

45. Standards of practice, nutrition support dietitians. *Nutr Clin Pract.* 1990;5:74–78.

46. ASPEN Nutrition Support Practice Manual. Silver Spring, MD: American Society for Parenteral and Enteral Nutrition; 1997.

47. Winkler MF. Standards of practice for the nutrition support dietitian: importance and value to practitioners. *J Am Diet Assoc.* 1993;93:1113–1116.

48. Wade J. Role of a clinical dietitian specialist on a nutrition support service. *J Am Diet Assoc.* 1977;70:185–189.

49. Skipper A, Perlmutter S. Function and role of the dietitian on the nutritional support team. *Nutrition.* 1992;8:391–394.

50. Skipper A, Winkler MF. The changing role of the dietitian in clinical practice. *Nutr Clin Pract.* 1992;7:S5–S8.

51. Schwartz DB. Nutritional support dietetics: past, present, and future. *Nutrition.* 1991;10:1–3.

52. Davis AM, Baker SS, Leary RA. Advancing clinical privileges for nutrition support practitioners: the dietitian as a model. *Nutr Clin Pract.* 1995;10:98–103.

53. Dowling R. Role expansion for dietetics professionals. *J Am Diet Assoc.* 1996;96:1001–1002.

CHAPTER 24

Nutrition Support in Home Care

Nancy H. Westbrook

INTRODUCTION

The trend in health care delivery is to move patients out of costly, acute care facilities into alternate care sites—such as subacute or rehabilitation facilities, skilled or intermediate long-term care facilities, outpatient centers, and the home—so that care can be provided in a cost-effective setting. With this shift in thinking, the alternate site providers have adapted their services to accommodate the new demands on their respective industries. Medically complex patients, patients who are dependent on technology, and patients who are facing long-term rehabilitation from an illness or injury are commonly referred to alternate site care. Managers and clinicians who are employed by alternate site providers face many challenges to offer the clinical expertise necessary to care for a diverse patient population, usually without the immediate technological support available in hospitals, while still maintaining costs within the expected reimbursement limits.

Based on industry surveys, estimated expenditures for home health care in 1996 were $36 billion dollars.[1] Although this figure represents less than 4% of the total amount spent on personal health care during the same period, home care is the most rapidly growing arena for the delivery of health care services. Funding sources for home care are identified in Exhibit 24–1.

TRENDS IN THE HOME CARE INDUSTRY

As home care providers serve the current needs of home care customers and prepare to compete in the future, the following trends have emerged:

- *Monitoring of the use of resources.* Management is looking carefully at staff productivity. With reduced payments per patient visit and limitations on the number of visits allowed by many managed care payers, clinicians are ex-

Exhibit 24–1 Sources of Payment for Home Care, 1996

Medicare—37.8%
Private pay out of pocket—31.4%
Medicaid—24.7%
Private insurance—5.5%
Other—0.6%

Source: Courtesy of National Association for Home Care, Washington, D.C.

pected to manage their time and perform their skills effectively. Multiskilled staff are valuable.

- *Technological advances.* Technology is replacing direct care whenever possible. Electronic communication to home care patients reduces travel costs. Communication via phone, facsimile, and modem is common practice in home care.
- *Outcomes assessment.* Outcomes are being measured and evaluated. The home care industry and payers are working together to develop definitions and measurement tools for clinical and financial outcomes. Also important to both industries are the opinions of their customers. Satisfaction surveys are often collected and published by consumer groups as a way of educating the public.
- *Merging and networking.* Home care providers are merging and networking with other providers to develop comprehensive health care delivery systems. Home care is seen as an essential component in the continuum of health care services. Hospitals frequently lead in the formation of a network of affiliated providers, by acquisition or development of new services such as home health care. Individual home care providers may develop business relationships or merge with other home care providers to offer a more comprehensive menu of home care services (including skilled services, equipment, infusion, or hospice services).
- *Interdisciplinary care.* Providers are developing an interdisciplinary team approach to clinical care. To meet the demands of customers, payers, and regulatory bodies, providers are developing service programs that involve several clinical disciplines and support staff. Nurses, home health aides, therapists, and pharmacists continue to provide the majority of services, but dietitians are becoming a valuable team member for many providers.
- *Clinical pathways and disease management programs.* These tools allow home care providers and payers to identify individuals who have chronic health care problems or a catastrophic event. Through education and close monitoring of their conditions, the cost of providing health care may be re-

duced, perhaps extending the benefit dollars and time for which the individual can remain covered under the insurance plan.

- *Joint Commission Accreditation.* The Joint Commission on Accreditation of Healthcare Organizations (Joint Commission) began voluntary accreditation of home health care organizations in 1988. This accreditation is now used as a quality indicator by managed care organizations when choosing providers.

TYPES OF HOME CARE ORGANIZATIONS

The home care industry is composed of four basic "product lines." Organizations may choose to provide only one, or they may offer a combination of services under one company name.

1. *Home health services.* This term generically describes the services provided by home health agencies, including skilled nursing in the home, and usually other related services such as home health aides, therapy services (physical, speech, and occupational), medical social work, and possibly companion and homemaker services. All agencies must be licensed in the state in which they provide services. Home health agencies may specialize in certain types of nursing services, such as private duty or "shift" staffing, or offer specialty programs for pediatric or human immunodeficiency virus/acquired immune deficiency syndrome patients. Agencies that wish to provide services to Medicare beneficiaries must agree to comply with Medicare's Conditions of Participation, which clearly define the reimbursed services and the numerous regulations for the provision of these services. Many states regulate the number of agencies that can participate in the Medicare program by requiring a Certificate of Need for an agency to become a Medicare-certified home health agency.

2. *Home infusion pharmacy.* A home infusion provider must hold a valid pharmacy license and meet the local and state requirements to operate as a pharmacy dispensing intravenous (IV) medications. Home IV therapies typically include IV antibiotics, parenteral nutrition, enteral nutrition, chemotherapy, blood and blood products, hydration therapy, various injectable medications such as vitamins, and biological response modifiers. Most home infusion pharmacies ship or deliver the medications and supplies to the patient's home, coordinating with a local home health agency to provide a nurse to administer the medication or teach the patient. A home infusion pharmacy must have a pharmacist on staff, and may have nurses and other professional staff who provide direct patient care services. Frequently, home infusion nurses and other professional staff serve as resources to the other clinicians, patients, and referral sources.

3. *Home medical equipment providers or durable medical equipment providers.* These companies provide hospital beds, wheelchairs, respiratory equipment, and other supplies to individuals at home. Most home medical equipment companies also provide enteral nutrition therapy, since a pharmacy license is not required.
4. *Hospice services.* A hospice organization is dedicated to providing skilled and supportive services to the terminally ill and their families. The focus is generally on palliative care and coping mechanisms rather than complex, invasive therapies.

PAYERS OF HOME CARE SERVICES

It is essential for home care providers to understand the reimbursement systems for the products and services. Medicare is the largest single payer of home health care services and products. Payment occurs under two sections: Medicare Part A and Medicare Part B.

Medicare Part A (Hospital Insurance) pays for the home health services that are provided by a certified home health agency: skilled nursing, therapy, home health aide, and medical social worker services. Criteria for provision of services and qualification of the patients are defined by the Conditions of Participation.

- The patient must be homebound.
- The patient must require a skilled service rather than custodial care.
- There must be a defined goal for services, and the patient must demonstrate reasonable progress toward achievement.

The amount reimbursed to the agency for the services rendered is based on the direct cost of the staff labor and an additional amount to cover the overhead costs of the agency. Through a complex accounting process, agencies can recoup a portion of the cost of their office space, equipment, office supplies, and other related support services that contribute to the cost of providing care to the Medicare population. The cost of a dietitian's services can be included in this overhead cost. However, the agency may only include the cost of the services that are provided to Medicare patients. The dietitian can assist the agency by accurately documenting the amount of time spent on Medicare and non-Medicare patients.

Medicare Part B is optional, and individuals who choose this option pay a monthly premium for coverage of physician visits, durable medical equipment, and prosthetic devices (including parenteral and enteral nutrition products and supplies). Reimbursement under Part B is only 80% of the allowed amount, established by the Health Care Financing Administration (HCFA). The remaining 20% must be paid by the patient, or another insurance company. The guidelines for reimbursement of home parenteral and enteral nutrition (HPEN) are defined in Exhibits 24–2, 24–3, and 24–4.[2] It is the responsibility of the provider to screen and qualify patients who are referred for HPEN.

Exhibit 24-2 Medicare Guidelines for Reimbursement of Home Parenteral and Enteral Nutrition

---

Diagnostic Criteria

1. The diagnosis must meet the test of permanence. Criteria for Medicare reimbursement for both parenteral and enteral nutrition include documentation of a diagnosis that causes a permanent (ie, expected to last at least 90 days) impairment or dysfunction of the gastrointestinal tract, precluding the patient from obtaining sufficient nutrients to maintain weight and strength commensurate with the patient's overall health status. This does not mean that the patient must have a diagnosis with no hope of recovery—just that the condition is expected to last at least 90 days.

2. The diagnosis must be supported. The diagnosis used for HPEN qualification must be supported in the medical record of the hospital or physician's office by documentation of testing or qualified expert opinion of the physician. The home care provider should request copies of the diagnostic evaluations and physicians' statements for the home care record in case the information is requested by the payer. The payer may ask for clinical information to clarify a specific patient's claim, or they may request information on several patients for a specific time frame if the provider is selected to undergo an audit by HCFA. In either case, several months, or even years, may have passed since the patient began HPEN therapy, and the provider may not be able to obtain the needed documentation at that time. Inability to provide the supporting clinical information may result in denial of payment or penalties for fraudulent billing of Medicare.

3. The diagnosis(es) should be specific to the gastrointestinal tract and support the need for specialized nutrition support.

Source: Reprinted from *DMERC Medicare Advisory,* April 1996, Health Care Financing Administration.

The nutrient content of the formula must also meet reimbursement guidelines, which are based on the recommendations of experts in the field of nutrition support. The prescribing physician must provide clinical justification for nutrient amounts under the circumstances listed in Exhibit 24–5.

The majority of patients who require total parenteral nutrition (TPN) at home fall within the Medicare guidelines. However, providers value the services of a clinical nutrition support expert who can evaluate the prescribed formulas and ensure that appropriate documentation is provided. Some patients have nutritional requirements that justify nutrients outside of the prescribed ranges, such as patients who are extremely obese or patients with high nitrogen losses; reimbursement may be limited or denied if appropriate clinical justification is not provided.

Patients referred for enteral nutrition must also meet the diagnostic criteria listed in Exhibits 24–2 and 24–3. They must have a diagnosis that impairs the

Exhibit 24–3 Specific Guidelines for Enteral Nutrition

---

1. The diagnosis must affect the function of the structures that permit food to reach the small bowel, such as the oral cavity, esophagus, and stomach. ICD-9 (*International Classification of Diseases,* 9th edition) codes are used to describe the qualifying diagnoses. The provider should be sure that all appropriate ICD-9 codes are included, since the qualifying HPEN diagnosis may be a secondary diagnosis. For example, cancer of the lung will not qualify a patient for enteral nutrition because there is no evidence of gastrointestinal (GI) involvement. However, if the lung tumor is pressing on the esophagus and causing an esophageal stricture, and this is documented, this diagnosis will qualify the patient for enteral nutrition because it clearly identifies the impairment of the upper GI tract.
2. Enteral nutrition is also covered if there is an impairment of the intestinal tract that impairs digestion and absorption of an oral diet. This qualification is an expansion of the benefit, which became effective April 1996. Until that time, the benefit limited coverage of enteral nutrition to conditions that affected ingestion of nutrients; this did not allow reimbursement of enteral feedings for conditions such as pancreatitis, Crohn's disease, or enteropathies. With the advances in nutrition support science and new delivery technologies, HCFA has realized that many diseases of the endocrine glands and small bowel can be cost-effectively treated with enteral nutrition. Under the previous guidelines, diseases of the small bowel were considered appropriate for TPN only.
3. Enteral nutrition is not covered for patients with a functional GI tract who are unable to consume oral nutrition for reasons of anorexia or nausea.

Source: Reprinted from *DMERC Medicare Advisory,* April 1996, Health Care Financing Administration.

---

ability to ingest, digest, or absorb nutrients taken orally. In addition, the formula prescription and delivery methods must be the simplest, least expensive means of adequately providing appropriate nutrition support. For reimbursement purposes, Medicare has categorized the delivery of supplies into "kits," identified by the delivery method. Definitions of delivery methods are provided in Exhibit 24–6. Supplies are reimbursed on a per diem basis, meaning that the provider is paid a specific amount for each day that the patient infuses the feedings. Medicare does not specify exactly what supplies should be provided to the patient to administer the feedings. However, the provider is expected to provide everything the patient should reasonably need to administer the feeding safely and to care for the insertion site of the feeding tube or nasal or ostomy site. Patients may be instructed to clean supplies and reuse them, if this is safe and accepted practice.

Exhibit 24–4 Specific Guidelines for Parenteral Nutrition

The patient must have:

a. a diagnosis involving the small intestine or exocrine glands that significantly impairs the absorption of nutrients, or

b. a disease of the stomach or intestinal tract that is a motility disorder and impairs the ability of the nutrients to be transported through the GI tract

It is the responsibility of the provider to obtain objective evidence of the clinical diagnosis to support the need for parenteral nutrition. There must also be evidence that attempts were made to provide modified enteral nutrition through a trial of an elemental or defined-formula diet, and that appropriate pharmacological agents were also used to enhance digestion and/or absorption.

The guidelines for reimbursement for total parenteral nutrition (TPN) specifically exclude reimbursement for patients whose need for parenteral nutrition is due to:

a. a swallowing disorder

b. a temporary defect in gastric emptying such as a metabolic or electrolyte disorder

c. a psychological disorder impairing food intake, such as depression

d. a metabolic disorder inducing anorexia, such as cancer or chemotherapy

e. a physical disorder impairing food intake such as the dyspnea of severe pulmonary or cardiac disease

f. a side effect of a medication

g. renal failure and/or dialysis

To qualify a patient for reimbursement for parenteral nutrition, the provider's record should indicate that appropriate nutritional and pharmacological efforts were made to wean the patient off TPN, such as:

a. that the patient was unable to maintain weight and strength using specialized enteral diets to improve absorption (ie, elemental diets, or those with MCT oils, hydrolyzed proteins, or free amino acids)

b. that appropriate pharmacological agents were utilized to enhance digestion (ie, pancreatic enzymes or bile salts) or alter intestinal motility to maximize absorption, such as prokinetic agents

Clinical Diagnoses Appropriate for Parenteral Nutrition

Clinical diagnoses considered appropriate for parenteral nutrition support include:

a. recent small-bowel resection leaving < 5 ft of small bowel beyond the ligament of Treitz

b. short-bowel syndrome severe enough to create a negative fluid balance

c. a bowel condition severe enough to require at least 3 months of bowel rest such as pancreatitis, pseudocyst, enteritis, or an enterocutaneous fistula located where feeding distal to the fistula is not possible

d. a mechanical small-bowel obstruction

continues

Exhibit 24–4 continued

> e. severe malabsorption syndrome resulting in significant malnutrition
> f. a proven motility disorder, unresponsive to prokinetic medication, which results in severe malnutrition when the patient does not receive parenteral nutrition
>
> For the above diagnoses, documentation that confirms the presence of the diagnoses should be included in the home care record.
>
> Other diagnoses may be considered for reimbursement of parenteral nutrition support, but only if the patient is clinically malnourished, the patient is unable to be maintained on a modified oral diet or specialized enteral nutrition support, and pharmacological interventions have been unsuccessful. Such other diagnoses may include:
>
> a. moderate malabsorption syndrome
> b. gastroparesis
> c. small-bowel resection with > 5 feet of small bowel beyond the ligament of Treitz
> d. short-bowel syndrome without severe symptoms of malnutrition
> e. mild to moderate enteritis, or enterocutaneous fistula
> f. partial small-bowel obstruction, where surgery is not an option
>
> For qualification of reimbursement using these diagnoses, the home care record should include confirmation of the diagnoses, as well as clinical and diagnostic information documenting the need for TPN. Examples of such documentation include:
>
> a. results of tests for malabsorption, such as fecal fat, Sudan stain, or D-xylose testing
> b. radiographic, scintigraphic, or manometric studies showing altered motility of the stomach or small bowel
> c. documentation of a true failed enteral tube trial, including attempts to feed postpylorically, with a controlled infusion, and with pharmacological management of symptoms of intolerance
> d. evidence of malnutrition (when/or if TPN is not provided) through lab values, weight changes, and other indicators of malnutrition
>
> *Source:* Reprinted from *DMERC Medicare Advisory,* April 1996, Health Care Financing Administration.

Enteral Formula Reimbursement

Enteral formulas are divided into six categories, based on their nutrient composition (see Exhibit 24–7). All categories of formula are reimbursed by the 100-calorie unit. The reimbursement received by the provider is based on the number of calories the physician orders for the patient on the Certificate of Medical Necessity (CMN). Codes and reimbursement levels for enteral nutrition supplies, tubes, and formulas are found in Exhibit 24–7.[3]

Exhibit 24–5 Clinical Justification for Nutrient Amounts

1. Total daily caloric intake outside the range of 20 to 35 kcal/kg/day (For patients who receive TPN less than daily, formula calories should be totaled on a weekly basis, and divided by 7 to give the average number of calories provided by the TPN on a daily basis.)
2. Protein outside the range of 0.8–1.5 g/kg/day
3. Dextrose concentration of < 10% final concentration
4. Lipid concentration that will require a cumulative monthly total of greater than 15 500-cc bottles of 20% or 30 500-cc bottles of 10% intravenous lipid emulsions
5. Use of specialty amino acid formulas, such as those specifically designed for hepatic and renal failure and metabolic stress

Source: Reprinted from *DMERC Medicare Advisory,* April 1996, Health Care Financing Administration.

Medicare expects clinicians and providers to use the most cost-effective means of providing nutrition support. Consequently, orders for products other than those included in categories B4150 and B4152 require additional clinical justification on the CMN. If justification is not included or is inappropriate, reimbursement will be adjusted to allowance for category B4150. Examples of justification appear in Exhibit 24–8.

Medicare Reimbursement for Parenteral Nutrition

Reimbursement for TPN is divided into payment for formula components, supply kits, and equipment. Different rates have been established for formula mixed at home (although this is no longer a commonly prescribed practice) and for formula compounded by a pharmacy and shipped to the patient premixed. The categories for reimbursement are listed Exhibit 24–9.

As with the enteral nutrition, Medicare expects clinicians to prescribe the most cost-effective parenteral nutrition formula to meet the patient's needs. Justification must be submitted when certain prescribed formula components exceed generally accepted practice standards, such as those listed in Exhibit 24–10.

DOCUMENTATION

Documentation of the Need for Nutrition Support

Under Medicare guidelines, it is the responsibility of the provider to obtain and maintain a clinical record of patients receiving enteral or parenteral nutrition (see

Exhibit 24–6 Definitions for Enteral Feeding Delivery Methods

Delivery methods, listed below from least to most expensive, are defined as:
- **Syringe or bolus delivery:** This is the simplest and least expensive delivery method. It involves attaching a large (60-cc) syringe directly to the feeding tube, using it as a funnel to administer the formula over a period of several minutes. The tube is flushed before and after feedings to ensure patency and to clear the tube of residue. Feedings are usually administered several times per day, with the frequency and volume designed to meet the nutritional and fluid goals of the patient. This method of feeding is less restrictive for patients who are able to tolerate the volume needed for meeting nutrient needs. The supplies needed by the patient for bolus feedings include syringes (60-cc for feedings and smaller syringes for flushing, if needed) and dressing supplies and tape for the tube insertion site.
- **Gravity delivery:** This involves a slow, manually regulated infusion of formula. A prescribed amount of formula is hung in a formula reservoir (bag or bottle) on an IV pole, higher than the insertion site of the feeding tube. The roller clamp on the tubing is used to adjust the flow rate of the formula. Feedings may take from several minutes to hours, depending on the tolerance of the patient. The flow rate may vary throughout the feeding as the patient shifts positions, or if gastric pressure rises. The frequency and volume of feedings are designed to meet the patient's nutritional and fluid requirements. Supplies needed for gravity administration include feeding reservoirs large enough to hold the prescribed volume for one feeding, syringes for flushing the feeding tube, dressings and tape for care of the tube insertion site, and an IV pole.
- **Pump delivery:** The formula is delivered at a prescribed rate, continuously, over several hours of the day or night using a stationary or ambulatory pump. The formula is held in a reservoir container, which is refilled or replaced when empty. The supplies needed for pump delivery include the reservoir containers (bag or bottle), syringes for flushing the feeding tube, dressing supplies and tape for the tube insertion site, IV pole (if using a stationary pump), and the enteral feeding pump (either stationary or ambulatory). Under the Medicare guidelines, the use of a pump to administer the feedings must be justified by physiologic intolerance to bolus or gravity administration to qualify for reimbursement. Examples of conditions requiring pump administration include documented incidents of reflux and/ or aspiration, severe diarrhea, dumping syndrome, and other conditions that necessitate a precise flow rate (such as circulatory overload or blood glucose fluctuations). If justification for use of a pump is not provided, the reimbursement for the pump may be denied, and the reimbursement for the supplies will be reduced to the amount for gravity or syringe supply kit.

Exhibit 24–11 and Exhibit 24–12). A nutrition support clinician can evaluate the clinical information available to the provider when the patient is referred, and assist the referral source and provider by recommending appropriate therapy modifications and monitoring parameters.

Exhibit 24–7 Medicare Coding for Enteral Nutrition Supplies, Tubes, and Formula

ENTERAL NUTRITION SUPPLIES

	Allowed Amount
B4034—Enteral supplies for syringe feedings	$5.39 per day
B4035—Enteral supplies for gravity feedings	$7.74 per day
B4036—Enteral supplies for pump feedings	$11.30 per day
B9000—Enteral infusion pump, without alarm	$106.19 per month
B9002—Enteral infusion pump, with alarm	$111.92 per month
E0776—IV pole	$24.33 per month

ENTERAL FEEDING TUBES

	Allowed Amount
B4081—nasogastric tubing, with stylet	$20.00
B4082—nasogastric tubing, without stylet	$15.59 each
B4083—stomach tube, levine type	$2.38 each
B4084—gastrostomy/jejunostomy tubing	$17.50
B4085—gastrostomy tube, silicone, with sliding ring	$39.68

For gastrostomy/jejunostomy tubes, justification required for > 1 every 3 months

For nasogastric tubes, justification required for > 3 per month

ENTERAL FORMULAS

The formula categories are listed below, along with the reimbursement levels effective March 1997.

Category	**Allowed Amount**
Category 1 (HCPC code B4150)—semisynthetic intact protein/isolates, most provide 1.0–1.5 kcal/cc, and provide balanced total nutrition support (eg, Osmolite, Sustacal, Jevity, Isocal, Nutren 1.0)	$0.65 per 100-kcal unit
Category 1-B (HCPC code B4151)—Natural protein/protein isolates, most provide 1.0–1.5 kcal/cc; also known as blenderized nutritional formulas (eg, Compleat B, Vitaneed, Compleat Modified)	$1.51 per 100-kcal unit
Category 2 (HCPC code B4152)—Calorically dense intact protein/protein isolate, 1.5–2.0 kcal/cc (eg, Nutren 2.0, Deliver 2.0, Ensure Plus)	$0.54 per 100-kcal unit

continues

Exhibit 24–7 continued

Category 3 (HCPC code B4153)—Hydrolyzed protein/amino acid formula, also known as elemental formula (eg, Criticare, Vivonex T.E.N., Vital HN)	$1.84 per 100-kcal unit
Category 4 (HCPC code B4154)—Includes a variety of formulas with nutrient composition designed to meet specific metabolic needs; reimbursement varies for each formula	Indiv. considered
Category 5 (HCPC code B4155)—Modular nutrient components; reimbursement varies for each formula (eg, Polycose, Promix, MCT oil)	Indiv. considered
Category 6 (HCPC code B4156)—Standardized nutrients (eg, Tolerex, Precision LR, Travasorb STD)	$1.27 per 100-kcal unit

Source: Reprinted from 1997 *Region C DMEPOS Fee Schedule Catalog,* Health Care Financing Administration.

For providers of HPEN, compliance with Medicare guidelines is critical. Noncompliance, whether intentional or not, can result in delayed or denied payments, or, in extreme cases, prosecution for fraudulent billing of Medicare. When a patient is referred to the provider for home enteral or parenteral nutrition, the burden is upon the provider to obtain complete and accurate documentation of the clinical diagnoses, and to ensure that the prescribed formula meets the patient's needs and is within the prescribed guidelines established by Medicare. If the prescription is not within the guidelines, the provider can intervene by working with the prescribing physician to revise the nutrition care plan or obtain the needed supporting documentation so that the nutrition care plan is clinically appropriate, well-justified, and reimbursable. If that is not possible, the provider should inform the patient and physician that the prescribed nutrition formula is not within the Medicare guidelines and may not be reimbursed, which means the patient is financially responsible for the cost.

The provider can offer suggestions to reduce the cost of the nutrition support plan or offer nutrition counseling to improve the patient's oral intake and absorption.

To work with a prescribing physician or other referral source, it is essential to have an understanding of the Medicare guidelines and the myriad of options available to administer enteral and parenteral nutrition safely. The home nutrition support clinician may be able to offer options for home care that are not available in the hospital. Many formulas made by different manufacturers have similar nutrient composition, and formulas can easily be substituted to reduce the price, or

Exhibit 24–8 Justification for Specialized Enteral Products, by Category

---

For B4151—Excessive diarrhea on a synthetic formula, or uncontrolled blood glucose fluctuations in a diabetic patient using synthetic formula

For B4153—Maldigestion or malabsorption of a synthetic, intact nutrient formula, resulting in uncontrolled diarrhea or dumping syndrome

For B4154—A specific diagnosis that corresponds to the design of the formula and documentation that patient's nutritional needs cannot be appropriately or safely met with a less expensive formula

For B4155—Documented need for the use of modular nutrient components to develop or supplement an enteral formula

For B4156—Intolerance to intact nutrient formulas

---

improve the convenience to the patient. Ambulatory pumps and simplified administration supplies are also desirable for many home patients. When patients begin home enteral therapy, an initial assessment and training period should occur. At this time, the supply needs should be determined and arrangements made to provide the supplies and formula on a regular, usually monthly, basis.

Documentation for Reimbursement

The billing of enteral and parenteral nutrition to Medicare requires the submission of two documents to the fiscal intermediary: the CMN (see Exhibits 24–13 and 24–14) and the HCFA 1500 (see Exhibit 24–15). The physician verifies the home care orders and the medical necessity for the home nutrition support on the CMN. The CMN is required when the initial claim is submitted for either enteral or parenteral nutrition.

Recertification requirements differ for enteral and parenteral nutrition. For *enteral nutrition,* recertification is required under the following circumstances:

- when the prescription changes to include formula or supplies that were not previously certified
- if the patient resumes enteral nutrition after a break in service of more than 2 months

For *parenteral nutrition,* recertification is required under the following circumstances:

- after 6 months of continuous therapy, to recertify the need for continued home TPN

Exhibit 24–9 Medicare Reimbursement for Parenteral Nutrition

FOR PATIENTS WHO MIX THEIR OWN TPN AT HOME (HOME MIX)

	Allowed amount
Amino acid solutions—reimbursed per 500-cc unit.	
Specify concentration of amino acid solution.	
B4168—3.5%	Indiv. considered
B4172—5.5%–7.0%	Indiv. considered
B4176—7.0%–8.5%	$34.73
B4178—> 8.5%	$52.47
Dextrose solutions—reimbursed per 500-cc unit.	
Specify concentration of dextrose.	
B4164—≤ 50% solution	$15.96
B4180—> 50% solution	$22.88
Lipid emulsions—reimbursed per 500-cc unit.	
Includes administration set. Specify concentration of lipid.	
B4184—10% solution	$75.03
B4186—20% solution	$100.13
Formula additives—reimbursed per infusion for all additives	
B4216—includes vitamins, trace elements,	
heparin, electrolytes	$7.04
Home mix supplies—one supply kit allowed per infusion	
B4222—includes syringes, needles, sterile wipes,	
etc. needed to compound formula and additives	$7.71

FOR PATIENTS WHO RECEIVE PREMIXED FORMULA

Reimbursement is for the compounded formula including the amino acids, dextrose, electrolytes, vitamins, and trace elements. The reimbursement amount is based on the grams of protein administered per day. Lipids are reimbursed separately, using the same codes listed for home mix.

Parenteral nutrition formula	**Allowed amount**
B4189—10–51 grams of protein per day	$166.94
B4193—52–73 grams of protein per day	$215.72
B4197—74–100 grams of protein per day	$254.94
B4199—Over 100 grams of protein per day	$283.73
Premix supplies—one supply kit per infusion	
B4220—includes needles, syringes, sterile wipes	
to add vitamins and other prescribed additives	$7.51

continues

Exhibit 24–9 continued

SPECIALIZED FORMULAS FOR ORGAN FAILURE AND TRAUMA

Reimbursement is contingent upon documentation supporting the need for specialized nutrition support and evidence that traditional nutrition support does not adequately meet the needs of the patient. Reimbursement is for compounded formula including specialized amino acid solution, dextrose, vitamins, and trace elements.

Specialized formulas—reimbursed per gram of

protein	**Allowed amount**
B5000—renal failure formula, any strength	$10.84
B5100—hepatic failure formula, any strength	$4.36
B5200—stress formula, high branched chain, any strength	Indiv. considered

SUPPLIES

For both home mix and premix patients:	**Allowed amount**
Administration supplies—one supply kit per infusion	
B4224—includes gloves, sterile wipes, filters, tubing, and other ancillary supplies needed to connect and administer the infusion	$23.50
Equipment	
B9004—portable infusion pump (includes carrying case)	$364.93 per month
B9006—stationary infusion pump	$364.93 per month
E0776—IV pole	$24.33 per month

Source: Reprinted from *1997 Region C DMEPOS Fee Schedule Catalog,* Health Care Financing Administration.

- when the prescription changes so that nutrient component billing codes differ from those previously certified
- when the number of infusion days per week is increased
- if the patient resumes therapy after a break in service of 2 months or more, another initial certification is required, and the recertification schedule begins again

The provider is allowed to complete the patient information in CMN Section A and the description and financial information about the prescribed items in Section C. The physician or his/her designee must complete Sections B and D. Anyone with a financial relationship to the provider is prohibited from completing the CMN Section B. However, most providers send a cover letter with a reminder of

Exhibit 24–10 Situations Requiring Additional Justification for Prescribed TPN Formula

1. Total prescribed calories are not within 20–35 kcal/kg/day
2. Amount of lipids prescribed exceeds 15 500-cc bottles of 20% lipid or 30 500-cc bottles of 10% lipid on a monthly basis
3. Amount of protein is outside the range of 0.8–1.5 g/kg/day
4. Use of a special organ failure or stress amino acid formula
5. Final dextrose concentration is < 10%

Source: Reprinted from *1997 Region C DMEPOS Fee Schedule Catalog,* Health Care Financing Administration.

the diagnosis and the prescribed nutrition care plan to assist in the completion of the CMN (see Exhibits 24–13 and 24–14).

The HCFA 1500 form is the actual bill that includes the amount and type of supplies delivered to the patient. Items billed should be expressed in the Medicare billing language (ie, using HCPCS codes, per diem billing, calorie units, etc) (see Exhibit 24–15).

Exhibit 24–11 Intake Screening for Enteral Nutrition Therapy

For patients referred for enteral nutrition, the clinician should review the initial referral information for the following:

1. **Diagnosis.** Is impairment of ingestion, digestion, or absorption evident? If not, pursue investigation of secondary diagnoses that are documented in the medical record or can be confirmed by the physician.
2. **Permanence.** Is the qualifying diagnosis expected to last at least 90 days?
3. **Condition.** If a continuous or cycled infusion with a pump is prescribed, does the patient have a condition that requires a pump? If not, has/or could a trial of bolus or gravity feedings be attempted?
4. **Height, weight, and amount of calories prescribed.** Does the prescribed amount provide 20–35 kcal/kg/day? If not, can justification be documented?
5. **Oral intake.** Is the patient taking oral nutrients? If so, is the amount ingested and absorbed providing only minimal nutritional value, with the enteral nutrition support providing the majority of daily nutrients?
6. **Special formulas.** For any formula not in the B4150 or B4152 category, a diagnosis or condition should be documented that justifies use of a specialized enteral formula.

Exhibit 24–12 Intake Screening for Parenteral Nutrition Patients

For patients referred for total parenteral nutrition therapy, the clinician should review the following:

1. Has a trial of enteral feedings been attempted?
2. **Diagnosis.** Is impairment of digestion and/or absorption evident? (see Exhibit 24–4)
3. **Permanence.** Is the qualifying diagnosis expected to last at least 90 days?
4. **Medicare parameters.** Is the prescribed formula within the accepted parameters allowed by Medicare? (see Exhibit 24–5)
5. **Oral intake.** Is the patient taking oral nutrients? If so, is the absorbed amount providing only minimal contribution to the daily nutritional requirements?
6. **Nutritional status.** Is there evidence that malnutrition exists or existed when the patient was not receiving TPN?
7. **Specialized formulas.** If a specialized formula is ordered, are appropriate diagnoses present? Is there evidence that traditional nutrition support was ineffective?

OTHER PAYERS OF HOME NUTRITION SUPPORT

Medicaid and most private insurance companies also pay for nutrition support at home. Medicaid programs are funded by both federal and state monies and administered at the state level. Therefore, the reimbursement guidelines and qualifying criteria differ from state to state. Many states pay for nutrition support products. A local Medicaid office can offer guidance on how to obtain specific information about Medicaid benefits for home nutrition support.

Private insurance companies are all different and constantly changing. Most home care providers have a policy of verifying insurance benefits before initiating services. This process involves calling the insurance company to find out the following information:

- Is the patient covered by this policy?
- Does the policy provide coverage of home care? More specifically, does this policy include coverage for nutrition support products? Clinical services?
- What documentation is needed to ensure coverage of the prescribed home care services?
- Is there a case manager who needs to be kept informed of the patient's progress at home or who will be issuing authorizations for services on a periodic basis?
- What percentage of the charges will be covered by the insurance company, and what portion will be the patient's responsibility?

Exhibit 24–13 Certificate of Medical Necessity

U.S. DEPARTMENT OF HEALTH & HUMAN SERVICES
HEALTH CARE FINANCING ADMINISTRATION

CERTIFICATE OF MEDICAL NECESSITY
PARENTERAL NUTRITION

FORM APPROVED
OMB NO. 0938-0679
DMERC 10.02A

SECTION A	Certification Type/Date:	INITIAL	REVISED	RECERTIFICATION

PATIENT NAME, ADDRESS, TELEPHONE and HIC NUMBER

SUPPLIER NAME, ADDRESS, TELEPHONE and NSC NUMBER

HICN #

NSC #

PLACE OF SERVICE

NAME and ADDRESS of FACILITY if applicable
(See Reverse):

HCPCS CODES

PT DOB   ; SEX   (M/F); HT.   (in.);WT.   (lbs.)

PHYSICIAN NAME, ADDRESS (Printed or Typed)

PHYSICIAN'S UPIN:

PHYSICIAN'S TELEPHONE #:

SECTION B	Information In This Section May Not Be Completed by the Supplier of the Items/Supplies.

EST. LENGTH OF NEED (# OF MONTHS):   1-99 (99= LIFETIME)   DIAGNOSIS CODES (ICD-9):

ANSWERS

ANSWERS QUESTIONS 1, AND 3 - 5 FOR PARENTERAL NUTRITION.
(Circle **Y** for Yes, **N** for No, or **D** for Does No Apply, Unless Otherwise Noted)

Question 2 reserved for other or future use.

Y   N

1. Does the patient have severe permanent disease of the gastrointestinal tract causing malabsorption severe enough to prevent maintenance of weight and strength commensurate with the patient's overall health status?

3. Days per week infused? (Enter 1-7)

4. Formula Components:

Amino Acid	_____ (ml/day)	_____ Concentration %	_____ gms protein/day
Dextrose	_____ (ml/day)	_____ concentration %	
Lipids	_____ (ml/day)	_____ days/week	_____ concentration %

1 3 7

5. Circle the number for the route of administration.   2,4,5,6 - Reserved for other or future use.
1- Central Line   **3-** Hemodialysis Access Line;   **7-** Peripherally Inserted Catheter (PIC)

NAME OF PERSON ANSWERING SECTION B QUESTIONS, IF OTHER THAN PHYSICIAN (Please Print):

NAME: TITLE: EMPLOYER:

SECTION C	Narrative Description Of Equipment And Cost

(1) Narrative description of all items, accessories and options ordered; (2) Supplier's charge; and (3) Medicare Fee Schedule Allowance for each item, accessory, and option. *(See Instructions On Back)*

SECTION D	Physician Attestation and Signature/Date

I certify that I am the physician identified in Section A of this form. I have received Sections A, B, and C of the Certificate of Medical Necessity (including charges for items ordered). Any statement on my letterhead attached hereto, has been reviewed and signed by me. I certify that the medical necessity information in Section B is true, accurate and complete, to the best of my knowledge, and I understand that any falsification, omission, or concealment of material fact in that section may subject me to civil or criminal liability.

PHYSICIAN'S SIGNATURE   DATE   (SIGNATURE AND DATE STAMPS ARE NOT ACCEPTABLE)

SCS.10.02A (8/96) FORM HCFA 852 (4/96)   To Reorder Call ProForma-UniSource: 800-280-8877   Rev. 8-01-96

continues

Exhibit 24–13 continued

SECTION A:	**(May be completed by the supplier)**
CERTIFICATION TYPE/DATE:	If this is an initial certification for this patient, indicate this by placing date (MM/DD/YY) needed initially in the space marked "INITIAL." If this is a revised certification (to be completed when the physician changes the order, based on the patient's changing clinical needs), indicate the initial date needed in the space marked "INITIAL," and also indicate the recertification date in the space marked "REVISED." If this is a recertification, indicate the initial date needed in the space marked "INITIAL," and also indicate the recertification date in the space marked "RECERTIFICATION." Whether submitting a REVISED or a RECERTIFIED CMN, be sure to always furnish the INITIAL date as well as the REVISED or RECERTIFICATION date.
PATIENT INFORMATION:	Indicate the patient's name, permanent legal address, telephone number and his/her health insurance claim number (HICN) as it appears on his/her Medicare card and on the claim form.
SUPPLIER INFORMATION:	Indicate the name of your company (supplier name), address and telephone number along with the Medicare Supplier Number assigned to you by the National Supplier Clearinghouse (NSC).
PLACE OF SERVICE:	Indicate the place in which the item is being used, i.e., patient's home is 12, skilled nursing facility (SNF) is 31, End Stage Renal Disease (ESRD) facility is 65, etc. Refer to the DMERC supplier manual for a complete list.
FACILITY NAME:	If the place of service is a facility, indicate the name and complete address of the facility.
HCPCS CODES:	List all HCPCS procedure codes for items ordered that require a CMN. Procedure codes that do not require certification should not be listed on the CMN.
PATIENT DOB, HEIGHT, WEIGHT AND SEX:	Indicate patient's date of birth (MM/DD/YY) and sex (male or female); height in inches and weight in pounds, if requested.
PHYSICIAN NAME, ADDRESS:	Indicate the physician's name and complete mailing address.
UPIN:	Accurately indicate the ordering physician's Unique Physician Identification Number (UPIN).
PHYSICIAN'S TELEPHONE NO:	Indicate the telephone number where the physician can be contacted (preferably where records would be accessible pertaining to this patient) if more information is needed.
SECTION B:	**(May not be completed by the supplier. While this section may be completed by a non-physician clinician, or a physician employee, it must be reviewed, and the CMN signed (in Section D) by the ordering physician.)**
EST. LENGTH OF NEED:	Indicate the estimated length of need (the length of time the physician expects the patient to require use of the ordered item) by filling in the appropriate number of months. If the physician expects that the patient will require the item for the duration of his/her life, then enter 99.
DIAGNOSIS CODES:	In the first space, list the ICD9 code that represents the primary reason for ordering this item. List any additional ICD9 codes that would further describe the medical need for the item (up to 3 codes).
QUESTION SECTION:	This section is used to gather clinical information to determine medical necessity. Answer each question which applies to the items ordered, circling "Y" for yes, "N" for no, "D" for does not apply, a number if this is offered as an answer option, or fill in the blank if other information is requested.
NAME OF PERSON ANSWERING SECTION B QUESTIONS:	If a clinical professional other than the ordering physician (e.g., home health nurse, physical therapist, dietician) or a physician employee answers the questions of Section B, he/she must print his/her name, give his/her professional title and the name of his/her employer where indicated. If the physician is answering the questions, this space may be left blank.
SECTION C:	**(To be completed by the supplier)**
NARRATIVE DESCRIPTION OF EQUIPMENT & COST:	Supplier gives (1) a narrative description of the item(s) ordered, as well as all options, accessories, supplies and drugs; (2) the supplier's charge for each item, option, accessory, supply and drug; and (3) the Medicare fee schedule allowance for each item/option/accessory/supply/drug, if applicable.
SECTION D:	**(To be completed by the physician)**
PHYSICIAN ATTESTATION:	The physician's signature certifies (1) the CMN which he/she is reviewing includes Sections A, B, C and D; (2) the answers in Section B are correct; and (3) the self-identifying information in Section A is correct.
PHYSICIAN SIGNATURE AND DATE:	After completion and/or review by the physician of Sections A, B and C, the physician must sign and date the CMN in Section D, verifying the Attestation appearing in this Section. The physician's signature also certifies the items ordered are medically necessary for this patient. Signature and date stamps are not acceptable.

According to the Paperwork Reduction Act of 1995, no persons are required to respond to a collection of information unless it displays a valid OMB control number. The valid OMB control number for this information collection is 0938-0679. The time required to complete this information collection is estimated to average 15 minutes per response, including the time to review instructions, search existing resources, gather the data needed, and complete and review the information collection. If you have any comments concerning the accuracy of the time estimate or suggestions for improving this form, please write to HCFA, P.O. Box 26684, Baltimore, Maryland 21207 and to the Office of Information and Regulatory Affairs, Office of Management and Budget, Washington, D.C. 20503.

Source: Reprinted from Health Care Financing Administration.

Exhibit 24–14 Certificate of Medical Necessity

U.S. DEPARTMENT OF HEALTH & HUMAN SERVICES HEALTH CARE FINANCING ADMINISTRATION	**CERTIFICATE OF MEDICAL NECESSITY** ENTERAL NUTRITION	FORM APPROVED OMB NO. 0938-0679 **DMERC 10.02B**

SECTION A	Certification Type/Date: INITIAL	REVISED	RECERTIFICATION

PATIENT NAME, ADDRESS, TELEPHONE and HIC NUMBER	SUPPLIER NAME, ADDRESS, TELEPHONE and NSC NUMBER
HICN #	NSC #

PLACE OF SERVICE		HCPCS CODES	PT DOB ; SEX (M/F); HT. (in.);WT. (lbs.)
NAME and ADDRESS of FACILITY if applicable (See Reverse):			PHYSICIAN NAME, ADDRESS (Printed or Typed) PHYSICIAN'S UPIN: PHYSICIAN'S TELEPHONE #:

SECTION B	Information In This Section May Not Be Completed by the Supplier of the Items/Supplies.

EST. LENGTH OF NEED (# OF MONTHS): 1-99 (99= LIFETIME)	DIAGNOSIS CODES (ICD-9):

ANSWERS	ANSWERS QUESTIONS 7, 8, AND 10 - 15 FOR ENTERAL NUTRITION. (Circle **Y** for Yes, **N** for No, or **D** for Does No Apply, Unless Otherwise Noted)
	Questions 1-6, and 9, reserved for other or future use.
Y N	7. Does the patient have permanent non-function or disease of the structures that normally permit food to reach or be absorbed from the small bowel?
Y N	8. Does the patient require tube feedings to provide sufficient nutrients to maintain weight and strength commensurate with the patient's overall health status?
A) B)	10. Print product name(s)
A) B)	11. Calories per day for each product?
	12. Days per week administered? (Enter 1 - 7)
1 2 3 4	13. Circle the number for method of administration? **1** - Syringe **2** - Gravity **3** - Pump **4** - Does not apply
Y N D	14. Does the patient have a documented allergy or intolerance to semi-synthetic nutrients?
	15. Additional information when required by policy:

NAME OF PERSON ANSWERING SECTION B QUESTIONS, IF OTHER THAN PHYSICIAN (Please Print):
NAME: TITLE: EMPLOYER:

SECTION C	Narrative Description Of Equipment And Cost
(1) Narrative description of all items, accessories and options ordered; (2) Supplier's charge; and (3) Medicare Fee Schedule Allowance for each item, accessory, and option. (See Instructions On Back)	

SECTION D	Physician Attestation and Signature/Date

I certify that I am the physician identified in Section A of this form. I have received Sections A, B, and C of the Certificate of Medical Necessity (including charges for items ordered). Any statement on my letterhead attached hereto, has been reviewed and signed by me. I certify that the medical necessity information in Section B is true, accurate and complete, to the best of my knowledge, and I understand that any falsification, omission, or concealment of material fact in that section may subject me to civil or criminal liability.

PHYSICIAN'S SIGNATURE	DATE	(SIGNATURE AND DATE STAMPS ARE NOT ACCEPTABLE)

SCS.10.02B (8/96) FORM HCFA 853 (4/96)   To Reorder Call ProForma-UniSource: 800-280-8877   Rev. 8-01-96

continues

Exhibit 24–14 continued

SECTION A:	**(May be completed by the supplier)**
CERTIFICATION TYPE/DATE:	If this is an initial certification for this patient, indicate this by placing date (MM/DD/YY) needed initially in the space marked "INITIAL." If this is a revised certification (to be completed when the physician changes the order, based on the patient's changing clinical needs), indicate the initial date needed in the space marked "INITIAL," <u>and also</u> indicate the recertification date in the space marked "REVISED." If this is a recertification, indicate the initial date needed in the space marked "INITIAL," <u>and also</u> indicate the recertification date in the space marked "RECERTIFICATION." Whether submitting a REVISED or a RECERTIFIED CMN, be sure to always furnish the INITIAL date as well as the REVISED <u>or</u> RECERTIFICATION date.
PATIENT INFORMATION:	Indicate the patient's name, permanent legal address, telephone number and his/her health insurance claim number (HICN) as it appears on his/her Medicare card and on the claim form.
SUPPLIER INFORMATION:	Indicate the name of your company (supplier name), address and telephone number along with the Medicare Supplier Number assigned to you by the National Supplier Clearinghouse (NSC).
PLACE OF SERVICE:	Indicate the place in which the item is being used, i.e., patient's home is 12, skilled nursing facility (SNF) is 31, End Stage Renal Disease (ESRD) facility is 65, etc. Refer to the DMERC supplier manual for a complete list.
FACILITY NAME:	If the place of service is a facility, indicate the name and complete address of the facility.
HCPCS CODES:	List all HCPCS procedure codes for items ordered that require a CMN. Procedure codes that do not require certification should not be listed on the CMN.
PATIENT DOB, HEIGHT, WEIGHT AND SEX:	Indicate patient's date of birth (MM/DD/YY) and sex (male or female); height in inches and weight in pounds, if requested.
PHYSICIAN NAME, ADDRESS:	Indicate the physician's name and complete mailing address.
UPIN:	Accurately indicate the ordering physician's Unique Physician Identification Number (UPIN).
PHYSICIAN'S TELEPHONE NO:	Indicate the telephone number where the physician can be contacted (preferably where records would be accessible pertaining to this patient) if more information is needed.
SECTION B:	**(May not be completed by the supplier. While this section may be completed by a non-physician clinician, or a physician employee, it must be reviewed, and the CMN signed (in Section D) by the ordering physician.)**
EST. LENGTH OF NEED:	Indicate the estimated length of need (the length of time the physician expects the patient to require use of the ordered item) by filling in the appropriate number of months. If the physician expects that the patient will require the item for the duration of his/her life, then enter 99.
DIAGNOSIS CODES:	In the first space, list the ICD9 code that represents the primary reason for ordering this item. List any additional ICD9 codes that would further describe the medical need for the item (up to 3 codes).
QUESTION SECTION:	This section is used to gather clinical information to determine medical necessity. Answer each question which applies to the items ordered, circling "Y" for yes, "N" for no, "D" for does not apply, a number if this is offered as an answer option, or fill in the blank if other information is requested.
NAME OF PERSON ANSWERING SECTION B QUESTIONS:	If a clinical professional other than the ordering physician (e.g., home health nurse, physical therapist, dietician) or a physician employee answers the questions of Section B, he/she must <u>print</u> his/her name, give his/her professional title and the name of his/her employer where indicated. If the <u>physician</u> is answering the questions, this space may be left blank.
SECTION C:	**(To be completed by the supplier)**
NARRATIVE DESCRIPTION OF EQUIPMENT & COST:	Supplier gives **(1)** a narrative description of the item(s) ordered, as well as all options, accessories, supplies and drugs; **(2)** the supplier's charge for each item, option, accessory, supply and drug; and **(3)** the Medicare fee schedule allowance for each item/option/accessory/supply/drug, if applicable.
SECTION D:	**(To be completed by the physician)**
PHYSICIAN ATTESTATION:	The physician's signature certifies **(1)** the CMN which he/she is reviewing includes Sections A, B, C and D; **(2)** the answers in Section B are correct; and **(3)** the self-identifying information in Section A is correct.
PHYSICIAN SIGNATURE AND DATE:	After completion and/or review <u>by the physician</u> of Sections A, B and C, the physician must sign and date the CMN in Section D, verifying the Attestation appearing in this Section. The physician's signature also certifies the items ordered are medically necessary for this patient. Signature and date stamps are not acceptable.

According to the Paperwork Reduction Act of 1995, no persons are required to respond to a collection of information unless it displays a valid OMB control number. The valid OMB control number for this information collection is 0938-0679. The time required to complete this information collection is estimated to average 15 minutes per response, including the time to review instructions, search existing resources, gather the data needed, and complete and review the information collection. If you have any comments concerning the accuracy of the time estimate or suggestions for improving this form, please write to HCFA, P.O. Box 26684, Baltimore, Maryland 21207 and to the Office of Information and Regulatory Affairs, Office of Management and Budget, Washington, D.C. 20503.

Source: Reprinted from Health Care Financing Administration.

Exhibit 24–15 Health Insurance Claim Form (HCFA 1500)

PLEASE DO NOT STAPLE IN THIS AREA

CARRIER

PICA

HEALTH INSURANCE CLAIM FORM

PICA

1. MEDICARE ☐ (Medicare #)   MEDICAID ☐ (Medicaid #)   CHAMPUS ☐ (Sponsor's SSN)   CHAMPVA ☐ (VA File #)   GROUP HEALTH PLAN ☐ (SSN or ID)   FECA BLK LUNG ☐ (SSN)   OTHER ☐ (ID)   1a. INSURED'S I.D. NUMBER   (FOR PROGRAM IN ITEM 1)

2. PATIENT'S NAME (Last Name, First Name, Middle Initial)

3. PATIENT'S BIRTH DATE   MM DD YY   SEX   M ☐   F ☐

4. INSURED'S NAME (Last Name, First Name, Middle Initial)

5. PATIENT'S ADDRESS (No., Street)

6. PATIENT RELATIONSHIP TO INSURED   Self ☐   Spouse ☐   Child ☐   Other ☐

7. INSURED'S ADDRESS (No., Street)

CITY   STATE

8. PATIENT STATUS   Single ☐   Married ☐   Other ☐   Employed ☐   Full-Time Student ☐   Part-Time Student ☐

CITY   STATE

ZIP CODE   TELEPHONE (Include Area Code)   (   )

ZIP CODE   TELEPHONE (INCLUDE AREA CODE)   (   )

9. OTHER INSURED'S NAME (Last Name, First Name, Middle Initial)

10. IS PATIENT'S CONDITION RELATED TO:

11. INSURED'S POLICY GROUP OR FECA NUMBER

a. OTHER INSURED'S POLICY OR GROUP NUMBER

a. EMPLOYMENT? (CURRENT OR PREVIOUS)   YES ☐   NO ☐

a. INSURED'S DATE OF BIRTH   MM DD YY   SEX   M ☐   F ☐

b. OTHER INSURED'S DATE OF BIRTH   MM DD YY   SEX   M ☐   F ☐

b. AUTO ACCIDENT?   PLACE (State)   YES ☐   NO ☐

b. EMPLOYER'S NAME OR SCHOOL NAME

c. EMPLOYER'S NAME OR SCHOOL NAME

c. OTHER ACCIDENT?   YES ☐   NO ☐

c. INSURANCE PLAN NAME OR PROGRAM NAME

d. INSURANCE PLAN NAME OR PROGRAM NAME

10d. RESERVED FOR LOCAL USE

d. IS THERE ANOTHER HEALTH BENEFIT PLAN?   YES ☐   NO ☐   *If yes*, return to and complete item 9 a-d.

READ BACK OF FORM BEFORE COMPLETING & SIGNING THIS FORM.

12. PATIENT'S OR AUTHORIZED PERSON'S SIGNATURE. I authorize the release of any medical or other information necessary to process this claim. I also request payment of government benefits either to myself or to the party who accepts assignment below.

SIGNED _____   DATE _____

13. INSURED'S OR AUTHORIZED PERSON'S SIGNATURE. I authorize payment of medical benefits to the undersigned physician or supplier for services described below.

SIGNED _____

14. DATE OF CURRENT: MM DD YY   ILLNESS (First symptom) OR INJURY (Accident) OR PREGNANCY(LMP)

15. IF PATIENT HAS HAD SAME OR SIMILAR ILLNESS. GIVE FIRST DATE   MM DD YY

16. DATES PATIENT UNABLE TO WORK IN CURRENT OCCUPATION   MM DD YY   FROM   TO   MM DD YY

17. NAME OF REFERRING PHYSICIAN OR OTHER SOURCE

17a. I.D. NUMBER OF REFERRING PHYSICIAN

18. HOSPITALIZATION DATES RELATED TO CURRENT SERVICES   MM DD YY   FROM   TO   MM DD YY

19. RESERVED FOR LOCAL USE

20. OUTSIDE LAB?   YES ☐   NO ☐ $ CHARGES

21. DIAGNOSIS OR NATURE OF ILLNESS OR INJURY. (RELATE ITEMS 1,2,3 OR 4 TO ITEM 24E BY LINE)

1. L___ . ___   3. L___ . ___

2. L___ . ___   4. L___ . ___

22. MEDICAID RESUBMISSION CODE   ORIGINAL REF. NO.

23. PRIOR AUTHORIZATION NUMBER

24. A DATE(S) OF SERVICE						B Place of Service	C Type of Service	D PROCEDURES, SERVICES, OR SUPPLIES (Explain Unusual Circumstances) CPT/HCPCS	MODIFIER	E DIAGNOSIS CODE	F $ CHARGES	G DAYS OR UNITS	H EPSDT Family Plan	I EMG	J COB	K RESERVED FOR LOCAL USE
MM	DD	YY	MM	DD	YY											
1																
2																
3																
4																
5																
6																

25. FEDERAL TAX I.D. NUMBER   SSN ☐   EIN ☐

26. PATIENT'S ACCOUNT NO.

27. ACCEPT ASSIGNMENT? (For govt. claims, see back)   YES ☐   NO ☐

28. TOTAL CHARGE $

29. AMOUNT PAID $

30. BALANCE DUE $

31. SIGNATURE OF PHYSICIAN OR SUPPLIER INCLUDING DEGREES OR CREDENTIALS (I certify that the statements on the reverse apply to this bill and are made a part thereof.)

SIGNED _____   DATE _____

32. NAME AND ADDRESS OF FACILITY WHERE SERVICES WERE RENDERED (If other than home or office)

33. PHYSICIAN'S, SUPPLIER'S BILLING NAME, ADDRESS, ZIP CODE & PHONE #

PIN#   GRP#

(APPROVED BY AMA COUNCIL ON MEDICAL SERVICE 8/88)   APPROVED OMB-0938-0008

PLEASE PRINT OR TYPE

FORM HCFA-1500 (12-90)   FORM OWCP-1500   FORM RRB-1500

PATIENT AND INSURED INFORMATION

PHYSICIAN OR SUPPLIER INFORMATION

By getting all of this information before home therapy is started, the provider is able to inform the patient of his or her financial responsibility and alert the organization's clinical and billing departments about what is expected so that the organization can be reimbursed in a timely manner. Once a patient is started on home nutrition support, it is the responsibility of the provider to ensure that the clinical information requested by the insurance company is communicated to the appropriate individual. Any clinical changes, especially those that impact the nutrition support orders, should be communicated immediately to ensure that the authorization for services corresponds to the services provided. Failure to do so may jeopardize payment for the services.

MAINTAINING THE HOME CARE CLINICAL RECORD

Experienced nutrition support clinicians usually find that the information required for appropriate clinical monitoring of the patient is very similar to that required for financial justification of the therapy. For patients who are receiving nutrition support, the home care medical record should minimally include the following clinical information:

- referral information (including origin of referral to home care, contact person for obtaining more information, and payer requirements)
- standard paperwork for admission to home care services (informed consent for therapy, financial disclosure, rights and responsibilities of patient/ caregiver, advance directives, emergency plans)
- an initial nutritional assessment that documents the primary diagnosis, other relevant diagnoses or conditions, and baseline nutritional status parameters
- a brief past medical history, if relevant, and history of present illness
- description of any recent surgeries or medical treatments, especially if related to the need for nutrition support
- medication profile
- description of psychosocial status of patient and patient's home environment (related to patient's ability to safely store, prepare, and administer the feedings at home)
- outline of the nutritional care plan, including guidelines for implementation of the feedings, patient education strategies, guidelines for monitoring the progress of the patient, and quantifiable goals of therapy
- names and contact numbers for other providers involved in the patient's care who should be informed or involved when changes to the nutrition care plan are made

- documentation of follow-up, as described in the care plan, showing evidence of the patient's progress and adjustments to care plan as needed
- physician's orders for the implementation of therapy and for changes in therapy as needed
- evidence of communication and coordination of care between all involved providers, the physician, the patient, and other caregivers

Nutritional care goals, implementation plans, and monitoring parameters for home care should be realistic. Home care clinicians should involve the patient and caregivers in the development of the plan to ensure that the patient understands what is expected and will be able to comply with the plan. Consideration must be given to the patient's literacy level, willingness and ability to participate in his or her care, access to measurement tools such as scales and labeled measuring cups, and access to follow-up care after leaving the referring facility. Efforts should be made to coordinate follow-up with other providers so that the information can be shared.

Reasonable parameters for follow-up include the following:

- *Patient's weight.* The family may have a scale, or weight can be obtained when the patient goes to the physician's office for follow-up. If it is not possible to obtain the patient's weight, measurements of girth or estimates based on how clothing fits may be all that can be documented.
- *Laboratory tests.* Laboratory values are essential when monitoring TPN. Frequent lab tests may be required when TPN is initiated, but stable, long-term patients may have lab tests done monthly or even quarterly. Lab panels, which include many standard parameters, are usually more cost-effective than requesting several individual parameters. The home care provider can request information from local labs to determine which panels can provide the most valuable information for monitoring TPN cost-effectively.
- *Oral nutritional intake.* Patients, family members, and caregivers can be instructed to monitor the patient's oral intake, and they can be given simple tools for collecting and documenting this information. Long-term documentation of oral intake can become overwhelming, especially if the family is documenting other care parameters as well (such as urine outputs, blood sugars, temperatures). A periodic 3-day nutrient intake, combined with a phone diet history by a registered dietitian, generally provides a good estimate of the patient's oral intake and tolerance. More detail may be needed when the patient is making the transition from one mode of feeding to another.
- *Documentation of tolerance to prescribed feeding and progress toward established goals.* Caregivers should be instructed on how to recognize signs and symptoms of intolerance and how to respond to minor problems. Major problems could require immediate assistance by a home care professional. Periodic follow-up by the nutrition support clinician should always include a

review of all problems experienced. If continued problems appear to interfere with the progress toward goals, changes in the care plan or feeding regimen may be indicated.

Ideally, the home care medical record should reflect an interdisciplinary approach to care. For services provided through a home infusion company, pharmacists and nurses usually provide the majority of clinical services and documentation. Home health agencies usually employ nursing, therapies (physical, speech, and occupational), medical social workers, and home health aides, all of whom document in the medical record when their services are included in the plan of care ordered by the physician.

Registered dietitians may be employed by the home care agency or the infusion company. When dietitians are asked to assess and make recommendations for a patient receiving nutrition support, it is important to know the following:

- Who is the provider of the enteral or parenteral nutrition products? (This is the provider who will need the clinical information related to the billing of the products.)
- Who is the provider of the direct clinical, hands-on care? (This is the provider who needs information on patient education, physical assessment, and monitoring parameters related to nutritional status.)

In some cases, one company may be providing both the nutrition support product and the nutrition support services. Frequently, though, there are two separate providers, and coordination of information and services is critical to the successful implementation and monitoring of the nutrition support plan. The dietitian may be asked to provide clinical information and recommendations and to coordinate services between the two providers.

PROVISION OF NUTRITION PRODUCTS TO THE HOME CARE PATIENT

Home care providers are responsible for delivering the nutrition therapy products and supplies to the patient. Most providers use a combination of company-owned delivery systems, commercial courier services, and commercial shipping services. The type of delivery system chosen will depend on the urgency of the delivery, the weight of the products, the stability of the product, and the location of the patient's home.

Enteral nutrition products and supplies are usually shipped on a monthly basis. Once a patient is stabilized on an appropriate feeding plan, usage of product is predictable, and the amount of formula and administration supplies needed can be estimated fairly easily. Patients should be educated on how to store their enteral products and supplies properly, how to check for expiration dates, and how to rotate stock. Most suppliers conduct a monthly phone assessment and inventory of home supplies with each patient to determine if the patient's needs have changed before shipping out the next month's order. Any variance from the prescribed amount is reported to a home care clinician, who can follow up to determine if adjustments to the feeding plan are needed.

Total parenteral nutrition products and supplies are not usually shipped together. Once a patient has been trained and is stable on the infusion schedule, supplies can be shipped out on a monthly basis. Regular follow-up by the home care nurse or pharmacist can identify changes in supply needs. Most suppliers telephone the patient prior to shipping supplies to determine the patient's home inventory to avoid over- or understocking the patient. TPN formulas are usually shipped weekly or biweekly. They are shipped more frequently if the patient is unstable or if lab work is scheduled, which might necessitate a change in formulation. Temperature-controlled packaging is necessary, and quality assurance monitoring should be performed regularly to ensure that products maintain their integrity. Patients should be instructed on how to store their TPN formula and supplies properly and how to rotate stock. For patients with limited refrigeration space, providers may have to give the patient a small refrigerator to ensure safe storage of the TPN formula and other related medications. Patients should be educated on how to examine their TPN formula prior to infusion to identify any crystals, sediment, discoloring, or separation of the formula. Three-in-one mixtures (those with lipids added to the amino acid and dextrose base formula) are opaque, and patients cannot easily identify sediment. Therefore, most providers routinely use in-line, 1.2-micron filters to infuse three-in-one TPN formula at home.

ROLE OF NUTRITION SUPPORT PROFESSIONALS

Registered dietitians with nutrition support expertise are well qualified to provide a valuable service to home care patients and providers. A dietitian should evaluate patients before and during HPEN therapy to ensure that clinical criteria are met, that documentation is correct, and that appropriate therapy is rendered. Because of reimbursement limitations and limitations on scope of practice in some states, nurses are frequently the main providers of direct care to patients. Pharmacists are usually the primary contact for the physicians of patients who receive home infusion therapies. A dietitian may be employed—often as a part-time employee or consultant—to provide guidance to the nurse or pharmacist on how to develop, implement, and monitor the nutrition support care plan. The role of dietitians depends on availability; organizational policies and procedures; and professional relationships established with nurses, pharmacists, and physicians.

Suggestions for the role of the dietitian in home care are outlined below.

- Establish a screening tool to identify patients at high nutritional risk.
- Provide nutritional assessment and recommendations for patients who require nutritional interventions.

- Participate in interdisciplinary care planning and follow-up for high-risk patients or those receiving nutrition support.
- Provide education to home care staff, referral sources, and physicians directing home care on the regulations, products, reimbursement qualifications, and standards of practice related to home nutrition support.
- Provide direct patient care for patients requiring nutrition support for assessment, teaching, and monitoring of nutritional progress.
- Develop standard policies and procedures for developing, implementing, and monitoring nutrition support–related therapies.
- Participate in the development of disease management programs and standard care maps for diagnoses that are likely to benefit from appropriate nutrition support.

JOINT COMMISSION STANDARDS

In 1995, the Joint Commission on Accreditation of Healthcare Organizations (Joint Commission) began evaluating how home care providers serve the nutritional needs of home health clients. All home care providers who consider nutrition within the scope of their services must meet the standards relating to the nutrition care process. The standards apply to home health agencies, home infusion providers, hospice organizations, and providers of home medical equipment. *Nutrition care,* as defined by the Joint Commission, is "Interventions and counseling of individuals on appropriate nutrition intake by integrating information from the nutrition assessment with information on food and other sources of nutrients and meal preparation consistent with cultural background and socioeconomic status. Nutrition therapy, a component of medical treatment, includes enteral and parenteral nutrition."[4] Nutrition care standards are found in the "Care, Treatment and Service" chapter of the Joint Commission's *Comprehensive Accreditation Manual for Home Care.*[4] Several other chapters also include standards related to the provision of nutrition care, such as those found in the "Assessment" and "Education" chapters. Nutrition care and other related standards are listed in Exhibit 24–16.

The nutrition care process begins with the screening of all patients admitted to home care to identify those who have nutritional needs and those who are at high risk to develop nutrition-related problems. Each organization should have a screening process, defined by the organization's policies and procedures. When the nutrition screening process identifies a patient at high risk, the organization should designate a qualified professional to initiate an in-depth nutritional assessment and develop an interdisciplinary nutrition care plan that identifies appropriate interventions and goals to address nutritional aspects of care. If the organization is not able to provide the nutrition care services, it should refer the patient to another organization or qualified professional who can assess and manage the level of nutrition care required. This expectation is consistent with the standards

Exhibit 24–16 Joint Commission Standards for Nutrition Care

Care, Treatment, and Service

TX.8: Interdisciplinary nutrition care planning is performed, as appropriate.

TX.8.1: Authorized individuals prescribe or order nutrition therapies.

TX.8.2: Responsibilities for preparing, storing, distributing, and administering nutrition therapy are identified and assigned.

TX.8.3: Each patient's nutrition therapy is distributed in a safe, accurate, and timely manner.

TX.8.4: Each patient's nutrition therapy is administered in a safe, accurate, and timely manner.

TX.8.5: Each patient's nutrition status is monitored on an ongoing basis.

TX.8.6: The organization provides appropriate nutrition therapy when diets or diet schedules are altered.

Assessment

PE.2.5: The organization identifies patients who are at nutritional risk.

Education

PF.4.10: The patient receives counseling on potential drug-food interactions, nutrition intervention, and modified diets, when applicable.

Source: © 1997 *Comprehensive Accreditation Manual for Home Care, 1997-1998.* The Joint Commission on Accreditation of Healthcare Organizations, 1996. Reprinted with permission.

---

found in the "Continuum of Care" chapter.[4] Providers of enteral and parenteral nutrition are expected to perform the nutrition care process. For providers who do not provide parenteral nutrition, only standards TX.8 through TX.8.3 apply; standards TX.8.0 through TX.8.6 apply to providers of parenteral nutrition.

The Joint Commission standards emphasize the importance of interdisciplinary care. However, they recognize the special skills of a qualified nutritional professional for the delivery of high-level nutritional services such as nutritional assessments, nutrition support, staff education, and development of organizational policies and procedures related to nutrition care. The dietitian is the most accepted professional to provide these services.

CONCLUSIONS

Home health care is the fastest-growing segment of the health care delivery continuum. Registered dietitians are becoming essential members of the interdisciplinary team of professionals working for home health agencies, home infusion pharmacies, and other home care providers. Successful practice in home care requires good clinical knowledge and skills and ability to collaborate with other professionals, such as nurses and pharmacists. Home health care also presents clinicians with the opportunity to become involved with issues of reimbursement. Registered dietitians with the right combination of clinical knowledge, expertise in nutrition support reimbursement, and an understanding of the regulatory standards for nutrition care will be considered a valuable resource to home care providers.

REFERENCES

1. National Association for Home Care. *Basic Statistics about Home Care.* Washington, DC: National Association for Home Care; 1996.
2. Palmetto Government Benefits Administrators. *DMERC Medicare Advisory.* Columbia, SC: Palmetto Government Benefits Administrators; April 1996.
3. Palmetto Government Benefits Administrators. *1997 Region C DMEPOS Fee Schedule Catalog.* Columbia, SC: Palmetto Government Benefits Administrators; 1997.
4. Joint Commission on Accreditation of Healthcare Organizations. *Comprehensive Accreditation Manual for Home Care, 1997–1998.* Oakbrook Terrace, IL: Joint Commission on Accreditation of Healthcare Organizations; 1996.

Index